The Fallopian Tube

Basic Studies and Clinical Contributions

edited by **Alvin M. Siegler, M.D., D.Sc.**

Clinical Professor
Department of Obstetrics and Gynecology
State University of New York
Health Science Center
Brooklyn, New York

Associate Editor
Amir H. Ansari, M.D., F.R.C.S.(C.)
Clinical Professor
Department of Obstetrics and Gynecology
Medical College of Georgia
Director
Department of Obstetrics and Gynecology
Georgia Baptist Medical Center
Atlanta, Georgia

Editorial Assistant
Leon C. Chesley, Ph.D.
Professor Emeritus
Department of Obstetrics and Gynecology
State University of New York
Health Science Center
Brooklyn, New York

FUTURA PUBLISHING COMPANY, INC.
Mount Kisco, New York
1986

Library of Congress Cataloging-in-Publication Data

The Fallopian tube.

Bibliography: p.
Includes index.
1. Fallopian tubes—Diseases. 2. Fallopian tubes—Surgery. 3. Fallopian tubes—Anatomy. I. Siegler, Alvin M. II. Ansari, Amir H.
RG421.F35 1986 618.1'2 85-45881
ISBN 0-87993-283-X

Published by
Futura Publishing Company, Inc.
295 Main Street, P.O. Box 330
Mount Kisco, New York 10549

L.C. no. 85-45881
ISBN no. 0-87993-283-X

Contributors

Sneh Anand, M.D.
Assistant Professor, Center for Biomedical Engineering, Indian Institute of Technology and All Indian Institute of Medical Sciences, New Delhi, India

John F. Angle, M.D.
Fertility Center of North Texas Gynecological Microsurgical Institute, Dallas, Texas

Shawky Z. A. Badawy, M.D.
Professor, Department of Obstetrics and Gynecology, Upstate Medical Center, Syracuse, New York

B. Norman Barwin, M.D.
Associate Professor, Department of Obstetrics and Gynecology, University of Ottawa, School of Medicine, Ottawa, Ontario, Canada

Uziel Beller, M.D.
Department of Obstetrics and Gynecology, Hadassah University Hospital, Jerusalem, Israel

Yoram Beyth, M.D.
Professor, Department of Obstetrics and Gynecology, Hadassah University Hospital, Jerusalem, Israel

Steven P. Bondell, M.D.
Associate Pathologist, Georgia Baptist Medical Center, Atlanta, Georgia

Geoffrey Chamberlain, M.D.
Professor, Department of Obstetrics and Gynecology, St. George's Hospital Medical School, University of London, London, England

Ettore Cittadini, M.D.
Professor, Department of Obstetrics and Gynecology, University of Palermo, Palermo, Italy

Brian Cohen, M.B.Ch.B., M.D.
Fertility Center of North Texas, Gynecological Microsurgical Institute, Dallas, Texas

Gene L. Colborn, Ph.D.
Director, Medical Gross Anatomy, Medical College of Georgia, Augusta, Georgia

Edgard Cornier, M.D.
Chief of Services, Department of Obstetrics and Gynecology, L'hôpital De Neuilly, Paris, France

Günter Corts-Kleinwort, M.D.
Department of Obstetrics and Gynecology, Michaelis Midwifery School, University of Kiel, Kiel, West Germany

Ernelando Cosmi, M.D.
Assistant Professor, Department of Obstetrics and Gynecology, University of Perugia, Perugia, Italy

Alan H. DeCherney, M.D.
Professor, Department of Obstetrics and Gynecology, Director, Division of Reproductive Endocrinology, School of Medicine, Yale University, New Haven, Connecticut

Frank DeStefano, M.D.
Epidemiologic Studies Branch, Division of Reproductive Health, Center for Health Promotion and Education, Centers for Disease Control, Atlanta, Georgia

Luigi Devoto, M.D.
Department of Obstetrics and Gynecology, University of Chile and Institute of Clinical Investigation, Paula Jaraquernada Hospital, Santiago, Chile

Izu Eibschitz, M.D.
Department of Obstetrics and Gynecology, Haifa City Medical Center (Rothschild), Faculty of Medicine, Technion, Haifa, Israel

Sándor L. Erdö, Ph.D.
Pharmacological Research Center, Chemical Works of Gedeon Richter Ltd., Budapest, Hungary

Tommy Evans, M.D.
Professor, Vice-chairman, Department of Obstetrics and Gynecology, University of Colorado Health Science Center, Denver, Colorado

Jamil A. Fayez, M.D.
Professor, Department of Obstetrics and Gynecology, Bowman Gray School of Medicine, Winston-Salem, North Carolina

Christopher M. Fredericks, Ph.D.
Professor of Physiology, Medical Uneversity of South Carolina, Charleston, South Carolina

Franco Gasparri, M.D.
Department of Obstetrics and Gynecology, University of Florence, Florence, Italy

Gary S. Grubb, M.D., M.P.H.
Epidemiologic Studies Branch, Division of Reproductive Health, Center for Health Promotion and Education, Centers for Disease Control, Atlanta, Georgia

W. David Hager, M.D.
Associate Professor, Department of Obstetrics and Gynecology, University of Kentucky, School of Medicine, Lexington, Kentucky

Jacques Hamou, M.D.
Hospital Tenon, Paris, France

Göran Helm, M.D.
Department of Obstetrics and Gynecology, University of Lund, Lund, Sweden

Gary Holtz, M.D.
Department of Obstetrics and Gynecology, Medical University of South Carolina, Charleston, South Carolina

Abdol H. Hosseinian, M.D.
Professor and Chairman, Department of Obstetrics and Gynecology, The Chicago Medical School, Chicago, Illinois

Randal C. Jaffe, Ph.D.
Department of Physiology and Biophysics, University of Illinois, Health Sciences Center, Chicago, Illinois

Anthony Johns, Ph.D.
Assistant Professor, Department of Obstetrics and Gynecology, The University of Texas Health Science Center, San Antonio, Texas

Jurgen Kleinstein, Ph.D.
Director Frauenklinik, Giesen University, Giesen, West Germany

Robert W. Kelly, M.D.
Associate Professor, Department of Obstetrics and Gynecology, University of Kansas, Wichita, Kansas

Bertil Larsson, M.D.
Associate Professor, Department of Obstetrics and Gynecology, Huddinge University Hospital, Karoloinska Institute, Huddinge, Sweden

Neri Laufer, M.D.
Mellon Fellow, Yale University School of Medicine, Hadassah University School of Medicine, Jerusalem, Israel

Arthur Leader, M.D.
Assistant Professor, Department of Obstetrics and Gynecology, University of Calgary, Calgary, Alberta, Canada

Bo Lindblom, M.D., Ph.D.
Department of Obstetrics and Gynecology, University of Göteborg, Göteborg, Sweden

Jaroslav J. Marik, M.D.
Clinical Assistant Professor, Department of Obstetrics and Gynecology, University of Southern California, Los Angeles, California

John Marlow, M.D.
Clinical Assistant Professor, Department of Obstetrics and Gynecology, George Washington University School of Medicine, Washington, District of Columbia

Dan C. Martin, M.D.
Clinical Assistant Professor, Department of Obstetrics and Gynecology, University of Tennessee Center for the Health Sciences, Memphis, Tennessee

John A. McLachlan, M.D.
Developmental Endocrinology and Pharmacology Section, National Institutes of Health, National Institute of Environmental Health Sciences, Research Triangle Park, North Carolina

C. Irving Meeker, M.D.
Professor, Department of Obstetrics and Gynecology, University of Vermont, College of Medicine, Burlington, Vermont

Luca Mencaglia, M.D.
Assistant Professor, Department of Obstetrics and Gynecology, University of Florence, Florence, Italy

John G. Moore, M.D.
Chief Resident, Department of Obstetrics and Gynecology, Georgia Baptist Medical Center, Atlanta, Georgia

Shlomo Mor-Yosef, M.D.
Associate Professor, Department of Obstetrics and Gynecology, Hadassah University Hospital, Jerusalem, Israel

Retha R. Newbold, M.D.
Developmental Endocrinology and Pharmacology Section, National Institutes of Health, National Institute of Environmental Health Sciences, Research Triangle Park, North Carolina

Anders Norström, M.D., Ph.D.
Department of Obstetrics and Gynecology, University of Göteborg, Göteborg, Sweden

Francis B. O'Brien, M.D.
Associate Director, Clinical Research in Obstetrics and Gynecology, G.D. Searle & Co., Skokie, Illinois

Gene Oliphant, Ph.D.
Associate Professor, Department of Anatomy, University of Virginia School of Medicine, Charlottesville, Virginia

Jardena Ovadia, M.D.
Professor and Chairman, Department of Obstetrics and Gynecology, Beilinson Medical Center, Tel Aviv University, Sackler School of Medicine

Earl Owen, M.D.
Medical Director, Microresearch Foundation of Australia, Sydney, Australia

Christer Owman, M.D., Ph.D.
Professor and Dean, Department of Histology, University of Lund, Lund, Sweden

Antonio Perino, M.D.
Assistant Professor, Department of Obstetrics and Gynecology, University of Palermo, Palermo, Italy

Herbert B. Peterson, M.D.
Deputy Chief, Epidemiologic Studies Branch, Division of Reproductive Health, Center for Health Promotion and Education, Centers for Disease Control, Atlanta, Georgia

Ana María Pino, Ph.D.
Division of Basic Science, University of Chile, Santiago, Chile

Donald E. Pittaway, M.D., Ph.D.
Associate Professor, Department of Obstetrics and Gynecology, Bowman Gray School of Medicine, Winston-Salem, North Carolina

Hans-Harald Riedel, M.D.
Department of Obstetrics and Gynecology, Michaelis Midwifery School, University of Kiel, Kiel, West Germany

Maxwell Roland, M.D.
Honorary Gynecologist, Department of Obstetrics and Gynecology, Booth Memorial Hospital, Flushing, New York

Wilfred Roth, Ph.D
Professor of Electrical Engineering, University of Vermont, Burlington, Vermont

George L. Rubin, M.D.
Chief, Epidemiologic Studies Branch, Division of Reproductive Health, Center for Health Promotion and Education, Centers for Disease Control, Atlanta, Georgia

Gianfranco Scarselli, M.D.
Associate Professor, Department of Obstetrics and Gynecology, University of Florence, Florence, Italy

Alexander Sedlis, M.D.
Professor, Department of Obstetrics and Gynecology, State University of New York, Health Science Center, Brooklyn, New York

Kurt Semm, M.D., D.V.M.
Professor, Michaelis Midwifery School, University of Kiel, Kiel, West Germany

Mordechai Sharf, M.D.
Associate Professor and Head, Department of Obstetrics and Gynecology, Haifa City Medical Center (Rothschild), Faculty of Medicine, Technion, Haifa, Israel

Nils-Otto Sjöberg, M.D.
Professor, Department of Obstetrics and Gynecology, University of Lund, Lund, Sweden

H. Randall Squires, M.D.
Chief Resident, Department of Obstetrics and Gynecology, Georgia Baptist Medical Center, Atlanta, Georgia

William C. Stewart, M.D.
Director, Clinical Research in Obstetrics and Gynecology, G.D. Searle & Co., Skokie, Illinois

Barbara J. Struthers, Ph.D.
Associate Director, Office of Scientific Affairs, G.D. Searle & Co., Skokie, Illinois

Yona Tadir, M.D.
Clinical Instructor, Department of Obstetrics and Gynecology, Beilinson Medical Center, Tel Aviv University, Sackler School of Medicine, Tel Aviv, Israel

Patrick J. Taylor, M.B., F.R.C.S.
Professor, Department of Obstetrics and Gynecology, University of Calgary, Calgary, Alberta, Canada

Christopher J. Verco, M.D.
Senior Staff Specialist and Visiting Scholar, Department of Obstetrics and Gynecology, Modbury Hospital, Modbury, South Australia

Harold G. Verhage, Ph.D.
Associate Professor, Department of Obstetrics and Gynecology, University of Illinois, Health Sciences Center, Chicago, Illinois

Karl de Vries, M.D.
Clinical Instructor, Department of Obstetrics and Gynecology, Haifa City Medical Center (Rothschild), Haifa, Israel

Bengt Walles, Ph.D.
Department of Histology, University of Lund, Lund, Sweden

Foreword

I am doubly pleased to write the foreword to this monograph. The subject has long been of scholarly interest to me, and I have numbered Dr. Alvin M.Siegler among my mentors and friends since the start of my residency training, nearly three decades ago. In fact, I performed my first tuboplasty under his guidance.

Several monographs on the oviduct and fallopian tube are already in print. Yet, I believe that there is a place for this one, because it presents some new material and because Drs. Siegler and Ansari have the experience and perception to bring the basic science contributions into clinical perspective. The editors have assembled a group of acknowledged authorities about basic and applied aspects of tubal structure and function.

Before reviewing some specifics of the monograph, I will take advantage of the broad license that Dr. Siegler graciously offered me, to share with the reader some questions about the fallopian tube that I believe are critical. These questions are grouped under categories that reflect those into which this monograph is organized.

I. Tubal Anatomy and Physiology

1. How does the tube transport the ovum from the abdominal ostium toward the uterus, while at the same time transporting spermatozoa from the uterus toward the abdominal ostium? Although this question has intrigued many scientists, a definitive answer has not been written.

2. What control systems regulate gamete transport through the tube? How crucial is the detailed time-course of ovum transport to successful reproduction in the human? In our species, as in other primates but unlike the rabbit, the fertilized egg spends the bulk of its sojourn in the tube within the ampulla. Passage through the isthmus is quite rapid. Is there biological significance to this time-course?

3. How critical is exposure to the tubal environment to successful implantation in the human? Are the success rates of in-vitro fertilization (IVF) limited by lack of exposure to the tubal environment? We have found that early exposure of IVF-produced monkey embryos to the tubal

environment enhances subsequent development in vivo.

4. How critical is embryo-uterine synchrony to reproduction in the human? Although it is well known that synchrony is important to implantation in the rabbit, this question has not been systematically examined in the human or in other primates.

5. Is it possible to develop techniques to evaluate the integrity of some of the physiological functions of the fallopian tube? As noted by Dr. Siegler, present diagnostic techniques do not measure any aspects of tubal function. In our laboratories, we have developed a radioactive microsphere that measures the ability of the rabbit oviduct to transport ova. We are now attempting to modify the system for use in primates.

II. *Tubal Pathology*

1. Precisely how does tubal disease interfere with fertility? For example, salpingitis isthmic nodosa is associated with infertility, but it is unclear whether or not the relationship is causal. In a similar vein, pregnancy rates after apparently successful reparative surgery of diseased tubes are still significantly reduced.

2. Why do humans develop tubal pregnancy? The answer to this question has major biological, as well as clinical, implications. The problem goes beyond the question usually addressed, "What arrests the fertilized egg in the tube?" Rather, we must ask, "Why can the human embryo implant, when arrested in the tube?" Tubal pregnancy is extremely rare in other primates and is nonexistent in infraprimates. In the latter species, if the fertilized egg is arrested in the oviduct, it never develops beyond the blastocyst stage. At this stage or earlier, the embryo dies. Is the human embryo different from that of infraprimates? Or is the human tubal environment different?

3. Is it possible to rationally select the best surgical approach to a given tubal pregnancy, based on the intraoperative findings?

4. How does minimal endometriosis affect fertility? It is not entirely clear whether endometriosis interferes with ovulation, ovum pick-up, ovum transport, or other critical steps in the reproductive process.

III. *Sterilization*

1. Do we need new sterilization techniques or do we have enough choices now? Although tubal sterilization is now the leading method of contraception in much of the world, we still do not have an ideal method. The ideal sterilization technique would be inexpensive, simple to perform, require no anesthesia, have no side effects, be 100% effective, and readily reversible. Millions of dollars have been expended in attempts to develop methods that satisfy these criteria. To date, our efforts have achieved only limited success.

2. Should we desist in these efforts until new technology warrants new attempts?

3. Does the tubal ligation syndrome exist? In addition to the limitations of current methods, the popularity of tubal sterilization has given rise to a putative new illness: the tubal ligation syndrome. At this moment it is not certain whether or not the tubal ligation syndrome actually exists. If it does exist, we must ask:

4. What is the underlying pathophysiology?

5. Which women are at high risk to develop the syndrome?

6. Is the syndrome associated with any particular method of sterilization?

IV. *Tuboplasty*

1. Which regions of the tube are essential to optimize the success rates of tuboplasty?

2. What is the appropriate role of the laser in tuboplasty?

3. Can we offer patients a realistic prognosis based on the procedure per-

formed and the condition of the repaired tubes at completion of the operation?

With these questions in mind, let us turn our attention to *The Fallopian Tube: Basic Studies and Clinical Contributions.* In perusing the monograph, readers will find at least tentative answers to many of these questions, and will no doubt frame new questions of their own. The book is organized into four parts: Tubal Anatomy and Physiology, Tubal Pathology, Sterilization, and Tuboplasty. Each section is preceded by an editorial summary that reviews the material covered in the section and highlights areas in which more information is needed.

Part I, Tubal Anatomy and Physiology, contains 13 chapters that deal with the anatomical components of the tube, the mechanisms for control of tubal functions, and the ovum pick-up function of the tube. The individual contributions should provide a reference source for years to come. Clinicians will be interested in the wealth of information concerning the basics of tubal anatomy and function. As I read the contributions, several ideas for future research projects came to mind. I was intrigued to see work done in our own laboratories placed into context by the individual essayists, many of whom are my friends and colleagues.

Part II, Tubal Pathology, is made up of 11 chapters that cover such diverse subjects as the effects of intrauterine exposure to diethylstilbestrol, infections, ectopic pregnancy, intrauterine devices, endometriosis and tumors on the tube. These contributions reflect the level of current knowledge and, perhaps equally important, demonstrate areas in which we are still ignorant.

The seven chapters in Part III are devoted to sterilization. The contributors discuss the history of sterilization, various techniques for sterilization, and the complications of sterilization.

The final section, Part IV, is comprised of nine chapters concerned with various aspects of tuboplasty. The first chapter of this segment offers a historical review of tuboplasty. The remainder of the chapters are devoted to technical aspects of tuboplasty, including a classification of tuboplastic operations.

The Fallopian Tube: Basic Studies and Clinical Contributions deserves a thorough reading by clinicians and scientists who are interested in reproduction and infertility. In addition, it warrants a place in one's library, as a reference source for laboratory projects and for clinical problems.

CARL J. PAUERSTEIN, M.D.
Professor and Chairman
Department of Obstetrics and Gynecology
The University of Texas
Health Science Center at San Antonio
San Antonio, Texas

Preface and Acknowledgments

"and fleshy through its red colour and its end is torn and ragged like the fringe of well-worn garments."

Since its classic description by Gabriele Falloppio in 1661, the physiology of the fallopian tube has intrigued many investigators. Until the advent of in-vitro fertilization and embryo transfer, an intrauterine pregnancy could not occur without a fallopian tube. It is a paradox that although its physiology is quite complex, each segment acting in a different and important manner, most portions of the oviduct are not essential for pregnancy.

As clinicians editing this book, we have been intrigued by the experimental studies described in the first section on tubal anatomy and physiology. The contributors to this section are recognized authorities in their fields and, indeed, it has been a privilege to have them participate in this project. The information should serve as a reservoir of important facts for the gynecologic surgeon who deals with infertility and tubal disorders.

The second part of this book concerns abnormalities such as tubal endometriosis, tubal tuberculosis, and salpingitis isthmica nodosa. The first clue to these three conditions comes from the hysterosalpingogram; the differential diagnosis is essential but sometimes difficult. Obviously, books could be written about salpingitis and tubal pregnancy. We have limited the contributions to specific areas such as making an accurate early diagnosis, conservative surgical management, and the effects of IUDs relative to these two entities.

Although perinatal exposure to diethylstilbestrol has caused significant uterine changes, few authors have noted the effect on oviductal development. We learn of some of these changes from the report by Newbold and McLachlan.

The section on sterilization includes the history of this fascinating operation and current developments in hysteroscopic methods. The quest for a reversible technique continues, as does the interest in a simple, safe, effective outpatient procedure. Laparoscopic methods and the Pomeroy technique continue to be most popular and reliable. No operation is without complications, morbidity and even mortality. A detailed analysis of this aspect has been described by Peterson and his coworkers.

Methods for repairing damaged fallopian tubes continue to intrigue gynecologic surgeons. It is important to emphasize that the required judgment and skill concerning tuboplasty develop gradually.

Only by continued practice can higher standards be achieved. The number of term pregnancies following tuboplasty has shown some improvement with the advent of better selection of patients and microsurgical techniques. Aside from the gratifying results from reversing sterilization operations, salpingoneostomy, anastomosis, and implantation for occlusion caused by disease have been mostly unsuccessful.

In the section on tuboplasty, chapters on ampullofibroscopy describe one method of possibly predicting which patient has a better chance of becoming pregnant postoperatively. Here is another endoscopic instrument, as yet difficult to use, but certainly the information as revealed by Hamou and Cornier is exciting.

How can postoperative adhesions be avoided? Is the laser an instrument that reproductive surgeons must learn to use? What are the limitations of therapeutic laparoscopy in regard to tuboplasty? Some answers to these difficult questions are given by the authors of chapters in this section.

Overall, the editors have tried to avoid excessive duplication but in a multiauthored book of this size, the task was not always easy. This book represents a survey of laboratory and clinical studies relating to the oviduct. It was our wish to bring together in one volume representative works of the experimentalists, pathologists, and research clinicians. We sincerely thank our contributors for giving us the license to edit their contributions so that our combined efforts would make a readable, informative book. One person, Doctor Leon Chesley, was indomitable in this task. Indeed, he read, edited, and reread these chapters and without a doubt, his caring made our task an easier one. We also wish to express our sincere appreciation to Mrs. Shawn Simpson-Haynes and Ms. Lynn Tolbert, who carefully typed and willingly retyped these manuscripts. Last but not least, we wish to thank Mr. Steven Korn of Futura Publishing Company for urging us to write this book and for his conscientious efforts in moving it toward completion.

ALVIN M. SIEGLER, M.D.
Editor

AMIR H. ANSARI, M.D.
Associate Editor

Contents

Part II. Tubal Pathology

Part III: Sterilization

Part IV: Tuboplasty

I

Tubal Anatomy and Physiology

Editorial Comments

These chapters on the anatomical and physiological aspects of the fallopian tube include fundamental and exciting new information of interest to basic scientists and clinicians who are concerned with conservative management of the adnexa and reparative surgical procedures.

The proper functioning of the fallopian tube would seem to be a prerequisite for normal transport of gametes, fertilization, and passage of the fertilized ovum into the uterine cavity. When there is complete tubal occlusion, the relationship between infertility and tubal disease is obvious.

Thus far, the clinician has not been able to measure tubal function in women by any specific or simple test. Tubal patency and luminal shadows can be fairly well defined but ciliary activity, oviductal secretions, myosalpingeal contractility, and the method of fimbrial pickup cannot be measured nonoperatively.

Capacitation of spermatozoa in the female reproductive tract was thought to be indispensible for fertilization. It is now quite obvious that incubation in a precise medium also can accomplish this phenomenon.

Attempts to modify tubal function pharmacologically are described in several of these chapters. The methods discussed include altering levels of steroid hormones, modification of adrenergic innervation, and treatment with prostaglandins. Lindblom and Norström show that denervation of the tube does not disrupt ovum transport.

The effects on fertility after extirpation of various tubal segments in experimental animals have been studied extensively. The clinician knows that the absence of almost any tubal segment is compatible with an intrauterine pregnancy. Patients become pregnant with only the presence of a contralateral tube and ovary, or absent uterotubal or ampullary-isthmic junctions; the isthmus is not crucial and even the fimbria are not indispensible for pregnancy to occur. The ampulla, however, appears to be essential.

Mitotic activity of the tubal endosalpinx is low and not cyclic, unlike the changes in the endometrium. With scanning electron microscopy, Fredericks has clearly delineated the cyclic changes in ciliated and secretory cells. The secretory cells are at their height during ovulation. Especially impressive is the observation of the discharge of the cytoplasmic con-

The Fallopian Tube: Basic Studies and Clinical Contributions, edited by Alvin M. Siegler, M.D. Mount Kisco, New York: Futura Publishing Company, Inc.

tents of the secretory cells into the tubal lumen. Controversy still surrounds the mode of release of secretory products and the biochemical nature of the product packaged in the electron-dense secretory granules.

The basic tonic supply of estrogen is sufficient to maintain tubal activity and it is enhanced by the added estrogen present in the proliferative phase of the cycle. This observation may have clinical implications regarding the choice for a repair in the proliferative phase and estrogen supplementation for all patients having tubal reconstruction. It makes more clinical sense than prophylactic antibiotics and hydropertubation. DeVoto and Pino describe and illustrate the steroid influence on the tubal epithelium, indicating that many of the changes are estrogen-dependent.

Verhage and Jaffe report in detail the sensitive steroid gradient of responses of fimbrial, ampullary, and isthmic ciliated and secretory cells using cell height, percentage of ciliation, and the presence of secretory granules as quantitative indicators. They also note that the height and the number of ciliated cells are greatest during ovulation. Although some cilia are normally shed, they are renewed in each cycle.

Lindblom describes experiments on the effect of prostaglandins on the tube. In essence, the E series relaxes or inhibits contractility of the myosalpinx, while the F series stimulates, although they do not accelerate ovum transport. Some of these results can also be of value to those interested in contraceptive technology because it may be possible to interfere with gamete transportation and fertilization in the tubal environment. The response of the oviduct to prostaglandins appears to depend on the steroid levels associated with the reproductive cycle. PGF_2 seems to have no effect on the tube during the follicular phase but causes contractions just prior to ovulation. The role of prostaglandins in the regulation of tubal motility is still not completely resolved.

Oviductal fluid apparently does not pass through the uterotubal junction but exits into the peritoneal cavity. Alteration of the endosalpinx with deciliation, loss of rugae, and decrease in estrogen receptors, occurs with increased intratubal pressure in the distally obstructed tube. In the absence of significant infection, these processes are reversible following fimbrioplasty or salpingoneostomy. Apparently one milliliter of fluid is produced daily but the volume is affected by the level of steroids. Oliphant describes the unique characteristics of this special fluid so that so-called unexplained infertility might possibly be caused by abnormal quality or quantity of tubal fluid.

Pickup of the ovum under normal circumstances in experimental situations is described by Beyth and Mor-Yosef. In women, ovulated eggs with their cumuli are drawn into the tube by muscular movements and fimbrial cilia. In humans and monkeys, the cilia have a unidirectional beat toward the uterus. The ciliary activity, along with to-and-fro tubal contractions, account for transport of the ovum.

Transmigration of gametes and zygotes has been documented. In patients who have been sterilized, a fistula can occur in the proximal segment; spermatozoa can travel into the peritoneal cavity from this opening and to the distal segment of the contralateral tube, and can fertilize an egg picked up by that tubal segment. A zygote fertilized in a proximal segment also could pass through a fistula and be swept into the distal segment of the opposite tube. An ovum released from one side could enter the proximal segment of the opposite tube, become fertilized, and then migrate back to the opposite distal fimbriated end. The first possibility is most likely. Indeed, it is rare for a tubal pregnancy ever to occur in the proximal segment of a patient previously sterilized.

1

The Anatomy of the Fallopian Tube

Gene L. Colborn

Embryologic Development

Early urogenital events

In the discussion that follows, attention will be directed to those aspects of embryologic development that pertain most specifically to the development of the uterine tubes; little will be said regarding the formation of the uterus and the vagina. The major steps in the development of the female reproductive system are accomplished quite early in the gestational period[1] and are inextricably interrelated with the formation of the early rudiments of the urinary excretory system. Although the finer details of development of the urinary system do not fall within the confines of this discussion, mention will be made of those features that assist in understanding the sequences of events leading to the final disposition and form of the tubes.

The intermediate mesoderm and the nephrogenic cords

The urogenital system is derived largely from the intermediate cell mass and the adjacent epithelium of the coelom. The migration of intermediate mesoderm from its parasomitic site of origin to a more ventral location on the dorsal wall of the coelomic cavity gives rise to bilateral urogenital ridges. These ridges initially extend from the upper cervical region to the cloaca caudally.[2–5]

The intermediate mesoderm within the urogenital ridges is at first segmented, but shortly fuses into nephrogenic cords which provide origin for the renal tubules of the kidneys. From the nephrogenic tissue three successive sets of excretory organs develop in serial fashion, in cranial to caudal orientation: the pronephric kidney, the mesonephric kidney, and the metanephric kidney (Fig. 1:1).

The Fallopian Tube: Basic Studies and Clinical Contributions, edited by Alvin M. Siegler, M.D. Mount Kisco, New York: Futura Publishing Company, Inc. © 1986.

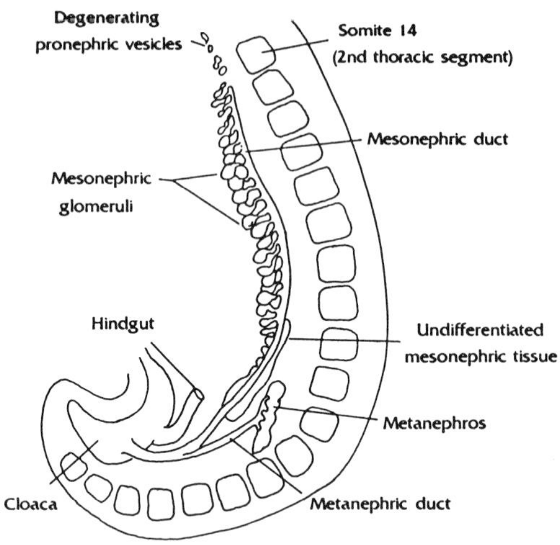

FIGURE 1:1—*Schematic representation of the development of the pronephros, nephros, metanephros, and their ducts at about the 5 mm stage.*

Pronephros

The pronephric kidney and its duct develop early in the fourth week of embryonic life. This kidney, which is nonfunctional in humans, appears in the cervical region as a half-dozen or so tubules that end at the pronephric duct. The pronephric duct terminates caudally in the cloaca. The pronephric renal elements degenerate rapidly and the pronephric duct is assimilated by the mesonephric kidney late in the fourth week and becomes the mesonephric (wolffian) duct.

Mesonephros

By the end of the somite period, the mesonephros has differentiated to the level of the third lumbar segment and is suspended from the body wall by a thick mesonephric mesentery. The mesonephric kidney probably functions to some degree in humans, forming and excreting a very dilute form of urine.[2,5,6] By birth, the mesonephros has disappeared for the most part. The mesonephric duct and a few tubules are retained as genital ducts in the male; in the female, there are only vestigial remnants (Table 1:1). The mesonephric duct is nevertheless essential to the appearance and proper development of the primordium of much of the definitive female reproductive system.[5,7]

Metanephros

The metanephric kidney, which ultimately develops into the definitive excretory organ, makes its appearance early in the fifth week. Its formation involves a diverticulation of the caudal end of the mesonephric duct, the ureteric bud. The ureteric bud grows cranially from its point of emergence on the dorsal aspect of the mesonephric duct to reach the metanephric blastema, from which arise the nephrons of the definitive kidney.

Formation of the ovary

During the fifth week of embryonic development a thickening of coelomic epithelium makes its appearance on the medial aspect of the urogenital ridge. Further proliferation of the epithelial cells there, together with multiplication of the underlying mesenchymal cells, results in the formation of the gonadal ridge. It is here that the formation of the ovary will take place. The germ cells of the ovary, however, do not appear here initially. The primitive germ cells develop in the endodermal layer of the yolk sac during the third week; subsequently, after transverse folding of the embryo leads to the incorporation of portions of the yolk sac by the embryo, the germ cells migrate along the dorsal mesentery of the hindgut to the gonadal ridges, bilaterally. The germ cells then invade the underlying mesenchyme, becoming incorporated into the primary sex cords (which, in the female, later degenerate and disappear).

At about ten weeks the ovarian cortex makes its appearance and secondary cortical cords invade the mesenchyme from the germinal epithelium, incorporating the primordial germ cells. Subsequently, these cords separate into primordial follicles, each consisting of a central primordial germ cell (oogonium) and a peripheral

Table 1:1
*Developmental Remnants in the Female**

Vestige	*Position*	*Origin*	*Disorder*
Hydatid of Morgagni	On fimbria	Accessory müllerian orifice	Spontaneous torsion
Appendix vesiculosa (sessile hydatid)	Infundibular region	Blind cranial end of wolffian duct	Cyst
Epoophoron (Rosenmüller's organ)	Tubules in lateral third of mesovarium; duct in mesosalpinx, close to oviduct	Cranial mesonephric duct and tubules	—
Paroophoron (tubes of Kobelt)	Caudal to lateral half of ovary—seen in infants	Caudal mesonephric tubules	—
Ductus epoophori longitudinalis (Gartner's canal)	Cervical and vaginal wall	Caudal wolffian duct	Cysts; ectopic ureter

*Based on Gray and Skandalakis.[5]

layer of flattened follicular cells derived from the cortical cords. Mitoses of the oogonia occur during the fetal period. Enlargement of the oogonia into primary oocytes, together with the addition of one or more layers of follicular cells, leads to the formation of the primary ovarian follicles.[4,5] The mesenchymal cells surrounding the primary follicles form the stroma of the ovaries.

The cells of the germinal epithelial layer flatten after birth to form a layer of cuboidal cells which is continuous at the hilum of the ovary with the peritoneal mesothelium. The ovary is suspended by a peritoneal mesentery, the mesovarium, part of the broad ligament.

Formation and fate of the müllerian duct

During the sixth week (10 mm) the coelomic epithelium on the lateral aspect of the mesonephric portion of the urogenital ridge at the level of the third thoracic somite becomes thickened and then invaginates. Further ingrowth of the blindly ending paramesonephric duct then ensues in a caudal direction through the mesenchyme of the mesonephros. Formation and development of the paramesonephric duct occurs close to, and is apparently dependent on, the mesonephric duct, since interruption of the latter will cause failure of development of the former.[5,7] The initial site of invagination, the funnel field, is retained definitively as the abdominal ostium of the uterine tube. Supernumerary sites of ostia can form; these may be retained as hydatid cysts or as oviductal appendages.

The uterine tubes, the uterus, and the broad ligaments

As the two urogenital ridges approach the cloaca caudally, they swing toward the midline of the embryo and fuse into the genital cord. Cranially, the urogenital ridges become increasingly displaced more laterally by the developing suprarenal glands and kidneys (Fig. 1:2).[8] Thus, cranial vertical, intermediate hori-

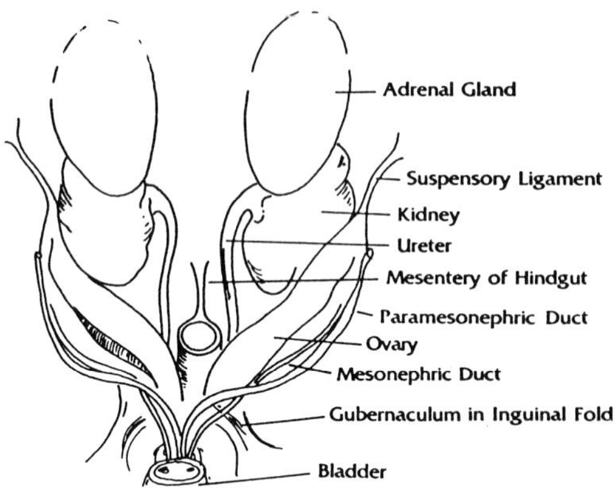

FIGURE 1:2—*Appearance of the posterior abdominal wall in a 26 mm embryo to show the relationships of the various components of the urogenital system.*

zontal, and caudal vertical portions of the urogenital ridges and their associated anlage are soon established.

In its proximal segment the paramesonephric duct lies lateral to, and courses parallel with the mesonephric duct; the intermediate portion crosses ventral to the mesonephric duct; the distal segment courses caudally once more, medial to the mesonephric duct. By the eighth week, therefore, the rostral vertical, middle transverse, and caudal vertical portions of the paramesonephric duct are evident.[7] The mesonephric and paramesonephric ducts are both enclosed in urogenital folds of peritoneum which contribute later to the formation of the broad ligament of the uterus.

As the caudal vertical segments of the paramesonephric ducts grow toward the urogenital sinus within the genital cord, they approach one another in the midline and fuse to form the uterovaginal canal. At nine weeks the caudal limit of this fusion is evident as the blindly ending Müller's tubercle, a median protuberance projecting from the dorsal wall of the urogenital sinus (Fig. 1:3).[8] Subsequently, this canal will form the uterus and contribute to the formation of the superior portion of the vagina. Fusion of the paramesonephric ducts brings together the peritoneal mesenteries of the transverse intermediate segments of the ducts, forming the right and left broad ligaments. Further proliferation and differentiation of mesenchyme between the two peritoneal layers of each broad ligament gives rise to the loose connective tissue and smooth-muscle fibers of the parametrium.

The cranial vertical and intermediate transverse portions of the paramesonephric ducts, now the formative oviducts, increase in prominence as the mesonephric system degenerates. The open, cranial end soon develops a fringe of fimbriae. Originally, the future site of the junction of the fundus and body of the uterus is represented by the transverse portions of the paramesonephric ducts (Fig. 1:3). After a time the cranial aspects of these parts of the ducts bulge upward, so that their original angular junction becomes a convex dome. The definitive fundus and body of the uterus are formed in this way. The uterine cervix arises probably from the more cranial portion of the fused lower vertical duct segments. In the eighth month, the oviducts increase in length and subsequently in tortuosity.

The ovarian gubernaculum

At about 15 mm the gonad is attached to the body wall by the cranial and caudal ligaments of the degenerating mesonephros[3] as the ovary outgrows the mesonephros. By 26 mm the cranial pole of the developing ovary is attached (through the degenerating mesonephros) to the posterior coelomic wall by a suspensory ligament (Fig. 1:2). The caudal pole of the gonad is continuous with a band of mesenchyme that extends along the urogenital ridge, crosses the umbilical artery, and ends in the inguinal region. This band of mesenchyme is the gubernaculum of the ovary. The gubernaculum becomes attached to the uterovaginal canal just inferior to the junction of the canal with the uterine tube. The portion of the gubernaculum between the ovary and the uterus becomes the proper ligament of the ovary; the dis-

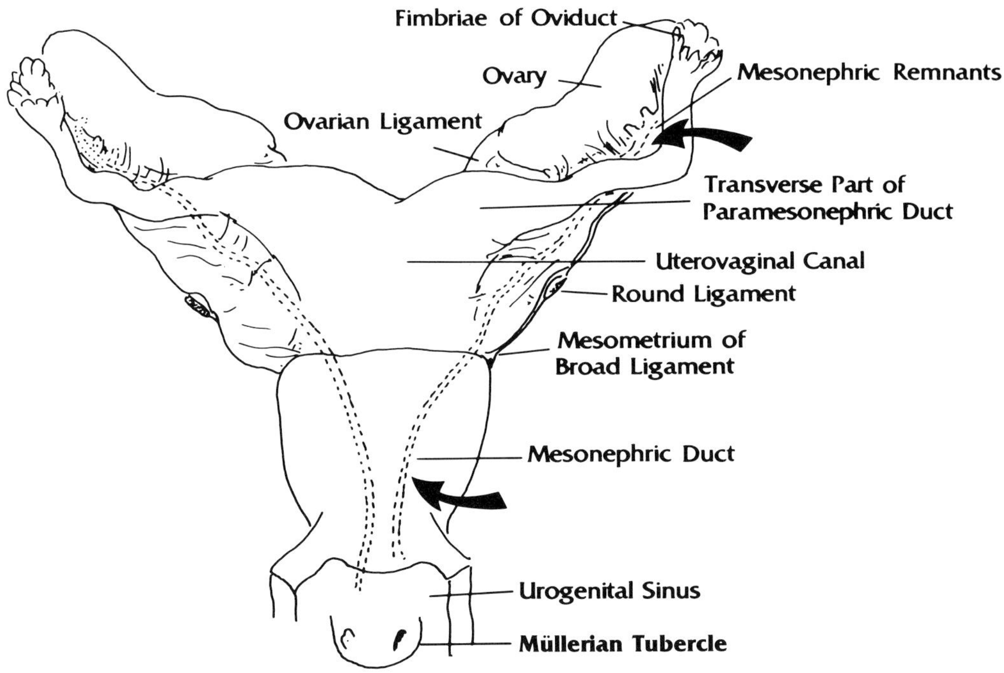

FIGURE 1:3—*Anterior view of the appearance of the genital ducts in a 48 mm female embryo. The mesonephros and the mesonephric duct in part are represented by interrupted lines (arrows).*

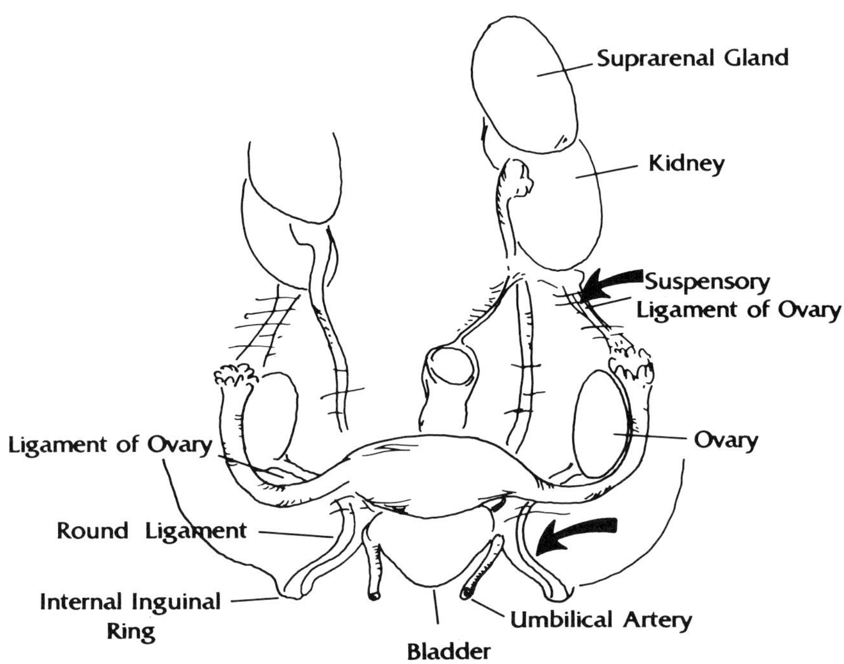

FIGURE 1:4—*The posterior abdominal wall in a 70 mm human female embryo demonstrating the definitive female organs and the fate of the gubernaculum (arrows).*

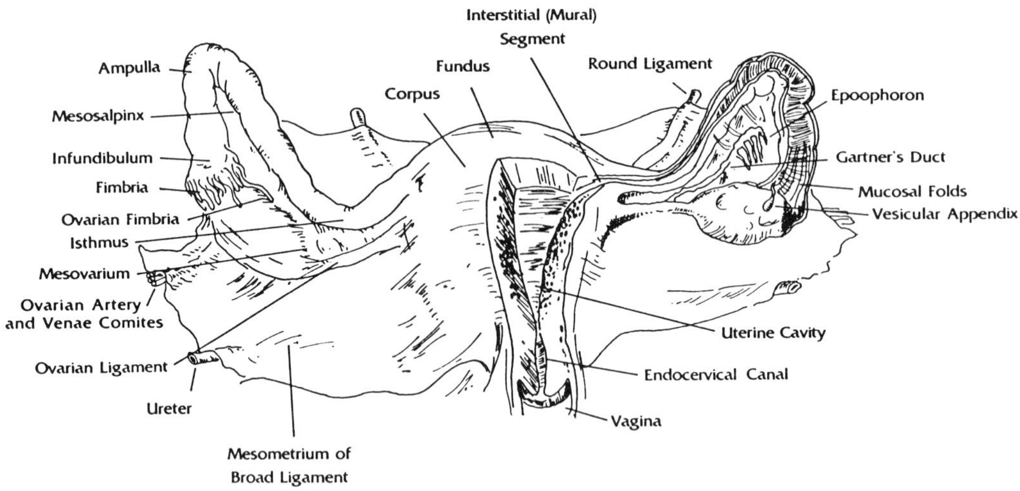

FIGURE 1:5—*Posterior view of uterus and adnexa.*

tal part of the gubernaculum, extending from the uterus to the labium majus, forms the round ligament of the uterus (Fig. 1:4).

The attachment of the gubernaculum to the uterus presumably prevents the external passage of the ovary. The ovary, thus, descends into the true pelvis and rotates such that the original caudal ovarian pole becomes directed medially and the original cranial pole becomes directed laterally. From its initial position medial to the urogenital mesentery, the ovary now comes to occupy a dorsal relationship to that structure (now the broad ligament) and the uterine tube.

Gross Anatomy

The two oviducts are enclosed by the mesosalpingeal portions of the broad ligaments of the uterus (Fig. 1:5) In general form, as traced laterally from the uterus, each tube passes at first horizontally, laterally, and posteriorly along the uterine pole of the ovary. After ascending the wall of the true pelvis, often tortuously, it passes along the mesovarial border of the ovary to the tubal pole of the ovary, arching over it and descending to its free border. There, the fimbriated end approaches the medial surface of the ovary. In the adult the oviducts are about 10 cm long, with variations in length from 7 to 14 cm.[9,10] Considering the tube as the ovary's "excretory duct," its parts are described below, beginning with its lateral extremity, the fimbriated infundibulum.

Infundibulum

The opening of the relaxed abdominal tubal ostium is about 3 mm in diameter. The infundibulum is funnel-shaped and its circumference is characterized by the presence of numerous irregularly slender processes called fimbriae.

The internal surface of the fimbriae is covered with mucous membrane which is continuous with that within the tube. The mucosal surface of some of the broader fimbriae possesses longitudinal foldings continuous with foldings within the lateral end of the tube. One such fimbria, the ovarian fimbria, is longer, reaching to the tubal pole of the ovary, to which it is closely applied.

The infundibulum possesses only a thin intramural musculature. It is continuous with the thin-walled ampullary portion of the uterine tube.

Ampulla

The ampulla provides about half of the length of the tube and, in some individuals, is quite tortuous in configuration. It is typically 5 to 8 cm long. The lateral end of the ampulla has a luminal diameter of about one centimeter. This dimension narrows considerably, medially, to the 1 to 2 mm width at the ampullary-isthmic junction. The ampulla possesses a poorly defined internal longitudinal musculature dispersed within its mucosal folds. A circular layer of smooth muscle can be seen, although this layer is often interrupted by fascicles of outer longitudinal muscle fibers.[11] The ampulla is succeeded by the narrow, thick-walled isthmic section.

Isthmus

The isthmus, which is 2 to 3 cm long, provides about one-third of the length of the tube. A line drawn between the cornual terminations of the two uterine tubes is conventionally used to demarcate the uterine corpus and fundus. The medial attachment of the isthmic segment is situated just cephalad to the uterine attachments of the ovarian ligament and the round ligament. The muscle layers of the isthmus are the thickest and most clearly defined of the major segments of the tube and consist of inner and outer longitudinal layers and a middle circular layer. The inner longitudinal layer, which is well defined at its uterine end, begins to be less distinct approximately 1 cm medial to the ampullary-isthmic junction. The thickness of the middle circular layer increases progressively from its ampullary end to the uterine end. The lumen of the isthmus varies between 230 μm and 2 mm in diameter.[11]

Intramural segment

The intramural (or interstitial) segment of each uterine tube is about 1 cm long and varies from 0.2 to 0.4 mm in diameter; it extends through the wall of the uterus from the end of the isthmic segment to its ostium, opening into the superior angle of the uterine cavity. There is an ampulla-like dilatation of the intramural segment just proximal to its termination. The intramural portion may take a rather simple, straight course through the uterine wall, or it may take an irregular pathway.[11,12] The three layers of musculature of the oviduct are continuous with those of the uterine wall.

Arterial supply

The arterial supply of the tube is derived from both the ovarian artery and the uterine artery. The ovarian arteries arise from the ventral aspect of the abdominal aorta just below the origin of the renal arteries. They descend obliquely in an inferolateral direction, reaching the brim of the true (lesser) pelvis. The ovarian artery crosses the external iliac artery and vein and the ureter, then courses through the connective tissue of the infundibulopelvic fold (ligament), which provides the lateral fifth of the broad ligament.

Subsequently, the ovarian vessels pass between the two peritoneal layers of the broad ligament inferior to the oviduct and inward through the mesovarium to reach the ovary. In its course to the mesovarium, the ovarian artery divides into ovarian and tubal branches. The tubal branch supplies the lateral third of the tube,[10,11] anastomosing thereafter with tubal branches of the uterine artery. The ovarian artery, in addition to supplying the ovary, provides one or two collateral branches to the oviduct and anastomoses with the ovarian branch of the uterine artery.

The uterine artery arises from the anterior division of the internal iliac (hypogastric) artery; it then passes medially from the wall of the lesser pelvis, on the fascia covering the levator ani muscle of the pelvic floor, thereafter entering the caudal portion of the broad ligament. Coursing through the parametrium, the uterine artery crosses the ureter approximately 2 cm from the cervix, gives off the vaginal artery, and then ascends the lateral aspect of the cervix and body of the uterus, supplying these by numerous branches.

Near the uterine cornu, the uterine artery gives off a stem that divides into ovarian and tubal arterial branches which pass laterally into the mesovarium and mesosalpinx, respectively.[13,14] The ovarian branch passes within the mesovarium to supply the ovary; it anastomoses with the ovarian artery and may provide a collateral branch to the oviduct. The tubal artery supplies the medial two-thirds of the oviduct,[10,11] and anastomoses with the tubal branch of the ovarian artery. The terminal part of the uterine artery supplies the cornual region, the intramural part of the oviduct, and the tissues of the upper uterus.

Venous drainage

The venous vessels of the tube accompany the arterial supply. The plexus of ovarian veins in the broad ligament communicates with the uterine venous plexus. The right ovarian vein drains into the inferior vena cava just below the renal veins; the left ovarian vein drains to the left renal vein. The uterine veins pass through the lateral ligaments (of Mackenrodt) to attain the internal iliac veins.

Lymphatic drainage

The lymph vessels of the tube pass with those of the ovary and uterus to para-aortic and lumbar lymph nodes. Tubal vessels pass within the mesosalpinx to enter a network below the hilum of the ovary. This drainage appears to be totally separate from that of the uterus.[15]

Innervation

The nerve supply of the uterine tube reaches it largely on the ovarian and uterine arteries. Parasympathetic supply to the lateral half of the tube is derived from vagal fibers; pelvic splanchnic fibers from the S2–S4 segments of the spinal cord supply the medial half of the oviduct. The secondary cell bodies on which the vagal and pelvic splanchnic fibers synapse are probably in paracervical ganglia, since no ganglionic cell bodies are seen adjacent to the uterine tube.[10]

The preganglionic sympathetic supply for the tube arises largely from the intermediolateral cell column of spinal cord segments T10–L2. Secondary, postganglionic fibers arise in celiac, preaortic, renal, inferior mesenteric and hypogastric ganglia. The ampullary region is supplied by sympathetic fibers that accompany the ovarian artery and pass into the ovarian plexus; the isthmic region is supplied by fibers that pass through the hypogastric plexus. The afferent nerve fibers for pain for the oviducts accompany the sympathetic innervation; the majority of these sensory fibers enter the T10 and T11 spinal cord levels, with some input also to the L1 and L2 segments.[11]

References

1. Price D, Zaaiijer JJ, and Ortiz E: Prenatal development in vivo and in vitro. In Hafez ESE and Blandau R (Eds): *The Mammalian Oviduct.* Chicago: University of Chicago Press, 1969: 29.
2. Hamilton WJ, Boyd JD, and Mossman HW: *Human Embryology*, 3d ed. Baltimore: Williams & Wilkins, 1962: 267.
3. Allan FD: *Essentials of Human Embryology*. New York: Oxford University Press, 1960: 108.
4. Moore KL: *The Developing Human*, 2d ed. Philadelphia: W.B. Saunders, 1977: 220.
5. Gray SW and Skandalakis JE: *Embryology for Surgeons: The Embryological Basis for the Treatment of Congenital Defects*. Philadelphia: W.B. Saunders, 1972: 443.
6. Gersh I: The correlation of structure and function in the mesonephros and metanephros. *Contrib Embryol Carneg Inst*, 26:33, 1937.
7. O'Rahilly R: Prenatal human develop-

ment. In Wynn RM (Ed): *Biology of the Uterus*. New York: Plenum Press, 1977: 35.

8. Arey LB: *Developmental Anatomy*, 7th ed. Philadelphia: W.B. Saunders, 1965: 295.
9. Markee JE: The urogenital system. In Anson BJ (Ed): *Morris' Human Anatomy*, 12th ed. New York: McGraw-Hill, 1966: 1457.
10. Warwick R, and Williams PL: *Gray's Anatomy*, 35th Br. ed. Philadelphia: W.B. Saunders, 1973: 1354.
11. Pauerstein CJ: *The Fallopian Tube—A Reappraisal*. Philadelphia: Lea and Febiger, 1974.
12. Hafez ESE, and Black DL: The mammalian uterotubal junction. In Hafez ESE and Blandau RJ (Eds): *The Mammalian Oviduct: Comparative Biology and Methodology*. Chicago: The University of Chicago Press, 1969: 85.
13. McVay CB: *Surgical Anatomy*, Vol. II, 6th ed. Philadelphia: W.B. Saunders, 1984: 844.
14. Goss CM: *Gray's Anatomy of the Human Body*, 29th ed. Philadelphia: Lea and Febiger, 1973: 1321.
15. Rodbard S, McMahon NJ, and Denk M: Uterine structure and lymphatics. *Obstet Gynecol* 38: 171, 1971. (Cited by Pauerstein.[11])

2

The Smooth-Muscle Architecture of the Human Fallopian Tube

Bo Lindblom and
Anders Norström

The mammalian oviduct is comprised of two easily distinguishable parts, the wide ampulla and the narrow isthmus. The ampulla terminates at the distal abdominal opening, the infundibulum with its finger-like processes, the fimbriae. The term "ampullary-isthmic junction" (AIJ) denotes the border between the isthmus and ampulla, considered to be of special importance in the regulation of ovum transport. The proximal part of the oviduct, constituting the junction between the uterus and the tube, is often referred to as the "uterotubal junction" (UTJ) (Fig. 2:1). In primates and most laboratory animals, smooth muscle is the dominant tissue in the isthmus, whereas the mucosa is more prominent in the ampullary portion.

Except for the myosalpinx, the motile properties of the oviduct may be influenced by contractile activity in adjacent structures—primarily the mesosalpinx but also the ovarian ligaments, the ovarian pedicle, and the uterus. The smooth muscular coat surrounding the oviductal lumen is arranged in more or less distinct layers with different directions. In the UTJ at least three muscular layers can be distinguished: the innermost longitudinal, the intermediate circular, and the outer longitudinal ("uterine") layer with mixed fiber direction. The latter layers appear to continue into the circular and outer (longitudinal or mixed) layers of the isthmus and the ampulla, whereas the inner longitudinal layer disappears in the middle part of the isthmus.

In all mammalian species studied so far, the circular muscular layer is the most constant and prominent, having a thickness exceeding the luminal diameter in the isthmus and UTJ. In the human fallopian tube, the narrowest part has an inner diameter of less than 0.3 mm, although an exact estimation of the luminal size is imprecise because of the presence of mucosal folds and tubal secretions. In the proximal ampulla, the diameter is in the area of 5 mm and at the infundibular end it

The Fallopian Tube: Basic Studies and Clinical Contributions, edited by Alvin M. Siegler, M.D. Mount Kisco, New York: Futura Publishing Company, Inc. © 1986.

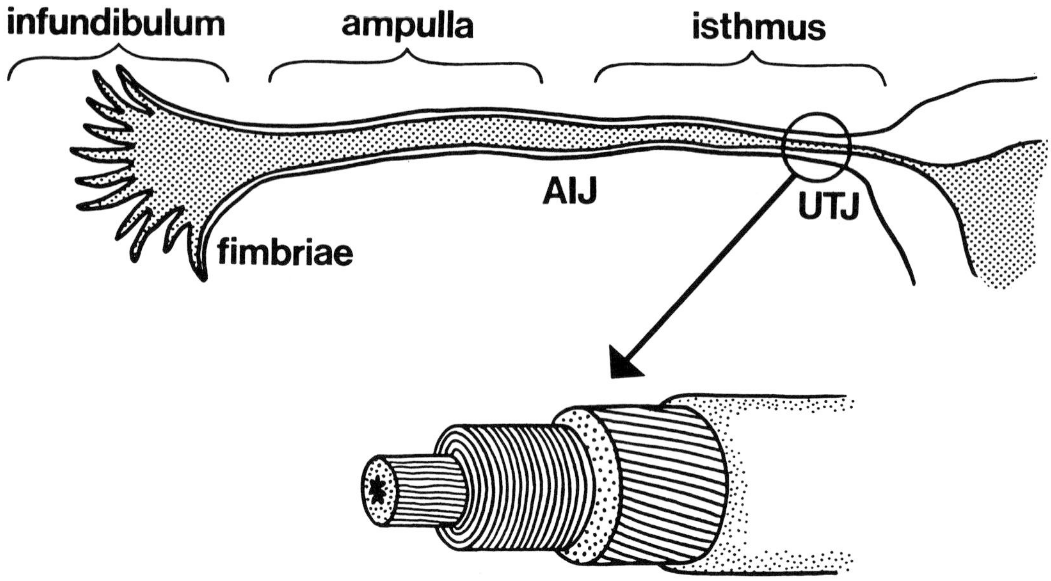

FIGURE 2:1—*The anatomy of the human fallopian tube (semi-schematic). AIJ = ampullary-isthmic junction; UTJ = uterotubal junction, which is comprised of an interstitial and an intramural part. In the proximal isthmus, three muscle layers can be identified: (at arrow) an outer longitudinal or spiral-shaped, an intermediate circular, and an innermost longitudinal layer. (Reproduced by permission from Lindblom et al.)*[10]

measures about 10 mm. Concomitantly with the increase in luminal size, there is gradually increased number and height of mucosal folds (Table 2:1). As the musculature becomes comparatively less abundant in ovarian direction, lumen ratio is gradually decreased, from 15 at the UTJ to less than 0.2 at the infundibulum (Figs. 2:1, 2:2, and 2:3).

While the frequency of contractions appears to be under hormonal influence,[1,2] the duration of contraction does not.[3] However, the duration of contraction varies in a specific manner among the various tubal muscular layers and in different tubal segments. The longest duration of contraction is encountered in the most proximal region and in the outer zones (Table 2:2). In these areas, the pattern of contraction shows striking similarities to the activity of uterine muscle, i.e., slow frequency, long duration. Daniel et al.[4] studied the anatomy of the human oviduct by both light microscopy and electron microscopy. Their studies revealed close apposition between muscle cells in both the isthmus and ampulla and also in between various muscular layers. However, no cell-to-cell contacts fulfilling the criteria of "gap junctions" could be demonstrated in any of the layers. The isthmic muscle cells appeared more densely distributed and also were equipped with a more dense innervation.

The Muscular Layers

The outer longitudinal layer is not as distinct as the other layers of the tubal wall. Daniel et al.[5] prefer to use the term "mixed" to describe the direction of the muscle fibers in the outer zone. Other investigators, however, agree that the fibers run longitudinally or in a spiral.[6,8] In the isthmus, the circular and outer layers are separated by a collagenous part containing the blood vessels of the tubal wall (Fig. 2:2). The longitudinal muscular layer extends to the thin serosal epithelium and

Table 2:1

Criteria Used for the Identification of the Ampullary-Isthmic Junction (AIJ) of the Human Oviduct[8]

Property	*UTJ*	*AIJ*	*Ampulla*
Luminal diameter (mm)	0.2–0.5	0.4–1.3	1.5–5.0
Distance from the uterine wall (mm)	0	25–35	>35
Number of mucosal folds	3–5	6–8	> 8
Inner longitudinal layer	distinct	infrequent	absent

Table 2:2

*Mean Duration of Contraction in Different Muscle Layers of Various Tubal Regions (Time in Seconds)**

	Muscle layer			
Region	*Inner longitudinal*	*Middle circular*	*Outer longitudinal*	*Reference*
UTJ	8	18	46	Wilhelsson et al.[4]
AIJ	—	17	31	Lindblom et al.[9]
Ampulla	—	12.5	15	Caschetto et al.[2]

*The time from the rise of the contraction to the return of the tension to the baseline.

during dissection it may be accidentally removed together with the peritoneum.

Muscle strips dissected from the outer longitudinal layer exhibit a typical contractile pattern when mounted in an organ bath.[9,10] The contractions are usually of phasic character but episodic "bursts" of activity may also be observed, especially when the size of the piece is increased. The frequency of contraction is in the area of 20 per 10 minutes and the mean duration is about 25 seconds.[10] By using big suction electrodes a similar spike frequency may be recorded from the outer surface of the tube after removal of the serosa.[11] Interestingly, early studies using whole oviduct segments suspended in organ baths showed a similar frequency of mechanical activity.[12] One may assume from this that: (1) mounting of gross tubal segments in organ baths will imply recording of activity from the outer longitudinal layer mainly; and (2) electrodes placed on the external side of the tubal wall will lead to recording from the outer longitudinal layer only.

The circular layer

The intermediate circular layer exhibits a higher contractile frequency in vitro than the outer longitudinal layer (Fig. 2:4), and the duration of contraction is significantly shorter. The phasic character is still more prominent when compared with

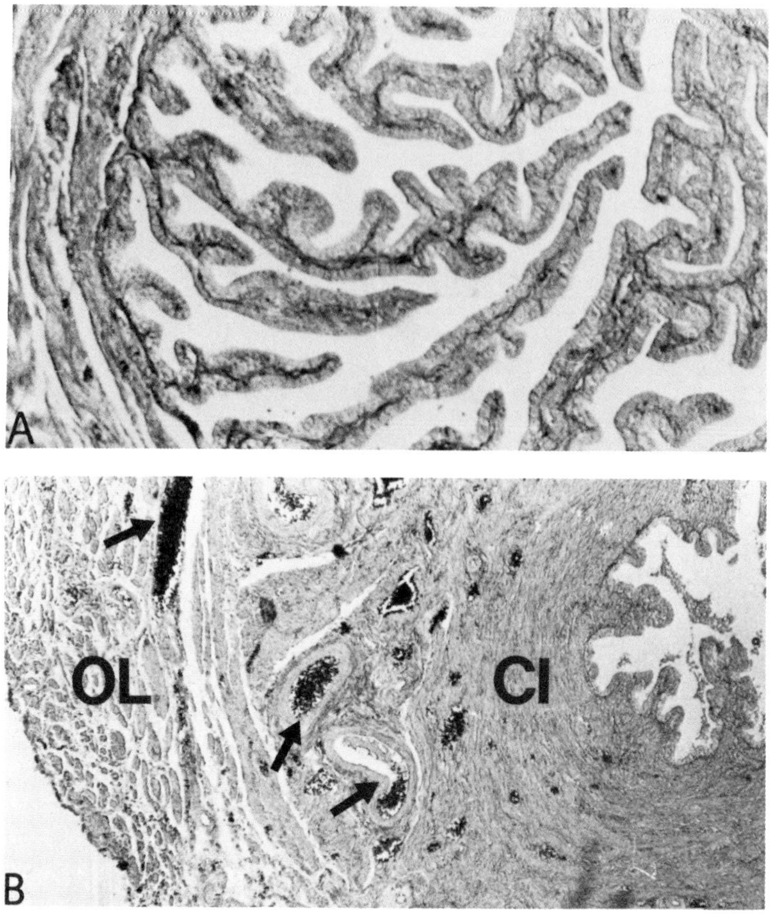

FIGURE 2:2—*Transverse sections.* A. *The ampullary portion of the human oviduct, showing the deep mucosal infoldings within the tubal lumen. (× 42)* B. *The distal isthmus corresponding to the AIJ. CI = circular intermediate layer; OL = outer longitudinal layer. Arrows indicate blood vessels. (Original magnification, × 24) (Mallory-Azan.)*

the outer longitudinal layer, and at the time of ovulation the contractile frequency is significantly increased.[3] By using the intact segment of the distal portion of the isthmus, action potentials of similar frequency can be picked up by small suction electrodes from the inner surface after removal of the mucosa (Lindblom and Talo, unpublished observations).

The inner longitudinal layer

As mentioned before, the innermost longitudinal layer is absent in the distal part of the isthmus but may, at least in some individuals, be identified in the mid-isthmus. However, in this area, this layer often covers only part of the circumference. In the proximal part of the isthmus and in the intramural portion, the inner longitudinal layer is clearly distinguishable along the whole circumference (Fig. 2:3).

Lisa et al.[13] investigated the anatomy of the interstitial portion of the human oviduct, using a large clinical material and standard histologic techniques. They found that the inner longitudinal layer at this region was a continuation of the sub-

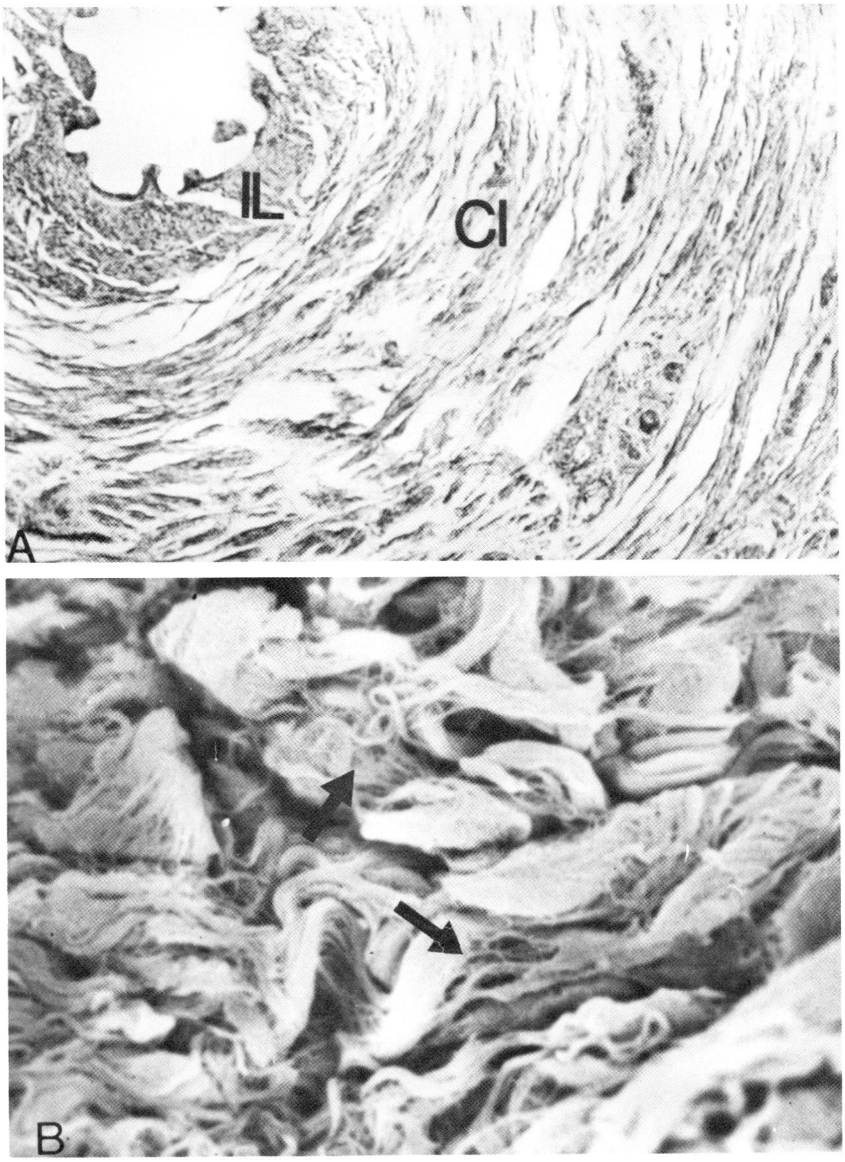

FIGURE 2:3—A. *Transverse section of the proximal isthmus adjacent to the UTJ. IL = inner longitudinal layer; CI = circular intermediate layer.* (× 42)(*van Gieson.*) B. *Scanning electron micrograph of a muscle strip from the outer longitudinal layer of the isthmus. Thin collagen fibers (arrows) intermingle among the smooth muscle cells.* (× 3000)

endometrial layer of the uterus. They also showed that the medial part of the narrow gate between the tube and the uterus was not equipped with tubal but with uterine epithelium and preferred to call this region the "uterine funnel." Later, David and Czernobilsky[6] made a comparative study of the uterotubal junction in the rabbit, rhesus monkey, and human. Although the patient material was very small, their study included the important observation that the inner longitudinal layer was present also in the isthmic part of the tube. Interestingly, this layer appeared to consist of hyalinized connective tissue in the monkey, but was clearly muscular in

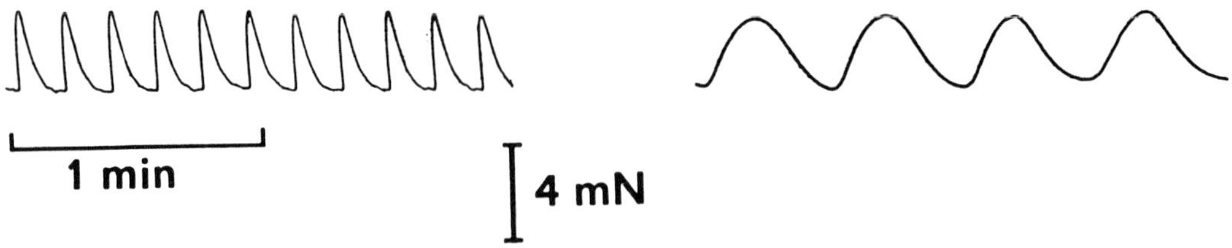

FIGURE 2:4—*Spontaneous rhythmic activity of strips isolated from the circular (left tracing) and outer longitudinal (right tracing) muscle layers at the ampullary-isthmic junction of the human oviduct. Note the regularity of contractions and the difference in contraction frequency between the circular and longitudinal muscle.*

the woman. The layer was compact and occupied all or most of the lamina propria area. Based on their findings, David and Czernobilsky suggested that a sphincter action may result from the contraction of the inner longitudinal and the circular layers. Like the circular and outer longitudinal layers, the inner longitudinal layer exhibits regular spontaneous activity, and the frequency is significantly higher than in the other layers.[14]

The interstitial portion constitutes the narrowest part of the tube, with a luminal diameter varying between 0.2 and 0.5 mm. The muscle fibers of the inner longitudinal layer typically run inside the mucosal folds. This interesting observation has not been further explored in terms of its significance for closure of the tubal lumen. Without any sharp limit, the muscle layers of the interstitial portion continue into the myometrial layers: the outer longitudinal, the intermediate spiral-shaped, and the subendometrial longitudinal.[15] This similarity between tubal and uterine layers does not seem surprising in view of the common embryological origin of the organs, i.e. the müllerian ducts.

General Features of Tubal Smooth Muscle

Tubal musculature has the capacity of maintaining rhythmic spontaneous activity when deprived of its external innervation and should therefore be classified as a single unit type of smooth muscle. Conductivity is comparatively slow: estimated velocity of spread ranges from 1 to 9 mm/sec.[5,11] Whereas Daniel et al.[5] stated that the electrical activity in the tube only travels very short distances, Talo and Pulkkinen[11] quoted that the potentials often spread along the entire length of the oviduct. This discrepancy can probably be explained by the fact that the latter investigators used big suction electrodes which will cover a greater surface and this will increase the probability of picking up signals spread randomly. Each contraction is accompanied by only one action potential and "burst activity" does not occur.[16]

The mesosalpinx

The mesosalpingeal muscle elements are least investigated but are probably of great importance for the gross movements during the ovum pickup, when the fimbriae are in contact with the ovulatory site of the ovarian surface. The mesosalpingeal muscle also seems to be responsible for the twisting appearance of the oviduct. Sterin-Speziale et al.[17] studied the activity of isolated strips from the human tubo-ovarian ligament and fimbriae, and found evidence for a steroid dependent change in their activity and response to specific agents. However, in general, the contractile properties of the mesosalpinx and other supporting structures of the oviducts have attracted comparatively little interest in tubal physiological research.

The fimbriae

The anatomic configuration of the infundibulum and its fimbriae varies greatly among species and very little information is available concerning the muscle elements of the human fimbriae. At the midcycle, however, the human fimbriae are remarkably fringed and fluted, with numerous lanciform extensions. When the entire human fimbriae are observed in a tissue culture medium in vitro, one may see a slow pendulum-like movement of the various lappets.[18] At ovulation, the fimbriae come into close contact with the surface of the ovary and move back and forth over the ovulatory follicle to remove the viscous mass of the oocyte and corona cells.

Concluding Remarks

In summary, the human oviduct is equipped with a developed smooth muscle of the single unit type. Most of the musculature is arranged in defined muscle layers whereas some of the contractile elements are dispersed in thin strands with ill-defined structure.

The smooth-muscle tissue serves its purpose of promoting transport of ova and spermatozoa by a complex pattern of integrated movements. The basic pattern of activity in various muscle layers and tubal segments have been explored but knowledge is still lacking about some fundamental principles of interaction between adjacent areas. Such insight may probably best be attained by delicate electrophysiological studies. This knowledge, together with an exploration of the role of the mesosalpinx and the adjacent myogenic structures, seems essential for a better understanding of tubal motility and its importance in the function and dysfunction of the organ.

References

1. Lindblom B, Wilhelmsson L, Wikland M, et al: Prostaglandins and oviductal function. *Acta Obstet Gynecol Scand*, 113:43, 1983.
2. Caschetto S, Lindblom B, Wiqvist N, et al: Prostaglandins and the contractile function of the human oviductal ampulla. *Gynecol Obstet Invest*, 10:212, 1979.
3. Lindblom B, Ljung B, and Hamberger L: Adrenergic and novel nonadrenergic neuronal mechanisms in the control of smooth muscle activity in the human oviduct. *Acta Physiol Scand*, 106:215, 1979.
4. Daniel EE, Posey VA, and Paton DM: A structural analysis of the myogenic control systems of the human fallopian tube. *Am J Obstet Gynecol*, 121:1054, 1975.
5. Daniel EE, Lucien P, Posey VA, et al: A functional analysis of the myogenic control systems of the human fallopian tube. *Am J Obstet Gynecol*, 121:1046, 1975.
6. David A, and Czernobilsky B: A comparative histologic study of the uterotubal junction in the rabbit, rhesus monkey, and human female. *Am J Obstet Gynecol* 101:417, 1968.
7. Hafez ESE, and Black DL: The mammalian uterotubal junction. In Hafez ESE, and Blandau RJ (Eds): *The Mammalian Oviduct*. Chicago: University of Chicago, Press, 1969.
8. Lindblom B: Hormonal and neuronal control of human oviductal contractility. Thesis, University of Göteborg, Sweden, 1979.
9. Lindblom G, Hamberger L, and Wiqvist N: Differntiated contractile effects of prostaglandins E and F on the isolated circular and longitudinal smooth muscle of the human oviduct. *Fertil Steril*, 30:553, 1978.
10. Lindblom B, Hamberger L, and Ljung B: Contractile patterns of isolated smooth muscle under different hormonal conditions. *Fertil Steril*, 33:283, 1980.
11. Talo A, and Pulkkinen MO: Electrical activity in the human oviduct during the menstrual cycle. *Am J Obstet Gynecol*, 142:135, 1982.
12. Sandberg F, Ingelman-Sundberg A, Lindgren L, et al: In vitro studies of the motility of the human fallopian tube (part I). *Acta Obstet Gynecol Scand*, 39:506, 1960.
13. Lisa JR, Gioia JD, and Rubin IC: Observations on the interstitial portion of the fallopian tube. *Surg Gynecol Obstet*, 99:159, 1954.

14. Wilhelmsson L, Lindblom B, and Wiqvist N: The human uterotubal junction: Contractile patterns of different smooth muscle layers and the influence of prostaglandin E_2, prostglandin F and prostaglandin I_2 in vitro. *Fertil Steril* 32:303, 1979.
15. Wetzstein R: Der Uterusmuskel: Morphologie. *Arch Gynäkol,* 202:1, 1965.
16. Lindblom B, and Wikland M: Simultaneous recording of electrical and mechanical activity in isolated smooth muscle of the human oviduct. *Biol Reprod,* 27:393, 1982.
17. Sterin-Speziale N, Gimeno MF, Zapata C, et al: The effect of neurotransmitters, bradykinin, prostaglandins, and follicular fluid on spontaneous contractile characteristics of human fimbriae and tubo-ovarian ligaments isolated during different stages of the sexual cycle. *Int J Fertil,* 23:1, 1978.

3

Tubal Vasculature

Christopher J. Verco

The anatomy of the arterial and venous vessels of the fallopian tube is well described in women and in laboratory animals. The arteries are derived from the ovarian and uterine stems; the relative contribution of these vessels, however, or variations in the contribution of each with, for example, the menstrual cycle in women or during the estrus cycle and ovum transport in laboratory animals, is unknown. In addition, there are few coherent data on the microvasculature of the reproductive organs available in current texts of reproductive medicine and, indeed, this subject does not yet warrant a chapter in the latest texts on the microcirculation.

Human Tubal Vasculature

Human fallopian tube arterial blood supply is derived from the uterine and ovarian arteries. The uterine artery ascends closely applied to the myometrium and, near the uterine cornu, branches to supply the cornu and the interstitial portion of the tube. The uterine artery then divides into two trunks. One supplies the medial portion of the tube. The other courses through the mesosalpinx just beneath and along the entire length of the tube[1] and anastomoses with the ovarian artery; this anastomosis may be in the ovarian ligament.[2] The ovarian artery divides into two trunks. One supplies the ovary and anastomoses with the ovarian branch of the uterine artery and the other supplies the distal portion of the tube. Either the uterine or ovarian arteries may send a second trunk to the tube.[1,3] There is considerable variation in the contribution of the uterine and ovarian arteries; however, branches of the uterine artery in general supply the isthmus, and branches of the ovarian artery the remaining parts of the tube.[3] Either artery alone, however, may supply the whole tube.[3] In-vivo arteriography revealed that the tubal arterial supply may be derived entirely from either the ovarian or uterine arteries or from an admixture of the two.[4] The venous drainage follows that of the arterial supply.[1,3] Venous drainage from the tube in the ovarian vein is particularly interesting, since the ovarian vein and artery are closely related in the human ovarian pedicle.[5] Areas of contact between the ovarian artery and vein are characterized by thin-

The Fallopian Tube: Basic Studies and Clinical Contributions, edited by Alvin M. Siegler, M.D. Mount Kisco, New York: Futura Publishing Company, Inc. © 1986.

ning of the ovarian vein wall.[5,6] This anatomical arrangement is consistent with the hypothesis that there is a countercurrent transfer of factors from the ovarian veins to arteries.[5–7]

Human Tubal Microvasculature

Human fallopian tube microvasculature has been studied in 200 postmortem specimens; the tubal vaculature was injected with china ink and gelatin and the tubes were cleared and examined by stereo and light microscopy.[8–12] The tubal subserosa is supplied by arterioles that arise from a juxtatubal arterial arcade. The myosalpinx is supplied by tortuous arterioles that subsequently pass through the myosalpinx to give rise to the mucosal arterioles.[8–10] Mucosal arterioles, located at regular intervals of 0.3 to 0.5 mm,[9,10,13] are coiled and terminate in a dense submucosal capillary network; this capillary network subsequently drains to irregular caliber venules that pass parallel to each other and at right angles to the long axis of a mucosal fold,[8,11,12] to join deeper venules. Fimbrial angioarchitecture differs from that of the isthmic or ampullary mucosa in that arteries are more numerous than in isthmic or ampullary mucosa[9] and are located peripherally around a centrally located core venule.[8,10,11,13]

Tubal mucosal microvasculature varies with the menstrual cycle; during the proliferative phase, mucosal arterioles become increasingly coiled and this progresses, during the secretory phase, to a maximum at the time of menstruation.[9,10,12,13] These microvascular changes are most marked in the fimbria.[9,10] Mucosal venules are markedly dilated at the time of ovulation and maximally at the time of menstruation.[9,10,12] Mucosal arteriolar coils progressively tighten during pregnancy.[10,13] After the menopause, mucosal arterioles and venules dilate and mucosal arterioles are less tightly coiled.[10,13] Mucosal capillaries are normally 10 microns in diameter; premenstrually capillary diameters increase to 20 to 25 microns.[9] These morphological studies indicate that human tubal microvasculature varies with the menstrual cycle, pregnancy, and after the menopause; this suggests a sensitivity of the tubal microvasculature to ovarian and pregnancy hormones. The significance of these observations remains to be ascertained. Further study, preferably in tissue in which the vascular dimensions have been stabilized at normal distending pressures, is required to describe human tubal microvasculature adequately and to enable interpretation of the role of the tubal microvasculature in tubal function.

Animal Tubal Vasculature

The vasculature of tubal arterial supply and venous drainage has been described in a number of laboratory animals.[14–16] The rabbit is the laboratory animal most frequently used in the study of tubal morphology, physiology and pathology; for this reason, it is primarily the rabbit's oviductal vasculature that will be discussed.

The rabbit's tubal vasculature has been studied by a number of authors, and their descriptions generally are similar.[15,16] The ovarian arteries originate from the abdominal aorta, caudal to the origin of the renal arteries and cranial to the termination of the aorta; the right artery arises cranial to the origin of the left. The arteries pass ventrolaterally toward the ovary and about midway between their origin and the ovary, give off a long caudal branch, which runs about 2 cm from and substantially parallel to the tube.[16] This caudal branch in turn provides branches to the oviduct and the uterine horn.[15] The tubal branches divide, interconnect, and ramify over the tubal surface.[16] The caudal branch terminates by anastomosis with the terminal cranial end of the uterine artery.[15] The cranial branch divides to supply the ovary, infundibulum, and surrounding tissues. The uterine arteries arise from a branch of the internal iliac arteries and pass ventrally toward the cranial portion of the vagina and cervix, to run parallel to the caudal portion of the uterine horn and then divide into two prominent branches. The medial branch supplies the caudal portion of the uterine horn and ends by anastomosis with the contralateral uterine artery. The lateral branch provides branches that supply the cranial half of the uterine horn and the uterine tube. In vivo, in estrual rabbits, tubal blood flow is entirely derived from the ovarian artery; in vitro, however, tubal vasculature may be cast by infusion via either the uterine or the ovarian arteries.[16] The anatomy of the venous drainage is similar to that of the corresponding arteries. The right ovarian vein empties into the vena cava; the left empties into the lumbar vein.[15,16]

In rabbits and rhesus monkeys,[18] and in pigs and sheep,[19] the fimbriae are engorged with blood at the time of ovulation. Fimbrial "erection," aiding ovum capture was a widespread concept.[20] In addition, in the isthmus, when a contraction has subsided the previously contracted segment becomes engorged with blood.[21] This engorgement may cause some tubal sections to double their normal thickness; the relevance of this finding remains undetermined. Further investigation of tubal vasculature and the variations with changing hormone levels is clearly required. It would appear, however, that tubal vasculature varies with tubal activity and with the hormonal status of the animal.

The proximity of the utero-ovarian vein and ovarian artery in sheep resulted in the demonstration of the countercurrent transfer of prostaglandin $F_{2\alpha}$, the luteolysin in sheep, from the utero-ovarian vein to the ovarian artery and hence to the ovary.[22] A local transfer mechanism, for radioactive xenon, from the uterine horn to the ipsilateral ovary has been described in the mouse, hamster, and guinea pig, but not in the rabbit.[23] This was not observed in the rabbit, where the ovarian artery is not in close proximity to the uterine vein.[14,15,17,24] The countercurrent transfer of radioactive krypton from utero-ovarian vein to ovarian artery and thence to the ipsilateral tube and ovary was reported in sheep[25] and, in vivo from ovarian vein to ovarian artery in women.[26] These observations supported, but did not prove, the hypothesis that there was ovarian vein to artery countercurrent transfer of bioactive substances. The countercurrent transfer of progesterone (molecular weight 318) in the sheep utero-ovarian pedicle was later confirmed.[27] In addition, there is a countercurrent multiplier effect for [3H]-testosterone transfer from utero-ovarian vein to artery in the cow.[28] In vitro, there is a countercurrent transfer of progesterone and antipyrine between the ovarian veins and the ovarian artery in the human ovarian pedicule.[32] In the pig there is evidence of the countercurrent exchange between ovarian vein and artery of [3H]-testosterone, [3H]-progesterone, and [3H]-estradiol.[29,30] Such a countercurrent transfer of steroids and $PGF_{2\alpha}$ in pigs may influence isthmic function and therefore could influence tubal sperm transport.[7] Ovarian vein to artery exchange would enable the local regulation of uterine, tubal, and ovarian function with genital organs exposed to higher than central mixed venous or central arterial hormonal concentrations.[31,32]

Such an exchange mechanism renders quantification of ovarian steroids in peripheral blood interesting but of little value in predicting the genital end-organ effect. Countercurrent exchange between ovarian vein and artery, and perhaps between ovarian and tubal lymphatics and the ovarian vessels is of particular relevance to the study of tubo-ovarian physiology. The absorption of bioactive tubal factors could be readily transmitted to the ovary and may thereby signal, for example, the stage of embryonic development.

Animal Tubal Microvasculature

Fallopian tube microvascular architecture (MVA) has been ascertained by using the corrosion vascular cast scanning electron microscope (SEM) technique, in estrual rabbits.[33] By three-dimensional determination of vascular connections and easy distinction between arteries and veins, this technique

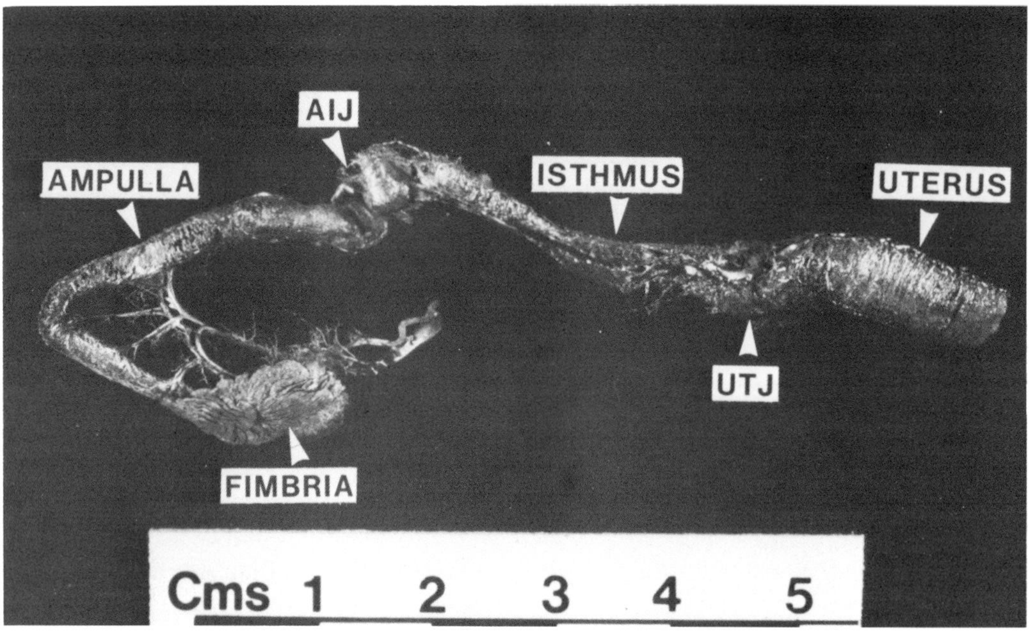

FIGURE 3:1—*A methylmethacrylate vascular corrosion cast of an estrual rabbit oviduct. UTJ = uterotubal junction; AIJ = ampullary-isthmic junction.*

of examining the microvasculature allows greater definition of the MVA. Vascular corrosion casts indicate the vasculature perfused and represent a vascular skeleton of the tissue at the time of casting. This technique compares favorably with vascular perfusion fixation with osmium tetroxide,[33] which is not associated with the tissue distortion that usually occurs with primary aldehyde fixation. In this technique, rabbits are anesthetized, the great vessels cannulated, and the blood washed from the vasculature. After blood washout, the vasculature is perfused with the casting medium, methylmethacrylate, which is allowed to polymerize under slight positive intravascular pressure.

Microscopically, the casts obtained (Fig. 3:1) are readily identified as oviducts. The uterotubal junction (UTJ), isthmus, ampullary-isthmic junction (AIJ), ampulla, and fimbria are easily located by their position along the tube and their characteristic morphological features. Tubal MVA, determined from vascular corrosion casts, varies characteristically along the length of the oviduct. The predominant differences are in the subserosal and submucosal microvasculature. In the isthmic subserosa there is an extensive interlocking venous plexus (Figs. 3:2 and 3:3); ampullary subserosal vasculature, in contrast, is comprised of parallel branching arteries and veins (Figs. 3:4 and 3:5). Isthmic plicae are well supplied with arterioles that branch little before terminal ramification, into capillaries, high in the plical core. Isthmic plical capillaries drain either down the fold or directly to centrally located plical core venules. Ampullary plical arterioles are less frequently observed and either branch low in a mucosal fold or pass to the top of a fold, along which they run before terminal ramification into capillaries. Ampullary plical capillaries drain to large venules that originate high in the plical core. Fimbrial arterioles and venules exhibit parallel branching; near the edge of a fimbrial fold the arterioles branch terminally into capillaries which

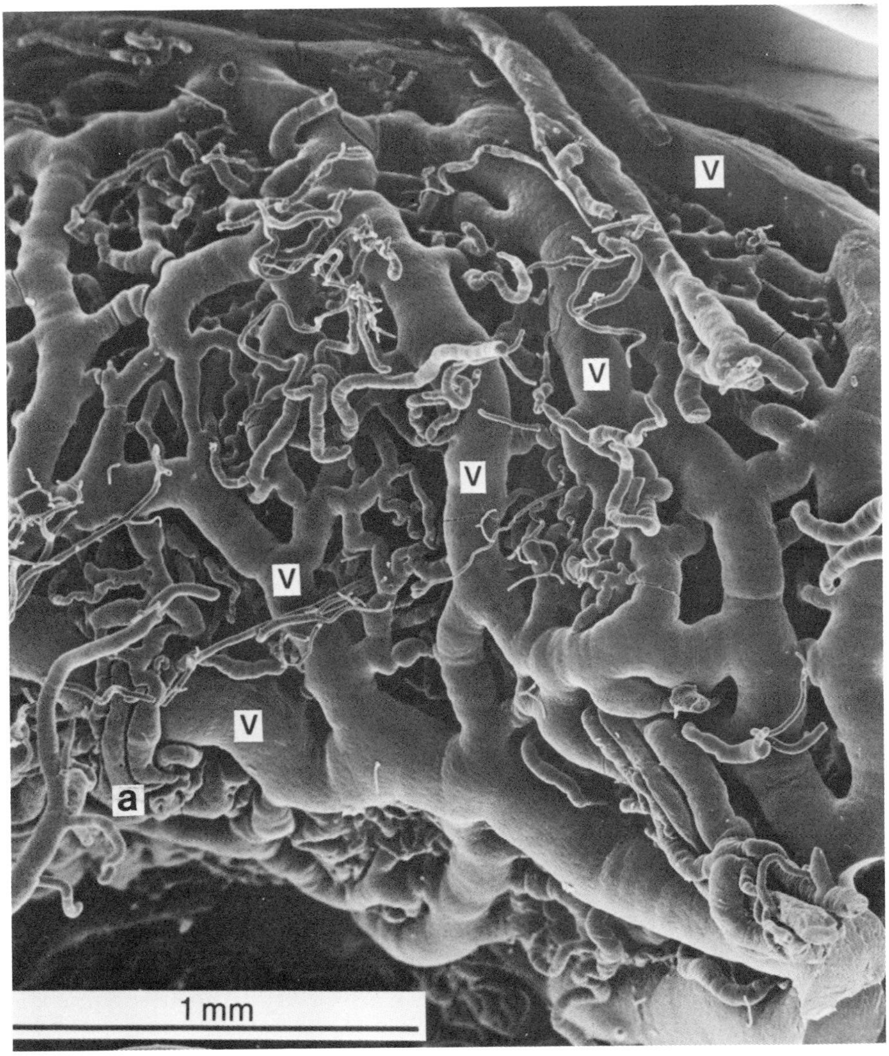

FIGURE 3:2—*A longitudinal segment of a methylmethacrylate vascular corrosion cast illustrating the isthmic subserosal venous plexus. v = vein; a = arteriole.*

drain to the large, frequently observed core venules.[33]

These studies suggest, first, that isthmic subserosal venous plexus dilatation (caused by either a rise in venous pressure or a fall in venous wall smooth-muscle tone) could, within the limiting perimeter of the serosal connective tissue occlude the isthmic lumen to ovum or embryo transport. Second, the observed differences in the MVA imply a greater blood delivery to the submucosal capillary network of the isthmus and a greater venous drainage capacity in the ampulla. This suggests that there may be a net movement of intravascular fluid to the interstitium and possibly thence to the tubal lumen in the isthmus, and a net movement of tubal fluid from the tubal lumen to the mucosal interstitium and thence to the subepithelial capillaries in the ampulla.[33] A pattern of tubal luminal fluid movement may thus be initiated or a preexisting pattern of fluid flow along the

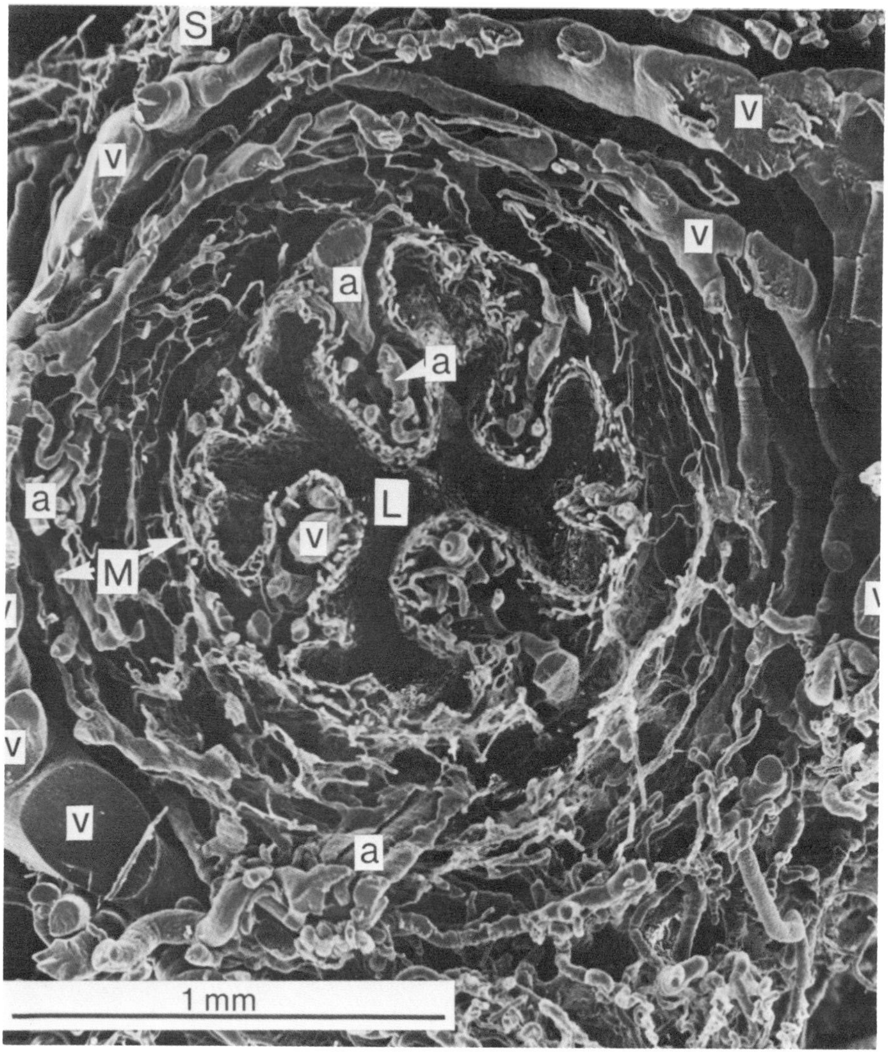

FIGURE 3:3—*A transverse section through a methylmethacrylate vascular corrosion cast of the isthmus. The small tubal luminal space and the extensive subserosal venous plexus, which surrounds the myosalpinx, are seen. L = luminal space; M = myosalpingeal microvasculature; a = arteriole; v = venule; s = serosal microvasculature.*

tube modified. This is consistent with the isthmic to ampullary tubal luminal fluid current previously described.[34,35]

Tubal MVA after Oophorectomy

Four weeks after bilateral oophorectomy, tubal microvascular connections in the rabbit were unaltered. When compared with controls, there was a decrease in the frequency and size of the large ampullary plical and fimbrial core venules; fimbrial subepithelial capillary density was reduced.[36] It is possible, then, that the ampullary "sump" for absorbing tubal luminal fluid suggested above is less efficient after oophorec-

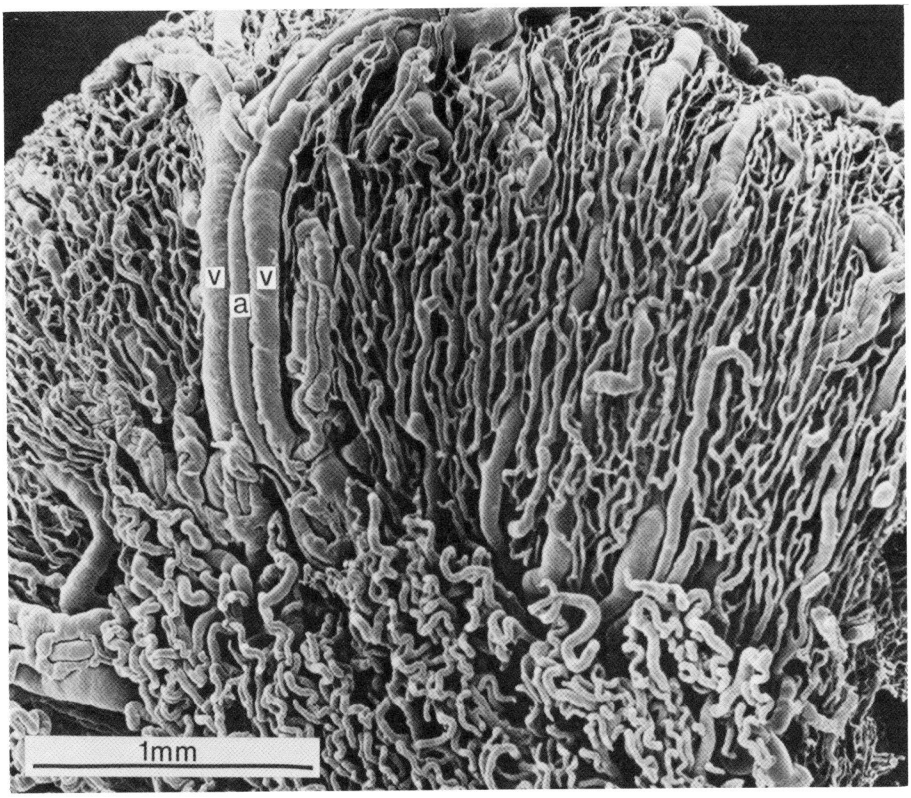

FIGURE 3:4—*A longitudinal segment of an ampullary methylmethacrylate vascular corrosion cast illustrating parallel branching of the subserosal arteries and veins. a = arteriole; v = venule.*

tomy; this correlates well with the poor ovum pickup and ampullary ovum retention observed after oophorectomy in rabbits.[37,38]

Tubal MVA in Mid-Pregnancy

Tubal microvasculature at two or three weeks of pregnancy in the rabbit is characterized by venous distension in the isthmic and ampullary subserosal veins and in the fimbrial core veins[39] when compared to those of control oviducts. The observations of tubal microvasculature after oophorectomy and in pregnancy imply that there is a sensitivity, and perhaps a dependence, of the tubal vasculature on local or circulating ovarian or placental hormones.[36,39,40] Tubal microvasculature may, thus, vary at the time of ovulation and tubal ovum transport. Such variations might include isthmic subserosal venous dilatation, with resultant isthmic luminal occlusion, thus preventing isthmic ovum transport.

Tubal MVA 12 and 36 Hours after Ovulation

To delineate further the role of the tubal MVA at the time of ovulation and tubal ovum transport, corrosion vascular casts were prepared 24 and 48 hours after ovulation was induced with intravenous HCG.[40] Ovulation occurs some 10 to 14 hours after HCG injection in rabbits,[41] ova would be at the AIJ 24 hours

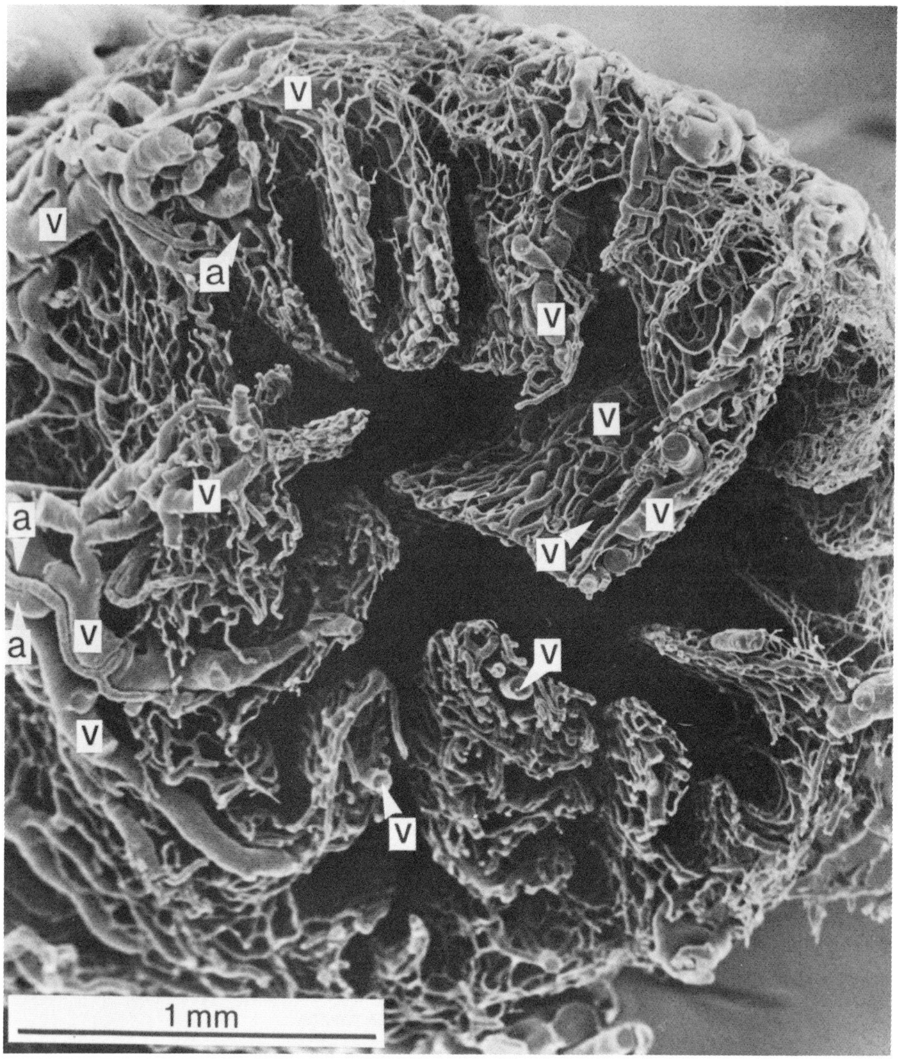

FIGURE 3:5—*A transverse section through a vascular corrosion cast of the ampulla. The extensive mucosal folding in the ampulla is demonstrated well by the plical vascular skeleton. a = arteriole; v = venule.*

and traversing the isthmus 48 hours after HCG injection.[42] Isthmic subserosal venous plexus dilatation is greater at 24 hours than either at 48 hours after HCG, or in controls. Isthmic subserosal venous plexus dilatation at 48 hours is less than that at 24 hours after HCG and is similar to that observed in controls. Isthmic luminal space in some tubal casts and in all tubal tissue segments after fixation by vascular perfusion with osmium tetroxide are of a similar area and are greater than observed in controls.[40] Isthmic subserosal venous plexus distention did not maintain isthmic luminal occlusion, as might have been expected. However, in the absence of any other coherent explanation for the pre-isthmic delay in ovum transport, it is reasonable to speculate that dilatation of the isthmic subserosal venous plexus limits isthmic wall distensibility and thus contributes to the known pre-isthmic delay in ovum transport.[40]

There is no evidence, despite fimbrial core venous distention, of fimbrial "erection." However, the casts prepared at 24 hours after HCG injection are prepared at least ten hours after ovum capture and therefore observation at the time of ovulation is required to determine the accuracy or inaccuracy of this suggested role for the fimbria.

Tubal MVA in the Mechanically Induced Hydrosalpinx in the Rabbit

Hydrosalpinges were induced by isthmic and ampullary occlusion with small tantalum clips. The resultant corrosion vascular casts exhibit isthmic and ampullary luminal dilatation, reduction in the extent of projection of the primary mucosal folds into the lumen, and loss of secondary mucosal folds.[43,44] Plical MVA is preserved; in contrast, interplical subepithelial capillaries are not cast (Figs. 3:6 and 3:7). Larger and more extensively branching interplical subepithelial arterioles are observed in both the isthmus and the ampulla.[43,44] Isthmic and ampullary subserosal venous distention is greater in the hydrosalpinx than in controls or in adjacent tubal segments.[43,44] The reduction in interplical subepithelial cast filling indicates poor perfusion in this region at the time of casting.[43,44] Subepithelial capillary perfusability and permeability to native rabbit and bovine serum albumin were reduced in the hydrosalpinx, particularly between plicae.[44,45] Poor interplical subepithelial capillary perfusion is probably the underlying mechanism of interplical deciliation, previously reported in this model.[46,47] Preservation of plical MVA, the absence of interplical subepithelial capillary filling, and reduced interplical subepithelial capillary perfusion indicate, since all mucosal subepithelial capillaries are exposed to the same increased tubal intraluminal hydrostatic pressure, that the microvascular changes are primarily due to stretching of the tubal wall.[43–45] The larger and more extensive mucosal arterioles of the hydrosalpinx suggest increased blood pressure in the hydrosalpinx. In addition, the subserosal venous dilatation observed in the hydrosalpinx implies superregulation of blood flow and thus increased blood flow in the hydrosalpinx. A net increase in capillary fluid outflow and a net decrease in capillary fluid absorption would therefore be predicted. Interstitial fluid in the hydrosalpinx could pass between the epithelial cells through "leaky" tight intercellular junctions (rendered more "leaky" by stretching of the epithelium), thus maintaining the hydrosalpinx.[44,45] The reduction in subepithelial capillary permeability to albumin, in the hydrosalpinx model, would increase osmotically driven absorption of luminal fluid and thus contribute to maintenance of the hydrosalpinx. Reduced human fertility after salpingoneostomy for hydrosalpinges may be due to persistence of the vascular changes similar to those described above.

Tubal MVA after Pomeroy Tubal Ligation

Dysmenorrhea or increased menstrual loss have been reported after human tubal sterilization[48] and more previously sterilized, compared to nonsterilized, women undergo hysterectomy.[49] Alteration of ovarian blood supply after tubal sterilization has been only one explanation of these observations,[48,50–52] which are by no means universal (Chapter 32). A direct effect of tubal sterilization on ovarian blood supply is unlikely, unless tubal damage occurs as a result of extensive electrocautery or destructive surgery. A more likely consequence is interference with tubal absorption of, say, early pregnancy factors or interference with the countercurrent exchange between the ovarian vein (which in the rabbit and human contains tubal venous blood) and the ovarian artery.

To determine alterations in tubal vasculature after sterilization, rabbit's tubal MVA was examined by the corrosion vascular cast SEM technique four weeks after midisthmic Pomeroy tubal ligation.[53]

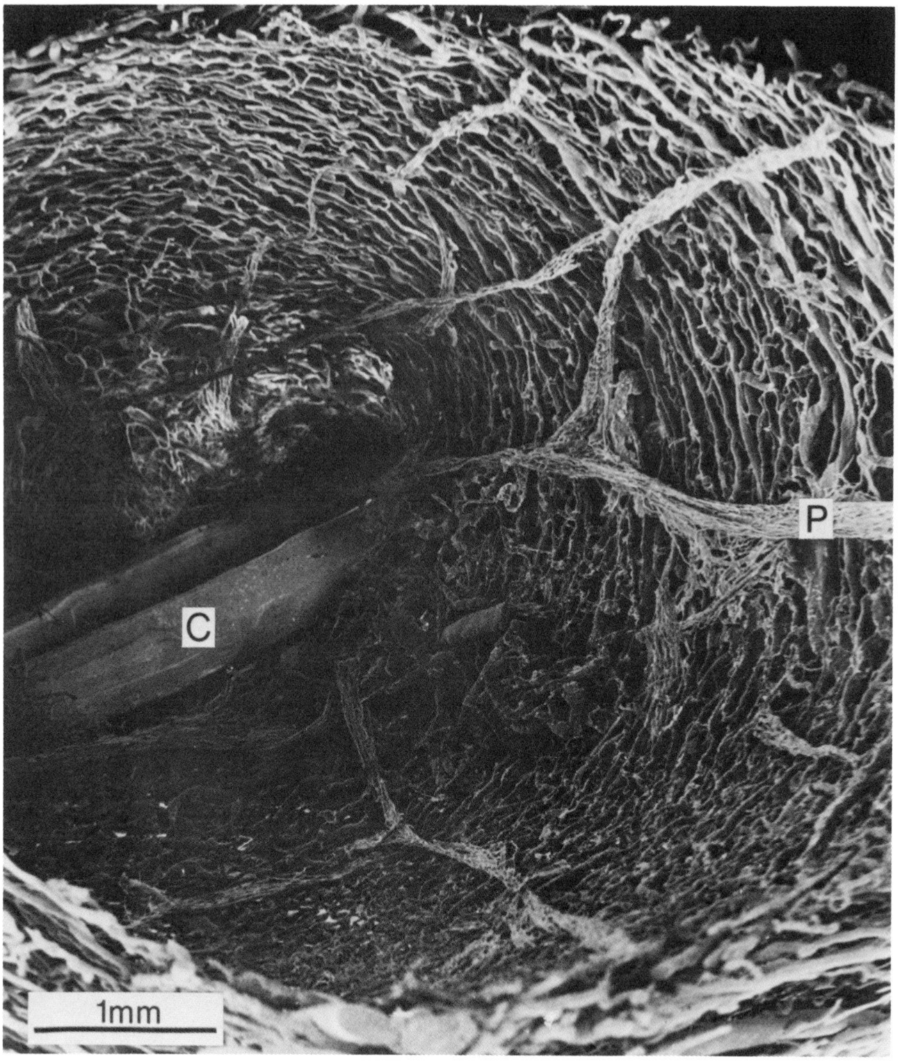

FIGURE 3:6—*An oblique section of a vascular corrosion cast of a mechanically induced hydrosalpinx isthmus. Plical subepithelial capillaries have been cast, whereas those between capillaries have failed to fill with casting medium. This implies poor interplical subepithelial capillary perfusion in the hydrosalpinx. P = plical microvasculature; C = hemoclip (used to occlude the tubal lumen).*

Tubal MVA, except within one millimeter of the site of tubal ligation, was similar to that observed in controls. The site of ligation was characterized by a randomly oriented vascular proliferation of fine vessels. This was interpreted as indicating the extent of proliferative tissue reaction to the surgery involved in tubal ligation. Pomeroy tubal ligation would be expected to have little effect on tubal, ovarian, or uterine vascular interelationships.

Tubal MVA after Tubal Microsurgery

Experimental tubal microsurgery is associated with a decrease in the number

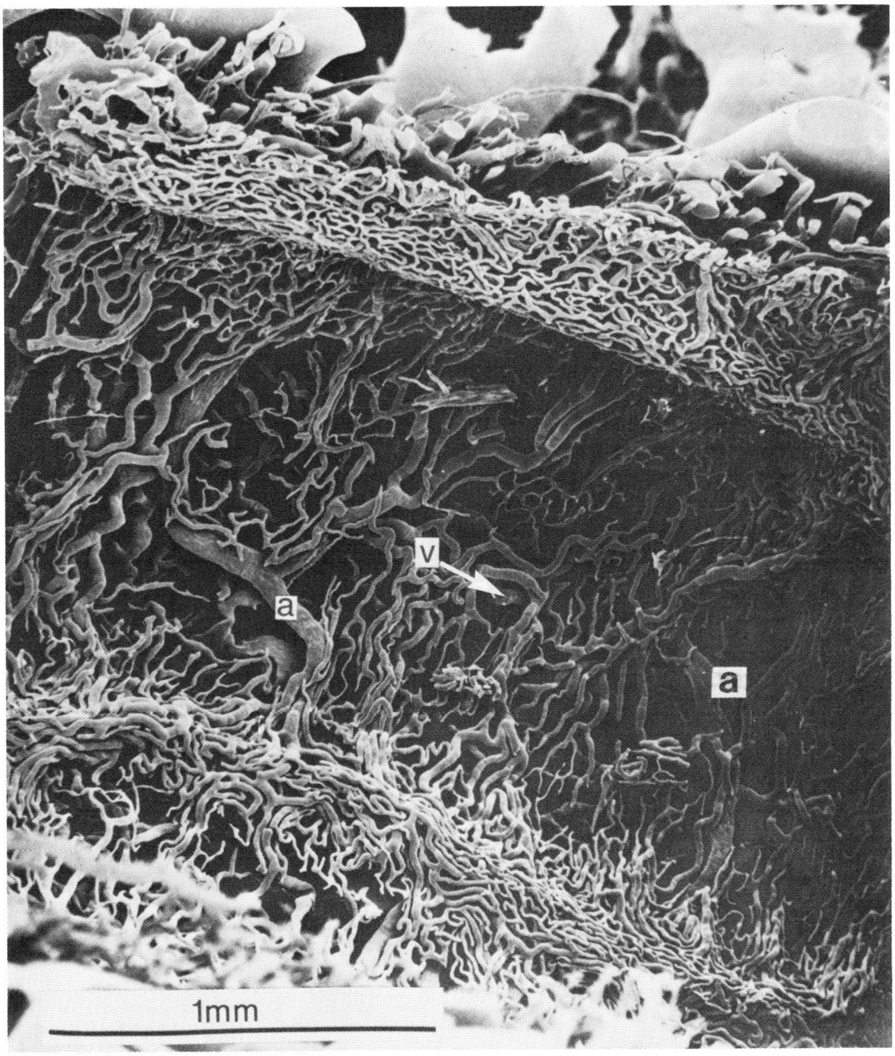

FIGURE 3:7—*A longitudinal section, the luminal aspect, of an isthmic hydrosalpinx vascular corrosion cast. Preservation of plicae, in contrast to interplical, subepithelial capillary casting, and dilated interplical mucosal vessels are shown. a = arteriole; v = venule.*

of corpora lutea on the operated side in rabbits [54–57] and in pigs.[58]

Tubal MVA was therefore examined in rabbits four weeks after transection and microsurgical anastomosis of the isthmus and the ampulla. Tubal morphology, except within one millimeter of the site of isthmic and within 150 microns of the site of ampullary anastomosis, is similar to that in control oviducts. The site of isthmic anastomosis is characterized by a serosal vascular proliferation;[59] this indicates the local tissue hyperplasia reported following isthmic anastomosis.[60,61] The site of ampullary anastomosis had little serosal "reaction";[62] transanastomotic interplical transluminal vascular bands were observed.[59] The vascular components of tubal function (except at and adjacent to the site of anastomosis) would vary little as a consequence of tubal microsurgery.[59] It is possible for tubal ovum transport to be delayed at the site of isthmic or ampullary anastomosis; in the isthmus, delay could be attributed to extraluminal restriction of isthmic distensibility and in the ampulla, to intraluminal adhesions limiting luminal diameter and distensibility. Delay in tubal embryo transport may result in embryonic degeneration in pigs[64] and in rabbits[65]; these data suggest an explanation of the reduction in nidation index after tubal surgery. Also, the sites of isthmic and ampullary anastomosis could be loci for ectopic gestation.

Suggested Areas for Further Examination of Tubal Microvasculature

Morphometric stereology of tubal vasculature

The corrosion vascular cast SEM studies referred to above rely on the subjective assessment of venous dilatation and vessel frequency. Morphometric stereology of thin, suitably prepared tissue sections (in which the microvascular dimensions have been stabilized at normal distending pressure before final fixation) is required for objective testing of the hypotheses proposed regarding the role of the tubal microvasculature in gamete transport.

Tubal capillary blood flow and hydraulic conductivity

Speculation (in the preceding discussion) suggested a specific and different role for the subepithelial capillaries in the isthmus and ampulla and in plicae and interplical capillaries in the hydrosalpinx model. Measurements of capillary blood flow and hydraulic conductivity in these locations and perhaps during the period of ovum transport would delineate the speculated fluid exchange from the mucosal subepithelial capillaries to the interstitium and tubal lumen. Tubal capillary blood flow and hydraulic conductivity may be calculated from observations obtained by video-television microscopy and either tubal transillumination or by incident light fluorescence.

Tubal interepithelial cell junctions

To extend the arguments developed above, it is necessary to ascertain the "leakiness" of the "tight" intercellular junctions in the tubal epithelium; this would ideally need to be performed in a variety of hormonal conditions. Methods by which this may be done include freeze-fracturing of the epithelium.[66]

Acknowledgments: The author wishes to thank Dr. B.J. Gannon for reviewing the manuscript and Ms. K.L. Shepherd who prepared the illustrations.

References

1. Diamond E: A microsurgical study of the blood supply to the uterine tube and ovary. In Phillips JM (Ed): *Microsurgery in Gynecology*. Downey, CA: AAGL Publications, 1977:69.
2. Watanabe A: Studies on the vascular system of human fallopian tube. *Acta Obstet Gynaecol Japonica*, 10:199, 1963.
3. Eddy CA, and Pauerstein CJ: Anatomy and physiology of the fallopian tube. *Clin Obstet Gynecol*, 23:1177, 1980.
4. Borell U, and Fernstrom I: The adnexal branches of the uterine artery. An arteriographic study in human subjects. *Acta Radiol*, 40:561, 1953.
5. Bendz A: The anatomical basis for a possible counter current exchange mechanism in the human adnexa. *Prostaglandins*, 13:355, 1977.
6. Bendz A, Hansson HA, Svendsen P, et al: On the extensive contact between veins and arteries in the human ovarian pedicle. *Acta Physiol Scand*, 115:179, 1982.
7. Hunter RHF, Cook B, and Poyser NL: Regulation of oviduct function in pigs by local transfer of ovarian steroids and prostaglandins: A mechanism to influ-

ence sperm transport. *Eur J Obstet Gynaecol Reprod Biol*, 14:225, 1983.
8. Koritke JG, and Gillet JY: La microvascularisation de la trompe utérine chez la femme. *Acta Anat*, 68:612, 1967.
9. Koritke JG, Gillet JY, and Leissner P: La microvascularisation de la muqueuse tubaire et ses variations au cours du cycle ovarien chez la femme. *Ztschr Zellforsch*, 88:48, 1968.
10. Koritke JG, Muller P, and Gillet JY: La vascularisation de la trompe utérine chez la femme. *Bull Fed Soc Gynecol Obstet*, 20:405, 1968.
11. Muller M, Koritke JC, and Gillet JY: L'architecture vasculaire de la trompe utérine chez la femme. *Bull Fed Soc Gynecol Obstet*, 20:407, 1968.
12. Gillet JY, and Leissner P: Les variations de la microvascularisation de la troupe utérine au cours du cycle ovarien chez la femme. *Acta Anat*, 68:608, 1967.
13. Gillet JY, and Koritke JG: Les artérioles spiraléeles de la muqueuse de la trompe utérine chez la femme. *Acta Anat*, 68:609, 1967.
14. Ginther OJ: Internal regulation of physiological processes through local venoarterial pathways. A review. *J Anim Sci*, 39:550, 1974.
15. Del Campo CH, and Ginther OJ: Vascular anatomy of the uterus and ovaries and the unilateral luteolytic effect of the uterus: Guinea pigs, rats, hamsters, rabbits. *Am J Vet Res*, 33:2561, 1972.
16. Dickson WM, Waldhalm SJ, and Amend N: Blood flow to the oviduct of the nonpregnant rabbit. *Biol Reprod*, 10:335, 1974.
17. Ginther OJ: Comparative anatomy of utero-ovarian vasculature. *Veterinary Scope*, 20(1):1, 1976. Kalamazoo, MI: Agricultural Division, The Upjohn Company.
18. Westman A: Investigations into the transit of ova in man. *J Obstet Gynaecol Br Emp*, 44:821, 1937.
19. Hunter RHF: Anatomy and physiology of the fallopian tube. In Chamberlain G, and Winston R (Eds): *Tubal Infertility, Diagnosis and Treatment*. Oxford: Blackwell Scientific Publications, 1982:1.
20. Andersen D: The rate of passage of the mammalian ovum through various portions of the fallopian tube. *Am J Physiol*, 82:557, 1927.
21. Hafez ESE: Tuboovarian mechanisms and ova reception in mammals. A comparative study. *Cornell Vet*, 49:459, 1959.
22. Barrett S, Blockley MAdeB, Brown JM, et al: Initiation of the oestrus cycle in the ewe by infusions of $PGF_{2\alpha}$ into the auto transplanted ovary. *J Reprod Fertil*, 24:136, 1971.
23. Einer-Jensen N: Local transfer of 133 Xe from the uterine horn to the ipsilateral ovary in the mouse, hamster and guinea pig. *J Reprod Fertil*, 40:479, 1974.
24. Janson PO, and Svendsen P: Angiographic studies of the extrinsic vasculature of the rabbit ovary. *J Reprod Fertil*, 42:175, 1975.
25. Einer-Jensen N, and McCracken JA: The effect of prostaglandin $F_{2\alpha}$ on the counter-current transfer of 85 krypton in the ovarian pedicle of the sheep. *Prostaglandins*, 13:763, 1977.
26. Bendz A, Einer-Jensen N, Lundgren O, et al: Exchange of krypton-85 between the blood vessels of the human uterine adnexa. *J Reprod Fertil*, 57:137, 1979.
27. Walsh SW, Yutrzenka GJ, and Davis JS: Local steroid concentrating mechanism in the reproductive vasculature of the ewe. *Biol Reprod*, 20:1167, 1979.
28. Kotwica J, Williams GL, and Marchello MJ: Countercurrent transfer of testosterone by the ovarian vascular pedicle of the cow: Relationship to follicular steroidogenesis. *Biol Reprod*, 24(Suppl. 1):144, 1981.
29. Kryzmowski T, Kotwica J, and Stefanczyk S: Venous-arterial counter-current transfer of (3H) testosterone in the vascular pedicle of the sow ovary. *J Reprod Fertil*, 61:317, 1981.
30. Kryzmowski T, Kotwica J, Stefanczyk S, et al: A subovarian exchange mechanism for the counter-current transfer of ovarian steroid hormones in the pig. *J Reprod Fertil*, 65:457, 1982.
31. Kryzmowski T, Kotwica J, Stefanczyk S, et al: Steroid transfer from the ovarian vein to the ovarian artery in the sow. *J Reprod Fertil*, 65:451, 1982.
32. Bendz A, Lundgren O, and Hamberger L: Countercurrent exchange of progesterone and antipyrine between human utero-ovarian vessels, and of antipyrine between the femoral vessels in the cat. *Acta Physiol Scand* 114:611, 1982.
33. Verco CJ, Gannon BJ, and Jones WR:

Fallopian tube microvasculature in the rabbit. *Aust J Exp Biol Med Sci*, 61:127, 1983.

34. Koester H: Ovum transport. In Gibian H, and Plotz EJ (Eds): *Mammalian Reproduction*. New York: Springer-Verlag, 1970:189.
35. Black DL, and Asdell SA: Transport through the rabbit oviduct. *Am J Physiol*, 192:63, 1958.
36. Verco CJ, Gannon BJ, and Jones WR: Fallopian tube microvascular architecture after oophorectomy in the rabbit. *Acta Anat*, 117:193, 1983.
37. Noyes RW, Adams CE, and Walton A: The transport of ova in relation to the dosage of oestrogen in ovariectomized rabbits. *J Endocrinol*, 18:108, 1959.
38. El-Banna AA, and Sacher B: Egg transport in ovariectomized rabbits as affected by different combinations of oestrogen and progesterone. *J Endocrinol*, 68:331, 1976.
39. Verco CJ, Gannon BJ, and Jones WR: Microvascular architecture of the pregnant rabbit oviduct. *Acta Anat*, 118:167, 1984.
40. Verco CJ, Gannon BJ, and Jones WR: Variations in rabbit oviduct microvascular architecture following gonadotrophin induced ovulation. *J Reprod Fertil*, 72:15, 1984.
41. Harper MJK: Ovulation in the rabbit: The time of follicular rupture and expulsion of the eggs, in relation to injection of luteinizing hormone. *J Endocrinol*, 26:307, 1963.
42. Pauerstein CJ, Anderson V, Chatkoff ML, et al: Effect of estrogen and progesterone on the time-course of tubal ovum transport in rabbits. *Am J Obstet Gynecol*, 120:299, 1974.
43. Verco CJ, Gannon BJ, and Jones W: Microvascular architecture of the mechanically induced hydrosalpinx in the rabbit. *Clin Reprod Fertil*, 1:311, 1982.
44. Verco CJ, and Gannon BJ: Rabbit hydrosalpinx microvascular architecture, vascular perfusability and macromolecular permeability. In Courtice FC, Garlick DG, and Perry MA (Eds): *Progress in Microcirculation Research*, 11:232, 1984. Sydney: Committee in Postgraduate Medical Education.
45. Verco CJ, and Gannon BJ: Vascular perfusability and capillary macromolecular permeability in the mechanically induced rabbit hydrosalpinx. *Acta Anat*, 122:126, 1985.
46. Vasquez G, Oberti C, Boeckx W, et al: The evolution of experimentally induced hydrosalpinges in rabbits. *Fertil Steril*, 35:342, 1981.
47. Kleinstein J, Neubuser D, and Mussmann J: Mechanically induced tube damage in the artificial hydrosalpinx. *Gynecol Obstet Invest*, 14:292, 1982.
48. Neil JR, Hammond GT, Noble AD, et al: Late complications of sterilization by laparoscopy and tubal ligation. *Lancet* 2:699, 1975.
49. Noble AD: Female sterilisation: long-term effects. In Sciarra JJ, Zatuchi GI, and Speidel JJ (Eds): *Risks, Benefits and Controversies in Fertility Control*. New York: Harper and Row, 1978:102.
50. Berger GS, Radwanska E, and Hammond JE: Possible ovulatory deficiency after tubal ligation. *Am J Obstet Gynecol*, 132:699, 1978.
51. Leading Article: Contraception by female sterilization. *Br Med J*, 280:1154, 1980.
52. Cattanach J: Oestrogen deficiency after tubal ligation. *Lancet*, 1: 847, 1985.
53. Verco CJ, Gannon BJ, and Jones WR: Rabbit oviduct microvascular architecture after tubal ligation. *Fertil Steril*, 40:127, 1983.
54. Eddy CA, and Bajpai VK: Healing and restoration of fertility following microsurgical transection and anastomosis of the rabbit oviduct. *Fertil Steril*, 38:354, 1982.
55. Beyth Y, and Winston RML: Ovum capture and fertility following microsurgical fimbriectomy in the rabbit. *Fertil Steril*, 35:464, 1981.
56. McComb PF, Bourdage RJ, and Halbert SA: Suppressed ovulatory function and oviductal microsurgery in the rabbit. *Fertil Steril*, 35:481, 1981.
57. Nerhoeven HC, Lott D, and Reichman J: Ovulatory function after tubal microsurgical procedures in the rabbit. *Am J Obstet Gynecol*, 143:835, 1982.
58. Paterson PJ, Downing B, Trounson AO, et al: Fertility and tubal morphology after microsurgical removal of segments of the porcine fallopian tube. *Fertil Steril*, 35:208, 1981.
59. Verco CJ, Gannon BJ, and Jones WR: Rabbit oviduct microvascular architecture after microsurgical transection and

anastomosis. *J. Obstet Gynaecol*, 6:68, 1985.

60. Halbert SA, McComb PF, and Bourdage RJ; The structural and functional impact of microsurgical anastomosis on the rabbit oviductal isthmus. *Fertil Steril*, 36:653, 1981.
61. Bernhardt-Huth D, Frantzen C, and Schlösser HW: Morphology of rabbit oviduct after microsurgical techniques for reanastomosis of the isthmus or ampulla. *Arch Gynäkol*, 230:251, 1981.
62. Patton DL, and Halbert SA: Electron microscope examination of the rabbit oviductal ampulla following microsurgical end-to-end anastomosis. *Fertil Steril*, 32:691, 1979.
63. McComb PF, Newman H, and Halbert SA: Reproduction in rabbits after excision of the oviductal isthmus, ampullary-isthmic junction and uteroisthmic junction. *Fertil Steril*, 36:669, 1981.
64. Murray FA, Bazer FW, Rundell JW, et al: Developmental failure of swine embryos restricted to the oviductal environment. *J Reprod Fertil*, 24:445, 191.
65. Adams CE: Egg development in the rabbit: The influence of post-coital ligation of the uterine tube and of ovariectomy. *J Endocrinol*, 16:283, 1958.
66. Murphy CR, Swift JG, Mukerjee TM, et al: Effects of ovarian hormones on cell membranes in the rat uterus. *Cell Biophysics*, 3:57, 1981.

4

Autonomic Neuromuscular Mechanisms in the Human Fallopian Tube

Christer Owman, Göran Helm, Nils-Otto Sjöberg, and Bengt Walles

Introduction

The transport of the ovum and blastocyst through the fallopian tube of man is a complex process. Although the pattern and time required for the transport are well established, the regulation of the transport process is still largely unknown. Knowledge of these regulatory mechanisms is important, not least in regard to the pharmacological possibilities of preventing or facilitating human fertility. Several factors may be involved in the ovum transport processes, such as the epithelial ciliary activity, oviductal secretions, the muscular contractions of the tubal wall, and its nerve supply.

After follicular rupture, the ovum is picked up by the oviductal fimbriae, which are brought in contact with the ovary by means of contraction of the myotube, the smooth muscle of the mesosalpinx, as well as of the tubo-ovarian ligaments. After fast passage of the ovum through the distal ampulla, which takes place in a pattern of to-and-fro movements, the ovum is retained in the proximal part of the ampullary region, near the ampullary-isthmic junction, for approximately 72 hours,[1] allowing fertilization to take place. In about 80 hours after ovulation the blastocyst reaches the uterine cavity.[2,3]

Most of the interest in the field of ovum transport has been focused on the muscular activity in the myosalpinx. The transient arrest of the ovum at the ampullary-isthmic junction, which seems to be crucial for successful conception to take place, may be an effect of a sphincter-like function.[4–6]

The Fallopian Tube: Basic Studies and Clinical Contributions, edited by Alvin M. Siegler, M.D. Mount Kisco, New York: Futura Publishing Company, Inc.

Recording of Smooth-Muscle Activity

Several methods have been used to study the tubal motility, with or without correlation to ovum transport. Perfusion of the oviduct with carbon dioxide or sa line solution has been used to obtain knowledge about the flow resistance.[4,7,8] The information from these experiments seems to have limitations. The site of resistance to flow cannot be ascertained, and other organ structures can influence the resistance. Moreover, the measurement requires a distending stimulus which may influence the recordings, and insufflation is often done in the isthmic-ampullary direction while the ovum moves from ampulla to isthmus. Intratubular pressure recordings have been performed by open-ended catheters or microballoon techniques.[9,10] This type of intraluminal monitoring also has limitations. Distention and occlusion of the oviduct will result in unreliable motor activity and the obstruction will prevent the study of normal gamete transport. The regional extension of the contractions is usually impossible to demonstrate with these methods, and contamination of extratubal smooth-muscle activity cannot be sorted out.

Transducer systems have been developed to measure the tubal muscular activity extraluminally. Among others, the miniature mercury strain gauges[11] and ultrasound transducers[12] have been used in vivo. Integrated circuit technology has led to smaller and highly sensitive transducers capable of simultaneously recording mechanical contractions, pressure waves, and electrical waves.[13] These techniques, together with electrical recording of tubal smooth-muscle activity,[14] are the most promising in-vivo approaches so far.

The in-vivo methods for registration of tubal muscular activity have a number of practical and ethical limitations, and they are difficult to standardize and evaluate appropriately for quantitative pharmacological analysis. In-vitro methods allow for more precisely controlled conditions and make pharmacological manipulation possible.[7,15–18] The influence of surrounding tissues can be avoided. On the other hand, it is impossible to evaluate the integrated activity of the smooth musculature in the tube and in adjoining peritoneal structures.

Depending on the aim of the study, essentially two types of smooth-muscle preparations have been used as in-vitro models. One consists of carefully microdissected and prepared smooth-muscle elements from the circular and longitudinal musculature.[19] In this method, the two major types of smooth musculature become well defined. Another type of preparation[17,20] uses segments from the entire intact wall of the oviduct, except for its connective tissue. This kind of preparation, with a preserved tubal wall architecture including close appositions between cells in the various muscle layers, has certain advantages. As a functional unit this preparation will more closely reflect conditions in situ.

Tubal Innervation: Histochemistry

The development of the FalckHillarp histofluorescence technique for visualization of adrenergic nerves[21,22] applied together with chemical measurements of norepinephrine as well as denervation experiments, have led to informative knowledge about the adrenergic innervation in the human female genital tract. It is now well established that the fallopian tube has a rich adrenergic nerve supply,[23–26] partly by means of so-called "short" adrenergic neurons which originate in ganglionic cells in the paracervical region.[27]

Adrenergic nerves

Fluorescence histochemical studies have shown that all norepinephrine in the human tube is present in nerves. As shown in Figure 4:1, most of the adrenergic nerve terminals in the isthmus are nonvascular and are primarily located in the smooth-muscle layers of the organ,

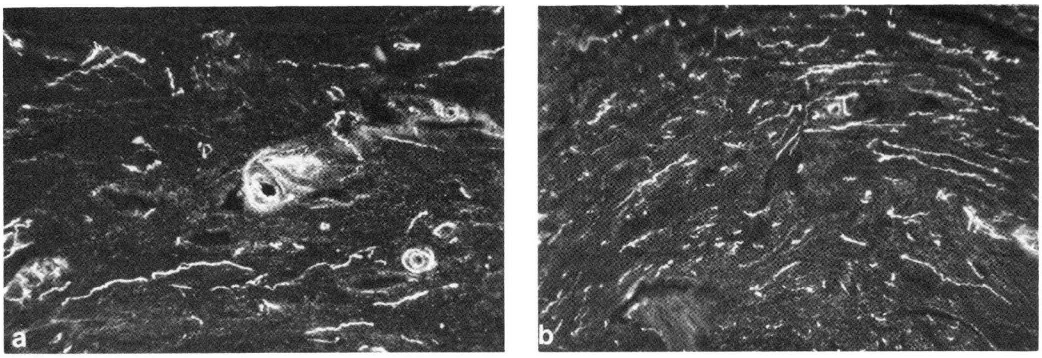

FIGURE 4:1—(a) *Section of ampulla proper. Only few fluorescent nerves are present, partly running in smooth muscles, partly enclosing blood vessels (autofluorescence in vessel walls). (Magnification × 70)*(b) *Transverse section of isthmus of uterine tube, mucosa toward left. Many fluorescent nerves are located mainly in prominent circular layer of smooth-muscle coat. (Magnification, × 70)*

whereas the adrenergic innervation in the ampullary and fimbriated regions to a major extent is related to blood vessels.[24,25,28] The small amount of dopamine found[29] may represent precursor levels present during the biosynthesis of norepinephrine.

Against the background of results ob tained on rat uterus,[30] it can be assumed that the minute levels of epinephrine measured in the tube [29] are not synthesized locally, but are taken up from the circulation and then stored extraneuronally, that is, diffusely in the smooth musculature. Since both the plasma epinephrine concentrations and the uterine binding of the amine in rats change independently during the estrous cycle, an explanation is offered for the lack of consistent cyclic variations in the tube of the kind found for dopamine and norepinephrine, as described below. In view of the lack of evidence that epinephrine in the tube is synthesized and stored in special cells, the higher concentrations present in the isthmic region[29] may simply be related to a more efficient binding to the smooth musculature, which is more prominent here than in the ampulla and fimbria.

The high concentration of norepinephrine found in the isthmus (Fig. 4:2), where the adrenergic nerves are primarily related to nonvascular smooth musculature, is consistent with the view that the musculature in this region may function as a sympathetically innervated sphincter mechanism. Although a tendency to a regional variation in the norepinephrine concentrations occurs in the isthmus,[29] it does not provide sufficient evidence that the sphincter function would be restricted to any particular portion of the isthmus (Fig. 4:2).

Cyclic changes in the adrenergic neurotransmitter

The sympathetic nerves belonging to the special system of short adrenergic neurons have a particular sensitivity to the effect of sex steroids.[27] There is evidence for such an influence also on the adrenergic nerves of the fallopian tube, although the results have not been unequivocal. Some authors[24,31] demonstrated with fluorometric methods a higher norepinephrine level in the secretory compared to the follicular phase, in contrast to Moawad et al.[25] who found that the concentration is higher in the follicular and lower during the luteal period, with the lowest values around the time of ovulation. Also, the data from fluorescence histochemical techniques are conflicting. Owman and Sjöberg[32] showed in rabbits that there is a marked increase in

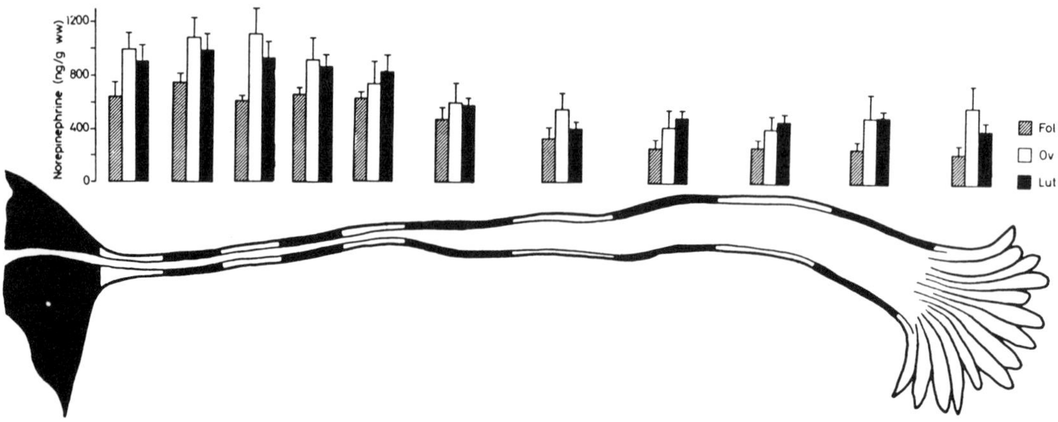

FIGURE 4:2—*Tissue concentrations of norepinephrine (ng/g wet weight) in consecutive parts throughout the length of the human fallopian tube (5 preparations of equal length from the isthmic and ampullary regions, respectively) during the follicular (Fol.;* n = *5 for isthmus and ampulla, 14 for fimbria), ovulatory (Ov.;* n = *6 for isthmus and ampulla, 7 for fimbria), and luteal (Lut.;* n = *14 for isthmus and ampulla, 13 for fimbria) phases of the menstrual cycle.*

the level of norepinephrine after administration of estrogen, and this was followed by a reduction to control levels when progesterone was added. The rate of turnover of catecholamines—an index of the functional state of sympathetic neurons in vivo—was higher in estrogen-treated rabbits.[33] Kennedy and Marshall,[34] giving 90 percent lower estrogen doses, did not reveal any difference between rabbits treated with estrogen and with estrogen in combination with progesterone. Thus, the level of plasma hormones, or rather the amount of steroid receptor available, may be of primary importance. Human oviducts have a larger number of fluorescent adrenergic terminals in the secretory phase compared to the follicular phase.[24] On the other hand, Moawad et al.[25] failed to demonstrate differences in adrenergic nerve fluorescence related to the hormonal phase.

The norepinephrine concentration in both isthmus and ampulla is higher in the luteal than in the follicular phase (Fig. 4:2), in both monkeys and women.[26,29,31] Thus, a high tubal norepinephrine concentration is associated with high plasma progesterone levels. A notable finding in regional determinations of norepinephrine is that ovulation (defined as the stagein the menstrual cycle when plasma estradiol concentration is maximal) is associated with a particularly high norepinephrine concentration in the isthmus, which is not the case in the ampullary region.[29]

The difference in tubal norepinephrine concentration during the menstrual cycle could simply have reflected changes in tissue weight due to, for example, altered water content. However, there are no significant cyclic variations in tissue wet weight, and the concentration of protein in the tube does not change to any significant extent.[35] Therefore, the higher norepinephrine concentrations measured during the ovulatory and luteal phases (Fig. 4:2) seem to represent a true increment in the neuronal transmitter level. The cyclic fluctuations in norepinephrine concentrations in the human tube are probably the net result of several biochemical processes in the adrenergic neurons, as investigated in some more detail for the uterine adrenergic innervation (cf. Owman[36]). Against the background of available information from this innervation system, it can be assumed that increasing levels of norepinephrine in the estrous or menstrual cycle reflect increased sympathetic nerve activity in the tube.

Exogenous norepinephrine is able to reduce tubal motor activity in vitro, to a similar extent during both the follicular and the luteal phases.[16,17,29] The uniformly higher transmitter level found in the tube during the luteal phase compared to the follicular phase may thus in functional terms suggest that the sympathomimetic inhibition of tubal motor activity in vivo is more prominent during the luteal phase. In line with this, the particularly high norepinephrine concentration in the isthmus during ovulation, in combination with the observation that norepinephrine increases isthmic motor activity in vitro at this stage,[16,17,29] suggests a special functional significance of the adrenergic innervation in the isthmus during a limited period of the entire ovulatory process. This is consistent with the involvement of an adrenergic component in the tube locking mechanism, which appears to have crucial importance for normal fertilization and transport of the blastocyst toward the site of implantation.[37]

Cholinergic nerves

Our knowledge about the cholinergic innervation of the female genital tract is limited, in part because of the lack of practically useful and specific histochemical methods. Acetylcholinesterase activity, although sparse, has been found to occur in the oviduct.[38,39] Cholinomimetic stimulation of the rabbit oviduct in vitro suggests that an adrenergic link may be involved in the motor effects.[40] However, the functional significance of the cholinergic system in tubal physiology is not clear.

Peptidergic nerves

Several polypeptides with possible neurotransmitter function have recently been shown to be widely distributed in peripheral organs. One of the most intensively studied is vasoactive intestinal polypeptide (VIP), a 28-amino-acid peptide chain that was originally isolated from porcine small intestine by Said and Mutt.[41] The sequence of the amino acids was also established by Mutt and Said[42] and the substance was then synthesized by Bodansky et al.[43] Evidence is accumulating that the peptide is a neurotransmitter,[44] although final proof for this is still lacking, mainly because an antagonist for the peptide is not yet available.

In immunohistochemical studies, VIP has been demonstrated to occur in the female genital tract of various animal species.[45–47] In human reproductive tissues (Table 4:1) the concentration of VIP is particularly high in the isthmus of the tube and in the cervical region.[48] VIP-immunoreactive nerve fibers in the human tube are found particularly in the smooth-muscle layers, but also beneath the epithelium of the isthmic part. In the ampullary region and in the fimbriated end, only scattered VIP terminals are observed. The content of VIP measured by radioimmunoassay (Table 4:1) was found to be significantly higher in the isthmus of the fallopian tube than in the rest of the tubal tissue,[48] showing a good correlation between the immunohistochemical and immunochemical findings.

Already at 18 to 23 weeks of pregnancy, VIP has been identified immunohistochemically in nerve cell bodies occurring in clusters in the paracervical tissue of the fetus. This suggests that uterovaginal VIP nerves may have a local origin, analogous to the previously mentioned short adrenergic neurons.[27] This is supported by denervation experiments in the cat, which have shown that VIP nerves originate from paracervical ganglia.[49]

Tubal Innervation: Electron Microscopy

With the triple fixation technique for electron microscopy,[50] it is possible to distinguish the adrenergic nerve terminals through their content of electron-dense synaptic vesicles. In human tubal preparations, adrenergic nerves can be identified both outside and within

Table 4:1

Distribution and Concentration of VIP, Measured by Radioimmunochemistry and Expressed as pmol/g Wet Weight, in the Human Female Reproductive Tract

Specimen	*Median*	(n)	*95% Confidence limits*	*Statistics*‡
Ovary	0.1	(6)	0– 2.4	
Fallopian tube: fimbria	1.0	(5)	0.1– 1.6	n.s.
ampulla	1.9	(27)	0.3– 2.8	p ≦ 0.05
isthmus	4.4	(26)	1.4– 7.2	n.s.
Uterine corpus myometrium	1.6	(30)	0.9– 2.7	p ≦ 0.05
Cervix: internal ostium	16.5	(10)	6.4–26.6	n.s.
external ostium	11.4	(8)	0.2–25.5	p≦ 0.05
Portio†	3.6	(6)	0.2–11.5	n.s.
Vagina	23.8	(6)	1.4–45.0	p ≦ 0.05
Uterine corpus endometrium	0.5	(18)	0– 0.8	n.s.
Cervical mucosa	1.7	(9)	0– 3.0	

†Transverse section of the portio.
‡Mann Whitney rank sum test.
n.s. = Nonsignificant.

smooth-muscle bundles.[51] Thus, nonmyelinated nerves are found in groups enclosed by a Schwann cell sheath and running in the connective tissue between the smooth-muscle layers. Closer to the smooth-muscle cells forming the circular layer of the tube, the Schwann cell ensheathing is partly broken up, and axonal varicosities characterized by numerous synaptic vesicles and mitochondria are seen. The adrenergic type of varicosities (Fig. 4:3a) is identified by their content of the highly electron-dense vesicles of 50 to 60 nm diameter together with 100 nm vesicles with a moderately dense content. Membrane-bound structures with a highly electron-dense core sometimes have a biconcave form. The naked part of the adrenergic nerve varicosities often approach the smooth-muscle cells (Fig. 4:3b) with a distance of approximately 200 nm, and sometimes the axonal membrane comes as close as 60 to 100 nm from the membrane of the muscle cell. These close contacts, containing only the basement membranes, usually occupy a considerable area of the naked varicosity, although membrane specializations are not seen on either the axonal or the muscular side.

Our observations on the human fallopian tube agree with the findings of Ishii.[52] A similar organization of the adrenergic nerves has been described for the rabbit[53] and the rat.[52] On the other hand, Daniel et al.[54] reported that nerves in the human tube are primarily present in the peripheral regions of the musculature, which contains chiefly collagen and blood vessels.

Although the minimal neuromuscular distance in many smooth-muscle tissues is 80 to 120 nm, transmitter released from nerves located 300 to 1000 nm or more away from smooth-muscle cells is likely to be effective,[55] which has been particularly well elucidated in sympathetically innervated vascular smooth musculature. Thus, the released norepinephrine probably reaches the smooth-muscle cells through diffusion, followed by myogenic spread of electrical activity by way of close appositions (rather than nexus formations) found between the muscle cells.[53,54] These cell-to-cell contacts also join smooth-muscle cells in different lay-

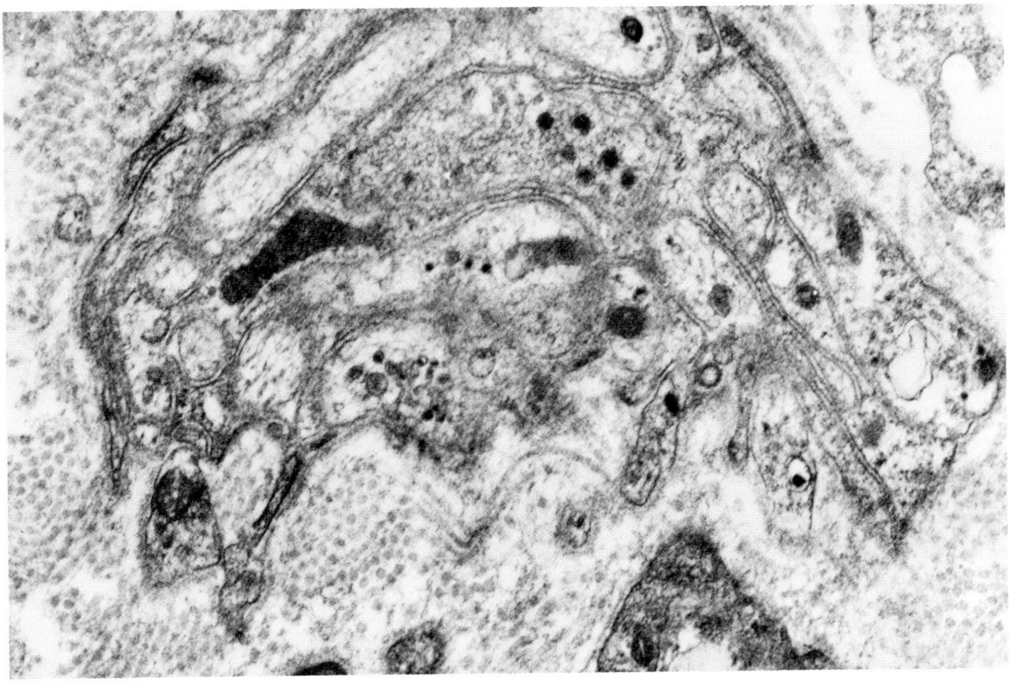

FIGURE 4:3a—*Several axons and axon varicosities enclosed by incomplete Schwann cell sheath. Such nerve bundles are found near the smooth-muscle cells. The adrenergic terminals are characterized by electron-dense synaptic vesicles with diameters of 50 to 60 nm. (× 32,000)*

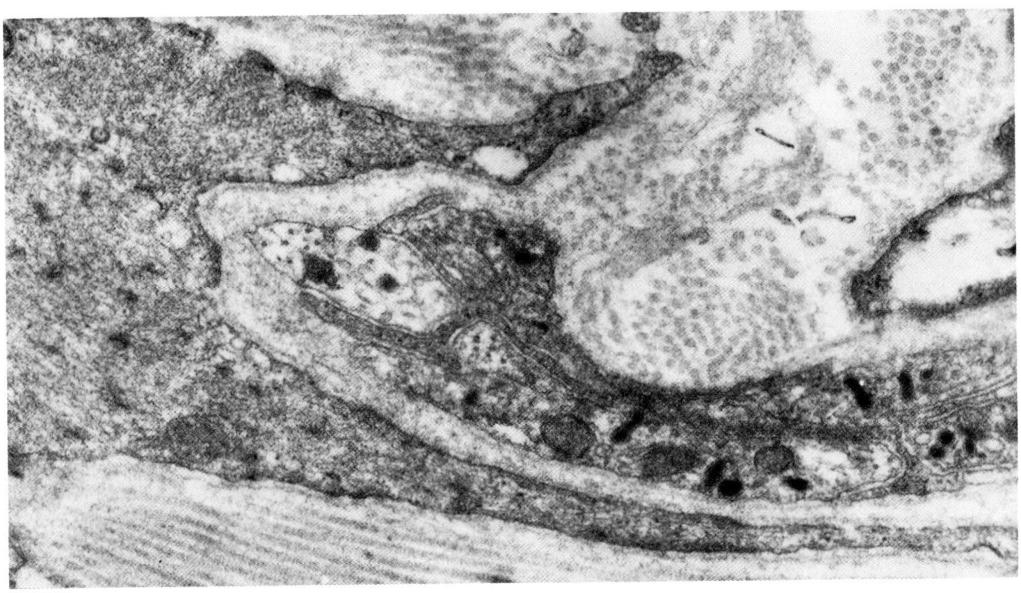

FIGURE 4:3b—*Adrenergic nerve terminal located 70 nm from the membrane of a smooth-muscle cell. The apposing membrane of the terminal is not covered by the Schwann cell. The size of the contact area is considerable. (× 35,000)*

ers of the tube,[54] which means that activity originating in those muscle cells being directly supplied with adrenergic nerve terminals will spread throughout the isthmus, involving not only the circular but also the longitudinally oriented muscle fibres.

Neuroeffector Pharmacology and Endocrinology

Electrical nerve stimulation

The ultrastructural observations are supported by pharmacological experiments in vitro,[51] showing that electrical stimulation of the nerves of the human tube releases a sufficient amount of norepinephrine to produce a frequency-dependent motor response in the isthmus. Electrical field stimulation results in an initial twitch contraction, with an amplitude clearly higher than that of the individual peaks in the phasic contractions present before stimulation. Immediately following the twitch contraction the tube relaxes, often in combination with a reduced or abolished phasic activity. After a one-minute stimulation period, the preparation returns to its normal activity in the course of another one to two minutes. This pattern of response is almost equal for the circular and longitudinal smooth-muscle preparations of the isthmus. The twitch contraction is frequency-dependent, with the highest amplitude at 8 to 16 Hz. When the two muscle layers are tested individually, it is evident that the contractile phase is more dominating in the longitudinal layer, whereas the inhibitory portion of the total response is most prominent in circular smooth musculature.[56]

Twenty minutes after the α-receptor antagonist, phentolamine, has been added to the organ bath, the twitch contraction during electric field stimulation is abolished.[51] The relaxation following the twitch, however, is not overtly altered. The twitch contraction during transmural electrical stimulation is also abolished in the presence of tetrodotoxin, which blocks the nerves by inhibiting the sodium transport across the axonal membrane. Tetrodotoxin, in addition, eliminates the relaxation following the twitch, but the phasic motor activity is not affected.

Thus, with the use of a model for pharmacological studies of the contractile neurogenic component in the human tube (avoiding differentiation between complex β-adrenergic and peptidergic components, which reduce tubal motor activity as described below) in combination with the ultrastructural observations, it seems clear that the adrenergic nerves do play a functional role in modifying contractile processes in the human fallopian tube.

Adrenergic receptors

In microdissected smooth-muscle preparations from the ampullary-isthmic junction of the human fallopian tube,[19] the α-receptor agonist, phenylephrine, stimulates both the circular and longitudinal musculature.[56] This is in contrast to norepinephrine and epinephrine which, although stimulating the longitudinally oriented musculature, inhibit the circular preparations in a concentration-dependent way. Isoprenaline blocks both types of smooth musculature. The findings indicate a variable dominance of α- and β-adrenoceptors in the two tubal layers.[56]

The β-adrenergic receptor

In order to elucidate in some more detail the pharmacological properties and the reactivity of the α- and β-adrenoceptors in the human fallopian tube, a quantitative pharmacological characterization of the receptors was carried out by Helm et al.[57] The relaxing effect of norepinephrine on the potassium-depolarized tubal smooth muscle was studied under conditions when the contractile response was inhibited by phenoxybenzamine (which also efficiently blocks the extraneuronal uptake of the transmitter) and the neuronal uptake of the amine was blocked by cocaine (cf. Furchgott[58]). The log concentration-response curve for the action of norepinephrine showed a parallel shift toward higher agonist concentrations in the presence of increasing concentrations of propranolol, confirming that the relaxation is mediated by β-adrenergic receptors. Under the standardized conditions used (cf. Furchgott[58]), this shift made it possible to calculate the dissociation constant for the complex between the β-receptor and propranolol (the K_B value) in different types of tubal preparations at various cyclic stages. The K_B values provide a powerful means to classify the receptor pharmacologically, since the value should be the same for a given receptor, irrespective of the type of preparation studied.[58] The K_B value for propranolol—that is, the affinity of this antagonist for the β-receptor in the tubal smooth musculature—resembled the value for the β-receptors mediating relaxation of the follicular smooth muscle in the human ovary.[59] There was no significant regional or cyclic variation in the affinity of propranolol for the tubal β-receptor.

The α-adrenergic receptor

The sympathomimetic contraction was studied under similar standardized conditions as the relaxation, using phenylephrine as agonist. Several of the preparations, especially from the circular smooth muscle, did not contract at all. This may be related to the particularly high proportion of β-receptor activity in this type of smooth musculature.[19] The responding preparations showed quite a varying degree of maximal contraction, and there was a tendency to reduced sensitivity during the ovulatory phase. Phentolamine inhibited the contractile response in a competitive manner, confirming the α-receptor nature of the response.

The affinity of phentolamine for the α-receptor showed a significant difference in the circular smooth musculature, related to low versus moderate to high plasma levels of sex steroids. Thus, the affinity was higher during the follicular phase than during the remainder of the menstrual cycle. No such difference was found for the longitudinal smooth muscle of the isthmus, whereas in the ampulla, the affinity was lower in the follicular phase.

It is established that α-receptors are also present prejunctionally in the sympathetic neuroeffector apparatus.[60,61] They have been designated α_2-receptors, in contrast to the traditional postjunctional receptors, which are named α_1-receptors. However, recent evidence suggests that the distinction "pre-" or "post-" synaptic is an oversimplification and both α_1 and α_2-adrenoreceptors may in fact be present postjunctionally.[62] The affinity of phentolamine for the postjunctional α-receptor has been found to be higher (pA_2 = 6.18).[63] It is notable that these two pA_2 values correspond in magnitude to the two populations of K_B values[57] obtained for the sympathomimetic contractile response of the fallopian tube at varying stages of the menstrual cycle (approximately 6×10^{-8} and 2×10^{-7}, respectively). It is thus conceivable that the two groups of K_B values reflect two subtypes of α-receptors, which may even be identical with the α_1- and α_2-receptors, each predominating during different parts of the menstrual cycle.

Adrenergic receptors and menstrual cycle

The sympathetic neurotransmitter has a decreased potency on the circular smooth musculature of the progesterone-dominated rabbit oviduct.[64,65] The effect of progesterone has been attributed to a decrease in α-receptor activity. This could not be verified by Rheaume and Paton,[66] who found that progesterone treatment increases the maximal inhibitory effect of isoproterenol on the β-receptor but does not alter the sensitivity to the agonist, suggesting a change in number of β-adrenoceptors rather than in receptor affinity. This is in accordance with the results of Martin et al.,[67] who observed enhanced β-receptor activity in the oviduct of progesterone-treated rabbits.

The relationship in the human tube of

the two types of postjunctional α-receptors to steroid levels is difficult to evaluate. Radioimmunoassays of plasma estradiol and progesterone[68] were used as markers to define different stages in the menstrual cycle.[57] It has been a general tendency when studying the effects of estradiol and progesterone on various female reproductive tissues to relate the results obtained to the concentration of sex hormones in the blood. However, it is more reasonable to assume that the biological activity will be governed rather by the concentration in the tissue or in the steroid receptors. Although there is a similarity in the general pattern of the cyclic fluctuations in mean steroid concentrations between tubal tissue and plasma, the correlation between these values in each individual patient has turned out to be poor.[35] This suggests that a more relevant parameter would be the ratio between tissue and plasma concentrations of the steroids which, particularly when the plasma levels are high, minimizes the error of nonspecific steroid accumulation in the tissue.

Radioimmunological measurements have shown that there is a much higher steroid level in the tubal tissue than in the plasma,[35] which confirms the presence of estrogen and progesterone receptors in the organ.[69–71] This indicates that the fallopian tube indeed can be considered as a target organ for ovarian steroids. Thus, the properties of adrenoceptors in different types of smooth musculature in different regions of the tube may be altered under the influence of sex steroids in a way that is not simply reflected in their plasma concentration.

It is thus evident from what has been discussed that the adrenergic neuromuscular mechanism in the human fallopian tube constitutes a functionally very complex entity. Adrenergic nerves innervate different types of smooth musculature in different tubal regions to different degrees. The function of the nerves is influenced by the menstrual cycle, which probably mediates effects of estrogen and progesterone on the nerves. Also the adrenergic receptors of the tubal smooth musculature are affected by these cyclic changes. The total response of a given portion of the tube to released norepinephrine transmitter under physiological conditions will vary during different stages of the menstrual cycle and also during pregnancy.

Sympathomimetic response and menstrual cycle

To illustrate the net response that might be expected from sympathetic neurotransmitter release in the human fallopian tube, the effect of norepinephrine on the motor activity has been studied in vitro. in the isthmic and ampullary parts.[20] A standard concentration of 3×10^{-6}M norepinephrine was chosen, since this turned out to induce an α-receptor-mediated effect that was between the half maximal and maximal responses. This concentration is in the region of the receptor in the same order of magnitude as the estimated instantaneous concentration of norepinephrine transmitter appearing in the synaptic cleft of a neuromuscular contact during the passage of a sympathetic nerve impulse.[55] The factors of particular interest reflecting motor activity are the frequency of the phasic contractions, as well as the area under the recorded curve. Also in this study,[20] the various stages in the menstrual cycle were defined on the basis of measurements of plasma estradiol and progesterone.[68] Samples from the "ovulatory phase" may be heterogeneous, consisting of not only material from women in the actual process of ovulation, but also preparations from the late follicular and probably also very early luteal stages.

When the adrenergic neurotransmitter was added to the organ bath, the frequency of the contractions in the circular smooth musculature of both isthmus and ampulla was lowered during the follicular and luteal phases, whereas little or no change occurred during the ovulatory period. To obtain a total picture of the composite changes in contractile activity of the fallopian tube, the surface area under

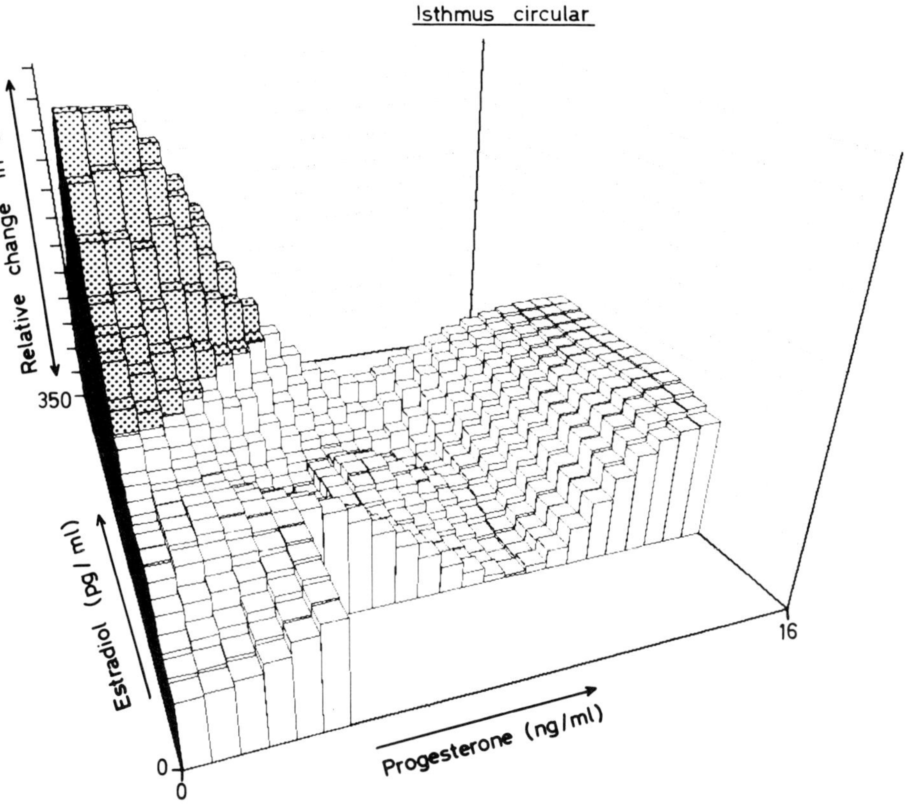

FIGURE 4:4—*Three-dimensional computer plot based on material from the circular isthmic smooth musculature* (n = *63), showing increase (shaded columns) or decrease (open columns) in area under curves of motor activity induced by* 3×10^{-6}*M norepinephrine, in relation to the plasma levels of estradiol and progesterone. The relative changes in area were measured planimetrically during equal time periods before and after administration of the amine.*

the recorded curve was measured during a three-minute period just before and after norepinephrine administration to the bath (Fig. 4:4). The baseline was defined as the lowest level of tone from which the individual deflections originated during the total six-minute measurement period.

A significant increase of contractile activity was found with norepinephrine around ovulation in all types of tubal preparations.[20] Also in the follicular phase there was an increase, although less pronounced, in contractile activity of the longitudinally oriented musculature. The circular musculature responded with reduced activity during this phase. In the luteal phase all preparations, except the isthmic longitudinal, responded to norepinephrine with a clear reduction. During menopause as well as during treatment with steroid contraceptives, or in pregnancy, norepinephrine always reduced tubal motor activity.

In general, not only the basal frequency but also the pattern of cyclic variations in frequency, and the difference by this factor between the circular and longitudinal smooth musculature in the composite type of preparations that we used were very similar to those recorded for microdissected smooth-muscle preparations from the human tube by Lindblom et al.[56] The results for women taking combined steroid-type oral contraceptives and for menopausal and pregnant women agree with what could be expected on the basis of the relationship found between plasma steroid levels and contraction frequency in patients with normal menstrual cycles (i.e., receiving no contraceptive pills). Administration of norepinephrine into the organ bath potentiated the difference in frequency of contractions during the ovulatory phase in comparison with the follicular and luteal phases.[20]

However, the contraction frequency represents only an isolated aspect of tubal motor activity. Planimetric measurement of the surface area under the recorded curve before and after the norepinephrine administration[20] confirmed that an α-receptor-mediated sympathomimetic increase in motor activity prevails during ovulation, whereas the contribution by a β-receptor-mediated reduction in motor activity is more prominent during the follicular and ovulatory phase.[16,57]

As mentioned above, there is ample evidence from studies on various laboratory animals that tubal motor activity is influenced by sex steroids—estradiol being associated with increased tubal contractility, whereas progesterone primarily seems to have an inhibitory effect. The biological activity of these steroids is probably governed by their concentrations in the tissue rather than in blood. Although there is a similarity in the general pattern of the cyclic fluctuations in the mean steroid concentrations between tubal tissue and plasma, the correlation between these values in each individual patient is poor.[35] The consistently high tubal motor activity, spontaneous and after sympathomimetic stimulation, found by Helm et al.,[20] corresponds with high progesterone receptor concentrations in the tissue.[35] Following ovulation, when the plasma progesterone levels rise, there is a drop in the specific tissue binding of progesterone, which is associated with a reduced motor activity in the oviduct after norepinephrine administration. The effect of norepinephrine is less consistent, particularly in the longitudinal smooth musculature, during the follicular phase. This may reflect a progressive increment in α-adrenoceptor activity in relation to the β-receptors during the follicular phase,[16] when there are high concentrations of estradiol and progesterone receptors.[35]

Peptidergic receptors

Two kinds of observations made in the course of our studies on the human fallopian tube have strongly indicated the existence of a nonconventional type of nerve-mediated motor inhibition in the tube. One was the previously mentioned presence of nerves containing VIP,[48] which was found to reduce the organ's contractile activity appreciably.[72] Another was the motor inhibition occurring during transmural nerve stimulation in spite of adrenergic and cholinergic blockade.[73] As described above, electrical field stimulation of composite preparations of tubal smooth muscle with short pulse duration evokes a motor response that is either an increase or a decrease in activity, or often a biphasic response. Initially, the stimulation often gives rise to a twitch contraction, which is the result of an α-adrenoceptor activation.[51] It is still possible to evoke the reduced motor activity in the presence of propranolol and atropine. Addition of the nerve-blocking agent, tetrodotoxin, abolished the α-adrenergic response and also the reduced motor activity, showing that both effects were mediated by stimulation of nerves in the preparations rather than a result of direct smooth-muscle activation. This is in agreement with the observation by Murcott and Carpenter,[74] who found evidence in the rat oviduct for a nonadrenergic inhibitory mechanism. Lindblom et al.[56] have confirmed the presence of a noncholinergic, nonadrenergic mechanism in the human oviduct.

Among the many known biological effects of VIP, it relaxes nonvascular smooth muscles. Exposure of smooth-muscle preparations from the human female reproductive tract to VIP induces a dose-dependent relaxation of the tubular isthmic smooth musculature (Fig. 4:5), in

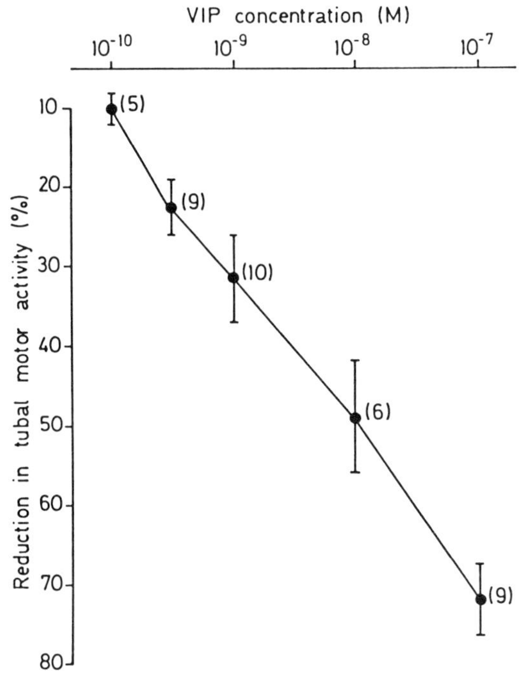

FIGURE 4:5—*Reduced contractile activity of the tubal isthmus (circular musculature) when increasing doses of VIP are added in a cumulative manner. The final mean concentrations in the bath are given; vertical bars show SEMs. Number of observations within parentheses.*

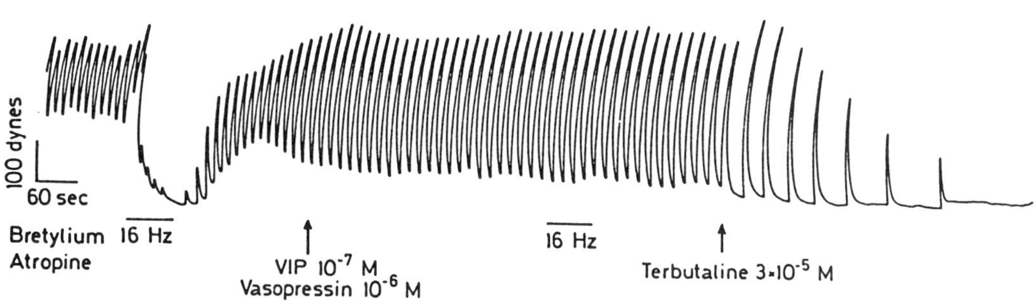

FIGURE 4:6—*A combination of VIP and vasopressin abolishes the neurogenic nonadrenergic, noncholinergic reduction of tubal motor activity (induced by 16 Hz nerve stimulation in the presence of 10^{-5}M bretylium and 10^{-5}M atropine). The peptides have not produced a nonspecific desensitization of the tube: reduced motor activity can still be induced by β-adrenergic stimulation with terbutaline. Vertical calibration, 100 dynes; horizontal calibration 60 sec.*

both circularly and longitudinally oriented preparations.[48,72] Also, the uterine cervical region, which like the tubal isthmus has a dense VIP innervation, shows a dose-dependent reduction in motor activity in the presence of exogenous VIP.[72] On the other hand, the poorly VIP-innervated corpus uteri does not react even to high doses of VIP.[48] Thus, the response of the tissue to exogenous VIP is well correlated to the local density of VIP-immunoreactive nerves, which suggests that VIP plays a role in the control of tubal smooth-muscle activity.

Administration of VIP to human tubal preparations in vitro induces a reduction in motor activity that is sometimes immediate, but in other instances the effect reaches its maximum more slowly.[73] The discrepancy between the immediate response during nerve stimulation and the sometimes more progressive change in motor activity following exogenous VIP administration might be caused by the relatively longer diffusion distance for the exogenous VIP, and does not contradict the possibility that the nerve-induced reduction in motor activity is the result of local VIP release.

For the lack of specific VIP-receptor blocking agents, another approach has been used (Fig. 4:6) to show that the nonadrenergic, noncholinergic motor inhibition of the tube is mediated by a VIP-receptor.[73] Thus, electrical field stimulation of the tubal nerves (in the presence of adrenergic and cholinergic antagonism) was carried out with a high concentration of VIP in the organ bath. The intention was to occupy the VIP-receptors and thereby block the effect of any nerve-released VIP on the smooth musculature. The decrease in tension obtained after addition of exogenous VIP was balanced by vasopressin in order to maintain the control level of tension before the transmural electric stimulation was started. Under these circumstances, nervous activation failed to reduce the smooth-muscle activity. It should be noted that vasopressin has not been found in tubal nerves and it does not in itself influence the nerve-induced nonadrenergic, noncholinergic reduction in motor activity.

The VIP-inhibitory effect did not seem to be nonspecific (e.g., involving desensitization), since the preparation still responded with a pronounced reduction in motor activity after addition of the β-receptor agonist, terbutaline. (Under these conditions, the adrenergic mechanisms were blocked by bretylium, which does not affect the adrenoceptors.) The experiments thus support our view that VIP is responsible for the neurogenic nonadrenergic, noncholinergic inhibition of motor activity in the isthmus of the human fallopian tube.

References

1. Cheviakoff S, Diaz S, Carril M, et al: Ovum transport in women. In Harper MJK, Pauerstein CJ, Adams CE, et al (Eds): *Ovum Transport and Fertility Regulation.* Copenhagen: Scriptor, 1976: 416.
2. Croxatto HB, Ortiz ME, Diaz S, et al: Studies on the duration of egg transport by the human oviduct. II. Ovum location at various intervals following luteinizing hormone peak. *Am J Obstet Gynecol,* 132:629, 1978.
3. Diaz S, Ortiz ME, and Croxatto HB: Studies on the duration of ovum transport by the human oviduct. III. Time interval between the luteinizing hormone peak and recovery of the ova by transcervical flushing of the uterus in normal women. *Am J Obstet Gynecol,* 137:116, 1980.
4. Brundin J: Distribution and function of the adrenergic nerves in the rabbit fallopian tube. *Acta Physiol Scand,* 66 (suppl):259, 1965.
5. Pauerstein CJ, Hodgson BJ, and Kramen MA: The anatomy and physiology of the oviduct. In Wynn RM (Ed): *Obstetrics and Gynecology Annual.* New York: Appleton-Century-Crofts, 1974: 137.
6. Harper MJK, Pauerstein CJ, Adams CE, et al (Eds): *Ovum Transport and Fertility Regulation.* Copenhagen: Scriptor, 1976.
7. Seitchik J, Goldberg E, Goldsmith J, et al: Pharmacodynamic studies of the human fallopian tube in vitro. *Am J Obstet Gynecol,* 102:727, 1968.
8. Levy B, and Lindner H: The effects of drugs on the rabbit oviduct. *Eur J Pharmacol,* 18:15, 1972.
9. Spilman CH, and Harper MJK: Comparison of the effects of adrenergic drugs and prostaglandins on rabbit oviduct motility. *Biol Reprod,* 10:549, 1974.
10. Maia H, and Coutinho EM: Motility of the human oviduct in vivo. In Harper

MJK, Pauerstein CJ, Adams CE, et al (Eds): *Ovum Transport and Fertility Regulation*. Copenhagen: Scriptor, 1976: 221.

11. Maistrello J: Extraluminal recording of oviductal contractions in the unanesthetized rabbit. *J Appl Physiol*, 31:768, 1971.
12. Hodgson BJ, Ware RW, Crosby RJ, et al: An ultrasonic transducer for recording of oviductal motility. *J Appl Physiol*, 34:873, 1973.
13. Nelsen T, Nunn T, and Angell J: Microminiature transducer for oviductal motor function. In Harper MJK, Pauerstein CJ, Adams CE, et al (Eds): *Ovum Transport and Fertility Regulation*. Copenhagen: Scriptor, 1976: 75.
14. Talo A: Myoelectrical activity and transport of unfertilized ova in the oviduct of mice in vitro. *J Reprod Fert*, 60:53, 1980.
15. Vastik-Fernandez J, Gimeno MF, Lima F, et al: Spontaneous motility and distribution of prostaglandins in different segments of human fallopian tubes. *Am J Obstet Gynecol*, 122:663, 1975.
16. Moawad AH, Hedquist P, and Kim MH: Correlation of plasma estrogens and progesterone levels with the in vitro adrenergic responses in the isthmus of the human oviduct. In Harper MJK, Pauerstein CJ, Adams CE, et al (Eds): *Ovum Transport and Fertility Regulation*. Copenhagen: Scriptor, 1976: 276.
17. Owman C, Falck B, Johansson EDB, et al: Autonomic nerves and related amine receptors mediating motor activity in the oviduct of monkey and man. A histochemical, chemical and pharmacological study. In Harper MJK, Pauerstein CJ, Adams CE, et al (Eds): *Ovum Transport and Fertility Regulation*. Copenhagen: Scriptor, 1976: 256.
18. Gimeno MF, Borda E, Sterin-Borda L, et al: In vitro spontaneous and norepinephrine induced contractions of ampulla, isthmus and mesosalpinx from human fallopian tubes. Effects of cocaine and indomethacin. *Int J Fertil*, 23:22, 1978.
19. Lindblom B: Hormonal and neuronal control of human oviductal contractility. (Thesis) University of Göteborg, Sweden, 1979.
20. Helm G, Owman C, Sjöberg NO, et al: Motor activity of the human fallopian tube in vitro in relation to plasma concentration of oestradiol and progesterone, and the influence of noradrenaline. *J Reprod Fert*, 64:233, 1982.
21. Falck B, Hillarp NA, Thieme G, et al: Fluorescence of catecholamines and related compounds condensed with formaldehyde. *J Histochem Cytochem*, 10:348, 1962.
22. Bjorklund A, Falck B, and Owman C: Fluorescence microscopic and microspectrofluorometric techniques for the cellular localization and characterization of biogenic amines. In Rall JE, and Kopin IJ (Eds): *Methods of Investigative and Diagnostic Endocrinology*, vol. 1, *The Thyroid and Biogenic Amines*. Amsterdam: North Holland Publishing Co., 1972: 318.
23. Nakanishi H, Wansbrough H, and Wood C: Postganglionic sympathetic nerves innervating human fallopian tube. *Am J Physiol*, 213:613, 1967.
24. Owman C, Rosengren E, and Sjöberg NO: Adrenergic innervation of the human female reproductive organs: A histochemical and chemical investigation. *Obstet Gynecol*, 30:763, 1967.
25. Moawad AH, Kim MH, Zuspan FP, et al: Effects of progesterone on the adrenergic mechanisms of the genital tract. *Ann NY Acad Sci*, 286:287, 1977.
26. Sjöberg NO, Johansson EDB, Owman C, et al: Cyclic fluctuation in noradrenaline transmitter of the monkey oviduct. *Acta Obstet Gynecol Scand*, 56:139, 1977.
27. Owman C, Alm P, and Sjöberg NO: Pelvic autonomic ganglia: Structure, transmitters, function and steroid influence. In Elfin LG (Ed): *Autonomic Ganglia*. New York: John Wiley, 1983: 125.
28. Kubo K, Kawano J, and Ishii S: Some observations on the autonomic innervation of the human oviduct. *Int J. Fertil*, 15:30, 1970.
29. Helm G, Owman C, Rosengren E, et al: Regional and cyclic variations in catecholamine concentration of the human fallopian tube. *Biol Reprod*, 26:553, 1982.
30. Wurtman RM, Axelrod J, and Potter LT: The disposition of catecholamines in the rat uterus and the effect of drugs and hormones. *J Pharmacol Exp Ther*, 144:150, 1964.
31. Dujovne AR, Laborde NP, Carril LM, et al: Correlation between catechol-

amine content of the human fallopian tube and the uterus and plasma levels of estradiol and progesterone. *Am J Obstet Gynecol*, 124:229, 1976.

32. Owman C, and Sjöberg NO: Influence of sex hormones on the amount of adrenergic transmitter in the rabbit oviduct. In Kumar A (Ed): *Neuroendocrine Regulation of Fertility. Int Symp Simla 1974.* Basel: Karger, 1976: 260.
33. Takeda H, and Doteuchi M: Adrenergic mechanisms and hormonal status of the oviduct. In Harper MJK, Pauerstein CJ, Adams CE, et al (Eds): *Ovum Transport and Fertility Regulation.* Copenhagen: Scriptor, 1976: 307.
34. Kennedy DR, and Marshall JM: Effect of adrenergic nerve stimulation on the rabbit oviduct: Correlation with norepinephrine content and turn-over rate. *Biol Reprod*, 16:200, 1977.
35. Batra S, Helm G, Owman C, et al: Female sex steroid concentrations in the ampullary and isthmic regions of the human fallopian tube and their relationship to the plasma concentrations during the menstrual cycle. *Am J Obstet Gynecol*, 136:986, 1980.
36. Owman C: Pregnancy induces degenerative and regenerative changes in the autonomic innervation of the female reproductive tract. In Elliot K, and Lawrenson G (Eds): *Development of the Autonomic Nervous System.* London: Pitman 1981: 252.
37. Pauerstein CJ, and Eddy CA: The role of the oviduct in reproduction; Our knowledge and our ignorance. *J Reprod Fertil*, 55:223, 1979.
38. Jacobowitz D, and Koelle G: Histochemical correlations of acetylcholinesters and catecholamines in postganglionic autonomic nerves of the cat, rabbit and guinea pig. *J Pharmacol Exp Ther*, 148:225, 1965.
39. Owman C, and Sjöberg NO: Adrenergic nerves in the female genital tract of the rabbit. With remarks on cholinesterase-containing structures. *Ztschr Zellforsch*, 74:182, 1966.
40. Howe GR: Cholinergic mechanisms, oviductal motility and ovum transport. In Harper MJK, Pauerstein CJ, Adams CE, et al (Eds): *Ovum Transport and Fertility Regulation*, Copenhagen: Scriptor, 1976: 342.
41. Said SI, and Mutt V: Polypeptide with broad biological activity: Isolation from small intestine. *Science*, 169:1217, 1970.
42. Mutt V, and Said SI: Structure of porcine vasoactive intestinal octacosapeptide. The aminoacid sequence. Use of kallikrein in its determination. *Eur J Biochem*, 42:581, 1974.
43. Bodansky M, Klausner YS, Yang Li C, et al: Synthesis of the vasoactive intestinal polypeptide (VIP). *J Am Chem Soc*, 96:4973, 1974.
44. Fahrenkrug J: Vasoactive intestinal polypeptide: Measurement, distribution and putative neurotransmitter function. *Digestion*, 19:149, 1979.
45. Alm P, Alumets J, Hakanson R, et al: Peptidergic (vasoactive intestinal peptide) nerves in the genito-urinary tract. *Neuroscience*, 2:751, 1977.
46. Larsson LI, Fahrenkrug J, and Schaffalitzky de Muckadell B: Vasoactive intestinal polypeptide occurs in nerves of the female genitourinary tract. *Science*, 197:1374, 1977.
47. Ottesen B, Larsen JJ, Fahrenkrug J, et al: Distribution and motor effect of VIP in female genital tract. *Am J Physiol*, 240:32, 1981.
48. Helm G, Ottesen B, Fahrenkrug J, et al: Vasoactive intestinal polypeptide (VIP) in the human female reproductive tract: Distribution and motor effects. *Biol Reprod*, 25:227, 1981.
49. Alm P, Alumets J, Hakanson R, et al: Origin and distribution of VIP (vasoactive intestinal polypeptide)—Nerves in the genito-urinary tract. *Cell Tissue Res*, 205:337, 1980.
50. Tranzer JP, and Richard JG: Ultrastructural cytochemistry of biogenic amines in nervous tissue: Methodologic improvements. *J Histochem Cytochem*, 24:1178, 1976.
51. Sporrong B, Helm G, Owman C, et al: Electron microscopic and pharamacological evidence for a functional adrenergic innervation of the smooth musculature in the human fallopian tube. *Brain Res Bull*, 9:695, 1982.
52. Ishii S: Autonomic innervation of human and rat oviducts with reference to its sympathetic innervation—An electron microscopic study. *Med J Osaka Univ*, 23:1, 1972.
53. Henderson RM, Johns A, and Paton DM: Cell contacts and distribution of nerves in the smooth muscle of estro-

gen-dominated rabbit oviduct. *Gynecol Invest*, 7:127, 1976.

54. Daniel EE, Posey VA, and Paton DM: A structural analysis of the myogenic control systems of the human fallopian tube. *Am J Obstet Gynecol*, 121:1054, 1975.
55. Bennett MR: *Autonomic Neuromuscular Transmission*. Cambridge University Press, 1972.
56. Lindblom, B, Ljung B, and Hamberger L: Adrenergic and nonadrenergic neuronal mechanisms in the control of smooth muscle activity in the human oviduct. *Acta Physiol Scand*, 106:215, 1979.
57. Helm G, Owman C, Sjöberg NO, et al: Quantitative pharmacological characterization of β-receptors mediating sympathomimetic smooth muscle response in the human fallopian tube at various cyclic stages. *Acta Physiol Scand*, 114:425, 1982.
58. Furchgott R: The classification of adrenoceptors (adrenergic receptors). An evaluation from the standpoint of receptor theory. In Blaschko H, and Muscholl E (Eds): *Handbook of Experimental Pharmacology*, vol. 33. New York: Springer-Verlag, 1972: 283.
59. Walles B, Falck B, Owman C, et al: Characterization of autonomic receptors in the smooth musculature of human graafian follicle. *Biol Reprod*, 17:423, 1977.
60. Starke K, Taube H, and Borowski E: Presynaptic receptor system in catecholaminergic transmission. *Biochem Pharmacol*, 26:259, 1977.
61. Langer SZ: Presynaptic receptors and modulation of neurotransmission: Pharmacological implications and therapeutic relevance. *Trends Neuroscience*, 3:110, 1980.
62. Lefkowitz R, and Hoffman B: Adrenergic receptors. *Cycl Nucl Res*, 12:37, 1980.
63. Starke K, Endo T, and Taube HD: Relative pre- and post-synaptic potencies of α-adrenoceptor agonists in the rabbit pulmonary artery. *Naunyn-Schmiedeberg's Arch Pharmacol*, 291:55, 1975.
64. Higgs G, and Moawad AH: The effect of ovarian hormones on the contractility of the rabbit oviductal isthmus. *Can J Physiol Pharmacol*, 52:74, 1974.
65. Rheaume DE, and Paton D: Effect of hormonal pretreatment on adrenoceptor sensitivity in the isthmus of the rabbit oviduct. *Proc West Pharmacol Soc*, 20:19, 1977.
66. Rheaume DE, and Paton D: Effect of progesterone on adrenoceptors in the isthmus of the rabbit oviduct. *Eur J Pharmacol*, 48:403, 1978.
67. Martin JE, Ware RW, Crosby RJ, et al: Demonstration of beta adrenergic receptors in the rabbit oviduct. *Gynecol Invest*, 1:82, 1976.
68. Mishell DR Jr, Nakamura RM, Crosignani PG, et al: Serum gonadotropin and steroid patterns during the normal menstrual cycle. *Am J Obstet Gynecol*, 111:60, 1971.
69. Robertson DM, Landgren BM, and Guerrero R: Oestradiol receptor levels in the human fallopian tube during the menstrual cycle. *Acta Endocrinol*, 80:705, 1975.
70. Meuchler EK, Flickinger GL, Mastroianni L Jr, et al: Progesterone binding in rabbit oviduct and uterus. *Proc Soc Exp Biol Med*, 150:275, 1976.
71. Verhage H, Akbar M, and Jaffe R: Cyclic changes in cytosol progesterone receptor of human fallopian tube. *J Clin Endocrinol Metab*, 51:776, 1980.
72. Walles B, Hakanson R, Helm G, et al: Relaxation of human female genital sphincters by the neuropeptide vasoactive intestinal polypeptide. *Am J Obstet Gynecol*, 138:337, 1980.
73. Helm G, Hakanson R, Leander S, et al: Neurogenic relaxation mediated by vasoactive intestinal polypeptide (VIP) in the isthmus of the human fallopian tube. *Regulatory Peptides*, 3:145, 1982.
74. Murcott CA, and Carpenter JR: Inhibition in the rat oviduct mediated by an unidentified transmitter. *Br J Pharmacol*, 61:498, 1977.

5

Tubal Innervation

Anthony Johns,
Jurgen Kleinstein, and
Sándor L. Erdö

Origin of the Efferent Tubal Innervation

The fallopian tube is dually innervated, receiving nerves from both the sympathetic and the parasympathetic divisions of the autonomic nervous system. The sympathetic nerves arise in the second to fifth lumbar regions and pass through the sympathetic chain to the inferior mesenteric ganglia. These ganglia in the rabbit and cat[1] are arranged in a group of four around the inferior mesenteric artery. The upper ganglionic pair send branches anteriorly to the superior mesenteric ganglia, while the hypogastric nerve emerges from the lower pair. Similar anatomical arrangements are found in the rat, guinea pig,[2] and dog.[3] In humans, however, the distinct hypogastric nerve of lower species is replaced by a diffuse plexus and Mitchell[4] suggested that the nerve supply to the human fallopian tube originates in the inferior hypogastric plexus, the ovarian nerve, and the superior hypogastric plexus. Owman and Sjöberg[5] showed that the sympathetic nerves synapse with adrenergic cells bodies close to or within the wall of the female genitalia of woman,[6] cat,[7] and dog.[8]

The parasympathetic nerves of the oviducts of rats, rabbits, cats, dogs, and humans arise in the second to fourth sacral roots or pass individually as the pelvic nerve or nerves (nervi ergentes) to the pelvic plexus ganglia. How many postganglionic fibers reach the oviduct, as well as their role, however, is uncertain.

In comparison to the sympathetic innervation, the parasympathetic innervation is slight.[9] Langley and Anderson[10] found that stimulation of the pelvic nerves in the cat and rabbit had no effect and did not modify the contractile response of the genitalia to hypogastric nerve stimulation; however, Schofield[11] stated that, in one-quarter of the animals she studied, stimulation of the nervi ergentes produced a contractile response of the genitalia.

Histochemical investigation of the parasympathetic innervation failed to

The Fallopian Tube: Basic Studies and Clinical Contributions, edited by Alvin M. Siegler, M.D. Mount Kisco, New York: Futura Publishing Company, Inc.

demonstrate cholinesterase-containing nerves that did not show catecholamine fluorescence.[5,12] However, using longer incubation times, Jacobowitz and Koelle[13] did show a few nerves that stained for cholinesterase without showing catecholamine fluorescence. Woodruff and Pauerstein[14] state, however, that in the human fallopian tube, there are nonfluorescent nerves that are presumably cholinergic.

Peptidergic nerves have been demonstrated in the tube but the role of these vasoactive intestinal polypeptide-containing fibers is not known. They may be modulators of adrenergic responses since they are destroyed by treatments thought to be specific for adrenergic nerves.

The fallopian tube may also have a well-developed afferent innervation. Theobald[15] reported that under local anesthetic, the fallopian tubes were the most sensitive structure in the abdominal cavity.

Distribution of Tubal Nerves

Several authors believed that the nerve cells in the oviduct were present as a plexus. Gawronsky[16] suggested that a plexus analogous to Meissner's plexus of the intestine exists in the human fallopian tube. Other authors using similar techniques reported that no nerve plexus was present in the oviduct.[16–19] The distribution of nerves within the fallopian tube was identified with heavy metal staining techniques that showed the nerves following the large subserosal blood vessels, then branching down along the smaller blood vessels, eventually forming a nerve network within the muscle layers.[19] The finest fibers (which may well be cholinergic fibers) were found in the submucosal region of the tube.

Brundin and Wirsen[20,21] were the first to apply the Falck-Hillarp technique[22] of localizing catecholamines in the tube. They found few fluorescent terminals in the ampulla and almost all of this fluorescence was associated with blood vessels. They also noted increased adrenergic terminals in the isthmic segment and a greater density of adrenergic terminals in the circular muscle than in the longitudinal muscle region. This work was considerably expanded by Owman and coworkers[23] who suggested that the greatest concentration of adrenergic terminals occurred at the ampullary-isthmic junction. Similar innervation patterns have been described in the oviduct of the rat,[24] cat,[7] dog,[8] cow,[24] and rhesus monkey.[23,25]

The few electron microscopy studies of the tubal innervation generally have confirmed the light microscopy results. Daniel et al.[26] showed that in human tubes, the nerves generally followed blood vessels and were largest in the subserosa. The nerve bundles themselves contained several axons that were surrounded by Schwann cell sheaths. When the nerves left the blood vessels, they usually paralleled the muscle fibers. Similar observations were reported for rabbits' and monkeys' oviducts,[27] as well as for baboons' oviducts.[28]

However, electron microscopic examination of the oviduct has failed to confirm the presence of sensory nerve endings or myelinated nerves in the oviduct described by Martinez and Perez[29] and Chiara[16] using light microscopy.

Relationship of Nerve Terminals to Smooth Muscle

Kushiya[30] found that the nerves were nonmyelinated in the rabbit's preovulatory ampulla and that they occurred in small bundles surrounded by a Schwann cell sheath, usually associated with blood vessels. Longitudinal sections of the nerves showed they were varicose and that these varicosities contained vesicles of different sizes in the same nerve terminal. The most common type of vesicle was the large dense core type (55 to 100 nm diameter). Although most varicosities were some distance from smooth-muscle cells, Kushiya[30] described a few nerves within 2 nm of smooth muscle with no intervening basement membrane. No specialization was seen in the apposing membrane of the smooth-muscle cell. Similar findings have also been reported in the estrogen-treated rabbit's oviduct.[31] Daniel et al.[26] discovered that the few nerves found in the ampulla of the human tube were usually associated with blood vessels. No varicosities free of Schwann cell sheath were reported. More nerves were seen in the isthmus compared to the ampulla and these nerves usually were associated with the circular muscle layer. The varicosities of these nerves contained small dense cored vesicles and a few nerves were seen making close contacts with muscle cells.

Kubo et al.[32] showed electron micrographs of nerve bundles in the human oviduct but gave little information concerning neuromuscular relationships. Ishii[33] found varicose nerves in rats' and human oviducts and stated that most of the varicosities contained small dense cored vesicles that could be depleted in rats by prior treatment with reserpine. He also reported that 20 nm gaps between nerve and muscle occurred rarely.

The monkey's oviduct has been shown to be less sensitive to norepinephrine[34] than the rabbit's oviduct,[35,36] and electron microscopic examination of these tissues has revealed fewer nerve bundles in the monkey than in the rabbit.[37] In the tissues studies, it was only in the rabbit's oviduct that axons free of their Schwann cell sheath were seen and only in the rabbit's oviduct were close contacts between nerve and muscle observed. In summary, the nerves present in the myosalpinx are typically adrenergic in appearance under the electron microscope in the submucosa; however, small nerves seen in bundles may be cholinergic nerves.[12]

Adrenergic Receptors in the Tube

Ultrastructural evidence

In principle it is possible to label α- and β-adrenergic receptors with fluorescent antibodies in their intact cell matrices and to show them histologically. Mapping of β-adrenergic receptors in the cerebellar cortex with the fluorescent adrenergic compound, 9-amino-acridin-propranolol (9-AAP), is stereospecifically blocked by (−) propranolol. Since foregoing destruction of adrenergic nerves with 6-hydroxydopamine does not prevent the binding of 9-AAP, postsynaptic β-adrenergic receptors could be demonstrated.[38] (+)Hydroxybenzylpindolol labeled with ^{125}I is a compound with a high affinity for β-adrenoceptors, and is useful for the autoradiographic demonstration of these receptors. It is also possible to make the adrenergic receptors microscopically visible using the immunocytochemical technique. To do this, antibodies against β_2-adrenergic receptors of frog erythrocytes were made visible using immunohistochemical staining with a peroxidase-antiperoxidase stain.[39] To date, these techniques could not be used in the ultrastructural demonstration of adrenergic receptors in the oviduct. Nevertheless, there are countless numbers of biochemical and pharmacological studies that provide evidence for the existence of these receptors in the oviduct.

Biochemical evidence

Despite the proven existence of the adrenergic nervous system in the oviduct, there are few studies that biochemically quantify the adrenergic receptors of the myosalpinx. The radioligand binding technique is the method of choice for the direct indentification of membrane-bound α- and β-adrenergic receptors. The procedure of this technique is as follows: catecholamine-sensitive tissue is homogenized and, as a crude membrane preparation, incubated with radioactively labeled adrenergic ligands. To find the amount of nonspecific binding, a control is also run, incubating the above products with an excess of nonradioactively labeled agonist or antagonist. The amount of nonspecific binding is represented by the fraction of membrane-bound radioactivity that cannot be displaced by the excess agonist or antagonist. Membrane-bound radioactivity is separated from non-membrane-bound radioactivity by filtration through a glass fiber filter. This technique may be used to demonstrate the adrenergic receptors in the oviduct. However, there are certain difficulties associated with the myosalpinx: (1) it possesses an inhomogeneous connective tissue fraction, which causes a relatively high nonspecific binding of 30 to 50 percent. In homogenizations in which nonspecific binding makes up more than 50 percent of the total membrane-bound radioactivity, calculations of binding kinetics using Scatchard analysis[40] become inaccurate. (2) The myosalpinx, compared to other catecholamine-sensitive tissues, such as heart, brain, or lung tissue, possesses one-tenth of adrenergic receptors per milligram of protein. To demonstrate these receptors, which are in such low concentrations, radioligands with a high specific binding activity are needed. These demands are not sufficiently met with ^{3}H-labeled adrenergic agonists and antagonists, whose specific activity is 20 to 50 Ci/mmole. Although binding sites for ^{3}H-norepinephrine have been documented[41] in the $105{,}000 \times g$ microsomal fraction of the rabbit's oviduct (4.5 pmol/unit microsomal fraction), nevertheless it is known that radioactively labeled adrenergic agonists bind nonspecifically, rather than to specific receptors. This is caused by their catechol component, which binds to the catechol-O-methyltransferase system or the catecholamine oxidizing system. Recently this disadvantage was abolished by using the ^{125}I-labeled β-adrenergic antagonist, (−)cyanopindolol (I-CYP). While I-CYP has a specific activity of over 2,200 Ci/mmole, it also has a few shortcomings that need to be considered. First, ^{125}I has a short half-life of only 60 days. Second, the ligands tend to radiolyse. Third, there are potential changes in the biological activity of the receptor molecule through iodination. Despite these restrictions, it was possible to characterize particular β-adrenergic receptors of oviductal smooth muscle in a radioreceptor assay with I-CYP.[42] Samples were taken from rabbits and women. The number of β-adrenergic receptors was 30 fmol I-CYP bound per mg protein. Binding affinity was high with a dissociation constant K_D between 20 and 60 pM. The distribution of β-adrenergic receptors in rabbit oviducts shows a predominance of these in the ampulla (55 to 77 percent), followed by 15 to 30 percent in the central portion of the tube and 10 to 15 percent in the proximal part (Fig. 5:1). Since the biological function of β-adrenergic receptors is smooth-muscle relaxation, their predominance in the isthmic-ampullary region of the tube could be responsible for the 24-hour arrest of rabbits' ova in this location.[43]

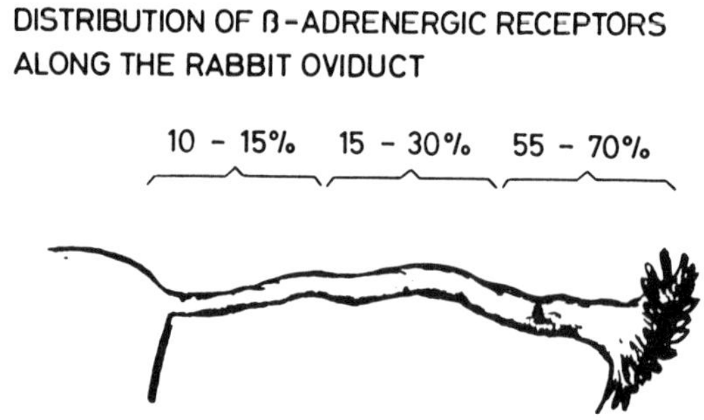

FIGURE 5.1—*Distribution of β-adrenergic receptor along the rabbit oviduct.*

Comparative results for the biochemical characterization of α-adrenergic receptors of myosalpinx do not exist. Several radioactively labeled α-adrenergic antagonists, such as ^{125}I-HEAT,[44] ^{3}H-prazosin,[45] and ^{3}H-rauwolscine,[46] are suitable for the demonstration of α-adrenergic receptors in the uterus. Results of the radioreceptor assay tests for oviductal α-adrenoceptors, bound to the above ligands, showed a high level of nonspecific binding (50 percent). Still, there was no proof of the ligand binding being saturated. The biochemical identification and characterization of adrenergic receptors of oviductal smooth muscle offer the possibility of ascertainng the activity of the adrenergic nervous system during ovum pickup and transport.

Pharmacological evidence

Numerous pharmacological studies reveal the existence and classification of adrenergic receptors in the oviduct. The following techniques were used: (1) in-vitro measurement of oviduct motility: the isolated parts of the oviduct were put into an organ bath and the muscular activity recorded with a transducer; and (2) in-vivo measurement of oviduct motility: in this case, different methods were used, namely, implantation or fixation of electrodes on the surface of the oviduct. These registered the electrical activity of the oviductal muscle.[47] The initiation of muscular contraction through transducer systems is often carried out together with perfusion or flow studies. Other studies register intraluminal pressure[48] and electrical impedance,[49] from which the contractility of myosalpinx is ascertained. In summary, these methods verified the existence of α- and β-adrenergic receptors in the oviduct muscle. The α-adrenergic agonists caused contraction of the oviductal smooth muscle, with the rank order of potencies epinephrine > norepinephrine > phenylephrine.[50] This rank order of potencies is typical because of the presence of α-adrenergic receptors.[51] The α-adrenergic antagonists such as phentolamine and phenosybenzamine cancel the effect of these adrenergic agonists.[52] There is evidence, as in the case of α-adrenergic receptors, that there are β-adrenergic receptors in the oviduct. In the rabbit, isoproterenol, a β-adrenergic agonist, depressed oviductal contractility of the isthmic musculature in vivo and in vitro. The β-adrenergic antagonist, propranolol, counteracted this effect.[53] The relaxation of the muscle through isoproterenol was more complete in rabbits treated with progesterone (10 mg/animal/day), compared to rabbits in estrus. As a result, it was concluded that progesterone increases the activity of the β-adrenergic receptors in the oviduct. Progesterone priming (5 mg/kg/day) for four days in rabbits reduces the number of β-adrenergic receptors in oviductal smooth muscle by 40 percent. On the other hand, estrogen priming (3 μg/kg/day) increases the number of β-adrenoceptors by a factor of 1.6.[43] The decrease in the number of β-adrenergic receptors under progesterone dominance is probably the cause of the more effective action of isoproterenol in the inhibition of oviductal contractility. Despite the pharmacologically proven existence of adrenergic receptors, it has thus far not been possible to use adrenergic antagonists as postcoital contraceptives.[54]

Classification of Tubal Adrenoceptor

Based on the characterization of α- and β-adrenergic receptors of the oviduct, a classification of these into subtypes was devised. Activation of α-adrenergic receptors by phenylephrine leads to contraction of the myosalpinx which is blocked by phentolamine. A comparison of the dissociation constants for the complex between α-adrenergic receptors and phentolamine in the circular and longitudinal muscle of the isthmus and the ampulla showed statistically significant differences that were dependent on the hormonal status. In the presence of a high sexual steroid level, the affinity of the α-adrenoceptors of the circular muscles is reduced for phentolamine, whereas that of the longitudinal ampullary muscles is inceased.[55] Because of these different affinities, it was concluded that there are two distinct α-adrenergic subtypes. These postulated subtypes could be identical with α-adrenergic postsynaptic and α_2-adrenergic presynaptic receptors. There is still evidence for the existence of distinct β-adrenergic subtypes. Beta-adrenergic agonists increase transisthmic flow in the sequence of potencies of terbutaline (β_2) > isoproterenol (β_1 + β_2) prenalterol (β_1), if they are applied transluminally.[56] Isthmic dilatation is mediated by β-adrenoceptors mainly of the β_2-subtype. Competitive binding experiments between ^{125}I-cyanopindolol, and α- and β-adrenergic substances for the binding to particulate membranes of the myosalpinx supported these findings. Beta-adrenergic drugs such as (−)propranolol and isoproterenol are more effective substances than α-adrenergic substances such as (−)phenylephrine and phentolamine (Fig. 5:2, left). Of the adrenergic antagonists, 32-468 HMO(β_2) is more effective than the β_1-antagonist, HI 42 BS (Fig. 5:2, right). It seems certain that α- and β-adrenergic receptors, with their subtypes, are found in the oviduct.

Presynaptic Receptors

Presynaptic receptors may have a function in the regulation of oviductal function. It is well documented that α_1-receptors are responsible for the contraction of smooth muscle whereas α_2-receptors reduce the nerve-induced output of norepinephrine from adrenergic nerve endings. Although direct evidence for the existence of both types of α-receptors with radioreceptor binding is not available, there is indirect evidence for their existence in the oviduct. Hedqvist and Moawad[57] showed that in the isthmic portion of the human fallopian tube incubated with ^{3}H-norepinephrine, α-agonists depressed nerve-induced release of norepinephrine and β-agonists increased norepinephrine release. These effects could be blocked by phenoxybenzamine and propranolol, respectively, demonstrating the existence of presynaptic control of norepinephrine release in the human fallopian tube.

Tubal Adrenoceptors and the Cyclic AMP Generating System

In smooth muscle a direct relationship between excitatory α-adrenergic receptors and cyclic AMP (cAMP) levels has never been demonstrated, whereas the β-adrenoceptors, mediating inhibitory responses, have generally been considered to be coupled to a cAMP-generating system. When an agonist binds to the β-adrenoceptor, a conformational change is produced that triggers the adenylate cyclase to increase its catalytic activity.

The early finding that the stimulation of β-adrenoceptors in the rabbit's oviduct by isproterenol induced a significant elevation of intracellular cAMP levels concomitant with its relaxing effect on contractility[58] has been reexamined as a function of hormonal status. It has been demonstrated that isoproterenol failed to influence significantly the tubal cAMP levels in estrual or estrogen-treated rabbits, but it caused a significant increase in the concentration of the second messenger under progesterone dominance.[59] The basal cAMP levels were highest under estrogen dominance and it is conceivable that the high cAMP concentrations during

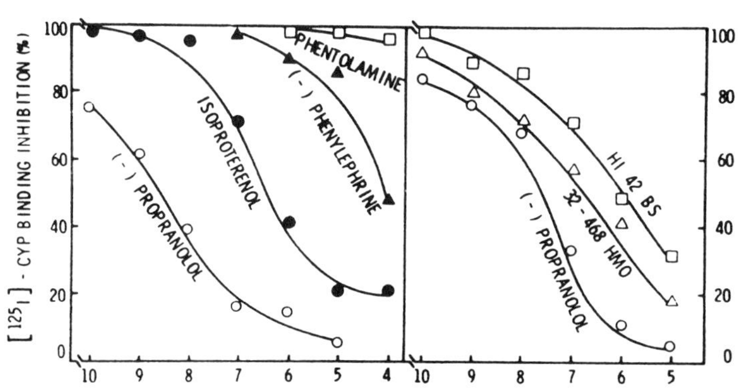

FIGURE 5.2—*Results of a competitive binding experiment with adrenergic drugs.*

estrus could not be further elevated by progesterone. On the other hand, the above finding may indicate that the responsiveness of the cAMP-generating system to β-adrenergic stimulation in the fallopian tube exhibits a considerable plasticity depending on hormonal status. This is in accord with the increased ability of isoproterenol to induce relaxation in oviducts from progesterone-dominant rabbits.[50]

In the human tube, the β-adrenoceptor agonist, isoproterenol, could not significantly influence the cAMP concentrations, even though it caused a significant inhibition of the contractility of both circular and longitudinal muscle preparations from the same specimens.[60] Thus, the altered tissue cAMP levels do not appear to be responsible for the inhibitory effects of β-adrenoceptor agonists.

The conflicting data with respect to the cAMP response to β-adrenergic stimulation in rabbit and human oviducts may partly be caused by species differences. It is also possible, however, that the human specimens used for the measurement of cAMP levels were obtained mainly from women under estrogen dominance, since the stage of the menstrual cycle was not specified in the study.[60] The lack of effect of isoproterenol on the cAMP levels of the human oviduct would therefore be consistent with findings in the rabbit's oviduct.[59]

Our knowledge of the interactions between the tubal β-adrenoceptors and the cAMP-generating system has been based on few studies. No attempts have been made to examine even the well-known subtypes of β-adrenoceptors regarding their relationship to this second messenger system. Nevertheless, it seems likely that the tubal β-adrenoceptors, or at least some of them, are coupled to a cAMP-generating system. The response of the adenylate cyclase/cAMP system to β-adrenergic stimulation, however, appears to depend on the animal's hormonal status. On the other hand, the ability of the β-adrenoceptor agonist, isoproterenol, to relax oviductal smooth muscle without changing cAMP levels may indicate that the contractile effects evoked by β-adrenoceptor stimulation are not always mediated by the cAMP-generating system.

Alteration of Sympathomimetic Responses in the Tube

The majority of data available concerning the changes of the adrenergic responses of the mammalian oviduct have been based on the measurement of the contractile response of the tube under the effect of various adrenergic model compounds or during adrenergic nerve stimulation. While α-excitatory and β-inhibitory receptor activity could be demonstrated in the oviducts of all species examined, the predominant response to adrenergic nerve stimulation varied. In rabbits, the action of norepinephrine on α-adrenoceptors predominates under all hormonal conditions; thus, norepinephrine always elicits contractions in the rabbit's oviduct; however, in other species, including humans, changes in hormonal dominance may lead to adrenergic reversal.[61]

In the early studies with women's and pigs' oviducts, epinephrine was found to evoke contraction in the luteal phase but relaxation during the follicular phase. In rabbits, the response of the oviduct to epinephrine was also reported to be hormonally dependent: the contractile response was maximal during estrus and was much smaller under progesterone dominance than under estrogen dominance.[62] A decreased stimulatory activity of norepinephrine on the rabbit's oviduct has also been observed during early gestation.[63] These findings served to draw attention to the dependency of oviductal adrenergic responses on hormonal status; however, they were unsuitable for providing direct information regarding the actual changes in α- and β-adrenergic responses, since in these experiments, epinephrine and norepinephrine interact with both α- and β-adrenoceptors and no α- or β-blockers were used to exclude interactions at the other adrenoceptor type. To avoid the undesirable interactions in later studies, α-adrenergic responses were studied under β-blockade, while β-adrenoceptor-mediated effects were examined in the presence of an α-adrenoceptor antagonist.

In the circular muscular layer of the rabbit isthmus, no significant alteration has been observed in the sensitivity of α-adrenoceptors during estrus or under progesterone dominance when β-adrenoceptors were blocked by propranolol.[50] Under α-blockade, the β-adrenergic response of the same preparation showed hormonally dependent changes. During progesterone dominance, the maximal inhibitory effect of isoproterenol increased but the sensitivity did not change. The authors concluded that there had been an increase in the number of β-adrenocep-tor s rather than a change in their affinity. This conclusion can be criticized, since these experiments were performed using cholinergic stimulation by a constant dose of acetylcholine under all hormonal conditions. Thus, alterations of cholinergic responses may also be involved in the above phenomena. Nevertheless, these results are in accord with the earlier observation that an increase of β-adrenoceptor activity occurred in the rabbit's isthmus under progesterone dominance.[64,65] The finding that the sensitivity of α-adrenoceptors failed to change with the hormonal status, however, contradicts the earlier proposal that α-adrenergic responsiveness of the rabbit's oviduct decreases under the effect of progesterone.[62,63]

In the guinea pig, norepinephrine induces contraction of the oviduct only during the follicular phase, but not during the luteal phase.[66] In the rat, the spontaneous contractility of the tube was inhibited by norepinephrine during proestrus and metestrus, but not during estrus.[67] Thus, in progesterone dominance, the β-adrenoceptors predominate in the oviducts of the rat and guinea pig. No information has accumulated that the increased β-adrenergic responses in these tissues are associated with the increases of the number or of the affinity of these receptors.

In the isolated human fallopian tube, norepinephrine and also transmural nerve stimulation produced a predominant inhibition of the spontaneous activity of ampulla and isthmus in all phases of the menstrual cycle, although excitatory α-responses could also be observed.[25,68]

The tissues from estrogen-dominant women (from the earlier part of the menstrual cycle) were less responsive to norepinephrine and to transmural stimulation than were those from the late phase of the cycle. These findings are inconsistent with certain earlier observations that norepinephrine exerts a predominantly excitatory response, or excitation followed by inhibition, in the human oviduct.[68] In another study, a reversal of β-inhibitory responses to norepinephrine during the late follicular phase (i.e., estrogen dominance) has been reported when responses became excitatory.[69] These studies did not attempt to characterize the changes of α- and β-adrenergic responses but they obviously demonstrated the hormonal dependency of adrenergic receptor sensitivity in the human fallopian tube.

In a recent study, the alteration of α-excitatory and β-inhibitory responses of the human oviduct has been characterized quantitatively at various cyclic stages.[55] No significant cyclic changes could be demonstrated in the affinity of β-adrenoceptors under α-adrenergic blockade. The affinity of α-adrenoceptors under β-blockade increased in the circular muscular layers of the ampulla and the isthmus but decreased in longitudinal ampulla during the follicular phase. In longitudinal isthmus, no change could be detected. These results provide information regarding the alteration of the affinity of α- and β-adrenoceptors but they do not reflect the possible changes in the number of these receptors as a function of hormonal status. In the light of these findings, no definite conclusion can be drawn; nevertheless, the variation of α- and β-adrenergic sensitivity in various muscular layers of the human oviduct during the menstrual cycle seems to be undoubted.

Functional Importance of Tubal Adrenoceptors

The early assumption that a hormonally dependent adrenergic sphincter is present at the ampullary-isthmic junction of the mammalian oviduct cannot be adequate for all species. The species differences in the responsiveness of the oviduct to norepinephrine and to adrenergic nerve stimulation definitely contradict this simplified hypothesis. The presumptive role of adrenoceptor-mediated effects in the regulation of ovum transport and fertility is also on a weak basis, since neither α- and β-adrenoceptor blockers nor chemical sympathectomy have been found to alter significantly the ovum transport and fertility in rabbits and mice. Nevertheless, it is conceivable that, in vivo, alterations in the release process through presynaptic mechanisms or other unidentified compensatory mechanisms may eliminate the effects of adrenoceptor blockers or adrenergic denervation on ovum transport and fertility. However, even if the adrenergic system does participate in the physiological regulation of these functions, the pharmacological manipulation of the tubal adrenoceptors cannot be suitable for efficient retardation or facilitation of ovum transport, particularly when the marked systemic effects of adrenergic drugs are taken into account.[61]

The accumulated information does not describe the exact role of adrenoceptors and adrenergic innervation in the oviductal function. Further studies demonstrating the common properties of the oviductal adrenergic systems in different species may lead to the better understanding of the functional importance of tubal adrenoceptors.

Conclusion

The fallopian tubes receive both sympathetic and parasympathetic postganglionic nerves, of which only the sympathetic nerves seem to be functionally important.

The adrenergic nerves innervate both the smooth muscle and blood vessels and are anatomically typical of adrenergic nerves innervating other tissues.

The adrenergic nerves rarely form close relationships with the smooth muscle.

The β-receptors of the tube are probably the β_2 subtype and both α_1 (postsynaptic) and α_2 (presynaptic) receptors have been demonstrated in the tube.

The β-adrenergic response is increased by progesterone pretreatment and reduced by estrogen treatment, probably by regulation of the number rather than of the affinity of the β-receptors. No hormonal effects on α-adrenergic receptors have been demonstrated.

The inhibitory motor effects of β-agonists are probably not mediated by the adenylate cyclase system.

There is no evidence that the adrenergic innervation is important in either ovum transport or normal fertility, but the changes in pharmacological responsiveness of the tube to adrenergic agonists could play an as yet undefined role in ovum transport and normal fertility of mammals.

References

1. Langley JN, and Anderson HK: The innervation of the pelvic and adjoining viscera. Part VII. Anatomical observations. *J Physiol* (London), 20:372, 1896.
2. Marshall JM: Adrenergic innervation of the female reproductive tract: Anatomy, physiology and pharmacology. *Ergeb Physiol*, 62:6, 1970.
3. Mizeres NJ: The anatomy of the autonomic nervous system of the dog. *Am J Anat*, 96:285, 1955.
4. Mitchell GAG: Innervation of the ovary, uterine tube, testes and epididymis. *J Anat*, 72:508, 1938.
5. Owman C, and Sjöberg NO: Adrenergic nerves in the female genital tract of the rabbit. With remarks on cholinesterase-containing structures. Ztschr Zellforsch, 74:182, 1966.
6. Owman C, Rosengren E, and Sjöberg

NO: Adrenergic innervation of the human female reproductive organs; A histochemical and chemical investigation. *Obstet Gynecol*, 30:763, 1967.
7. Rosengren E, and Sjöberg NO: Changes in the amount of adrenergic transmitter in the female genital tract of the rabbit during pregnancy. *Acta Physiol Scand*, 72:412, 1968.
8. Owman C, and Sjöberg NO: Adrenergic innervation of the female genital tract of the dog. *J Reprod Med*, 8:63, 1972.
9. Black DL: Neural control of oviductal musculature. In Johnson AD, Foley CW (Eds): *The Oviduct and Its Function*. New York: Academic Press, 1974: 66.
10. Langley JN, and Anderson HK: The innervation of the pelvic and adjoining viscera. Part IV. The internal generative organs. *J Physiol* (London), 20:372, 1895.
11. Schofield BM: The innervation of the cervix and cornu uteri in the rabbit. *J Physiol* (London), 117:317, 1952.
12. Jordan SM: Adrenergic and cholinergic innervation of the reproductive tract and ovary in the guinea-pig and rabbit. *J Physiol* (London), 210:115, 1970.
13. Jacobowitz D, and Koelle GB: Histochemical correlations of acetylcholinesterase and catecholamine in postganglionic autonomic nerves of the cat, rabbit and guinea-pig. *J Pharmacol Exp Ther*, 148:225, 1965.
14. Woodruff JD,and Pauerstein CJ: *The Fallopian Tube*. Baltimore: Williams and Wilkens, 1969.
15. Theobald GW: The role of the cerebral cortex in the appreciation of pain. *Lancet*, 2:41, 1949.
16. Gawronsky N: Ueber Verbreitung und Endigung der Nerven in den weiblichen Genitalien. *Arch Gynäkol*, 47:271, 1894.
17. Chiara F: Studio sulla fine innervazione dei genitali femminili tube. *Ann Ostet Ginecol*, 81:1161, 1959.
18. Damiani N, and Capadacqua A: Sull'-innervazione intrinseca della tuba. *Ann Ostet Ginecol*, 83:436, 1961.
19. Muller D: Zur Innervation des weiblichen Genitale mit besonderer Berucksichtigung der Pars intramuralis tubae. *Arch Gynäkol*, 194:395, 1961.
20. Brundin J, and Wirsen C: The distribution of adrenergic nerve terminals in the rabbit oviduct. *Acta Physiol Scand*, 61:203, 1964.
21. Brundin J, and Wirsen C: Adrenergic nerve terminals in the human fallopian tube examined by fluorescence microscopy. *Acta Physiol Scand*, 61:505, 1964.
22. Falck B, Hillarp WA, Thieme G, et al: Fluorescence of catecholamines and related compounds condensed with formaldehyde. *J Histochem Cytochem*, 10:348, 1966.
23. Owman C, Falck B, Johansson EDB, et al: Autonomic nerves and related amine receptors mediating motor activity in the oviduct of monkey and man. A histochemical, chemical and pharmacological study. In Harper MJK, Pauerstein CJ, Adams CE, et al (Eds): *Ovum Transport and Fertility Regulation*. Copenhagen: Scriptor, 1976:256.
24. Brundin J, Fredricsson B, Norberg KA, et al: The sympathetic innervation of the oviduct of the rat. *Acta Physiol Scand*, 75:69, 1969.
25. Cottle MKW, and Higgs GW: Adrenergic innervation of the fallopian tube of the monkey. *Histochem*, 5:143, 1973.
26. Daniel EE, Posey VA, and Paton DM: A structural analysis of the myogenic control systems of the human fallopian tube. *Am J Obstet Gynecol*, 121: 1054, 1975.
27. Widdicombe JH, and Paton DM: Fine structure of smooth muscle in the monkey oviduct. *Gynecol Obstet Invest*, 10:221, 1979.
28. Johns A: Unpublished studies.
29. Martinez MM,and Perez FP: Contribucion al conocimiento de la fina inervacion de la trompa de Falopia. *Acta Ginecol*, 9:365, 1958.
30. Kushiya I: An electron microscope study of the muscular coats in the ampulla of rabbit oviduct, with special reference to neuromuscular relationships. *J Electron Microsc* (Tokyo), 17:127, 1968.
31. Henderson RM, Johns A, and Paton DM: Cell contacts and distribution of nerves in smooth muscle of estrogen-dominated rabbit oviduct. *Gynecol Invest*, 7:121, 1976.
32. Kubo K, Kawano J, and Ishii S: Some observations on the autonomic innervation of the human oviduct. *Int J Fertil*, 15:30, 1970.
33. Ishii S: Autonomic innervation of human and rat oviducts with reference to

its sympathetic innervation. An electron microscopic study. *Med J Osaka Univ*, 23:1, 1972.

34. Widdicombe JH, Johns A, and Paton DM: Response of monkey oviduct to transmural stimulation and to drugs. *J Reprod Fertil*, 50:141, 1977.
35. Johns A, and Paton DM: Pharmacological characteristics of the response of rabbit oviduct to transmural stimulation. *Arch Int Pharmacodyn Ther*, 217:22, 1975.
36. Johns A, and Paton DM: Effects of cocaine and other drugs on the sensitivity of the oestrogen-dominated isthmus of rabbit oviduct to noradrenaline. *Can J Physiol Pharmacol*, 53:1172, 1975.
37. Widdicombe JH, and Paton DM: Fine structure of smooth muscle in the monkey oviduct. *Gynecol Obstet Invest*, 10:221, 1979.
38. Levitzki A: Catecholamine receptors. *Rev Physiol Biochem Pharmacol*, 82:13, 1978.
39. Strader CD, Pickel VM, Tong HJ, et al: Antibodies to the β-adrenergic receptor: Attenuation of catecholamine-sensitive adenylate cyclase and demonstration of postsynaptic receptor localization in brain. *Proc Natl Acad Sci* (USA), 80:1840, 1983.
40. Scatchard G: The attractions of proteins for small molecules and ions. *Ann NY Acad Sci*, 51:660, 1949.
41. Chatkoff ML, and Pauerstein CJ: Biochemistry of adrenergic receptors in ovum transport. *Gynecol Invest*, 6:43, 1975.
42. Kleinstein J: Binding properties of beta-adrenergic receptors in oviductal smooth muscle membranes. *Gynecol Obstet Invest*, 17:242, 1984.
43. Kleinstein J: Oviductal beta-adrenoceptor activity during ovulation and ovum transport. (Unpublished data), 1983.
44. Glossmann H, Lubbecke F, and Bellemann P: (^{125}I)-HEAT. A selective, high-affinity, high specific activity ligand for alpha$_1$-adrenoceptors. *Naunyn-Schmideberg's Arch Pharmacol*, 318:1, 1981.
45. Bottari SP, Vauquelin G, Lescrainier JP, et al: Identification and characterization of α-adrenergic receptors in human myometrium by (^{3}H)-prazosin binding. *Biochem Pharmacol*, 32:925, 1983.
46. Bottari SP, Volaer A, Kaivez E, et al: Identification and characterization of α_2-adrenergic receptors in human myometrium by (^{3}H) rauwolscine binding. *Am J Obstet Gynecol*, 146:639, 1983.
47. Talo A, and Brundin J: The functional connections and contractile function of the upper reproductive tract in female rabbits. *Biol Reprod*, 9:142, 1973.
48. Greenwald GS: In vivo recording of intraluminal pressure changes in the rabbit oviduct. *Fertil Steril*, 14:666, 1963.
49. Guha SK, Arand S, and Talwar GP: In vivo motility of the unobstructed fallopian tube. *J Appl Physiol*, 40:114, 1976.
50. Rheaume DE, and Paton DM: Effect of progesterone on adrenoceptors in the isthmus of the rabbit oviduct. *Eur J Pharmacol*, 48:403, 1978.
51. Alquist RP: Study of adrenotropic receptors. *Am J Physiol*, 153:586, 1948.
52. Ueda M, Mattos CER, and Cautinho EM: The influence of adrenergic activation and blockade on the motility of the circular and longitudinal muscle layers of the rabbit oviduct in vitro. *Fertil Steril*, 24:440, 1973.
53. Martin JE, Ware RW, Crosby RJ, et al: Demonstration of beta-adrenergic receptors in the rabbit oviduct. *Gynecol Invest*, 1:82, 1970.
54. Pauerstein CJ, Fremming DB, Hodgson BJ, et al: The promise of pharmacologic modification of ovum transport in contraceptive development. *Am J Obstet Gynecol*, 116:161, 1973.
55. Helm G, Owman C, Sjöberg NO, et al: Quantitative pharmacological characterization of beta-receptors and two types of alpha-receptors mediating sympathomimetic response in the human fallopian tube at various cyclic stages. *Acta Physiol Scand*, 114:425, 1982.
56. Strom C, Dahlstrom A, Lindblom B, et al: Effects of intraluminal administration of adrenoceptor agonists on transisthmic flow in the rabbit oviduct. *Biol Reprod*, 29:295, 1983.
57. Hedqvist P, and Moawad A: Presynaptic α- and β-adrenoceptor mediated control of noradrenaline release in human oviduct. *Acta Physiol Scand*, 95:494, 1975.
58. Brunton WJ: Adenylate cyclase activity in rabbit oviduct: Stimulation by isoproterenol and prostaglandins. *Biol Reprod*, 7:106, 1972.
59. Hodgson BJ, and Eddy CA: The autonomic nervous system and its relation-

ship to tubal ovum transport. A reappraisal. *Gynecol Invest*, 6:162, 1975.
60. Lindblom B, and Hamberger L: Cyclic AMP and human oviductal contractility. *Biol Reprod*, 22:173, 1980.
61. Paton DM, Widdicome JH, Rheaume DE, et al: The role of the adrenergic innervation of the oviduct in the regulation of mammalian ovum transport. *Pharmacol Rev*, 29:68, 1978.
62. Hunter DS, and Kendle KE: The influence of hormonal state on the responses of the isolated rabbit oviduct to catecholamines. *J Reprod Fertil*, 41:245, 1974.
63. Heilman RD, Reo RR, and Hahn DW: Changes in the sensitivity of adrenergic receptors in the oviduct during early gestation in the rabbit. *Fertil Steril*, 27:426, 1976.
64. Hodgson BJ, and Pauerstein CJ: The effect of ovulation on the responses of the rabbit oviduct to adrenergic agonists in vitro. *Biol Reprod*, 10:346, 1974.
65. Hodgson BJ, and Pauerstein CJ: Effects of hormonal treatments which alter ovum transport on beta-adrenoceptors of the rabbit oviduct. *Fertil Steril*, 26:573, 1975.
66. Gimeno MF, Borda ES, Sterin-Borda L, et al: Contractile activity of the oviduct and mesosalpinx isolated from guinea-pigs in different phases of the sex cycle. Effects of several pharmacological influences. *Int J Fertil*, 21:31, 1976.
67. Borda E, Sterin-Borda L, Gimeno MF, et al: Motility of the rat oviductal tract isolated in different stages of the sex cycle, effects of catecholamines. *Int J Fertil*, 20:170, 1975.
68. Molnar S, Johns A, Paton DM, et al: Characteristics of responses of isolated human fallopian tube to transmural stimulation and to sympathomimetic amines. *Arch Int Pharmacodyn Ther*, 220:205, 1976.
69. Moawad AH, Hedqvist P, and Kim M: Correlation of plasma estrogens and progesterone levels with the in vitro adrenergic responses in the isthmus of the human oviduct. In Harper MJK, Pauerstein CJ, Adams CE, et al (Eds): *Ovum Transport and Fertility Regulation*. Copenhagen: Scriptor, 1976: 276.

6

Morphological and Functional Aspects of the Oviductal Epithelium

Christopher M. Fredericks

The physiological functions of the fallopian tubes are complex and include facilitating gamete transport, supporting final gamete maturation and early embryonic development, and controlling embryo delivery to the uterus. The tubal epithelium is of fundamental importance in all of these processes. The overall physiological importance of this epithelial system is reflected in its responsiveness to the reproductive cycle, as well as its modification with aging and menopause. In addition, pathological alterations of epithelial structure and function contribute to human infertility.

Cell Types

The oviductal wall can be differentiated into four concentric layers by light microscopy. Innermost is a single-celled layer of columnar epithelium. Underlying this is a region of connective tissue, the lamina propria, which separates the epithelial cells from the tunica muscularis, the muscle layer that forms the bulk of the wall's thickness. The outermost layer (the tunica serosa) is again connective tissue.

The epithelial layer consists primarily of two types of cells: ciliated and secretory[1–10] (Figs. 6:1 and 6:2). It is now generally accepted that these cells are separate entities since no transitional forms have been identified by using the electron microscope.[1] Two other less common cells have also been described, an intercalary or "peg" cell, and an "indifferent" or basal cell.[11–13]

The epithelial ciliated cells are relatively cuboid in contour and contain a fine, granular cytoplasm. These cells are characterized by vesiculated endoplasmic reticulum, large mitochondria, and cytoplasmic droplets that may attain 800 nm in diameter. The nucleus, which is usually centrally located, is round or oval and is large in comparison with the cytoplasmic

The Fallopian Tube: Basic Studies and Clinical Contributions, edited by Alvin M. Siegler, M.D. Mount Kisco, New York: Futura Publishing Company, Inc. © 1986.

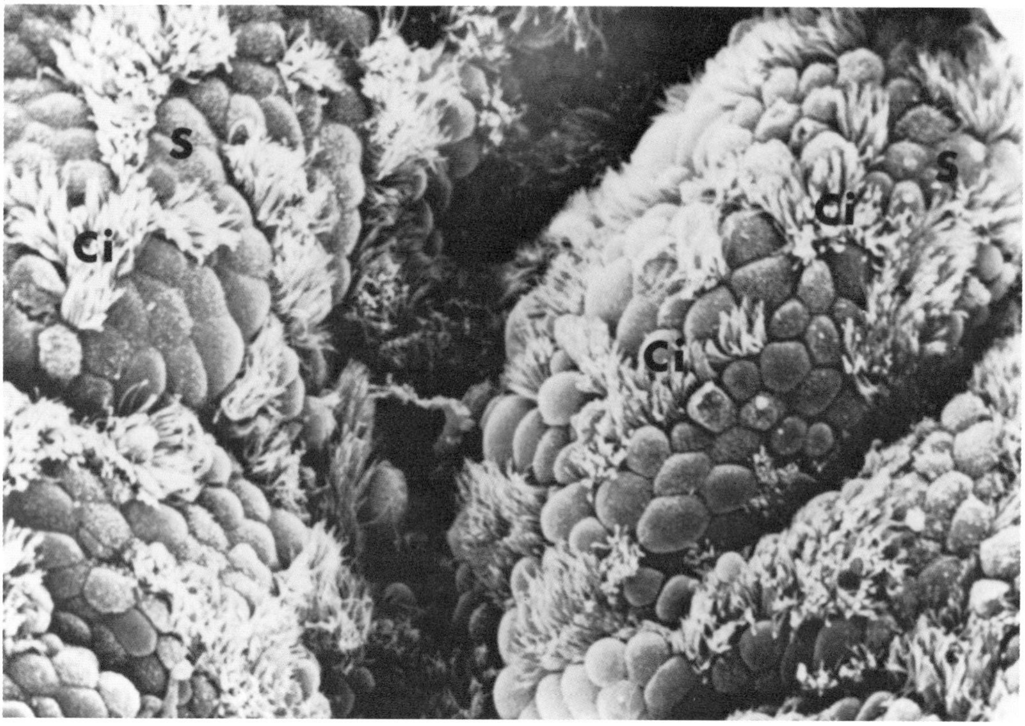

FIGURE 6:1—*Scanning electron micrograph of the summit of two adjacent ampullary folds, illustrating numerous clusters of ciliated cells (Ci) alternating with nonciliated dome-shaped secretory cells (S) (original magnification, ×2,000; Ferenczy and Richart[4]).*

volume. A perinuclear halo of clear cytoplasm is often prominent. The cilia are approximately seven microns long and are attached to a refractile row of basal granules beneath the cell membrane. The cilia are composed of two central filaments and nine double lateral filaments.[14,15] Small processes radiate from the central filaments to the ciliary membrane and may act as supports.

The secretory cells are distinguished by their more granular cytoplasm (secretory granules), well-developed endoplasmic reticulum, and Golgi bodies. The mitochondria appear smaller than those in ciliated cells. In the secretory cell the darker, oval nucleus is oriented with its long axis parallel to the long axis of the cell, although its position in the cell varies with the phase of the cycle.

The "peg" cells are thinner than either the ciliated or secretory cells and appear as long, slender, dark nuclei compressed between adjoinng cells. Only a small amount of cytoplasm surrounds the dark nucleus. Their function is unknown. Transitions between secretory cells and "peg" cells have been described, suggesting that the "peg" cells may be regressed or exhausted secretory cells or possibly a precursor of the secretory cell.

A smaller cell with a basal location, dark nucleus, rounded profile, and sparse cytoplasm with few organelles has also been described. Although there has been some debate about whether these cells are of epithelial origin, recent investigations suggest that these "indifferent" or basal cells are truly a fourth type of tubal epithelial cells.[11–13] These cells may act as granulocytes and increase in number during salpingitis.[13,16]

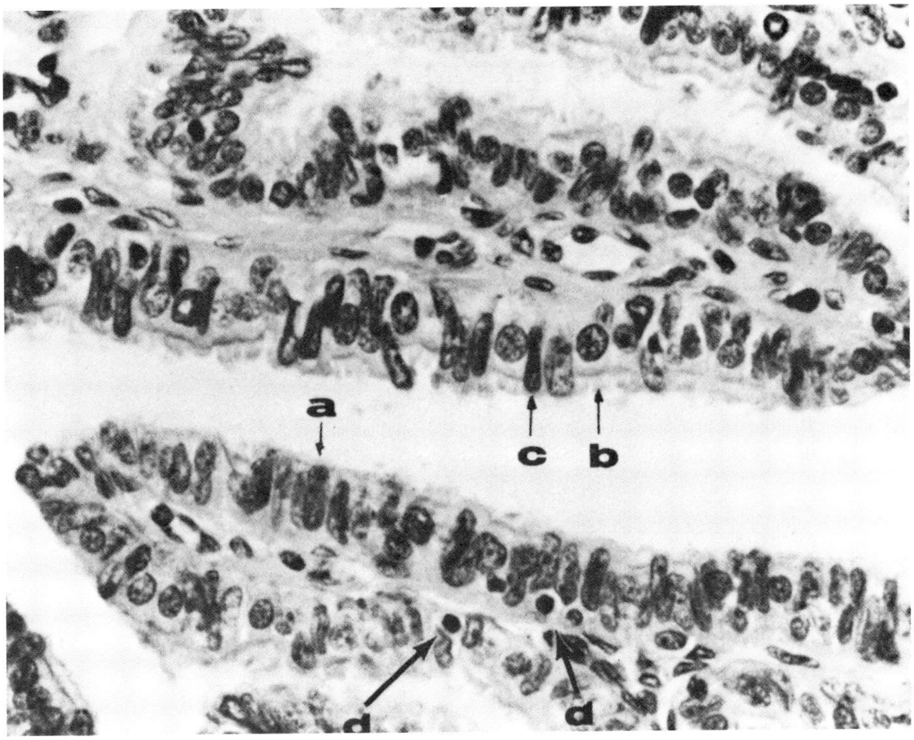

FIGURE 6:2—*Cells of the human tubal mucosa: a = secretory; b = ciliated; c = intercalary; and d = indifferent (Pauerstein et al.[3]).*

Regional Distribution of Cell Types

The mucosa of the oviducts is arranged in longitudinal folds that vary in their complexity along the length of the tube. In the thin-walled ampullary portion, the folds are highly developed with many secondary and tertiary folds superimposed on the primary ridges (Fig. 6:3). These highly ramified folds impinge strongly on the tubal lumen. In the isthmus, with its thicker, more muscular walls, the mucosal folds are much reduced. The lamina propria, underlying the epithelium, forms a supporting framework for these folds.

Ciliated cells are most frequently found on the apices of the mucosal folds, while nonciliated cells are found in greater numbers between and at the bases of the folds. Although some authors have reported a fairly uniform distribution of ciliated cells along the length of the tube, others report a progressive decrease in the proportion of ciliated cells from the fimbriae to the isthmus (Fig. 6:4).[17–19] About 70 percent of the cells of the fimbrial epithelium may be ciliated, decreasing to 50 percent nearing the ampullary-isthmic junction. Secretory cells are well distributed throughout the oviductal ampulla in higher mammals. However, there is some controversy as to the extent to which such cells are also found in the isthmus.[1]

Cyclic Changes

Although not as pronounced as those seen in the endometrium, morphological

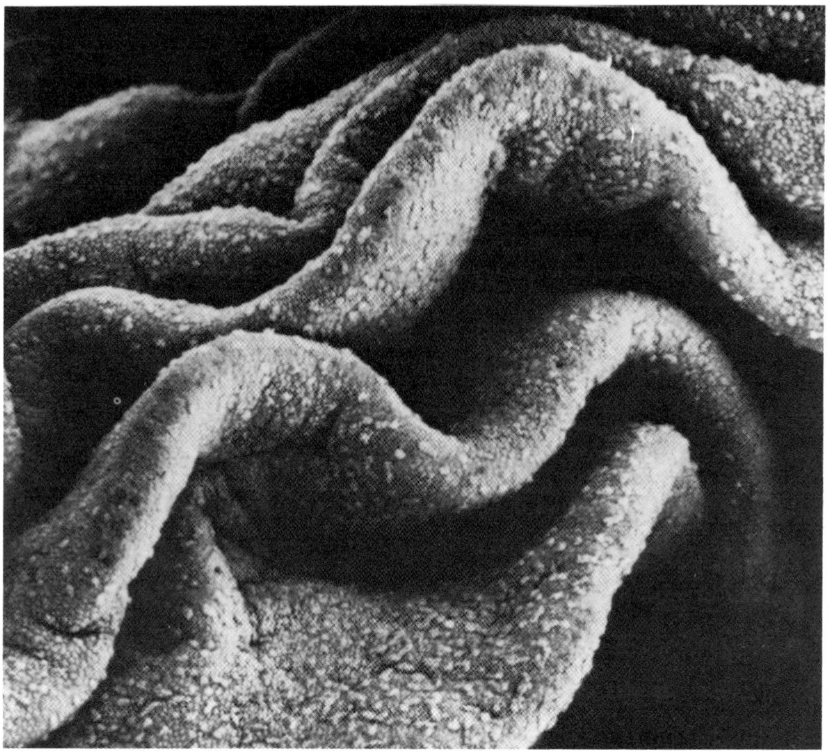

FIGURE 6:3—*Ampullary mucosa (day 11). Ampullary folds are covered by a relatively even distribution of bunches of ciliated cells (×200; Ludwig and Metzer[6]).*

and functional changes have been described in the epithelial cells in association with the hormonal fluctuations of the menstrual cycle (Figs. 6:5 and 6:6).[1–10] Disagreement remains, however, about the extent of these changes. There is general agreement that the changes in the secretory cells are the most pronounced and consistent.

During the *follicular phase,* cell heights increase, with epithelial thickening (30 microns) and secretory activity reaching a maximum close to the time of ovulation (Fig. 6:7). Both the secretory and ciliated cells reach equal heights, giving the luminal border of the epithelium a more regular appearance. Both cells are covered by well-shaped and regularly distributed microvilli. The individual villi are tall, and the cilia erect and vigorous. The microvilli of secretory cells may be swollen and adhere to each other in tufts or clumps. Some cells appear exhausted. It is possible that the mucus that adheres to the microvilli subserves some nutritional relationship between the ovum and the luminal structures. Considerable disagreement exists about whether an increase in the proportion of ciliated cells occurs during this phase.

During the *secretory phase,* the epithelium is somewhat lower. The ciliated cells become broader and lower, and the cilia may droop. The secretory cells enlarge and bulge into the lumen of the tube and are often taller than the ciliated cells, giving rise to a markedly irregular epithelial border. Their microvilli are less evenly distributed over their surface than during the proliferative period. "Peg" cells are often noted which appear as slightly elongated secretory cells in which the nucleus has migrated to an

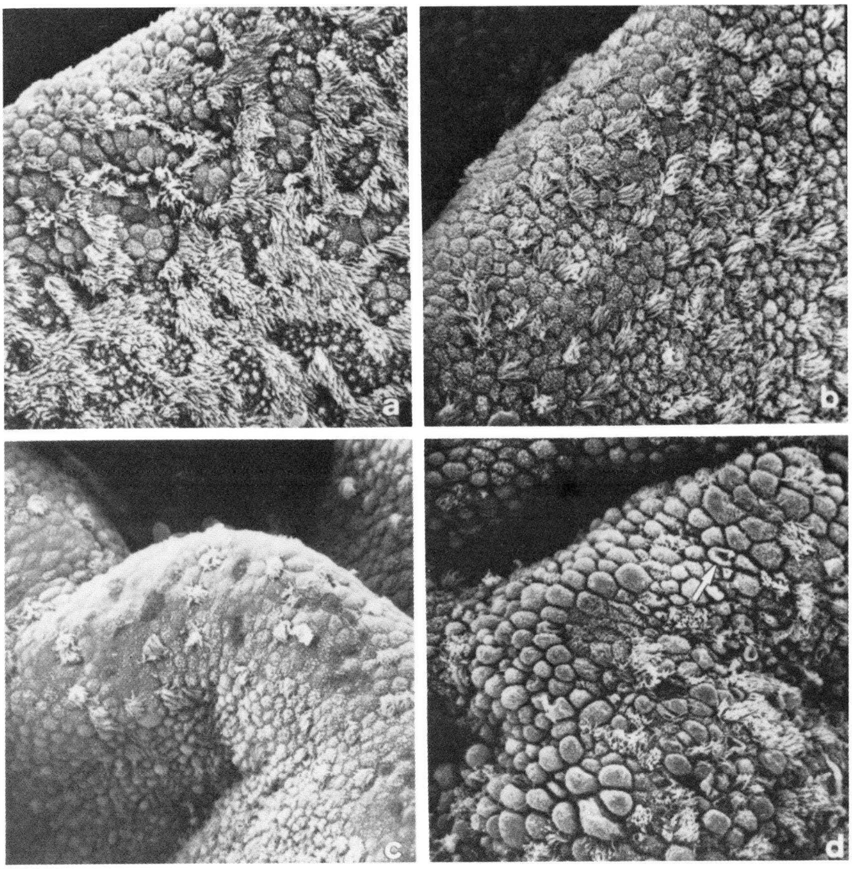

FIGURE 6:4—*Regional differences in tubal epithelium.* a. *Fimbriae. The majority of cells are ciliated, forming bunches arranged in tracts. The cellular boundaries of the ciliated cells cannot be identified despite their erected state, but presumably 4 to 6 cells are forming each group. The fields of nonciliated cells contain 6 to 10 cells along the declivity of the fold, but more along the crest. While groups of ciliated cells are connected to each other, nonciliated cell groups are divided by ciliated cell tracts.* b. *Ampulla. Fields of nonciliated cells are more extended and consist of more individual cells than at the fimbriae. These fields are composed of 10 to 20 single polyhedral cells. The ciliated cells in the ampulla are mostly solitary, but in places occur in pairs.* c. *Intermediary portion. The crest of the mucosal fold shown here exposes a remarkably denuded pattern that might be caused in part by deciliation. The nonciliated cells are flat and only a few intact ciliated cells are situated along the crest. In contrast, the declivity shows more ciliated cells interspersed among the fields of noncilated cells, each differentiated by the developed microvillous relief of its apical membrane.* d. *Isthmus. From a morphological point of view, the secretory activity of the nonciliated cells seems to be in an advanced state as compared to similar cells in the fimbriae or ampulla. Some of the cells look exhausted, possibly postsecretory. Ciliated cells are solitary or composed of small groups. These cells represent a striking minority within the pattern of the isthmic mucosal folds as compared to the fimbriae. (× 1,000; Ludwig and Metzer[6]).*

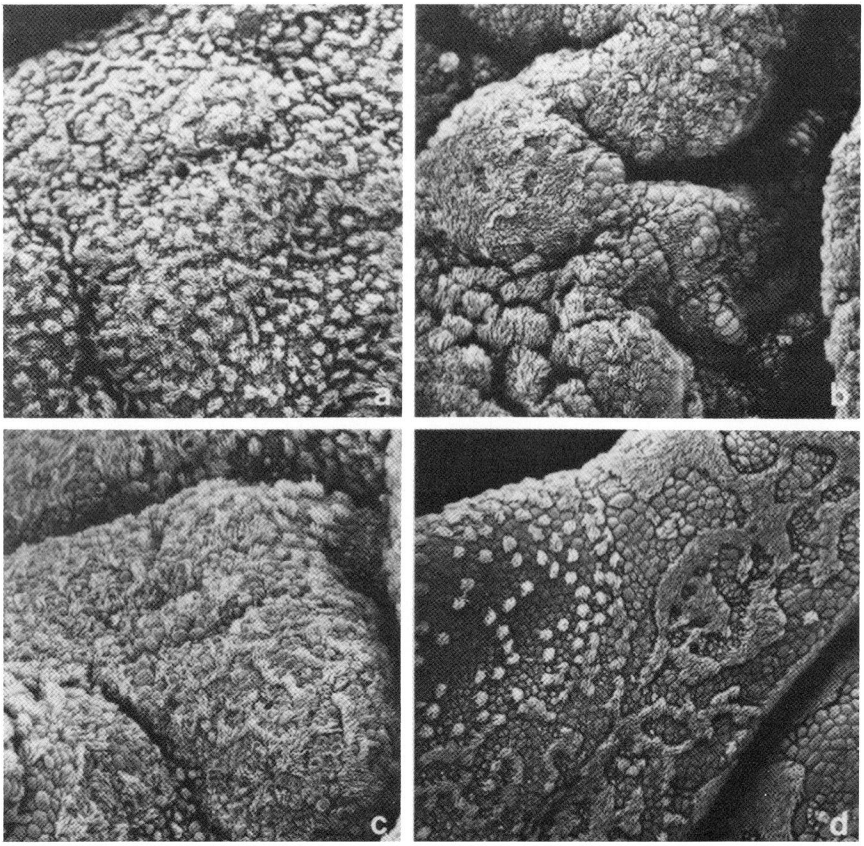

FIGURE 6:5—*Cyclic changes in ampullary epithelium.* a. *Postmenstrual. Ciliated and nonciliated cells are evenly distributed on the crest as well as on the declivity of the mucosal fold. The apices of the noncilated cells do not stick out between the ciliary bunches.* b. *Late proliferative phase. With the distention of the tops of nonciliated cells, the pattern has completely changed as compared to* a. *The original distribution of ciliated and nonciliated cells is maintained but groups of nonciliated cells bulge up to the level of the tips of the cilia.* c. *Midcycle (immediate postovulatory stage). The secretory nonciliated cells are distended, with a loss of microvilli and occasional apical membrane defects. The defects signify the release of secretory material which seems to culminate at the time of ovulation, with the secretory activity continuing up to the early luteal phase of the cycle.* d. *Premenstrual (late luteal phase). The tops of nonciliated cells have sunk to their previous level* (a)*. The tracts of ciliated cells are again the prominent structural sign together with separated bunches of those cells (× 500; Ludwig and Metzer[6]).*

apical position. They may represent exhausted secretory cells.

During *menstruation* the entire epithelium becomes much lower (10 to 15 microns), with both ciliated and nonciliated cells reduced in height. A few round secretory cells remain, however, appearing in clusters and bulging into the lumen as they did in the late secretory phase. Although the cilia are droopy, they are still present. There is no pronounced cyclic shedding of cilia in the oviduct, as is seen in the human endometrium or the infundibulum of the rhesus monkey's oviduct. The intercalary cell is most prominent during the premenstrual and menstrual period. Immediately after menstruation, secretory cells assume a narrow cylindri-

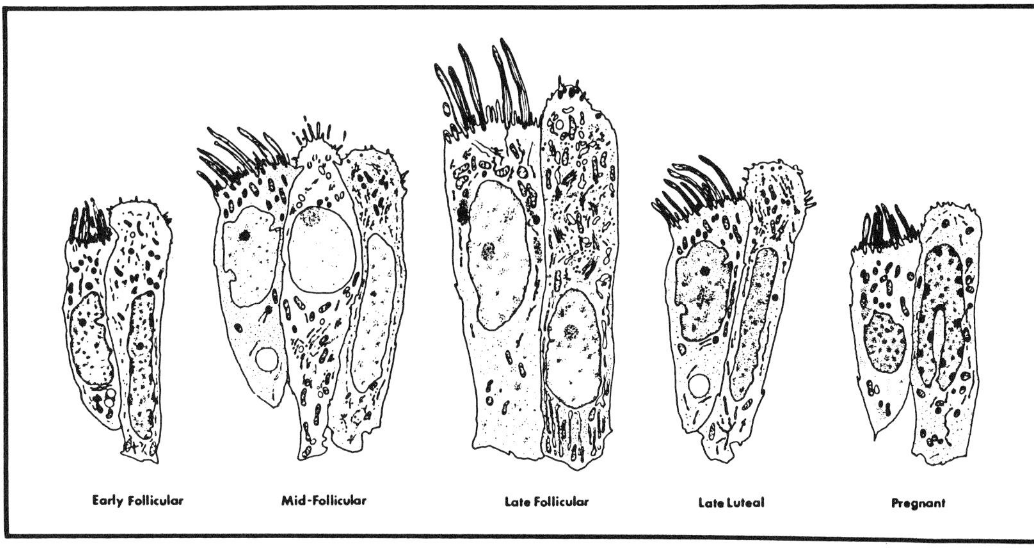

FIGURE 6:6—*Diagram illustrating the morphological appearance of the tubal epithelium at various stages of the menstrual cycle and after the first trimester of pregnancy. Hypertrophy and differentiation occur during the follicular phase and coincide with low serum levels of estradiol and essentially undetectable serum levels of progesterone. Atrophy and dedifferentiation begin during the luteal phase, continue into pregnancy, and coincide with elevated levels of serum progesterone. Ciliogenic cells are observed only during the midfollicular phase and a mature epithelium is present only at midcycle. Morphological alterations in the nuclei are as dramatic and characteristic as those that occur in the cytoplasm (Verhage et al.*[8]*).*

cal shape, so superficially they more closely resemble ciliated cells.

The secretory cells undergo definite ultrastructural changes during the ovarian cycle which seem to be associated with changing secretory activity.[7,8] Early in the proliferative phase, the secretory cells display a compact Golgi apparatus, a limited endoplasmic reticulum, and diminished mitochondria. Later, the mitochondria, endoplasmic reticulum, and Golgi apparatus become more prominent. On about day 10, Palade granules become numerous and the cells increase in height. At the end of this phase, the cell surface is domed and secretory granules appear beneath the cell membrane and near the lumen. During the luteal phase, the endoplasmic reticulum dilates and numerous secretory droplets and granules appear. The Golgi apparatus expands and the mitochondria decrease in number. In the midluteal phase, some secretory cells rupture and extrude their contents. Late in the cycle, liposomes appear in increased numbers.[7,8] Secretory function is more prominent in the isthmus than in the ampulla.

There is disagreement over the extent of change occurring in the ultrastructural morphology and distribution of the ciliated cells during the cycle. While the human tubal epithelium does not undergo cyclic ciliation-deciliation, some changes, such as increased size and number of cytoplasmic granules and mitrochondria, may occur as the cycle progresses. Some renewal of ciliated cells does occur, but there is little evidence for transformation of ciliated into secretory cells, or for cyclic desquamation of ciliated cells.[20] Verhage et al.[8] have reported that cyclic changes in ciliation were observed specifically in the human fimbria and ampulla during the menstrual cycle. In the fimbria, approximately 12 percent to 14 percent of the ciliated cells lost their cilia during the luteal phase and then regenerated them during the early follicular phase of the cycle. In women, as in several subhuman

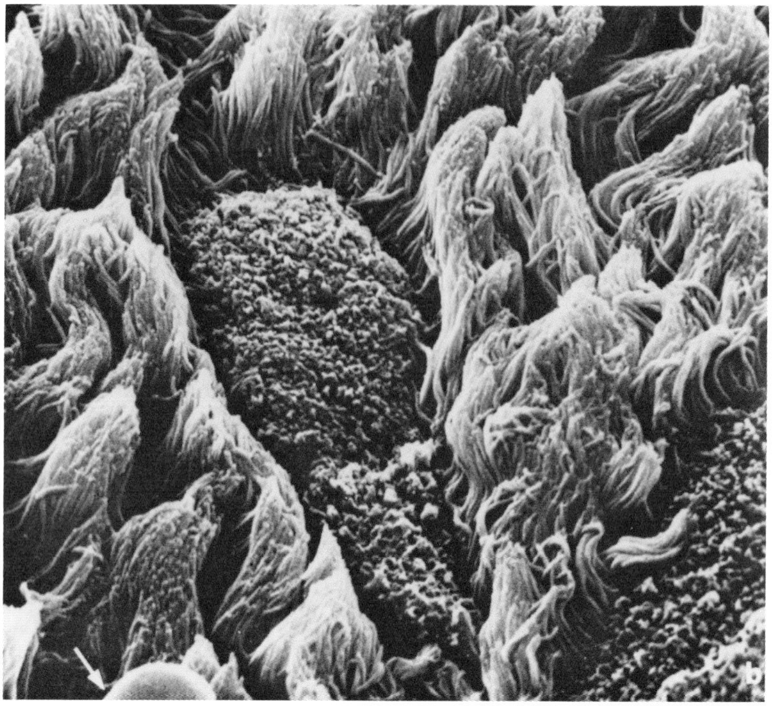

FIGURE 6:7A—*Late follicular phase tubal epithelium. Ciliated cells are tall and vigorous. The individual microvilli on the nonciliated cells are clearly visible; their shape is regular and they are evenly distributed over the cell surfaces. Several ciliated cells surround a few nonciliated cells without very clear cell borders.*

primates, progesterone may cause deciliation while estrogen supports ciliation of the epithelial cells. However, the extent to which the process occurs is much smaller in women than in other primates.

Pregnancy

In pregnancy the types of changes that occur at menstruation continue.[1–10] The epithelium remains low, the cilia droop, and the secretory cells are rounded and bulge into the tubal lumen. There is some evidence of extrusion of nuclei by nonciliated cells. Lipid droplets appear in ciliated cells, and secretory cells display further enlargement of the endoplasmic reticulum. Patek[21] reported no degeneration or decreased numbers of ciliated cells in late pregnancy or puerperium as have Seki[22] and Verhage.[8]

By two weeks after delivery, however, the epithelium resembles that of the late postmenopause with a lower epithelium and fewer and smaller ciliated cells. Exogenous estrogen antagonizes the puerperal changes, and within 48 hours induces proliferation of both ciliated and secretory cells. Progesterone alone does not change the normal puerperal histology, but when given in combination with estrogen, progesterone inhibits estrogen-induced growth.[21]

Menopause

The endocrine changes associated with the female climacteric are caused mainly by the loss of the cyclic secretion of 17-β estradiol. Cessation of 17-β estradiol secretion is attributed to a loss of follicular granulosal cells and to a decrease in their responsiveness to FSH.[23] The fallopian tubes contain estrogen re-

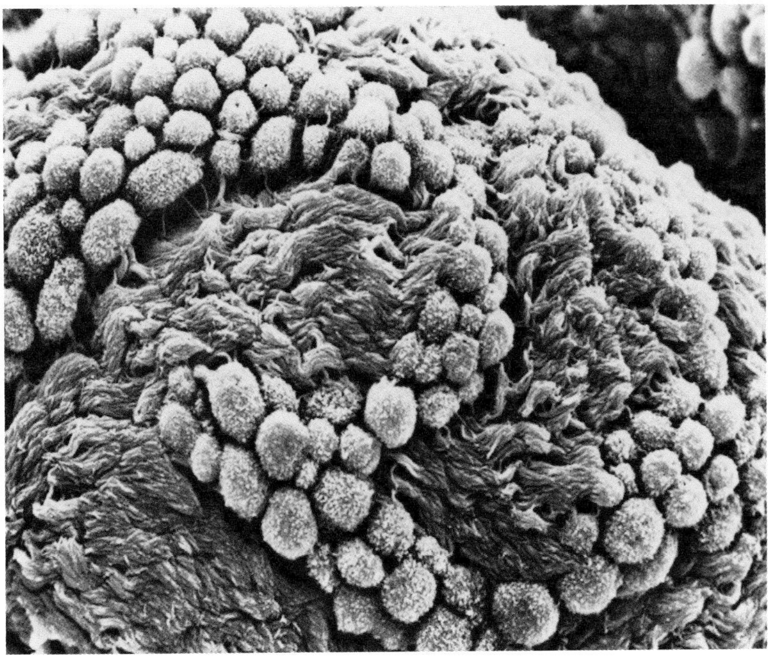

FIGURE 6:7B—*Luteal phase tubal epithelium. The epithelium is low. The secretory cells in the distal part of the tube have a rounded appearance and bulge into the lumen. The ciliae are often, but not always, drooping. The microvilli are shorter than before and are often irregularly scattered over the cell surfaces (Vasquez et al.*[31]*).*

ceptors and the postmenopausal changes parallel those in the uterus with epithelial and muscular atrophy (Fig. 6:8). The tube becomes shortened, the diameter decreases, and the mucosal folds become flattened or absent. Considerable disagreement exists, however, over the rate and extent of epithelial atrophy.[23–28]

Some reports have noted an early atrophy that affects both the ciliated and nonciliated cells, but others have noted little or no atrophic change until age 60.[6,28] Significant secretory function apparently ceases after the menopause but ciliated cells persist until the late postmenopause, when deciliation may become more evident, particularly on the fimbria. A study with the scanning electron microscope revealed no significant deciliation in tubes from women as much as 15 years postmenopausal.[28] It is possible that sufficient estrogen production to maintain the ciliated cells occurs in many postmenopausal women, although the nonciliated cells become inactive. Menopausal deciliation may be preventable or reversible with estrogen therapy.[27]

Secretory cells are generally very flat and atrophic. The microvilli are small and inactive with no signs of secretory activity. Peg cells, usually present in the tube, are significantly decreased.

Inflammation

Tubal damage accounts for at least 30 percent of female infertility, and most of this is a consequence of salpingitis.[29] Salpingitis results in varying degrees of mucosal damage, particularly in the fimbria.[30–33] The fimbriated folds may be agglutinated, show partial adhesions, or may be completely hidden by adhesions. Fimbrioplasty usually reveals a basically normal infundibulum, however, with its concentric folds leading to the ostium. The folds are densely ciliated, with more than

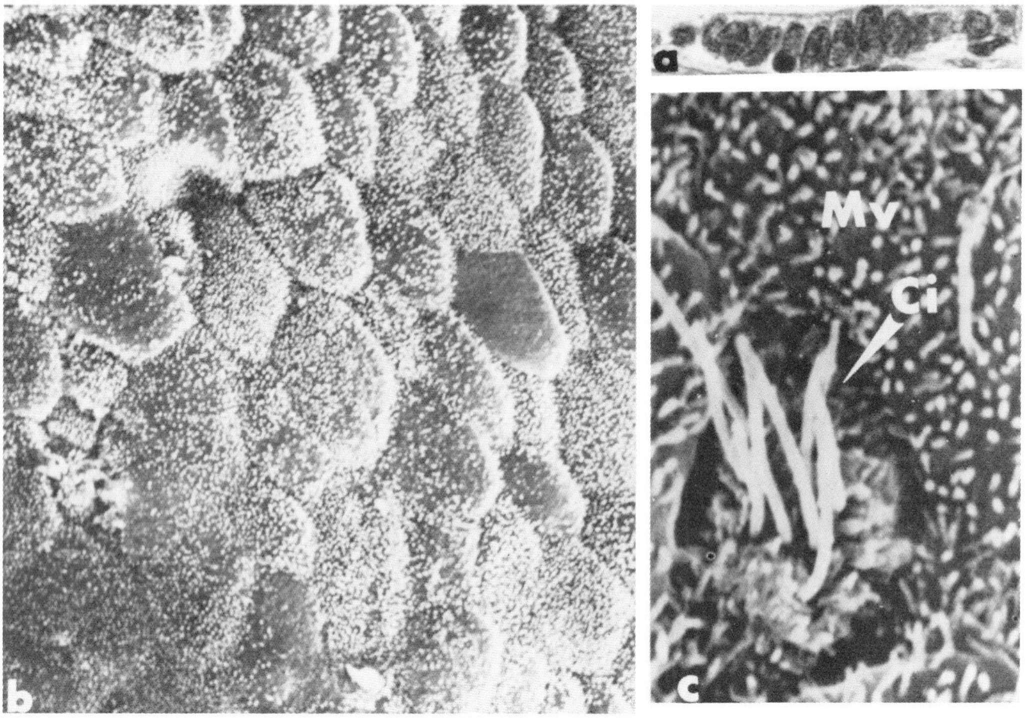

FIGURE 6:8—*Fallopian tube in menopause.* a. *Fimbria. In advanced menopause, epithelial atrophy is manifested by the presence of low columnar to low cuboidal epithelium, exhibiting a significant decrease in the cytoplasmic volume. Ciliated cells are absent (H&E stain; original magnification,* ×*120).* b. *Fimbria. With the scanning electron microscope, the surface of atrophic tubal epithelium has a monotonous cobblestone appearance because of the presence of flat-surfaced cells covered by short and sparse microvilli. Apocrine secretory activity is uniformly absent. (Original magnification* ×*1,600)* c. *Ampulla in advanced menopause. Scanning electron micrograph of a poorly developed ciliated cell (Ci) with few and short ciliary shafts. The surrounding cells have short and sparse microvillous (Mv) processes (original magnification,* × *8,000; Ferenczy and Richart[4]).*

50 percent of the surface being ciliated. The individual ciliated cells have long numerous cilia, and nonciliated cells have a rounded microvillous surface, not different from the normal. Occasional cells with long microvilli are found on biopsies taken during the follicular phase of the menstrual cycle. In a few biopsies, localized cell hyperplasia in the form of finger-like projections arising from the folds has been noted. When salpingitis gives rise to hydrosalpinx, mucosal changes become more evident.[32–33] The tubes show severe attenuation, discontinuity, or total absence of the ampullary folds. The mucosal surface is frequently interrupted by areas where epithelial cells are missing, corresponding to the desquamation of individual cells or larger areas of the mucosal surface. The epithelium shows a decreased population of ciliated cells with additional loss of ciliae from individual cells. Cells with a single cilium are common. It should be noted that other investigators have found relatively little change in the degree of ciliation in hydrosalpingitis.[34,35] Nonciliated cells vary greatly: they can be circular, polygonal, or extremely stretched, including giant forms with unclear cell boundaries. Fine microvilli cover most of the nonciliated cell surfaces, but areas with cells devoid of

microvilli or with decreased density of microvilli are frequent.

The use of microsurgical techniques has resulted in the restoration of tubal patency in more than 80 percent of such patients, but normal conception is still infrequent.[36] The ciliated epithelium is important for normal tubal physiology and it is possible that tubal surgery fails to result in more pregnancies because of irreversible damage to the tubal lining.[33]

Tubal Sterilization

Although histologic findings vary with the type of tubal sterilization, significant changes are noted in the mucosa of the proximal tubal segment in the majority of previously sterilized women.[31,37–39] Luminal dilation, flattening of the folds, deciliation, polyps, increased mitotic activity, epithelial inclusions, and focal endometriosis have all been reported with varying frequencies. Considerable controversy remains over the origins of these abnormalities. Tubal polyps, for example, may represent remnants of normal mucosa on atrophic folds, foci of acquired endometriosis, or a "reactive" process of the epithelium. The extent of these changes seems to be correlated with the degree of tissue destruction produced at ligation, and may have a prognostic value for the likelihood of successful reversal.

Ectopic Pregnancy

The cause of ectopic pregnancy remains obscure despite much investigation. Although fallopian tubes containing gestations often appear normal on macroscopic and routine histologic examination, abnormalities of the epithelium have been described.[40–46] While Samberg[46] found no change in the epithelial pattern and the same distribution of ciliated and nonciliated cells outside of the actual site of nidation, Vasquez[43] and Peretz et al.[45] have found a consistent pattern of tubal deciliation in a large series of biopsies. In patients with ectopic pregnancies or a history of ectopic pregnancy, the degree of deciliation was more than that seen in normal pregnant women at an equivalent gestational age. There were fewest ciliated cells when the pregnancy was implanted at the fimbriae or ampulla. Deciliation was less pronounced when implantation was at the ampullary-isthmic junction. The degree of deciliation was uniform, however, within the same tubal segment. It was noted also that some ciliated cells had fewer cilia per cell than normal. Nonciliated cells were hexagonal or rounded. Occasionally, these cells appeared to be very distended and the apical margin was frequently at a level with the tips of the cilia of adjacent ciliated cells. Microvilli were generally fine and numerous, and only occasionally scarce or absent. Groups of cells with larger, flatter surfaces, which resembled the squamoid transformation of the endometrium in pregnancy, were also common. Hexagonal spaces between cells were seen in all biopsies, generally close to the apices of mucosal folds. The cells may represent areas from which epithelial cells have been desquamated. Light microscopy showed that the epithelium was below normal height and often pseudostratified, and confirmed the relative frequency of distended secretory cells. Cell counts on light microscopy confirmed the decrease in ciliated cells.

The authors speculate that loss of ciliated cells from the ampulla may decrease the efficiency of ovum transport, leading to a delay in the ovum's entering the isthmus and subsequently the uterine cavity.[43,45] This delay could result in tubal implantation and explain why the mid-ampulla is probably the most common site for an ectopic pregnancy.[7,47] Deciliation[43] may also explain the increased incidence of ectopic pregnancy after tuboplasty despite tubal patency in most patients.

In addition to the abnormalities mentioned above, a variety of other pathological conditions may affect the tubal epithelium, including:

— metaplasias and neoplasms, recently classified and reviewed by Lauchian[48]
— deciliation and morphological changes in both ciliated and secretory cells associated with copper IUDs (see Chapter 21)
— ciliostatic effects and morphological changes associated with *N. gonorrhoeae*, *Mycoplasma hominis*, and other microorganisms.[49,50]

Conclusions

Important insights into the functional significance of the tubal epithelium are suggested by the morphological changes that occur in this system, both in association with the normal menstrual cycle and in association with various abnormalities.

Ciliary activity is responsible for the movement of ova into the fimbrial ostium and through the ampulla, as well as distribution of a tubal fluid rich in the mucoproteins, electrolytes, and enzymes that support gamete maturation and fertilization and facilitate gamete and embryo transport. Appropriately, ciliary activity is maximal at ovulation. Significant decreases occur in the atrophic postmenopausal tube, which suggests the endocrine dependence of ciliogenesis. The importance of ciliary activity is affirmed by the tubal dysfunction seen in association with the deciliation of tubal ligation, salpingitis, ectopic pregnancy, and IUDs. Questions are raised, however, by reports of normal fertility in women suffering from the immotile cilia syndrome (Kartagener's syndrome). This syndrome is characterized by a congenital defect in the dynein arms of the cilia,[51] and has been demonstrated in the tubal ciliated cells of fertile women.[52]

Secretory activity is also of fundamental importance in providing a supportive and nutritive environment for the spermatozoa, ovum, and embryo, as well as facilitating fertilization and transport. The secretory elements are also modified during the menstrual cycle. Early, the secretory cells are low and relatively inactive. As ovulation approaches, under the influence of estrogen, secretory cells become tall and columnar, and project beyond the ciliated cells, discharging secretions into the tubal lumen. The production of fluid within the fallopian tube seems greatest immediately before ovulation and may facilitate the overall transfer and sustenance of gametes.

References

1. Nilsson O, and Reinius S: Light and electron microscopic structure of the oviduct. In Hafez ESE, and Blandau RJ (Eds): *The Mammalian Oviduct*. Chicago: University of Chicago Press, 1969: 57.
2. Patek E: The epithelium of the human fallopian tube. A surface ultrastructural and cytochemical study. *Acta Obstet Gynecol Scand*, 53(Suppl. 31):1, 1974.
3. Pauerstein CJ, Hodgson BJ, and Kramen MA: The anatomy and physiology of the oviduct. *Obstet Gynecol Ann*, 3:137, 1974.
4. Ferenczy A, and Richart RM: Fallopian tube (oviduct). In Ferenczy A, and Richart RM (Eds): *Female Reproductive System: Dynamics of Scan and Transmission Electron Microscopy*. New York: John Wiley, 1974:213.
5. Patek E, and Nilsson L: The oviduct (man). In Hafez ESE (Ed): *Scanning Electron Microscopic Atlas of Mammalian Reproduction*. Tokoyo: Igaku Shoin Ltd., 1975: 156.
6. Ludwig H, and Metzer H: *The Human Female Reproductive Tract. A Scanning Electron Microscopic Atlas*. Heidelberg: Springer-Verlag, 1976: 80.
7. Pauerstein CJ, and Eddy CA: Morphology of the fallopian tube. In Beller FK, and Schumaker GFB (Eds): *The Biology of the Fluids of the Female Genital Tract*. Amsterdam: Elsevier/North Holland, 1979: 299.
8. Verhage HG, Bareither ML, Jaffe RC, et al: Cyclic changes in ciliation, secretion, and cell height of the oviductal epithelium in women. *Am J Anat*, 156:505, 1979.
9. Bonilla-Musoles F, Ferrer-Barriendos J, and Pellicer A: Cyclical changes in the epithelium of the fallopian tube. Studies with scanning electron micros-

copy (SEM). *Clin Exp Obstet Gynecol*, 10:79, 1983.

10. Martinek J: Cytological changes in human oviduct epithelium during the menstrual cycle. *Folia Morphol* (Praha), 32:398, 1984.
11. Pauerstein CJ, and Woodruff JD: The role of the "indifferent" cell of the tubal epithelium. *Am J Obstet Gynecol*, 98:121, 1967.
12. Odor DL: The question of "basal cells" in oviductal and endocervical epithelium. *Fertil Steril*, 25:1047, 1974.
13. Schulte BA, Rao KPP, Kreutner A, et al: Histochemical examination of glycoconjugate of epithelial cells in the human fallopian tube. *Lab Invest*, 52:207, 1985.
14. Clyman MJ: Electron microscopy of the human fallopian tube. *Fertil Steril*, 17:81, 1969.
15. Brenner RM: The biology of oviductal cilia. In Hafez ESE, and Blandau RJ (Eds): *The Mammalian Oviduct*. Chicago: University of Chicago Press, 1969: 203.
16. Van Bogaert LJ, Maldague P, and Staquet JP: The percentage of granulocyte-like cells in human oviduct epithelium. *Br J Obstet Gynaecol*, 85:373, 1978.
17. Ferenczy A, Richart RM, Agate FJ, et al: Scanning electron microscopy of the human fallopian tube. *Science*, 175:783, 1972.
18. Patek E, Nilsson L, and Johannisson E: Scanning electron microscopy of the human fallopian tube: Report I. The proliferative and secretory stages. *Fertil Steril*, 23:459, 1972.
19. Critoph FM, and Dennis KJ: The cellular composition of the human oviduct epithelium. *Br J Obstet Gynaecol*, 84:219, 1977.
20. Patek E, and Nilsson L: Scanning electron microscopic observations on the ciliogenesis of the infundibulum of the human fetal and adult fallopian tube epithelium. *Fertil Steril*, 24:819,1973.
21. Patek E, Nilsson L, and Hellema M: Scanning electron microscopic study of the human fallopian tube: Report IV. At term gestation and in the puerperium. The effect of a synthetic progestin on the postmenopausal tube. *Fertil Steril*, 24:832, 1973.
22. Seki K, Rawson J, Eddy CA, et al: Deciliation in the puerperal fallopian tube. *Fertil Steril*, 29:75, 1978.
23. Edman CD: The climacteric. In Buchsbaum HJ (Ed): *The Menopause*. New York: Springer-Verlag, 1983: 23.
24. Gaddum-Rosse P, Rumery RE, Blandau RJ, et al: Studies on the mucosa of postmenopausal oviducts: Surface appearance, ciliary activity, and the effect of estrogen treatment. *Fertil Steril*, 26:951, 1975.
25. Soriero AA: The aging uterus and fallopian tubes. In Schneider, EL (Ed): *The Aging Reproductive System*. New York: Raven Press, 1978: 85.
26. Voet RL: End organ response to estrogen deprivation. In Buchsbaum HJ (Ed): *The Menopause*. New York: Springer-Verlag, 1983: 9.
27. Donnez J, Casanas-Roux F, Ferin J, et al: Changes in ciliation and cell height in human tubal epithelium in the fertile and post-fertile years. *Maturitas*, 5:39, 1983.
28. Patek E, Nilsson L, and Johannisson E: Scanning electron microscopic study of the human fallopian tube: Report II. Fetal life, reproductive life, and postmenopause. *Fertil Steril*, 23:719, 1972.
29. Case AL, and Zuspan FP: Infertility. *Surg Clin North Am*, 49:121, 1969.
30. Brosens IA, and Vasquez G: Fimbrial microbiopsy. *J Reprod Med*, 16:171, 1976.
31. Vasquez G, Brosens IA, Gordts S, et al: The fallopian tube in infertility. In Hafez ESE, and Kenemans P (Eds): *Atlas of Human Reproduction by Scanning Electron Microscopy*. Boston: MTP Press Limited, 1982: 119.
32. Vasquez G, Winston RML, Boeckx W, et al: The epithelium of human hydrosalpinges: A light optical and scanning electron microscopic study. *Br J Obstet Gynaecol*, 90:764, 1983.
33. Donnez J, Casanas-Roux F, Ferin J, et al: Fimbrial ciliated cells percentage and epithelial height during and after salpingitis. *Eur J Obstet Gynecol Reprod Biol*, 17:293, 1984.
34. Patek E, and Nilsson L: Hydrosalpinx simplex as seen by the scanning electron microscope. *Fertil Steril*, 28:962, 1977.
35. Fedele L, Zamberletti D, Marchini M, et al: Degree of endosalpingeal deciliation (by S.E.M.) in hydrosalpinx is not prognostic for postsurgical fertility. *Acta Eur Fertil*, 15:199, 1984.

36. Winston RML: Microsurgery of the fallopian tube: From fantasy to reality. *Fertil Steril*, 34:521, 1980.
37. Donnez J, Casanas-Roux F, and Ferin J: Macroscopic and microscopic studies of fallopian tube after laparoscopic sterilization. *Contraception*, 20:497, 1979.
38. Vasquez G, Winston RML, Boeckx W, et al: Tubal lesions subsequent to sterilization and their relation to fertility after attempts at reversal. *Am J Obstet Gynecol*, 138:86, 1980.
39. Donnez J, Casanas-Roux F, Ferin J, et al: Tubal polyps, epithelial inclusions, and endometriosis after tubal sterilization. *Fertil Steril*, 41:564, 1984.
40. Bronson RD: Tubal pregnancy and infertility. *Fertil Steril*, 28:221, 1977.
41. Brenner PF, Roy S, and Mishell DR Jr: Ectopic pregnancy: A study of 300 surgically treated cases. *JAMA*, 243:673, 1980.
42. Budowick M, Johnson TRB, Genadry R, et al: The histopathology of the developing tubal ectopic pregnancy. *Fertil Steril*, 34:169, 1980.
43. Vasquez G, Winston RML, and Brosens IA: Tubal mucosa and ectopic pregnancy. *Br J Obstet Gynaecol*, 90:468, 1983.
44. Zamberletti D, Fedele L, Vercellini P, et al: The significance of scanning electron microscopy findings from the endosalpinx in tubal pregnancies. *Acta Eur Fertil*, 14:57, 1983.
45. Peretz BA, Lindenbaum ES, and Beach D: Ectopic pregnancy effects on the ipsilateral fallopian tube epithelium—An ultrastructural study. *Eur J Obstet Gynecol Reprod Biol*, 17:19, 1984.
46. Samberg I, Degani S, Zilberman A, et al: Scanning electron microscopy of human fallopian tube in ectopic pregnancy. *Gynecol Obstet Invest*, 16:65, 1983.
47. Pauerstein CJ: *The Fallopian Tube: A Reappraisal*. Philadelphia: Lea and Febiger, 1974: 92.
48. Lauchlan SC: Metaplasias and neoplasias of müllerian epithelium. *Histopathology*, 8:543, 1984.
49. Mardh PA, Baldetrop B, Hakansson CH, et al: Studies on ciliated epithelia of the human genital tract. III. Mucociliary wave activity in organ cultures of human fallopian tubes challenged with *Neisseria gonorrhoeae* and gonococcal endotoxin. *Br J Ven Dis*, 55:256, 1979.
50. Baldetrop B, Mardh PA, and Westrom L: Studies on ciliated epithelia of the human genital tract. IC mucociliary wave activity in organ cultures of human fallopian tubes challenged with *Mycoplasma hominis*. *Sex Trans Dis*, 11:363, 1983.
51. Afzelius BA, Camner P, and Mossberg B: On the function of cilia in the female reproductive tract. *Fertil Steril*, 29:72, 1978.
52. Jean Y, Langlais J, Roberts KD, et al: Fertility of a woman with nonfunctional ciliated cells in fallopian tubes. *Fertil Steril*, 31:349, 1979.

7

Tubal Myoelectrical Activity

Sneh Anand

Background

Electrical activity in smooth muscles of the uterus and ureter was demonstrated in 1910 by Fuchs.[1] Since definite correlations with mechanical contraction patterns could not be identified, electrical activity has been considered an incidental phenomenon.

This field of investigation developed very slowly. Brundin[2] mentioned electrical action in the fallopian tube but only the propagated signals from the adrenergic nerves were considered. Intrinsic potential generation in tubal cells independent of neurological stimuli was shown to exist by Zastowt[3] but the magnitude of resting and action potentials measured in the fallopian tube was far below those found in smooth muscles located elsewhere in the body. Many different animal species have been studied.[4–11]

Considerable variations in the recorded amplitude seem to arise with differing amounts of excision of the mesosalpinx surrounding the fallopian tube. The techniques and interpretation of results from the different methods require an understanding of the tissue-electrode interface problem. Following these clarifications, definite patterns in the electrical activity have been identified in coordination with other physiological phenomena. Research was not confined to monitoring of the electrical signals. Origin and control of signals were ascertained by using improved biomedical monitoring techniques.

Techniques of Measurement

In-vitro and in-vivo measurements have advantages and disadvantages. In-vitro methods have been used in several studies.[6,8,10,12,13] It is easier to position measuring electrodes at multiple points in vitro, as compared to in vivo, and environmental conditions can also be controlled. Nevertheless, several limitations arise. Although a well-oxygenated buffer solution maintained at body temperature is used for perfusion, the oxygen does not permeate to the deeper regions of the tissue.[14] Whether this lacuna alters the activity is not known. Further, the mechanical tethering of the tube is quite unlike that in vivo. There may be some excitation contraction coupling phenomenon in operation. The difference in the tether-

The Fallopian Tube: Basic Studies and Clinical Contributions, edited by Alvin M. Siegler, M.D. Mount Kisco, New York: Futura Publishing Company, Inc. © 1986.

ing leads to changes in the contraction patterns and as a consequence it also alters the electrical signals measured.

In-vivo preparations maintain the tube in a more normal physiological state. The tubal adventitia may affect the measured signals. Differences in the data can occur because of the nature of the experimental setup and the type of preparation.[3,15]

The simplest method for monitoring electrical activity involves two Ag/AgCl wire electrodes placed about 1 to 2 mm apart in contact with the tubal serosa.[16] These electrodes are connected to the active terminals of a high input impedance electronic differential amplifier; the common terminal of the amplifier is connected to an indifferent electrode placed at some other body site. With this configuration, the integrated activity of the cells is measured extracellularly. To achieve stable electrode polarization, conventional platinum/platinum black, silver/silver chloride, or platinum/platinum irridium electrodes have been used. Although stable, the magnitude of polarization potential is comparable to the phasic signal picked up. When the tube contracts, the electrode-tissue interface shift changes the charged bilayers, thus modifying the output. Such movement artifacts in the myoelectric activity are eliminated by signal processing.[8,12,17,18]

The standard double sucrose cup method has been used to record electrical activity from the fallopian tube with minimal polarization potential artifact. Sucrose cups with diameters of 0.2 to 0.5 mm were used in pairs separated by a distance of 1.5 mm. They were placed on the tubal serosa.[19] The information obtained pertains to the bulk of tissue in-between the cups.

Microelectrode techniques are suitable to obtain data from more localized zones. Microelectrodes varying from 50 to 80 microns in diameter are inserted into the tubal wall. Although the recording is still of the extracellular region, signals from different layers can be selectively monitored. Glass microelectrodes have been used to record the intracellular muscular layers of the guinea pig's fallopian tube.[18]

Suction cups are used to minimize motion artifact. A polymeric tubing incorporating the electrode wire is connected to a vacuum source. When the tubing is placed in contact with tissue, a small portion of tissue is sucked into the tube coming in firm contact with the metal electrode. The electrode also penetrates the tissue. With this method, fixation is of high quality and artifacts arising from movements are minimized.[20] On the other hand, the tissue is traumatized and some trauma potentials become superimposed on the tubal potential. Proper impalement helps to enhance the signal by increasing the extracellular shunt path resistance. Intracellular recordings have been attempted[3] but the results are imprecise.[15]

Microelectrodes measuring 50 microns in diameter have been inserted into the muscle cells and transmembrane potentials obtained. Even for as long as 15 minutes to one hour, the phasic potential does not stabilize.[9,13] Since observations beyond such a long period following cell membrane impalement are not very reliable, intracellular recordings have not as yet produced useful results.

Recently, Parkington[18] has attempted to pick up the transmembrane potentials in smooth muscles of guinea pig fallopian tube, using glass microelectrodes. Potentials were measured after 30 minutes of impalement. The magnitude of action potential was 40 to 80 mV and of 25 ms duration. The electrode impedance was of the order of 100 mV. Signals were fed into a high input impedance preamplifier and displayed on a dual-channel oscilloscope. Parkington reported a significant difference between the activity of cells in the longitudinal layer and that of cells in the circular layer. Reproducible reliable techniques to measure intracellular activity are needed and improvements in existing methods are evolving slowly.

Origin and Spread of Activity

The tubal myosalpinx has some unitary smooth-muscle characteristics and the electrical activity has many features in common with the smooth muscle of other organs (e.g., the intestines and the uterus). There are some specific differences. Cells in all parts of the fallopian tube have the intrinsic capability of autorhythmic potential generation. Intracellular electrode experimental data[3,13,16,18] revealed a slow localized depolarization of the cell membrane culminating in the reproduction of an action potential. At times, slow sinusoidal oscillations in the membrane potentials superimpose on the action potential.[16,19] When a series of surface electrodes is placed along the tube, electrical activity commences at one particular site.[15] Thereafter the electrical activity travels in both the abovarian and adovarian directions, as evidenced by the sequential time lag in the oscillations picked up by the electrodes at distances away from the site of initial signal generation.[8,20] As yet it has not been possible to ascertain the factors responsible for initiation of electrical waves at a particular site. At various times, commencement of the waves occurs at different locations. Functionally, these locations are termed as "pacemaker" in analogy with the cardiac pacemaker. In the fallopian tube, no characteristics of a pacemaker site can be identified morphologically although almost all sites can assume pacemaker functions.[7]

The extent of the ampullary-isthmic junction (AIJ) dominance varies during the course of the estrual or menstrual cycle.[4,7] The pattern of the pacemaker potential of the AIJ is the same as the pacemaker potential produced at other sites.[13] Talo and Brundin[7] removed the AIJ over a length of 10 mm from the rabbit's fallopian tube and showed that pacemaker functions shifted to the isthmus. The ampulla was rarely a site of such activity.

Character of the Electrical Potentials

Pacemaker potentials of varied patterns have been observed. One of them comprises a sharp positive deflection of amplitude, about 0.5 mV, followed by a number of rapid oscillations of such magnitude that the wave does not cross the baseline during the oscillations. Thereafter, the wave returns to the baseline. Oscillatory bursts varied from 0.7 to 1.5 seconds.[7] From the pacemaker site, the electrical signal propagated in the abovarian and adovarian directions at rates ranging from 2 to 17 mm/sec. Spread in the two directions was not symmetrical. Generally, the adovarian spread occurred more frequently, and often the abovarian spread either was not manifested or died out over a short distance.[12]

Besides the pattern described above, several other forms were noted. There was a burst of spikes more or less symmetrical about the baseline. Even during a particular experiment, considerable variability was seen. The number of spikes in a burst differed from time to time and spike amplitudes also differed (50 μV to 1 mV). Tomita and Watanabe[19] saw remarkably different patterns comprising slow waves that were almost sinusoidal in nature. These waves are very much akin to intestinal potential waves. Parkington[18] reported that transmembrane potential in longitudinal muscles rises steeply at a slope of 0.5 to 1 mV/sec to a magnitude of 40 to 80 mV, whereas the rise is extremely slow in circular muscle cells (0.01 to 0.1 mV/sec). Amplitudes for both layers were of a similar magnitude. The patterns of activity differed in the ampullary and isthmic cells in the same animal.

Changes commonly occurred during extended monitoring, with periods of intense activity alternating with relatively quiescent states. At one time at the AIJ of the mouse, the repetition rate of the bursts was 22 per minute and at other times they occurred at 15-second intervals.[21] Sometimes the entire tube became quiescent; occasionally, reduced activity at one site was associated with increased activity in another location.

Clearly, a spectrum of responses exists. Physiological variability monitoring techniques and equipment affect the patterns. For example, the return to and shift from the baseline is controlled by the time constant of the recorder as well as by the physiological event itself.

It is surprising that a wide spectrum of animal species has quite similar electrical responses. Table 7:1 summarizes the electrical characteristics in different animals. The similarity strongly suggests a functional association between the electrical activity and reproductive processes.

Myoelectric Signal Variations as Related to Reproductive Cycles

Polarization and depolarization of cells are membrane functions. Membrane properties are affected by hormonal status or by an excitation-energy coupling effect. Neurogenic stimulation by the autonomic nervous system also modifies the cell membrane characteristics and therefore the polarization-depolarization process. Besides the hormonal levels and neural excitation, other changes during the estrual and menstrual cycles, and factors such as environmental stress and smoking, affect the membrane function. Consequently, the electrical activity of the cells of the fallopian tube and the tube as a whole show a cyclicity in phase with the reproductive cycle.

Investigations in humans[6] and cows[22] showed that before ovulation (in the proliferative phase) the tube was quiescent. Electrical pulse bursts occurred, but after prolonged intervals. In the length of the tube, the sites of activity were few. Some diminution in the amplitude of the electrical signal has been reported but this feature was not a consistent finding.[4,5,8] The individual wave pattern remained the same during other times of the cycle.

Following ovulation a series of pattern alterations was noted. Talo[21] recorded the electrical activity at six different points in the rat's fallopian tube and at the same time observed the location of eggs. Elec-

Table 7:1

Characteristics of Electrical Activity in Various Species

Species	*Preparation*	*Pattern of spikes*	*Amplitude* (μV)	*Repetition rate/min.*	*Velocity of spread (mm/sec)*	*Reference*
Rat	in vitro	single & double	100	4–22	—	Talo[21]
Guinea pig	in vitro	single	40–80 action potential intracellular	9–18	—	Parkington[18]
Rabbit	in vitro	multiple, bursts	100–200	—	—	Ruckebusch[4]
Cow	in vivo	multiple	700	5–30	—	Ruckebusch, Bayard[22]
Ewe	in vivo	multiple	50	0.33–1	—	Ruckebusch, Bueno[25]
Sheep	in vivo	single	125–600	—	—	Larks et al.[5]
Baboon	in vitro	single	50	—	2–5	Johns, Coons[8]
Human	in vitro	single or multiple	200	2–4	1–3	Talo, Pulkkinen[23]
Human	in vitro	single or multiple	200	3	2–9	Daniel et al.[6]

trical activity began while the eggs were in the ampulla and the preferred site of commencement was over the eggs. Spread was in both directions but did not go beyond 0.5 to 1 mm in the ovarian direction; it was limited to the AIJ in the other direction. When the eggs were in the isthmic zone, there was considerable signal generation in the isthmus but the ampullary frequency remained high. The eggs moved just ahead of plateau waves.

In the rabbit the situation was different. The extent of apparent "randomness" was far greater than in a large number of points.[21] Ruckebusch and Bayard[22] observed in the cow that 48 hours before the onset of estrus the localized nonpropagating electrical waves switched to propagating forms. This transition coincided with the rapid decline in progesterone.

Human tubal functions during the menstrual cycle and various physiological states were assessed in vitro.[6,11,22,24] Initiation of mechanical and electrical activity began spontaneously in several cases while in others, a stretching force of 2 to 3 g had to be applied. No electrical activity prior to the onset of mechanical contractions was observed. Origin of electrical activity varied and originated at either the ampullary or the isthmic end. No consistent relationship between the hormonal status of the donor with the character of the electrical signal could be seen. In the mouse, there seems to be an independence in the activity of the ampulla from the isthmus. Results with the human fallopian tube did suggest such dissociation. In tubal pregnancy, the spread was toward the conceptus from both sides and the potentials had spikes with slow waves.[11]

Response to exogenous agents was variable. Ovulation induced by HCG altered the reaction of the fallopian tube to cigarette smoking. Prior to HCG administration only the muscle layers of the isthmus were activated on smoking. Following HCG-induced ovulation, the effect of cigarette smoking was more generalized and signal generation increased in the ampulla and isthmus. The tubal behavior toward sympathomimetic stimulation was different. Five micrograms of adrenaline or 10 μg of noradrenaline caused an increase in the electrical activity over the entire tube. This increase remained effective even if the hormonal state of the tube was changed by induction of ovulation by HCG or injection of 40 μg of estradiol benzoate. However, oxytocin caused a significant increase in the uterotubal junction activity, whereas the rest of tube remained unaffected.[4,22,25–28]

Correlation with Mechanical Contractions

Increasing evidence supports the view that electrical activity is correlated with mechanical contractions. For skeletal muscles, a definite cause and effect relationship exists although the situation is not so clear for smooth muscles. A low-amplitude electrical stimulation from an external source does not always produce a mechanical contraction in the smooth muscle, whereas a mechanical stretch can initiate electrical activity. Therefore, interpretation of the correlation between the electrical and mechanical activities for the fallopian tube differs from that applicable to other body tissue.

Data were obtained by monitoring mechanical contractions concurrently with the electrical signals.[28,29] An intraluminal balloon was connected to a pressure transducer. Although localized pressure waves were monitored, the balloon obstructed the passage of intraluminal fluid and ova, thereby altering the physiological state. Another method, transtubal electrical impedance, has now been established.[30] The tube remains open but the exact intraluminal pressure cannot be measured. In these techniques, the electrical signals are picked up by placing electrodes on the tube. With the advent of advanced semiconductor technology, it is possible to telemeter the electrical and mechanical activity in a conscious animal.[17]

The rhythmic, slow contractions caused by a combination of synchronized longitudinal and circular muscular movements are known as peristalsis. This propagative wave produces a pressure differential that leads to the movement of ova and other luminal contents.[31,32] A definite correlation was found to exist between ovum location and both electrical and mechanical activities in the rat's and the rabbit's fallopian tubes.[21,33] This correlation changed during the estrual cycle and along the length of the tube.[18] In isolated smooth-muscle fibers, the electrical and pressure waves propagated in both directions with velocity variations from 2 mm/sec to 9 mm/sec.[20] Johns and Coons[8] attributed this variation to the electrical signal pathway. Electrical transmission through longitudinal fibers was faster than through the circular fibers. Structural changes during estrus lead to change in conduction velocity and thus mechanical transport.

Another form of mechanical action is segmental contractions. Localized segmental contractions were observed by Black and Asdell,[34] and by Blandau,[35] and have also been confirmed by autoradiography and cinematography. Until recently no attempts had been made to correlate the segmental contractions with the electrical potentials. Arjamma and Talo[9,10] were able to record myoelectrical and mechanical activity simultaneously in the regions of segmental contractions. They found that in the vicinity of ovum, the stretching triggers electrical potential generation and contraction followed. Such triggering occurred in each subsequent location of the egg during its movement. Detailed experimental data in this area remain to be obtained.

Future Directions

At present, myoelectrical potentials are considered as a dominant factor in reproductive processes with possible significance in contraception. Although the pace of research has been accelerated, the major issues remain to be investigated and understood.

So far the cross-coupling between cells has not been considered in detail. Excitation of cell groups to produce an oscillatory state by current reentry, as observed in the heart, is a possibility that needs to be elucidated by theoretical analysis and experimental methods. Such an investigation will aid in the search for mechanisms of initiation of bioelectrical potentials.

There is an association between the electrical and mechanical behavior of the fallopian tube but the correlation has been drawn from data obtained during relatively brief experimental monitoring. Two apparently unrelated phenomena can appear over a short period but an extended time trend analysis will bring up the linking pattern. With the fallopian tube, continuous monitoring is needed over the entire reproductive cycle. Evaluation of the data by computer base trend analysis techniques can bring out subtle correlations. Adequate computer algorithms are now available.

Extended monitoring for computer analysis cannot be obtained by available techniques. Tissue-electrode interface problems must be better understood so that stable pickup electrodes can be prepared. New microminiaturized implantable pressure transducers are required. The methods now available do not permit a reliable assessment of the longitudinal contraction patterns of the tubal musculature. Soon very small semiconductor strain gauge elements may be implanted within the tubal wall to monitor longitudinal contractions. These devices will help in elucidating the possible effects of peritoneal folds and ligaments on tubal contractions.

While these studies are important, it must be remembered that the electrical potential and mechanical contractions result from some biochemical phenomena. It would be appropriate to study localized secretory activity synchronously with electrical signals. Emerging new chemical transducers will enable such investigations.

Acknowledgment: The author wishes to express her gratitude to Prof. Sujoy K. Guha for his guidance in preparation of the manuscript.

References

1. Fuchs RF: Die elektrischen Ercheinungen am glatten Muskel. *Arch Ges Physiol,* 136:54, 1910.
2. Brundin J: The distribution and function of adrenergic nerves in the rabbit fallopian tube. *Acta Physiol Scand,* 66(Suppl. 259):1, 1965.
3. Zastowt O: Bandania nad zjawiskami bioelectrycznmi blony komorkowej miesniowki jajowodow. *Gin Pol,* 40:371, 1969.
4. Ruckebusch Y: Relationship between the electrical activity of the oviduct and the uterus of the rabbit in vivo. *J Reprod Fert,* 45:43, 1975.
5. Larks SD, Lark GG, Hoffer RE, et al: Electrical activity of oviducts in vivo. *Nature* (Lond.), 234:556, 1971.
6. Daniel EE, Lucien P, Posey VA, et al: A functional analysis of the myogenic control systems of the human fallopian tube. *Am J Obstet Gynecol,* 121:1046, 1975.
7. Talo A, and Brundin J: Muscular activity in the rabbit oviduct. A combination of electric and mechanic recording. *Biol Reprod,* 5:67, 1970.
8. Johns A, and Coons LW: Physiological and pharmacological characteristics of baboon oviduct. *Biol Reprod,* 25:120, 1981.
9. Arjamma O, and Talo A: The membrane potential of the Japanese quail's oviductal smooth muscle during ovum transport. *Acta Physiol Scand,* 118:349, 1983.
10. Arjamma O, and Talo A: Smooth muscle of the quail oviduct function as a stretch receptor during ovum transport. *Biol Reprod,* 29:472, 1983.
11. Pulkkinen MO, and Talo A: Myoelectrical activity in human oviduct with tubal pregnancy. *Am J Obstet Gynecol,* 148:151, 1983.
12. Talo A: Electrical and mechanical activity of the rabbit oviduct in vitro before and after ovulation. *Biol Reprod,* 11:249, 1974.
13. Kishikawa T, and Kuriyama H: Electrical and mechanical activities recorded from smooth muscle cells of human fallopian tube. *Jpn J Physiol,* 31:417, 1981.
14. Kowalewski K, and Scharf R: Secretions of hydrochloric acid by in vivo isolated canine stomach. *J Gastroent,* 6:675, 1971.
15. Talo A: Electrophysiology of the oviduct. In Harper MJK, Pauerstein CJ, Adams CE, et al (Eds): *Ovum Transport and Fertility Regulation.* Copenhagen: Scriptor, 1976.
16. Nishimura T, Nakajima A, and Hayashi T: The basic pattern of electrical activities in the rabbit fallopian tube. *Acta Obstet Gynecol Jpn,* 16:97, 1969.
17. Nelson TS, Timothy AN, and Augell JB: Microminiature transducers for oviductal motor functions. In Harper MJK, Pauerstein CJ, Adams CE, et al (Eds): *Ovum Transport and Fertility Regulation.* Copenhagen: Scriptor, 1976:75.
18. Parkington HC: Intracellular recorded electrical activity of smooth muscles of guinea pig oviduct. *Am J Physiol,* 245:357, 1983.
19. Tomita T, and Watanabe H: Factors affecting myogenic activity in smooth muscle. *Phil Trans Roy Soc,* 265:73, 1973.
20. Talo A, and Pulkkinen MO: Electrical activity in the human oviduct during the menstrual cycle. *Am J Obstet Gynecol,* 142:135, 1982.
21. Talo A: Myoelectrical activity and transport of unfertilized ova in the oviduct of the mouse in vitro. *J Reprod Fertil,* 60:53, 1980.
22. Ruckebusch Y, and Bayard F: Motility of the oviduct and uterus of the cow during the oestrus cycle. *J Reprod Fert,* 43:23, 1975.
23. Talo A, and Pulkkinen MO: Electrical activity in human oviducts after menopause. *Maturitas,* 5:185, 1984.
24. Lindblom B, and Wikland M: Simultaneous recording of electrical and mechanical activity in isolated smooth muscles of the human oviduct. *Biol Reprod,* 31:417, 1982.
25. Ruckebusch Y, and Bueno L: An electromyographic study of uterotubal activity in the ewe. *J Reprod Fertil,* 47:221, 1976.
26. Sircar R: Action of contraceptives on the ovum transport in the oviduct. Thesis, All India Institute of Medical Sciences, New Delhi, 1980.
27. Ruckebusch Y, and Pichot D: Effects of adrenergic drugs on sheep oviduct motility. *J Pharmacol,* 33:193, 1975.
28. Manchanda SK, Roychoudhary R, Sengupta J, et al: Postovulatory motility

pattern on rabbit oviduct and effect of estradiol benzoate. In Talwar P (Ed): *Recent Advances in Reproduction and Regulation of Fertility*. Amsterdam, Elsevier/North Holland Biomedical, 1979:201.
29. Manchanda SK, Roychoudhary R, Sakhuja D, et al: Receptive relaxation and post ovulatory motility pattern of the oviduct in conscious rabbits. *Ind J Physiol Pharmacol*, 23:185, 1979.
30. Guha SK, Anand S, and Talwar GP: In vivo motility of unobstructed fallopian tube. *J Appl Physiol*, 40:114, 1976.
31. Maia H, and Coutinho EM: Peristalsis and antiperistalsis of the human fallopian tube during the menstrual cycle. *Biol Reprod*, 2:305, 1970.
32. Anand S, and Guha SK: Mechanics of transport of ovum in the oviduct. *Med Biol Eng Comput*, 16:256, 1978.
33. Hodgson BJ, Talo A, and Pauerstein CJ: Oviductal ovum surrogate movement: Interrelation with muscular activity. *Biol Reprod*, 16:394, 1977.
34. Black DL, and Asdell SA: Transport through the rabbit oviduct. *Am J Physiol*, 192:63, 1957.
35. Blandau RJ: Gamete transport. In Hafez ESE, and Blandau RJ (Eds): *Mammalian Oviduct*. Chicago: University of Chicago Press, 1969:169.

8

GABA-ergic System in the Fallopian Tube

Sándor L. Erdö

Since gamma-aminobutyric acid (GABA) was first identified in the mammalian brain,[1] increasing evidence has accumulated that GABA is a major inhibitory neurotransmitter in the invertebrate nervous system and in the central nervous system of vertebrates.[2,3] The high amount of GABA in neural tissue is synthesized from L-glutamic acid through decarboxylation catalyzed by the enzyme L-glutamate decarboxylase (GAD, E.C. 4.1.1.15). The major pathway of GABA metabolism in nervous tissue is its transamination by 4-aminobutyrate 2-oxoglutarate aminotransferase (GABA-T, E.C. 2.6.1.19) resulting in succinic semialdehyde formation, which is then rapidly converted to succinate by succinic semialdehyde dehydrogenase (SSA-DH, E.C. 1.2.1.16) (Fig. 8:1).

It has also been demonstrated that low levels of GABA and GAD are present in certain peripheral tissues of mammals.[4–11] Since the formation rate and the steady-state levels of GABA in the peripheral organs examined were rather low relative to the central nervous system, little attention was paid to a possible neurotransmitter role for the amino acid outside the mammalian brain. The finding that GABA, in addition to its neurotransmitter function, may be used as an energy source through the GABA shunt pathway[12] led to the general assumption that in so-called nonneural tissues, the importance of GABA would be minor, and that it is not a neurotransmitter.

Recently, high GABA concentrations and GAD activities have been found in certain peripheral tissues, such as the pancreatic islets of the rat and the human insulinoma,[13] and the ovary and fallopian tube of the rat.[14,15] The GABA levels in these tissues are in the same order of magnitude as in the brain. Moreover, increasing evidence has accumulated that GABA may possess a neurotransmitter function in the vertebrate peripheral nervous system, namely in the gut.[16–20] In light of these recent findings, increasing interest has been focused on peripheral GABA-ergic mechanisms, particularly in respect to the organs found to be the richest in GABA.

The Fallopian Tube: Basic Studies and Clinical Contributions, edited by Alvin M. Siegler, M.D. Mount Kisco, New York: Futura Publishing Company, Inc. © 1986.

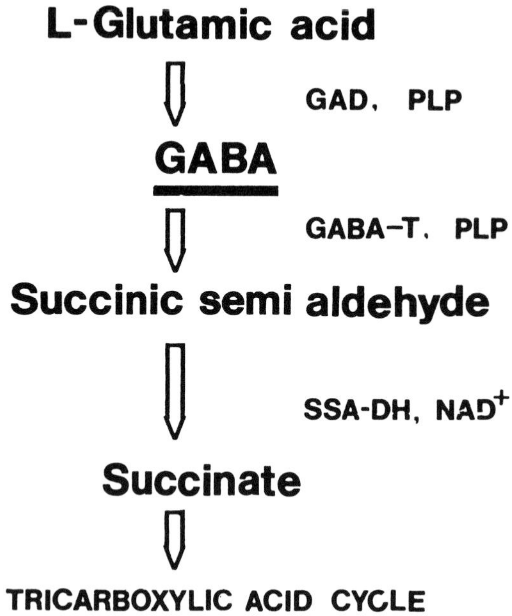

FIGURE 8:1—*Major metabolic pathways in the synthesis and further metabolism of GABA. Enzyme cofactors are indicated as PLP, pyridoxal phosphate, and NAD$^+$, oxidized nicotinamide adenine dinucleotide.*

In this study, the neurochemical characteristics of the GABA-ergic system in the fallopian tube are summarized. Furthermore, several recent data indicating the functional significance of this system in the oviduct are reviewed.

Occurrence and Distribution of the GABA-ergic System in the Tube

Two research groups, working independently, have recently reported the presence of extremely high GABA levels in the rat oviduct.[15,21] The consistent results obtained by different methods have demonstrated that the tubal GABA levels are more than double those in the whole rat brain. In other mammals, including humans, however, the GABA concentrations in the oviducts have been found to be considerably lower than in that organ of the rat.[21,22]

The GABA levels show an uneven distribution between the oviductal ampulla and isthmus of the rat and the rabbit: the ampulla is more than twice as rich in GABA as the isthmus (Table 8:1). In the human fallopian tube, the concentration of the amino acid is also lower in the isthmus than in the ampulla.[22]

The above findings suggest in-situ formation of GABA in the oviduct. The results obtained with the different species indicate the ubiquitous occurrence of GABA in the mammalian oviduct and draw attention to considerable species differences regarding tubal GABA levels (Table 8:1).

Biosynthesis and Metabolism of Tubal GABA

In crude homogenates of the rat oviduct, a significant rate of GABA formation from L-glutamic acid could be observed.[21] Also, dissected oviducts incubated with radiolabeled glutamate showed a considerable GAD activity.[23] The biosynthetic rate of GABA from glutamate appeared to be approximately 10 percent of that in the brain.

In vivo, after administration of ^{14}C-glutamic acid, about 6 percent of the tubal radioactivity was measured as ^{14}C-GABA.[24] Moreover, known inhibitors of cerebral GAD—i.e., isonicotinic acid hydrazide and thiosemicarbazide—significantly reduced GABA levels in the rat oviduct in a manner similar to that in the brain.[15]

The above results, obtained in vitro and in vivo, provide evidence for the formation of GABA in the rat oviduct; they also indicate that a similar biosynthetic pathway exists for cerebral and tubal GABA. Nevertheless, the formation of GABA in the oviduct from endogenous sources other than L-glutamate cannot be disregarded. In a preliminary report, research workers in Spain demonstrated that a significant amount of radiolabeled GABA could be extracted from oviducts of rats pretreated with ^{14}C-putrescine.[24] This suggests that tubal GABA may also

Table 8:1
Distribution of GABA Levels in the Oviduct

Tissue		GABA nmol/g frozen tissue	n
	Whole oviduct	4,933 + 254	8
Rat*	Ampulla	7,252 + 627	6
	Isthmus	3,117 + 276	6
	Whole oviduct	114 + 43	3
Rabbit*	Ampulla	174 + 35	4
	Isthmus	86 + 20	4
	Whole oviduct	177 + 54	4
Women†	Ampulla	224 + 54	4
	Isthmus	181 + 35	4

Each value is mean + SEM (n = 3–8).
*Erdö, unpublished data.
†Data from Erdö et al.[22]

be formed in situ from putrescine. Thus, two (or more) alternative biosynthetic pathways for GABA may exist in the oviduct.

The primary metabolic step of GABA in the brain is transamination by GABA-T. In vitro, GABA-T activity has been observed in a tissue homogenate of the rat's fallopian tube, which could be blocked significantly by aminooxyacetic acid, i.e., a carbonyl trapping agent known to block cerebral GABA-T.[21] Under in-vivo conditions, however, aminooxyacetic acid significantly reduced GABA levels in the tube, while cerebral GABA concentrations in the same rats showed a concomitant increase.[15,23] A possible explanation for the conflicting data of the in-vitro and in-vivo experiments is that aminooxyacetic acid, as a carbonyl trapping agent, is able to inhibit not only GABA-T but also GAD; both enzymes require pyridoxal phosphate as a coenzyme. If it is assumed that the compound has a much higher affinity for tubal GAD than for tubal GABA-T, the predominant blockade of GABA formation after aminooxyacetic acid administration may result in the diminution of GABA levels in the oviduct. In the brain tissue, however, this compound is about one thousand times as potent in inhibiting GABA-T as in blocking GAD.[25]

These results indicate that GABA-T is present in the mammalian oviduct, and this enzyme is probably responsible for the primary catabolic step of GABA degradation in this organ. On the other hand, the significant difference in the responsiveness of cerebral and tubal GABA-T to the same inhibitor in vivo should be emphasized.

GABA Receptors in the Tube

A widely used method for studying GABA receptors in neural tissues is the radioligand binding assay, when membranes are incubated in the presence of labeled GABA or GABA receptor agonists. Few attempts have been made, however, to identify GABA receptors in peripheral tissues of mammals by receptor binding assay.[22,26–28] On the other hand, numerous studies using pharmacological approaches, have indicated the presence of GABA receptors on components of the peripheral nervous system.[18,29–32] These experiments led to the distinction of two pharmacologically and functionally different GABA receptors. One of them is rather sensitive to muscimol and GABA, as agonists, and can be blocked by bicuculline ($GABA_A$); the other ($GABA_B$) can be stimulated by baclofen and GABA and cannot be blocked by bicuculline.[31,33]

In the rat's oviduct, a low density of bicuculline-sensitive ($GABA_A$) receptors has been identified by radioligand binding assay.[26] The tubal membranes used for this experiment were separated from rough tissue fragments by centrifugation. This method may result in a significant loss of the specific binding sites, since the muscle elements sedimented probably contain GABA receptors too. Thus, the density of the high affinity binding sites in the rat oviduct has been presumably underestimated (Table 8:2).

A very high concentration of high affinity and bicuculline sensitive GABA receptors has been demonstrated in the human fallopian tube.[22] The maximal binding capacity of 690 fmol/mg protein is over 40 times that in the rat oviduct and it is in the same order of magnitude as the number of high affinity GABA binding sites in the brain (Table 8:2). The rough tissue fragments of the homogenates from the human oviduct were removed by filtration through a fine mesh nylon screen, not by centrifugation. This procedure is unlikely to lead to a significant loss of specific binding sites.

Studies on the segmental distribution of GABA receptors have revealed that the human isthmus is about twice as rich in GABA receptors as the ampulla.[25] This finding indicates a reverse distribution of GABA levels and GABA receptors in the fallopian tube.

Under the conditions of the above receptor binding experiments, only $GABA_A$ receptors can be detected; thus, the presence of $GABA_B$ receptors in the oviduct cannot be disregarded. Interestingly, $GABA_B$-receptor-mediated stimulation of the spontaneous motility of the isolated rabbit oviduct could also be observed (Erdö and Riesz, unpublished data).

Table 8:2

Kinetic Parameters of ^{3}H-GABA Binding

Tissue	K^*_d nM	$B^\dagger_{max}$ fmol/mg protein
Rat oviduct[26]	52	17
Human oviduct[22]	40	690
Rat brain[34]	25	700

*Equilibrium dissociation constant.
†Maximal binding capacity.

GABA Receptors and Cyclic AMP in the Tube

The GABA receptors in the central nervous system are not coupled to a cyclic AMP generating system. Furthermore, no attempts have been made to examine a possible connection between peripheral GABA receptors and this second messenger in tissues other than the ovary and the fallopian tube.

In tissue slices of the rat's oviduct, GABA and the $GABA_A$ receptor agonist muscimol evoked significant increase in the intracellular cyclic AMP levels. These effects were completely antagonized by bicuculline and picrotoxin, which are both known blockers of GABA receptors.[26]

These findings may not necessarily prove the coupling of the tubal $GABA_A$ receptors to a cyclic AMP generating system, since it is also conceivable that the increase of the levels of the second messenger in the presence of GABA or muscimol is caused by secondary influences. The specific responsiveness of the oviduct tissue to GABA and GABA-mimetics, however, seems to be undoubted.

GABA Efflux from Tubal Slices

One of the most important postulations for a neurotransmitter candidate is that it should be released from nerve endings under the effect of various stimuli. For the in-vitro study of the release process, the measurement of the efflux of putative neurotransmitters from tissue slices is a widely used method. As a stimulus, high external potassium concentration in the incubation medium may be applied to induce depolarization of neuronal membranes.

The efflux of endogenous GABA from tissue slices of the rat oviduct was examined in the presence of high (30 mM) or low (4.7 mM) external potassium concentrations, in either a calcium-containing or a calcium-free modified Krebs-Henseleit bicarbonate buffer (pH = 7.4). The amount of the endogenous GABA released during the first five minutes of incubation at 37°C was about three times higher in the potassium-rich medium than in the buffer with a low potassium concentration, when calcium ions were present. In the calcium-free medium, however, even the high external potassium concentration failed to increase the efflux of GABA (Fig. 8:2).

The calcium dependence of the GABA efflux from slices of the oviduct represents a property similar to that of neuronal release mechanisms in the central nervous system.

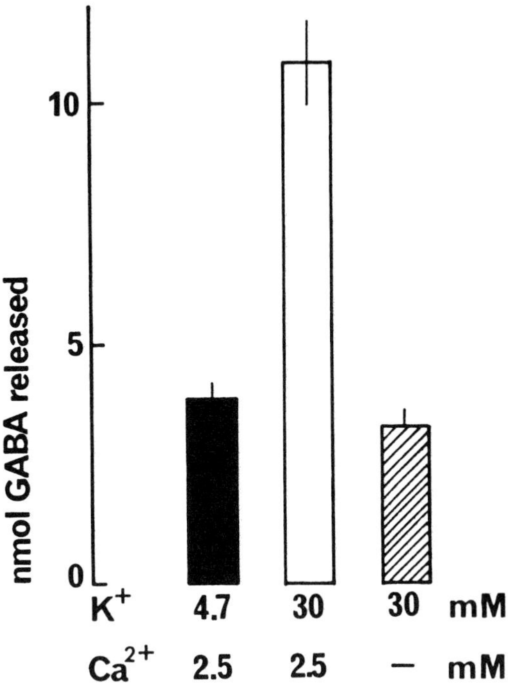

FIGURE 8:2—*Calcium-dependence of the endogenous GABA efflux from slices of the rat oviduct. Each column represents the mean amount of GABA released from slices of a pair organ, weighing 22.4 + 0.8 mg. Vertical bars represent SEM. Tissue slices were incubated for 5 min at 37°C, in normal or modified Krebs-Henseleit bicarbonate buffers, pH = 7.4 (Erdö, original data).*

GABA Uptake by Tubal Slices

The high affinity GABA uptake systems known to be present in cerebral nerve terminals and glia are needed for the inactivation and reuse of GABA.[35] High affinity GABA uptake by peripheral tissues, such as the thyroid and the ovary, has also been demonstrated.[36,37]

In vitro, the tissue slices of the rat oviduct have been found to be able to concentrate ^{3}H-GABA from an external medium with high affinity.[27] The tissue:-medium ratio of the labeled amino acid after 60 minutes incubation at 37°C was about 1.5 in these experiments (Erdö, unpublished data). This value is much lower than that demonstrated after incubation of cerebral slices, indicating that only a small number of tubal cells possesses the capacity to take up ^{3}H-GABA.[38] However, the poor penetration of the amino acid into the rat tubal slices may also be responsible for the low tissue:medium ratio. A significant portion of the high endogenous GABA levels can be spontaneously released from the rat oviduct during incubation and can partly block the uptake of the exogenous GABA under the conditions applied. The estimation of a tissue-:medium ratio of six after similar incubation of the rabbit ampulla, an organ containing about one-fortieth the endogenous GABA concentration than the rat oviduct (Erdö, unpublished data) may support the latter explanation.

The uptake of ^{3}H-GABA by slices of the rat's oviduct could be inhibited by unlabeled GABA, by well-known GABA uptake blockers, and by a metabolic inhibitor such as ouabain.[27]

The above findings provide evidence for the presence of an active GABA uptake system in the fallopian tube that is similar to that in the brain.

Alteration of Tubal GABA Levels with Functional Status

The neurochemical properties of a neurotransmitter system involved in the regulation of the function of an organ should generally reflect the alteration of the physiological status. In the mammalian oviduct, for instance, significant changes could be observed in the steady-state levels of noradrenaline under different hormonal conditions.[39–41]

The identification and characterization of the GABA-ergic system in the fallopian tube definitely indicate the functional significance of GABA in the oviduct. Thus, the alteration of GABA levels in the tube as a function of postnatal age, estrual cycle, or pregnancy may well be supposed.

In fact, the GABA content of the rat's oviduct gradually increases up to week 10 of postnatal life, indicating the maturation of the GABA-ergic system in the oviduct.[42]

In cyclic rats, the GABA concentration in the oviduct shows a maximal value during diestrus[21] or early proestrus, followed by a significant decrease at late proestrus.[42]

In pregnant rats, the tubal GABA concentration and the total amount of the amino acid showed significant diminution up to day 21 of gestation (Erdö, unpublished data).

Although the steady-state level of GABA may not be the most appropriate neurochemical marker characterizing the functional activity of the GABA-ergic system in the tube, the large variability of GABA concentrations in the rat oviduct as a function of the physiological status of the animals may confirm the functional significance of the GABA-ergic system in the fallopian tube.

Possible Role of GABA in the Tube: A Hypothesis

In light of the biochemical characteristics of the oviductal GABA-ergic system, it seems to be reasonable to assume that a GABA-ergic innervation is present in the fallopian tube. In the case of tubal GABA, all the important postulations for a neurotransmitter appear to be fulfilled. Namely, it is present in the target organ and shows an uneven distribution. Tubal GABA is formed in situ and can be released from its stores by a suitable stimulus. Also, specific receptor binding sites, mediating GABA-ergic responses, and an active uptake system for the amino acid that may inactivate and reuse GABA have been identified in the fallopian tube. All of these findings are consistent with the properties of the GABA-ergic system in the central nervous system (Table 8:3).

Still, there are some differences between the cerebral and tubal GABA-ergic systems at the neurochemical level. First, the responsiveness of GABA-T to various inhibitors differs in these two organs. Second, GABA mimetics can increase the cyclic AMP levels in the tube but not in the brain. The findings may provide the possibility of the selective pharmacological manipulation of GABA-ergic mechanisms in the oviduct. The poor penetration of GABA and certain GABA-ergic model compounds through the blood-brain barrier also indicates a possible way to influence the peripheral GABA-ergic system selectively by systemic administration of drugs.

Most of the biochemical results reviewed concerning the GABA-ergic system in the tube are in a preliminary stage. Even if more complete studies would be available, the results obtained by exclusively neurochemical methods are not definitive enough to provide sufficient evi-

Table 8:3

A Comparison of the Neurochemical Characteristics of Tubal and Cerebral GABA-ergic Systems

	Oviduct	*Brain*
GABA present	yes	yes
GABA uneven distribution	yes	yes
GAD present	yes	yes
GABA released	yes	yes
GABA recognition sites	yes	yes
GABA-ergic responses detected	yes	yes
GABA induces elevation of cyclic AMP levels	yes	no
GABA-T activity present	yes	yes
GABA-T blocked by aminooxyacetic acid, in vivo	no	yes
Active GABA uptake system	yes	yes

dence for the existence of tubal GABA-ergic innervation. Histochemical studies, namely the immunocytochemical identification of GABA containing cells and the autoradiographic localization of GABA recognition sites, are needed. Furthermore, the transmitter nature of GABA in the oviduct should be confirmed by pharmacological and electrophysiological methods. It should be proved that the same effect can be elicited by exogenous GABA administration and by the stimulation of the putative GABA-ergic nerves in the tube.

The physiological role of the hypothetical GABA-ergic innervation in the fallopian tube is not yet clear. Nevertheless, GABA, either as a neurotransmitter or not, may possess a functional importance in this organ. This statement can be supported by the following data: (1) GABA and model compounds known to act on $GABA_A$ receptors do influence the cyclic AMP levels in tubal tissue slices; (2) GABA and the $GABA_B$ receptor agonist baclofen stimulate the spontaneous contractility of the isolated rabbit oviduct; and (3) the GABA levels in the rat tube show significant alterations during postnatal development, the estrous cycle, and gestation.

The findings indicate that the GABA-ergic system may be involved in the regulation of oviductal contractility through $GABA_B$ receptors; consequently, GABA might influence the ovum transport and fertility under physiological conditions. The responses mediated by $GABA_A$ receptors, however, remain to be elucidated.

Concluding Remarks

During the last two years, increasing evidence has accumulated that a GABA-ergic system, showing many of the characteristics of a neuronal one, is present in the mammalian oviduct. Preliminary data indicate that this GABA-ergic system may play a part in the regulation of oviductal contractility. Thus, further in-vivo studies attempting to examine the effects of selective GABA-ergic model compounds on ovum transport and fertility may lead to a better understanding of tubal physiology and might also lead to the discovery of a novel site of action of drugs affecting fertility.

Acknowledgments: I wish to thank Mr. Bela Kiss, Mr. Miklos Riesz, and Dr. Laszlo Szporny for helpful discussion. Thanks are due also to Mrs. Maria Holeviczky for typing the manuscript.

References

1. Roberts E, and Frankel S: Gamma-aminobutyric acid in brain: Its formation from glutamic acid. *J Biol Chem*, 187:55, 1950.
2. Otsuka M: GABA in the crustacean nervous system: A historical review. In Roberts E, Chase TN, and Tower DB (Eds): *GABA in Nervous System Function*. New York: Raven Press, 1976: 245.
3. Krnjevic K: Chemical nature of synaptic transmission in vertebrates. *Physiol Rev*, 54:418, 1974.
4. Zachmann M, Tocci P, and Nyhan WL: The occurrence of gamma-aminobutyric acid in human tissues other than brain. *J Biol Chem*, 241:1355, 1966.
5. Whelan DT, Scriver CR, and Mohyaddin F: Glutamic acid decarboxylase and gamma-aminobutyric acid in mammalian kidney. *Nature* (Lond.), 224:916, 1969.
6. Haber B, Kuriyama K, and Roberts E: An anion stimulated 1-glutamic acid decarboxylase in non-neuronal tissues. *Biochem Pharmacol*, 19:1119, 1970.
7. Drummond RJ, and Phillips AT: L-glutamic acid decarboxylase in non-neural tissues of the mouse. *J Neurochem*, 23:1207, 1974.
8. MacDonnel P, and Greengard O: The distribution of glutamate decarboxylase in rate tissues; Isotopic vs. fluorimetric assays. *J Neurochem*, 24:615, 1975.
9. Wu JY: A comparative study of L-glutamate decarboxylase from brain and heart with purified preparations. *J Neurochem*, 28:1359, 1977.
10. Wu JY, Chude O, Wein J, et al: Distribution and tissue specificity of glutamate decarboxylase (EC 4.1.1.15). *J Neurochem*, 30:849, 1978.
11. Erdö SL, Nemet L, and Szporny L: The occurrence of GABA in vas deferens, prostate, epididymis, seminal vesicle and testicle of the rat. *Acta Biol Acad Sci*, 34:435, 1983.
12. Baxter CF: The nature of gamma-aminobutyric acid. In Lajtha A (Ed): *Handbook of Neurochemistry*, vol. 3. New York: Plenum Press, 1970:289.
13. Okada Y, Taniguchi H, and Shimida C: High concentration of GABA and high glutamate decarboxylase activity in rat pancreatic islets and human insulinoma. *Science*, 194:620, 1976.
14. Martin del Rio R, and Latorre Caballero A: Presence of gamma-aminobutyric acid in rat ovary. *J Neurochem*, 34:1584, 1980.
15. Erdö SL, Rosdy B, and Szporny L: Higher GABA concentrations in fallopian tube than in brain of the rat. *J Neurochem*, 38:1174, 1982.
16. Jenssen KR, Mirsky R, Dennison ME, et al: GABA may be a neurotransmitter in the vertebrate peripheral nervous system. *Nature* (Lond.), 281:71, 1979.
17. Taniyama K, Kusunoki M, Saito N, et al: Release of gamma-aminobutyric acid from cat colon. *Science*, 217:1038, 1982.
18. Giotti A, Iuizzi S, Spagnesi S, et al: $GABA_A$ and $GABA_B$ receptor-mediated effects in guinea pig ileum. *Br J Pharmacol*, 78:469, 1983.
19. Miki Y, Taniyama K, Tanaka C, et al: GABA, glutamic acid decarboxylase and GABA transaminase levels in the myenteric plexus in the intestine of humans and other mammals. *J Neurochem*, 40:861, 1983.
20. Ong J, and Kerr DIB: $GABA_A$ and $GABA_B$ receptor mediated modification of intestinal motility. *Eur J Pharmacol*, 86:9, 1983.
21. Martin del Rio R: Gamma-aminobutyric acid system in rat oviduct. *J Biol Chem*, 256:9816, 1981.
22. Erdö SL, Laszlo A, Szporny L, et al: High density of specific GABA binding sites in the human fallopian tube. *Neurosci Lett*, 42:155, 1983.
23. Martin del Rio R, and Sierra Lopez M: Effects of aminooxyacetic acid on in vivo gamma-aminobutyric acid system of rat oviduct. *Gen Pharmacol*, 14:281, 1983.
24. Orensanz LM, Fernandez I, and Martin del Rio R: On the origin and function of GABA in the rat fallopian tube. *Int J Fertil*, 28:11, 1983.
25. Baxter CF, and Roberts E: Elevation of gamma-aminobutyric acid in brain: Selective inhibition of gamma-aminobutyric acid gamma-ketoglutaric acid aminase. *J Biol Chem*, 236:3287, 1961.
26. Erdö SL, and Lapis E: Presence of GABA receptors in rat oviduct. *Neurosci Lett*, 33:275, 1982.
27. Erdö SL: Characterization of GABA-ergic system in the fallopian tube. *Int J Fertil*, 28:8, 1983.

28. Schaeffer JM, and Hsueh AJW: Identification of gamma-aminobutyric acid and its binding sites in the rat ovary. *Life Sci*, 30:1599, 1982.
29. Bowery NG, and Brown DA: Depolarizing actions of gamma-aminobutyric acid and related compounds on rat superior cervical ganglia in vitro. *Br J Pharmacol*, 50:205, 1974.
30. Brown DA, and Marsh S: Axonal GABA receptors in mammalian peripheral nerve trunks. *Brain Res*, 156:187, 1978.
31. Bowery NG, Doble A, Hill DR, et al: Bicuculline-insensitive GABA receptors on peripheral autonomic nerve terminals. *Eur J Pharmacol*, 71:53, 1981.
32. Hughes PR, Morgan PF, and Stone TW: Inhibitory action of gamma-aminobutyric acid on the excitatory but not inhibitory innervation of the rat anococcygeus muscle. *Br J Pharmacol*, 77:691, 1982.
33. Bowery NG, Hill DR, and Hudson AL: Characteristics of $GABA_B$ receptor binding sites on rat whole brain synaptic membranes. *Br J Pharmacol*, 78:191, 1983.
34. Olsen RW, Bergman MO, Van Ness PC, et al: Gamma-aminobutyric acid receptor binding in mammalian brain. Heterogeneity of binding sites. *Mol Pharmacol*, 19:217, 1981.
35. Iversen LL, and Kelly JS: Uptake and metabolism of gamma-aminobutyric acid by neurons and glial cells. *Biochem Pharmacol*, 24:933, 1975.
36. Gebauer H: GABA transport in the rat thyroid, *Naunyn-Schmiedeberg's Arch Pharmacol*, 317:61, 1981.
37. Erdö SL: High-affinity, sodium-dependent gamma-aminobutyric acid uptake by slices of rat ovary. *J Neurochem*, 40:572, 1983.
38. Taniguchi H, Okada Y, Hosoya Y, et al. Comparison of uptake of gamma-aminobutyric acid by pancreatic islets and by substantia nigra. *Biomed Res*, 1(Suppl):175, 1980.
39. Bodhke RR, and Harper MJK: Mechanism of egg transport: Changes in amount of adrenergic transmitter in the genital tract of normal and hormone-treated rabbits. In Segal SJ, Crozier R, Corfman PA, et al (Eds): *The Regulation of Mammalian Ovum Transport*. Springfield: Charles C Thomas, 1973:364.
40. Owman C, and Sjöberg NO: Influence of sex hormones on the amount of adrenergic transmitter in the rabbit oviduct. In Kumar A (Ed): *Neuroendocrine Regulation of Fertility*. Basel: Karger, 1976:260.
41. Helm G, Owman C, Rosengren E, et al: Regional and cyclic variations in catecholamine concentration of the human fallopian tube. *Biol Reprod*, 26:553, 1982.
42. Kiss B, Erdö SL, and Szporny L: Developmental and cyclic changes in noradrenaline and GABA contents of rat oviduct and ovary. In: *Supplement to Progress in Neuro-Psychopharmacology and Biological Psychiatry*. Oxford: Pergamon Press, 1983:190 (abstract 265).

9

Steroid Regulation of the Human Oviduct

Luigi Devoto and
Ana María Pino

Present knowledge of reproductive phenomena that take place in the oviduct is limited to a partial explanation of events such as ovum and sperm transport and early cleavage of the embryo.

The understanding of tubal function has increasing importance in clinical infertility, since it can lead to improvement in the treatment of iatrogenic or pathogenic tubal infertility[1] or to the development of new contraceptive strategies at the tubal level.[2]

The human oviduct undergoes morphological changes during the menstrual cycle. Tubal mucosal cells are highest and more ciliated during the later proliferative phase. At the late luteal phase, cells are flat and microvilli decrease in size as well as in number.[3] In addition to the morphological changes mentioned, tubal fluid secretions vary during the cycle, being heaviest during the follicular phase.[2]

These morphofunctional changes in the human oviduct in accordance with the ovarian cycle suggest that this tissue acts as a target organ for steroid hormone action. Steroid target tissues have specific hormone receptors, which are intracellular proteins that become "activated" by the binding of the proper hormone. The activated hormone-receptor complex translocates to the nucleus, where it promotes specific and characteristic changes of gene expression.[4]

Although the presence of specific estradiol and progesterone receptors in the human oviduct has been described,[5,6] some questions about steroid action on this tissue remain unanswered. This leads us to specify further the ovarian hormone action on this tissue, based on the following criteria: (1) measurement of tubal steroid concentration and its relationship with serum steroid content; (2) measurement of the steroid receptor content and its subcellular distribution throughout the menstrual cycle; and (3) measurement of a protein marker of the steroid action on the tissue.

The Fallopian Tube: Basic Studies and Clinical Contributions, edited by Alvin M. Siegler, M.D. Mount Kisco, New York: Futura Publishing Company, Inc. © 1986.

Methodology

Fertile patients requesting surgical sterilization in our institution were included in this study. Informed consent to remove one fallopian tube at operation was obtained from each patient. At laparotomy, the fallopian tube on the side of the corpus luteum or ripe follicle was removed, with careful attention given to preserving the ovarian blood supply. The tube was processed for the measurement of steroid tissue concentration, receptor determination, and 17-β estradiol dehydrogenase (17βHSDH) activity. Measurements were made in the total tube or in each anatomical segment (Figs. 9:1–9:4). In addition to the histologic data, the presumptive day of ovulation was ascertained by the plasma concentration of estradiol (E_2) and the LH peak. The samples were classified according to the following criteria: (a) early proliferative, before the beginning of the E_2 peak ($E_2 <$ 200 pg/ml); (b) late proliferative ($E_2 >$ 200 pg/ml); (c) early secretory, 24 to 96 hours after the LH peak; (d) late secretory, more than 96 hours after the LH peak.

Results and Discussion

Measurement of tubal steroid concentration

The earlier studies were focused on defining steroid retention by the human oviduct. We demonstrated that the three anatomical segments retain estradiol and progesterone at or above their plasma levels.[7] Our data demonstrated a lower tissue concentration of steroids in the fallopian tube as compared with those in human endometrium. In spite of the lack of variation in plasma estrone during the

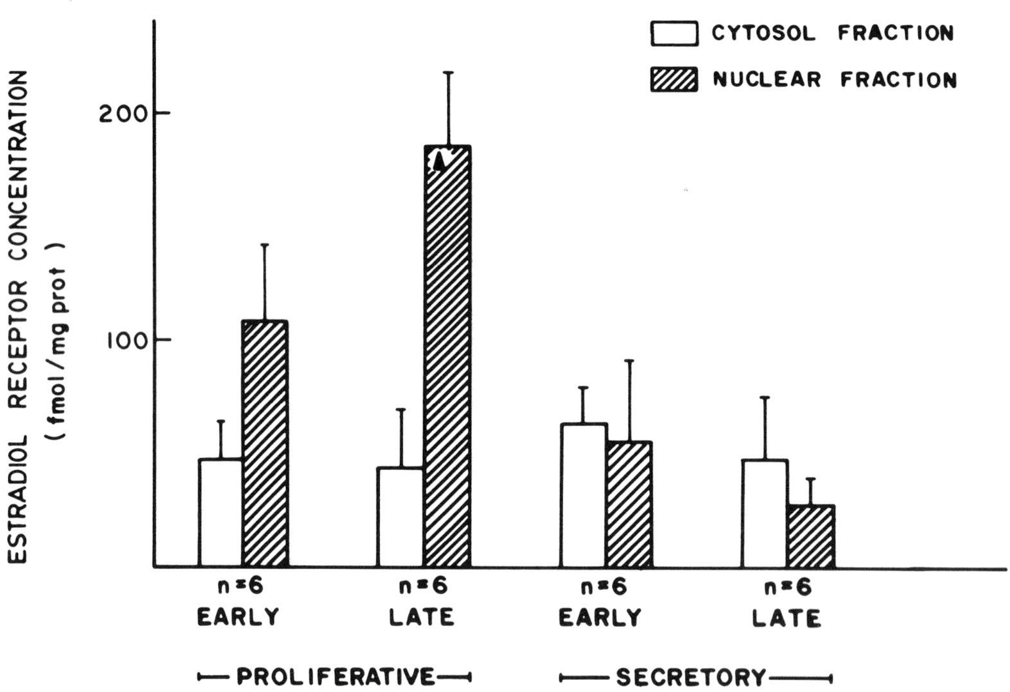

FIGURE 9:1—*Cytosolic and nuclear estradiol receptor concentrations of ampulla during the normal menstrual cycle. Each bar indicates the concentration (fmol/mg prot. ± SD) of cytosolic or nuclear receptors. Symbol (▲) indicates the probability of considered nuclear receptor concentration being significantly higher ($p < 0.05$)* than the corresponding concentration at the secretory stages.

Table 9:1

Unconjugated Estrone in the Fallopian Tube and Peripheral Blood during the Normal Menstrual Cycle

Stage of the Cycle	Plasma concentration pg/ml	Tissue concentration estrone (pg/g wt tissue)		
		Isthmus	Ampulla	Fimbria
Early proliferative $n = 3$	50 ± 10	100 ± 40	60 ± 30	70 ± 20
Late proliferative $n = 5$	70 ± 10	110 + 10	100 ± 8	110 ± 40
Early secretory $n = 8$	60 ± 10	190 ± 50	240 ± 60	310 ± 60
Late secretory $n = 6$	60 ± 8	120 ± 50	170 ± 50	150 ± 50

cycle, a significant increase was seen in oviductal tissue during the luteal phase. The results suggested an active process in estrone formation by the fallopian tube (Table 9:1).

Measurement of Specific Steroid Receptors and Protein Markers of Their Action

Our aim was to analyze not only the variations of receptor concentration through the menstrual cycle, but also to relate them to a hormone characteristic response. Therefore, as a response to estradiol action, the presence of the progesterone receptor was measured; since it has been proven with several tissues that estradiol priming is a requirement for progesterone receptor synthesis.[8] On the other hand, progesterone action on this tissue was related to the presence of 17β E_2 HSDH (hydroxy steroid dehydrogenase) activity; the latter enzyme is a protein synthesized after progesterone action in the human endometrium.[9]

Estradiol and progesterone concentrations were measured in the cytosol and nuclei of the three anatomical segments of the oviduct. The method employed has been previously described.[10,11]

The oviductal tissue bound estradiol with high affinity. The calculated KD for the ampullary protein was in close agreement with previous values obtained for the whole oviduct.[12]

Previous work on the human oviduct brought to light a lack of variation in the content of cytosolic estradiol receptor throughout the menstrual cycle[5] contrasting with the results obtained with the monkey's oviduct.[5,13] Our results confirmed the former finding (Fig. 9:1) and we further observed that this lack of variation was not from endogenous estradiol bound to the receptor, or to plasma steroid hormone binding globulin (SHBG) contamination, as heat exchange assays did not increase the estradiol binding and SHBG contamination proved to be constant during the cycle.

Nevertheless, plasma estradiol variation throughout the cycle was reflected by the changes in the content of the nuclear estradiol receptor. During the late proliferative stage, when plasma estradiol concentration reached a maximum, the highest content of the nuclear binding protein was found in all segments.

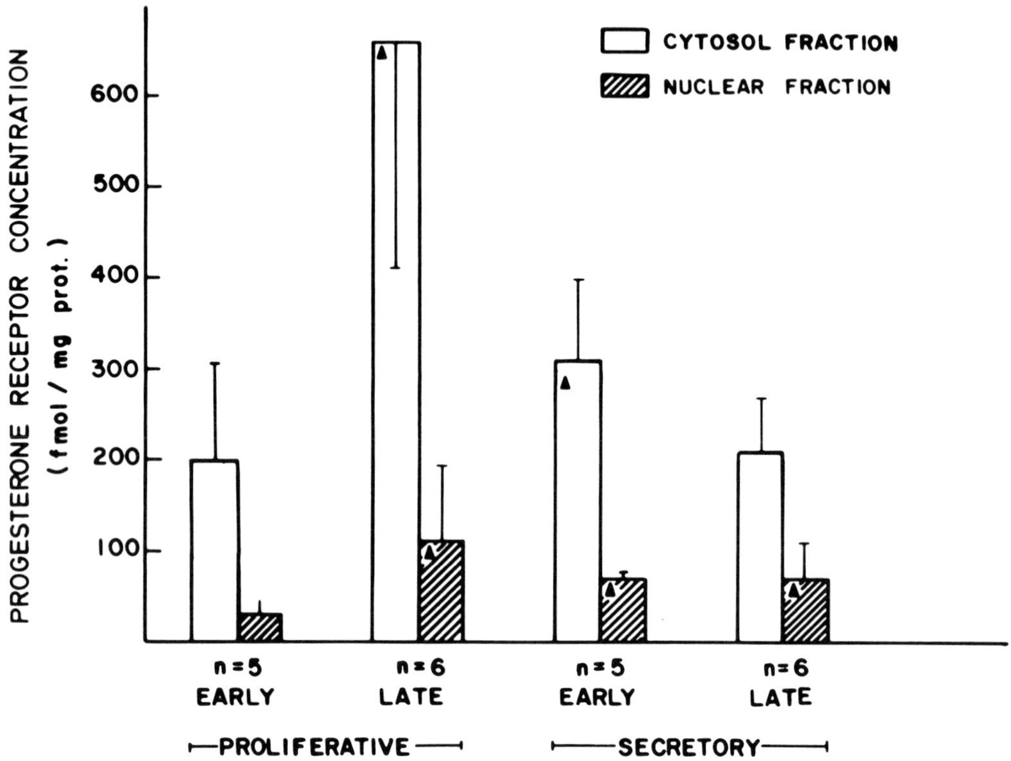

FIGURE 9:2—*Cytosolic and nuclear progestogen receptor concentrations of ampulla during the menstrual cycle. Values are mean ± SD for the number of samples indicated. The value is significantly higher* ($p < 0.05$) *than the corresponding concentration at the early proliferative stage.*

The isthmus showed a remarkable variation of its content during the transition of early to late proliferative stages. Although the ampulla and fimbria had a high nuclear estradiol receptor content at the early proliferative phase, a further increase was detected in the late proliferative stage. Figure 9:1 shows the variations observed in the ampulla.

During the transition through the secretory phases, a progressive decrease in the nuclear receptor content was observed in the three anatomical segments. These results strongly suggest that in this tissue, the concentration of estradiol receptor is regulated by changes in plasma concentration of estradiol and progesterone. In this sense, a good positive linear correlation was observed between the nuclear estradiol receptor content throughout the cycle and plasma estradiol concentration, while a negative linear correlation was observed with respect to plasma progesterone.[10]

This observation agrees with the opposite effect of those steroid hormones observed in experimental models[14,15] and shows that the same regulatory mechanism operates in a normal human tissue cycle. Thus, while the positive correlation found with plasma estradiol would be the consequence of cytosol receptor translocation to the nucleus, the negative one observed with progesterone could be the result of an inhibition of nuclear estradiol receptor retention, as proposed by Evans et al.[15]

The variation in the content of the progesterone receptors of the human oviduct has been described.[11,16–18] The observed variations (Fig. 9:2) suggest that

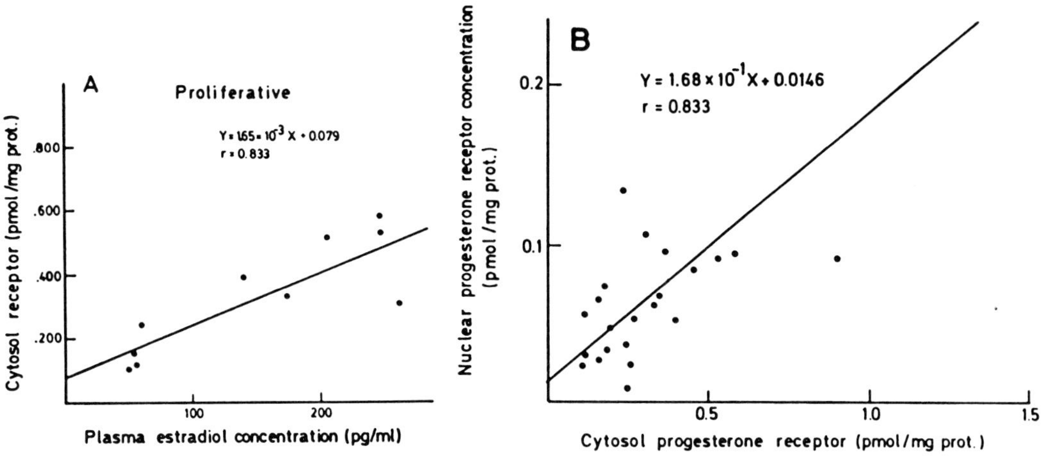

FIGURE 9:3—*Correlation between ampullary progestagen receptors (A) cytosol receptor and plasma estradiol concentration and (B) nuclear receptor and cytosol progestogen receptor.*

the progesterone receptor is under dual hormonal control, as reported by Vu Hai et al.[19] in animal and human tissues.

We infer from the good positive linear regression observed for plasma estradiol and cytosolic progestagen receptor content that estradiol stimulates the synthesis of the cytosolic progestogen receptor in the oviduct. The positive effect of estradiol was also shown for the nuclear progestagen receptor content throughout the whole cycle, suggesting that estradiol priming of the tissue is required to provide enough cytosolic receptor for translocation to the nucleus. This evidence supports the linear correlation found between cytosolic and nuclear progestagen receptor concentration (Fig. 9:3).

During the luteal stage, a decrease in the content of progesterone receptor was observed. This can be explained by translocation of cytosolic receptor to the nucleus[19] and a decrease in the stimulatory effect of estradiol.[15]

Finally, the oviductal response to progesterone action can be related to the increased activity of estradiol 17-β dehydrogenase observed during the secretory phase.[20] The increase in this enzyme activity, followed by an increased content of estrone during the secretory phase (Fig. 9:4), suggests that enhanced oxidation of estradiol occurs in the oviduct, as in the endometrium,[9,21] a long-term mechanism for progesterone antagonism of estradiol action.

Steroid Receptors in the Normal Tube

The low intrauterine pregnancy rates following restoration of tubal patency in a hydrosalpinx by microsurgery has been associated with the endosalpingeal damage caused by infection. We analyzed estradiol and progesterone receptors in cytosol and nuclear fractions from the hydrosalpinx of infertile patients.[22] The binding constants for these specific receptors were the same as those observed in normal tissues. However, the mean levels of estradiol receptors and progesterone cytosol receptors were significantly lower than those of the normal fallopian tube (Table 9:2). The decrease observed in the steroid receptor population of the damaged tube could be another cause of the poor pregnancy rates following salpingoneostomy.

In summary, the results presented in our study clearly demonstrate an accurate estradiol and progesterone interplay on the human oviduct. This is shown by the distribution observed in the content of receptors between cytosol and nuclear fractions and by the relationship between the

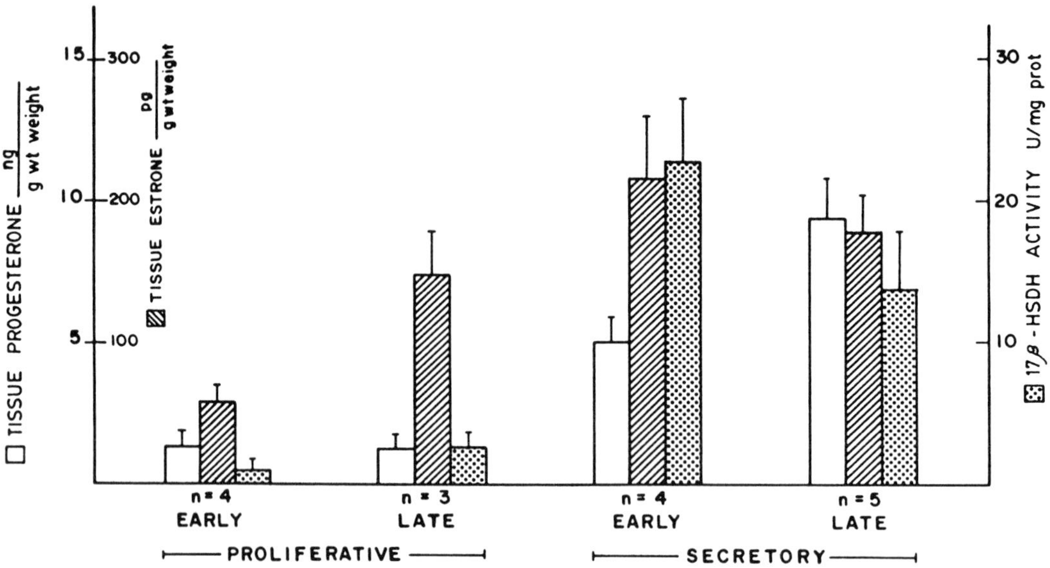

FIGURE 9:4—*Levels of 17 β-HSDH, estrone, and progesterone in oviduct at different stages of the menstrual cycle. The bars indicate the mean ± SEM of the number of samples indicated.*

Table 9:2

Comparison of Estradiol and Progesterone Receptor Content in Hydrosalpinx and Normal Tube

	Estradiol receptor		*Progesterone receptor (fmol/mg protein)*	
	Cytosol	*Nuclear*	*Cytosol*	*Nuclear*
Hydrosalpinx $n = 9$	$14.6 \pm 4.2^{\dagger}$	$43.6 \pm 8.6^{\dagger}$	$213 \pm 79^{\dagger}$	107 ± 24
Normal fallopian tube $n = 7$	60 ± 25	120 ± 30	465 ± 108	143 ± 25

*Mean ± standard error.
†Significantly different as compared with normal tube ($p < 0.05$).

tissue response to these hormones. Thus, estradiol action ensures subsequent progesterone action by promoting progesterone receptor synthesis. On the other hand, progesterone action provides an enzymatic activity that attenuates estradiol action.

Undoubtedly, these are not unique proteins that arise as a response to steroid action in this tissue. It would be interesting to identify other tissue-specific proteins that result from the action of ovarian hormones in controlling the physiological phenomena in the oviduct. The diminished steroid action in hydrosalpinx, expected as a consequence of a diminished steroid receptor content, could indicate a poorer oviductal milieu for the crucial processes that occur in the tube.

References

1. Winston RML: Microsurgery of the fallopian tube: From fantasy to reality. *Fertil Steril*, 34:521, 1980.
2. Aitken RJ: Tubal and uterine secretions, the possibilities for contraceptive attack. *J Reprod Fertil*, 55:247, 1979.
3. Verhage HG, Bareither ML, Jaffe RC, et al: Cyclic changes in ciliation, secretion and cell height of the oviductal epithelium in women. *Am J Anat*, 156:505, 1979.
4. Jensen EV, Green GL, Closs LE, et al: Receptors reconsidered: A 20 year perspective. *Recent Prog Horm Res*, 38:1, 1982.
5. Flickinger GL, Elsner C, Illingworth DV, et al: Estrogen and progesterone receptors in the female genital tract of humans and monkeys. *Ann NY Acad Sci*, 286:180, 1977.
6. Fuentealba B, Escudero G, and Swaneck G: Progesterone binding protein in cytosol fraction from human oviduct. In Harper MJK, Pauerstein CJ, Adams CE, et al (Eds): *Ovum Transport and Fertility Regulation*. Copenhagen: Scriptor, 1976:527.
7. DeVoto L, Soto E, Magofke AM, et al: Unconjugated steroids in the fallopian tube and peripheral blood during the normal menstrual cycle. *Fertil Steril*, 33:613, 1980.
8. Leavitt W, Chen TJ, and Allen TC: Regulation of progesterone receptor formation by estrogen action. *Ann NY Acad Sci*, 286:210, 1977.
9. Tseng L, and Gurpide E: Induction of human endometrial estradiol dehydrogenase by progestins. *Endocrinology*, 97:825, 1975.
10. Pino AM, DeVoto L, Soto E, et al: Changes in cytosolic and nuclear estradiol receptors of normal fallopian tube throughout the menstrual cycle. *J Steroid Biochem*, 16:193, 1982.
11. Pino AM, DeVoto L, Davila M, et al: Changes during the menstrual cycle in cytosolic and nuclear concentrations of progestogen receptor in the human fallopian tube. *J Reprod Fertil*, 70:481, 1974.
12. King RJB, and Mainwaring WIP: Oestrogens. In King RJ (Ed): *Steroid-Cell Interactions*. London: Butterworths, 1974:190, 248.
13. West NB, and Brenner RM: Estrogen receptor levels in the oviducts and endometria of cynomolgus macaques during the menstrual cycle. *Biol Reprod*, 29:1303, 1983.
14. Coulson PB, and Pavlik EJ: Effects of estrogen and progesterone on cytoplasmic estrogen receptor and rates of protein synthesis in rat uterus. *J Steroid Biochem*, 8:205, 1977.
15. Evans RW, Chen TJ, Hendry WJ III, et al: Progesterone regulation of estrogen receptor in the hamster uterus during the estrous cycle. *Endocrinology*, 107:383, 1980.
16. Verhage HG, Akbar M, and Jaffe RC: Cyclic changes in cytosol progesterone receptor of human fallopian tube. *J Clin Endocrinol Metab*, 51:776, 1980.
17. Runnonen R, and Lukola A: Binding of estrogen and progestin in the human fallopian tube. *Fertil Steril*, 36:610, 1981.
18. Pollow K, Inthraphuvasak J, Manz B, et al: A comparison of cytoplasmic and nuclear estradiol and progesterone receptors in human fallopian tube and endometrial tissue. *Fertil Steril*, 36:615, 1981.
19. Vu Hai MT, Logeat F, Warenbourg M, et al: Hormonal control of progesterone receptors. *Ann NY Acad Sci*, 286:199, 1977.
20. Sierralta W, Pino AM, Magofke AM, et al: Estradiol dehydrogenase activity in the fallopian tube during the normal menstrual cycle. *Arch Gynäkol*, 230: 189, 1981.
21. Tseng L, and Gurpide E. Estradiol and 20 L-dihydroprogesterone dehydrogenase activity in human endometrium during the menstrual cycle. *Endocrinology*, 94:419, 1974.
22. DeVoto L, Pino AM, Las Heras J, et al: Estradiol and progesterone nuclear and cytosol receptors of hydrosalpinx. American Fertility Society Meeting, San Francisco, California, April 1983.

10

Hormonal Control of the Mammalian Oviduct: Morphological Features and the Steroid Receptor Systems

Harold G. Verhage and
Randal C. Jaffe

The mammalian oviduct is a target tissue for the ovarian steroids, estrogen and progesterone. These hormones play an essential role in allowing the mammalian oviduct to provide an environment that supports the gametes, the process of fertilization, early embryonic development, and the delivery of a viable embryo to the uterus. Just as the ovarian steroids are synthesized and released in a cyclic nature, various morphological and biochemical changes of the oviduct also demonstrate a cyclic pattern. This is particularly true of the epithelium that lines the mammalian oviduct and the steroid receptor systems. It is our intent in this presentation to compare the cyclic nature of these changes in the carnivore and primate.

The Oviductal Epithelium

The epithelium of the mammalian oviduct is sensitive to the ovarian steroids; however, the degree to which this sensitivity is expressed morphologically depends on the species and the region of the oviduct studied. In the long-term ovariectomized cat (Table 10:1) and subhuman primate,[1,2] and in the anestrus dog[3] and cat,[4] the epithelial cells were cuboidal and lacked cilia and secretory granules. However, a significant number of cells remained ciliated in oviducts obtained from postmenopausal women (Table 10:2), a time when the ovary is quiescent. Even though a few ciliated cells persisted in the postmenopausal human tube, the cells

The Fallopian Tube: Basic Studies and Clinical Contributions, edited by Alvin M. Siegler, M.D. Mount Kisco, New York: Futura Publishing Company, Inc. © 1986.

Table 10:1

*Mitotic Index and Cell Height of the Oviductal Epithelium in the Ovariectomized Cat after Treatment with Estradiol (E_2) for up to 14 Days and Then with Estradiol and Progesterone for an Additional 7 Days**

Days E_2	*Mitotic index (%)*	*Cell height (μm)*
0	0	11
1	0	14
2	0.08	21
4	0.70	27
7	0.10	27
14	0.02	29
	14 days E_2 then days $E_2 + P$	
1	0	21
2	0	18
4	0	17
7	0	13

*All values are the mean of the results from three animals. Mitotic index was calculated by scanning 1,000 epithelial cells/animals, and the number of cells undergoing mitosis was counted. No mitotic index calculation was significantly different from zero. To determine the height, 15 secretory cells per oviduct were measured where the plane of section passed through the cell nucleus approximately parallel to the longitudinal axis of the cell. After one day of estradiol treatment, the cell heights were significantly different from those measured in the ovariectomized animals ($p < 0.005$). After one day of estradiol plus progesterone treatment, the cell heights were significantly different from those measured in the animals treated with estradiol for 14 days ($p < 0.005$).[7]

Table 10:2

*Cell Height and Ciliation of the Oviductal Epithelium at Various Reproductive Stages in the Human Oviduct**

	Cell height (μm)		*Ciliation (%)*	
Reproductive stage	*Fimbria*	*Ampulla*	*Fimbria*	*Ampulla*
Early follicular	24	23	49	35
Late follicular	31	29	57	41
Early luteal	26	25	51	40
Late luteal	24	23	50	43
Pregnant (10–12 wks)	21	20	41	37
Postpartum	21	21	25	25
Postmenopausal	**	17	**	21

*Values are the means of six measurements, except in the postmenopausal group where four measurements were made. Cell height was ascertained by measuring 30 cells from each oviduct where the plane of section clearly passed through the cell nucleus, parallel to the longitudinal axis of the cell. The percentage of ciliation was calculated by scanning 500 cells per oviduct.
**Not measured.[13]

were cuboidal and the nonciliated cells did not contain secretory organelles (Fig. 10:1).

Effect of Estradiol

Estradiol induced nuclear and cellular hypertrophy, hyperplasia, and the differentiation of ciliated and secretory cells in the carnivore[5] and primate oviduct.[2,6] In ovariectomized animals treated with estradiol, and all intact animals during estrus and the follicular phase thus far studied, the differentiation sequence followed the same temporal pattern. In the cat, nuclear[7] and cellular hypertrophy were evident within one day of estradiol treatment (Table 10:1), mitotic activity peaked on day four, ciliogenesis was maximal on days three through five, and mature ciliated and secretory cells were evident as early as day five.[5,7] This sequence of differentiation was also observed in cycling cynomolgus macaques if rigorous criteria were used to establish the reproductive stage.[6] The temporal pattern of differentiation induced by estradiol within the epithelium was predictable, yet the rate at which this occurred varied with the individual cell within a given region of the oviduct. For example, after being exposed to estradiol for the same length of time, cells at the base of a longitudinal mucosal fold may be at a more advanced stage of differentiation than those at the crests of the mucosal fold. Also, within the fully differentiated epithelium, patches of cells within a certain region may be mostly secretory whereas adjacent patches may consist mostly of ciliated cells. We have observed this type of regional variation in cat's[7] and human oviducts, and others have observed it in the oviducts of subhuman primates.[2,6,8] Ciliogenesis was first reported and described in detail in the rhesus monkey's oviduct.[9,10] A similar process of basal body and cilia formation has now been reported for oviducts of the mouse,[11] dog,[12] cat,[5] *Macaca nemestrina,*[2] and human fallopian tube.[13] Basal body precursors were first observed in large oval cells (Fig. 10:2), referred to as clear or electron lucent cells. Basal body precursors included fibrous granules, deuterosomes and procentrioles (Fig. 10:3). Both centriolar and acentriolar pathways of basal body formation have been observed in the oviducts of the rhesus monkey[10] and cat,[5] whereas only the acentriolar pathway was observed in the human oviduct.[13]

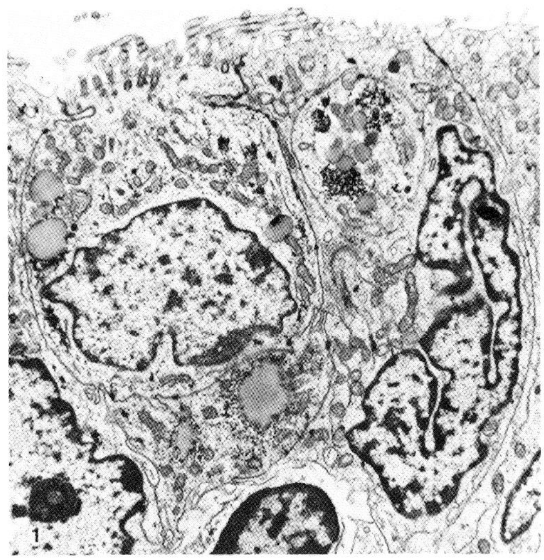

FIGURE 10:1—*Epithelium obtained from a 62-year-old postmenopausal woman. The ciliated cells still present are short and many have constricted apical borders. The nonciliated cells do not contain secretory granules. Note the lipid and glycogen deposits. The nuclear membrane forms deep folds within the nucleoplasm and the chromatin is condensed along the nuclear membrane. Ampulla, original magnification,* × *6,000.*

Controversy still surrounds the question of the extent to which the human oviduct responds to estradiol. In the cat's oviduct, estradiol treatment induced mitosis to such an extent that mitotic figures could be quantitated without using labeling techniques (Table 10:1). Mitotic figures were also observed in the human oviduct (Fig. 10:4); however, they occurred infrequently. We observed them most frequently within human tubes that also contained ciliogenic cells. In the fimbria and ampulla of subhuman primates, approximately 50 percent of the epithelial cells underwent ciliogenesis during the follicu-

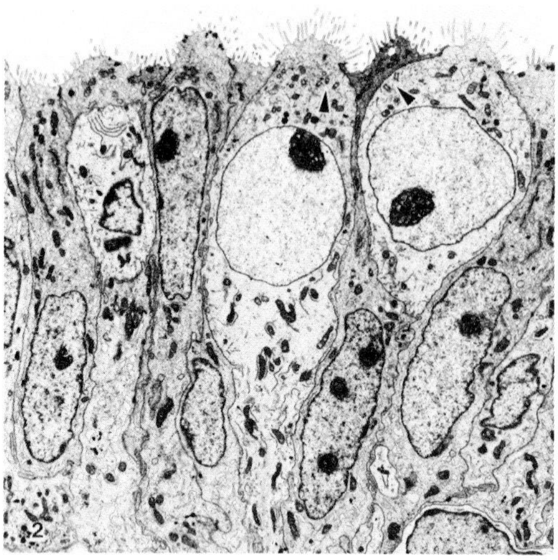

FIGURE 10:2—*Ciliogenic (clear or electron lucent) cells present in human epithelium during the follicular phase (day 8). Ciliogenic precursors (arrowheads) are present in the apical cytoplasm. Ciliogenic cells were observed as early as day 5 and as late as day 12 of the menstrual cycle. Ciliogenic cells were present in the fimbria and ampulla of 7 of the 16 oviducts examined during this stage of the menstrual cycle. Ampulla, original magnification,* × *3,400.*[13]

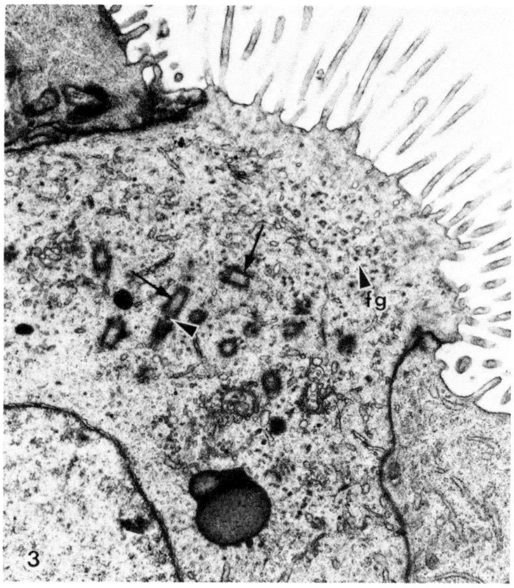

FIGURE 10:3—*Apical tip of a ciliogenic cell. Fibrous granules (fg), maturing basal bodies (procentrioles) (arrows), and a deuterosome (arrowhead) are present in the cytoplasm. Human ampulla, original magnification,* × *12,500.*[13]

lar phase,[2,6] while in human oviducts only 5 to 10 percent underwent ciliogenesis (Table 10:2). There is no known explanation for such species variation.

The appearance of the oviductal epithelium at the time of ovulation is remarkably similar in a variety of species. In the oviducts of the cat, subhuman primate,[2,6] and human fallopian tube, this included a similarity in epithelial cell height, the ratio of ciliated to secretory cells, and the ultrastructure of the ciliated and secretory cell (Tables 10:1–10:3). The greatest degree of variability was observed in the ultrastructural characteristics of the secretory granules. Electron-dense serous secretory granules were observed in dogs,[3,12] cats,[7] subhuman primates,[14] and women,[13] whereas electron lucent mucous secretory granules were observed in the rabbit's oviduct.[15] A lamellar substructure was observed in the secretory granules of sheep,[16,17] cattle,[18,19] and *Macaca nemestrina.*[14] Controversy still

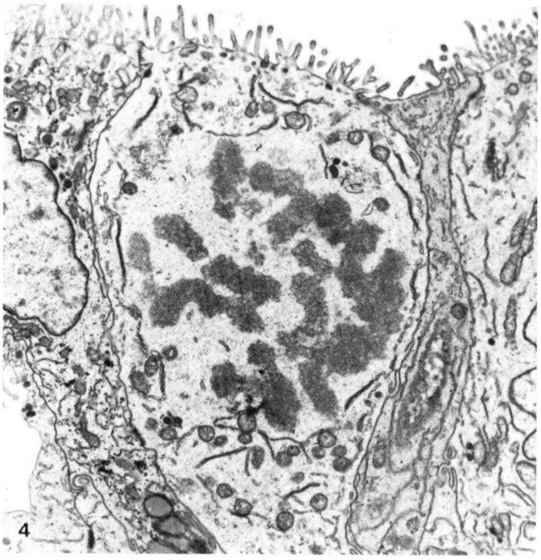

FIGURE 10:4—*Mitotic figure observed in human epithelium. Mitotic figures were most frequently observed within an epithelium that also contained ciliogenic cells. Ampulla, original magnification,* × *6,800.*

Table 10:3

*Cell Height, Ciliation, Progesterone Receptor Levels, and Serum Progesterone Levels in the Cat's Oviduct at Estrus and up to 14 days Postcoitus (PC)**

	Ampulla		*P-receptors*		
	Cell height (μm)	*Ciliation (%)*	*Cytosol (pmol/mg prot.)*	*Nuclear (fmol/μg DNA)*	*Serum P (ng/ml)*
Estrus	24 (3)	63 (3)	1.55 (4)	1.54 (4)	0.1 (5)
4 days PC	17 (3)	49 (3)	0.63 (3)	4.19 (3)	1.0 (3)
7 days PC	17 (3)	45 (3)	0.20 (3)	1.72 (2)	7.4 (3)
10–12 days PC	13 (2)	41 (2)	0.16 (3)	0.44 (3)	10.1 (3)
14 days PC	13 (3)	18 (3)	0.04 (3)	0.40 (3)	10.7 (3)

*Males were allowed to mate at least twice with each estrus queen and pregnancy was timed from the date of copulation. All values are the mean of the number of measurements shown in parentheses. Cell height was calculated from three different blocks of tissue per animal by measuring 45 cells per block. Percentage of ciliation was ascertained from three different blocks per animal by scanning 300 cells per block. Total cytosol receptor expressed as pmol ^{3}HP/mg protein and nuclear receptor expressed as fmol ^{3}H = R5020/μg DNA were quantitated by Scatchard analysis. Serum levels of progesterone were measured by RIA. The cell height was significantly reduced by day four postcoitus ($p < 0.05$). The percentage of ciliation at 14 days postcoitus was significantly different from that measured at all other times ($p < 0.05$). The cytosol receptor level measured at four days postcoitus was significantly different from that measured in estrus animals ($p < 0.05$).[24]

surrounds the mode of release of secretory products into the lumen. Release of secretory products is thought to occur by exocytosis in the cow,[18] ewe,[16,17] cat,[7] and *Macaca nemestrina.*[14] However, secretion of both apocrine[20,21] and holocrine[22] has been suggested for the human tubal secretory cell.

An important question that remains to be answered concerns the biochemical nature of the secretory product packaged in the electron-dense secretory granules. Recently, human tubal fluid was collected and several proteins were found to be present only during the periovulatory period.[23] It is not known whether these proteins are unique to human tubal fluid or if they are produced by the secretory cells.

Effect of Progesterone

Progesterone did not appear to have an effect on the morphology of the dedifferentiated epithelium in the dog's[12] and cat's oviduct. However, the effect of progesterone on the mature, fully differentiated epithelium was immediate and dramatic, even when elevated levels of estradiol were maintained. In both the dog's[25] and the cat's oviduct, treatment with progesterone resulted in atrophy, loss of cilia, and cessation of secretory activity. In the cat's oviduct, within one day of the elevation of progesterone in both the ovariectomized and intact animal, there was a significant reduction in cell height and the number of ciliated cells was reduced by 10 to 15 percent (Tables 10:1 and 10:3). After two to four days, electron-dense secretory granules were seldom observed. These regressive changes continued until the fully dedifferentiated state was reached.[7,24]

In both subhuman primates[2,6,14] and women,[13] the first morphological evidence for dedifferentiation occurred early in the luteal phase and included the formation of large patches of condensed chromatin along the margins of the nuclear membrane. The nuclear changes were followed by atrophy, deciliation, and cessation of secretory activity. These regressive changes were more evident in the fimbria and ampulla than in the isthmus, and were more dramatic with each menstrual cycle in oviducts from subhuman primates than in those from women. The rate of response to progesterone may just be slower in human oviducts since atrophy and deciliation continued throughout pregnancy (Table 10:2).

In both carnivore and primate oviducts, progesterone is responsible for inducing regression. Implicit within this process is the loss of cellular organelles, cytoplasm, and possibly individual cells or groups of cells. The older literature suggests that at least two mechanisms may be involved in regression: (1) the constriction and pinching off of the apical cell tips with subsequent loss of the apical cytoplasm and ciliary apparatus,[9] and (2) the loss of entire cells from the epithelium.[26] Several recent studies have reexamined the cytologic details of regression. In the dog's oviduct, morphological evidence was presented for the existence of both of these processes.[25] In addition, processes suggestive of resorption of basal bodies and cilia were observed, similar to reports in the subhuman primate's oviduct.[2] We observed an increase in lysosome-like structures and cellular death by the process of apoptosis in the cat's oviduct.[7,24] Apoptosis is a form of cell death characterized by extensive nuclear and cytoplasmic fragmentation.[27] In the cat's oviduct, apoptotic bodies were frequently observed three to four days after the elevation of serum progesterone. The early morphological stages of apoptosis were characterized by margination of the chromatin into dense masses beneath the nuclear envelope, and nuclear fragmentation (Fig. 10:5) More advanced apoptotic bodies included degenerative changes in cellular organelles and cytoplasmic fragmentation. The cellular fragments were apparently engulfed by another cell type, either a neighboring epithelial cell or possibly a macrophage (Fig. 10:6). Presumably the lysosomal system of the host cell was responsible for the further degeneration of the apoptotic bodies.[27] Apoptosis was not observed in the dog,[25] but was reported to occur in the cynomolgus macaque.[6]

We have looked for apoptotic bodies within the epithelium of the human tube. We have observed an increase in the number of macrophages, or some other type of reticuloendothelial cell, within the epithelium obtained during the luteal phase. These cells appeared identical to those reported in the cynomolgus macaque.[6] However, whether these cells are associated with the process of apoptosis still remains to be ascertained. Thus, whether apoptosis occurs as a process of oviductal cell death in a species other than the cat and possibly the cynomolgus macaque remains an open question.

In summary, several general conclusions seem appropriate based on the recent studies dealing with the cyclic nature of the oviductal epithelium in the carnivore and primate. (1) The oviductal epithelium is very sensitive to the ovarian steroids. Estradiol, when unopposed by progesterone, induces a mature epithelium consisting of ciliated and secretory cells. Progesterone, in the presence or absence of estradiol, induces atrophy and dedifferentiation. (2) A steroid sensitivity gradient exists such that the fimbria, when compared to the ampulla and isthmus, is the most sensitive when cell height, percentage ciliation, and presence of secretory granules are used as quantitative indicators. (3) The epithelium of the human tube demonstrates a slower rate of response to progesterone than the oviductal epithelium of the subhuman primate. This appears to be particularly true for the extent of deciliation, and thus reciliation, that occurs with each menstrual cycle. (4) Estradiol induces mitosis within the oviductal epithelium. Progesterone induces the loss of epithelial cells by sloughing, apoptosis, or possibly some other autolytic process during the regressive phase. Perhaps mitosis and cell loss are counterbalancing processes that assure the oviduct of a healthy population of epi-

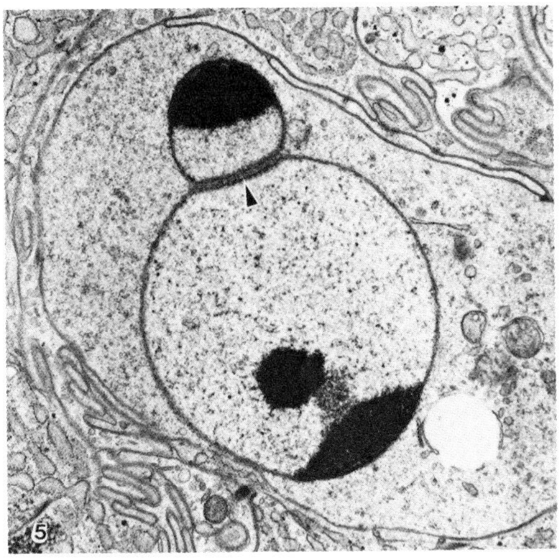

FIGURE 10:5—*An early stage of apoptotic degeneration observed in an ovariectomized cat treated for 14 days with estradiol, and then for 4 days with both estradiol and progesterone. Margination of the electron-dense chromatin is evident, and the nuclear membranes are still fused (arrowhead) between the nuclear fragments. Ampulla, original magnification,* × *15,400.*[7]

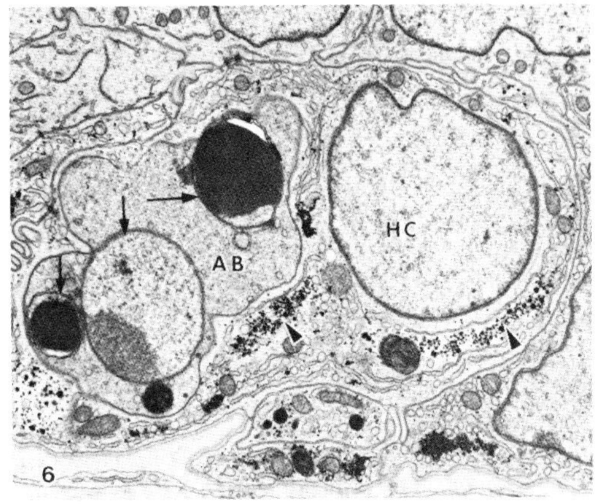

FIGURE 10:6—*An advanced stage in the process of apoptosis as observed in the ampulla obtained from a cat seven days after coitus (approximately six days after ovulation or about three to four days after progesterone begins to rise in the peripheral plasma). The apoptotic body (AB) appears to be within a host cell (HC). The host cell is probably an epithelial cell since it contains glycogen deposits (arrowheads), a characteristic of the epithelial cells at this stage. Arrows point to nuclear fragments. Original magnification,* × *9,700.*[24]

thelial cells capable of responding to the ovarian steroids. Further, these two processes may be a mechanism, inherent within the oviduct, capable of restoring damaged tubes. This mechanism may have important implications in tubal abnormalities, namely hydrosalpinx and salpingitis. Following treatment for the occlusion, the tube may be capable of restoring the mucosal lining during subsequent menstrual cycles.

The Steroid Receptor Systems

Both estrogen and progesterone receptors have been identified in the mammalian oviduct. Competition studies have shown that the estrogen receptors have a high affinity for estradiol and diethylstilbestrol[28,29] and that progesterone receptors have a high affinity for progesterone and R5020.[29–31] Both the estrogen and progesterone receptors had sedimentation coefficients of approximately 8 S in buffers of low ionic strength.[1,29,31] The binding affinity for estradiol ($K_A = 10^{10}$ M^{-1}),[32,33] and progesterone ($K_A = 10^{10}$ M^{-1})[28,29] by their respective receptors was high. Thus, the estrogen and progesterone receptors of the oviduct are very similar to those reported for the uterus and other steroid target tissues.

The steroid receptors are under the endocrine control of the ovarian steroids. Since the plasma concentrations of the ovarian steroids are dependent on the stage of the estrual or menstrual cycle, one would predict that the estrogen and progesterone receptors also exhibit stage-related variations. Several recent studies have corroborated such a pattern.

Control of the Estrogen Receptor System

In spayed macaques cytoplasmic estradiol receptor levels in the oviduct were increased during periods of estradiol treatment and these levels were suppressed when progesterone was added to the treatment regimen. When progesterone treatment was discontinued, the receptor levels were again elevated.[1] In a similar study in the cat's oviduct, estradiol treatment caused a dramatic elevation in the estradiol receptor content in both the cytoplasmic and nuclear compartments, while progesterone treatment again led to a reduction in the receptor levels in both the cytosol and nuclear compartments, even in animals continuously treated with estradiol. The degree to which the estrogen receptor was reduced following progesterone administration was similar to that observed with estrogen withdrawal.[34] These studies support the hypothesis that the synthesis of cytoplasmic estrogen receptors and their subsequent translocation to the nuclear compartment occurred during periods when the plasma levels of estradiol were elevated, and that progesterone, in the presence or absence of estradiol, suppressed the total estrogen receptor system. The suppression of the total estrogen receptor system was similar to what was observed in the spayed or estrogen-withdrawn animal.

The relationship between the estrogen receptor concentration in the oviduct and the plasma concentration of the ovarian steroids during the menstrual cycle in the cynomolgus macaque was shown to be consistent with that observed in the experimentally manipulated ovariectomized animal.[35] Cytoplasmic receptor levels were shown to be higher during the follicular phase than during the luteal phase. Nuclear receptor levels were increased during the follicular phase in parallel with the increase in serum estradiol concentrations and were significantly decreased during the luteal phase. These investigators hypothesized that the serum levels of estradiol were adequate during the entire macaque menstrual cycle to maintain elevated levels of the estradiol receptor system, and that the cyclic nature of this receptor system was caused by the rise in progesterone concentration which occurred during the luteal phase.

Several recent studies suggested that cyclicity occurs in the human oviduct also. Three groups reported that the nuclear receptor levels reached their zenith during the late follicular phase and then underwent a significant decline during the luteal phase.[28,29,32] In summary, the estrogen receptor system displays a cyclic nature during each menstrual cycle. Furthermore, progesterone appears to be the steroid responsible for the reduction seen in estrogen receptor levels during the luteal phase in both the cytoplasmic and the nuclear compartments.

Control of the Progesterone Receptor System

Estradiol induced the synthesis of the progesterone receptor in the immature dog's oviduct.[36] In estradiol-primed ovariectomized cat's oviducts, the intravenous infusion of progesterone resulted in a significant depletion of cytosol and marked elevation of nuclear progesterone receptor levels.[30] In oviducts of the cat, dog[37] and woman,[28,29] the cytosol progesterone receptor levels were elevated at estrus or during the follicular phase, a time when progesterone levels were low or undetectable, and depressed following coitus or during the luteal phase, a time when progesterone levels were elevated (Tables 10:3 and 10:4). We have observed a significant increase in nuclear receptor levels immediately after coitus in the cat's oviducts (Table 10:3) and during the early luteal phase in human oviducts (Table 10:4), although some investigators measured higher nuclear receptor levels during the follicular phase when compared to the luteal phase in human oviducts.[28,29] The increase in nuclear binding that we observed occurred when progesterone was first detected in peripheral plasma. Following the initial elevation of nuclear progesterone receptor levels, nuclear receptor levels were reduced if elevated levels of progesterone persisted (Tables 10:3 and 10:4). Both the cytosol and the nuclear progesterone receptor levels remained depressed during pregnancy and

Table 10:4

*Progesterone Receptor Levels and Serum Levels of Estradiol and Progesterone in the Human Oviduct**

Reproductive stage	Cytosol (pmol/mg Prot)	Nuclear (fmol/μg DNA)	E_2 (pg/ml)	P (ng/ml)
Early follicular	0.4 (3)	N.D. (3)	61 (3)	0.2 (3)
Late follicular	1.9 (4)	1.2 (5)	339 (4)	0.4 (4)
Early luteal	0.3 (5)	3.9 (3)	121 (4)	6.8 (5)
Late luteal	0.2 (5)	0.3 (5)	133 (4)	10.4 (4)
Pregnant (10–12 weeks)	0.2 (6)	0.1 (6)	$>$ 400 (5)	$>$ 150 (5)
Postpartum	0.5 (4)	N.D. (1)	205 (3)	5.5 (4)
Postmenopausal	N.D. (1)	N.D. (1)	**	**

*Values are the mean of the number of measurements shown in parentheses. Total cytosol receptor expressed as pmol ^{3}H-P/mg protein and nuclear receptor expressed as fmol ^{3}H-R5020/μg DNA were quantitated by Scatchard analysis. Serum levels of estradiol and progesterone were measured by RIA. The cytosol receptor level measured during the late follicular stage was significantly different from all other stages.
**Not measured.[31]
N.D. = nondetectable.

the postmenopausal period in human tubes (Table 10:4).

Although it is impossible to resolve the discrepancies in nuclear receptor levels which we (Tables 10:3 and 10:4) and others observed,[28,38] a couple of observations may account for some of the differences. First, the nuclear retention time of the progesterone receptor complex is very short.[39] Second, a continuous elevation in serum progesterone concentrations leads to the down regulation of the total receptor system (Tables 10:3 and 10:4).[40] Perhaps the nuclear receptor levels are elevated for only a brief time immediately following ovulation. Care must therefore be taken when one is determining the stage of the menstrual cycle since the level of receptor will vary, depending on how long progesterone concentrations were elevated.

The current data support the hypothesis that estradiol induces the synthesis of the progesterone receptor. Elevated levels of progesterone first result in the translocation and increased nuclear binding of the progesterone receptor and later these elevated levels result in the down regulation of the total receptor system. Thus, the steroid control of the progesterone receptor system in the mammalian oviduct is identical to that described for the mammalian uterus.

Conclusions

Clearly, estradiol is responsible for inducing a mature oviductal epithelium consisting of columnar ciliated and secretory cells. Progesterone is antiestrogenic. The response to progesterone appears to be similar in the epithelium of the subhuman and human oviduct when cell height and loss of secretory activity are used as comparative measurements. However, the human tube is more resistant to progesterone-induced deciliation.

Our studies, as well as those of others, have shown that the estrogen and progesterone receptor systems mediate the effects of the respective steroids on oviductal morphology. The changes in receptor levels are critical, along with hormone levels, in determining the functional state of the oviduct.

References

1. Brenner RM, Resko AJ, and West NB: Cyclic changes in oviductal morphology and residual cytoplasmic estradiol binding capacity induced by sequential estradiol-progesterone treatment of spayed rhesus monkeys. *Endocrinology,* 95:1094, 1974.
2. Odor DL, Gaddum-Rosse P, Rumery RE, et al: Cyclic variations in the oviductal ciliated cells during the menstrual cycle and after estrogen treatment in the pig-tailed monkey, *Macaca nemestrina. Anat Rec,* 198:35, 1980.
3. Verhage HG, Abel JH Jr, Tietz WJ Jr, et al: Development and maintenance of the oviductal epithelium during the estrous cycle in the bitch. *Biol Reprod,* 9:460, 1973.
4. West NB, Verhage HG, and Brenner RM: Changes in nuclear estradiol receptor and cell structure during estrous cycles and pregnancy in the oviduct and uterus of cats. *Biol Reprod,* 17:138, 1977.
5. Verhage HG, and Brenner RM: Estradiol-induced differentiation of the oviductal epithelium in ovariectomized cats. *Biol Reprod,* 13:104, 1975.
6. Brenner RM, Carlisle KS, Hess DL, et al: Morphology of the oviducts and endometria of cynomolgus macaques during the menstrual cycle. *Biol Reprod,* 29:1289, 1983.
7. Bareither ML, and Verhage HG: Control of the secretory cell cycle in cat oviduct by estradiol and progesterone. *Am J Anat,* 162:107, 1981.
8. Rumery RE, Gaddum-Rosse P, Blandau RJ, et al: Cyclic changes in ciliation of the oviductal epithelium in the pigtailed macaque *Macaca nemestrina. Am J Anat,* 153:345, 1978.
9. Brenner RM: Renewal of oviduct cilia during the menstrual cycle of the rhesus monkey. *Fertil Steril,* 20:599, 1969.
10. Anderson RGW, and Brenner RM: The formation of basal bodies (centrioles) in the rhesus monkey oviduct. *J Cell Biol,* 50:10, 1971.
11. Dirksen ER: Centriole morphogenesis in developing ciliated epithelium of the mouse oviduct. *J Cell Biol,* 51:286, 1971.
12. Verhage HG, Abel JH Jr, Tietz WJ Jr, et al: Estrogen-induced differentiation of the oviductal epithelium in prepubertal dogs. *Biol Reprod,* 9:475, 1973.
13. Verhage HG, Bareither ML, Jaffe RC, et al: Cyclic changes in ciliation, secretion and cell height of the oviductal epithelium in women. *Am J Anat,* 156:505, 1979.
14. Odor DL, Gaddum-Rosse P, and Rumery RE: Secretory cells of the oviduct of the pig-tailed monkey, *Macaca nemestrina,* during the menstrual cycle and after estrogen treatment. *Am J Anat,* 166:149, 1983.
15. Greenwald GS: Endocrinology of oviductal secretions. In Hafez ESE, and Blandau RJ (Eds): *The Mammalian Oviduct.* Chicago: University of Chicago Press, 1969:183.
16. Willemse AH, and Van Vorstenbosch CJ: The secretory activity of the epithelium of the ampulla tubae in cyclic ewes: An electron microscopical study. *Tijdschr Diergeneeskd,* 100:95, 1975.
17. Russe I, and Liebich HG: Maturation of secretory granules in the endosalpinx one to four days post-coitum in sheep. *Cell Tissue Res,* 201:145, 1979.
18. Bjorkman N, and Fredricsson B: The bovine oviduct epithelium and its secretory process as studied with the electron microscope and histochemical tests. *Ztschr Zellforsch,* 55:500, 1961.
19. Nayak RK, and Ellington EF: Ultrastructural and ultracytochemical cyclic changes in the bovine uterine tube (oviduct) epithelium. *Am J Vet Res,* 38:157, 1977.
20. Overbeck L: Die Feinstruktur des Tubenepithels im mensuellen Zyklus. *Ztschr Geburtsh Gynäkol,* 171:241, 1969.
21. Ferenczy A, and Richart RM: Scanning electron microscopy of human female genital tract. *NY State J Med,* 74:794, 1974.
22. Clyman MJ: Electron microscopy of the human fallopian tube. *Fertil Steril,* 17:281, 1966.
23. Lippes J, Krasner J, Alfonso LA, et al: Human oviductal fluid proteins. *Fertil Steril,* 36:623, 1981.
24. Verhage HG, Murray MK, Boomsma RA, et al: The postovulatory cat oviduct and uterus: Correlation of morphological features with progesterone receptor levels. *Anat Rec,* 208:521, 1984.
25. Sawyer HR, Olson PN, and Gorell TA: Effects of progesterone on the oviductal

epithelium in estrogen-primed prepubertal beagles: Light and electron microscopic observations. *Am J Anat,* 169:75, 1984.
26. Flerko B: Die Epithelia des Eileiters und ihre hormonalen Reaktionen. *Ztsch Mikr Anat Forsch,* 61:99, 1956.
27. Wyllie AH, Kerr JF, and Currie AR: Cell death: The significance of apoptosis. *Int Rev Cytol,* 68:251, 1980.
28. Punnonen R, and Lukola A: Binding of estrogen and progestin in the human fallopian tube. *Fertil Steril,* 36:610, 1981.
29. Pollow K, Inthraphuvaska J, Grill HJ, et al: Estradiol and progesterone binding components in the cytosol of normal human fallopian tubes. *J Steroid Biochem,* 16:429, 1982.
30. Verhage HG, Akbar M, and Jaffe RC: Cytosol and nuclear progesterone receptor in cat uterus and oviduct. *J Steroid Biochem,* 11:1121, 1979.
31. Verhage HG, Akbar M, and Jaffe RC: Cyclic changes in cytosol progesterone receptor of human fallopian tube. *J Clin Endocrinol Metab,* 51:776, 1980.
32. Pino AM, DeVoto L, Soto E, et al: Changes in cytosolic and nuclear estradiol receptors of normal fallopian tube through the menstrual cycle. *J Steroid Biochem,* 16:193, 1982.
33. Muechler EK, and Cary D: Further characterization of estrogen receptors in the human oviduct. *Fertil Steril,* 39:819, 1983.
34. West NB, Verhage HG, and Brenner RM: Suppression of the estradiol receptor system by progesterone in the oviduct and uterus of the cat. *Endocrinology,* 99:1010, 1976.
35. West NB, and Brenner RM: Estrogen receptor levels in the oviducts and endometria of cynomolgus macaques during the menstrual cycle. *Biol Reprod,* 29:1303, 1983.
36. Lessey BA, and Gorell TA: Analysis of the progesterone receptor in the beagle uterus and oviduct. *J Steroid Biochem,* 13:1173, 1980.
37. Lessey BA, Wahawisan R, and Gorell TA: Hormonal regulation of cytoplasmic estrogen and progesterone receptors in the beagle uterus and oviduct. *Mol Cell Endocrinol,* 21:171, 1981.
38. Pollow K, Intraphuvask J, Manz B, et al: A comparison of cytoplasmic and nuclear estradiol and progesterone receptors in human fallopian tube and endometrial tissue. *Fertil Steril,* 36:615, 1981.
39. Verhage, HG, Boomsma RA, Murray MK, et al: Subcellular compartmentalization of the progesterone receptor in cat uteri following the acute administration of progesterone. *Biol Reprod,* 28:545, 1983.
40. Boomsma RA, Jaffe RC, and Verhage HG: The uterine progestational response in cats: Changes in morphology and progesterone receptors during chronic administration of progesterone to estradiol-primed and nonprimed animals. *Biol Reprod,* 26:511, 1982.

11

Prostaglandins and Tubal Functions

Bo Lindblom

The prostaglandins (PGs) are a family of biologically active lipids; because they are characterized by an action close to the site of production, they have been looked on as "local hormones." More recently, PGs were considered as messengers or modulators of hormonal and neuronal effects in various organs and tissues. The number of biological systems known to involve PGs is constantly increasing, especially since new pathways in the metabolism of the PG precursor, arachidonic acid, are still being discovered. This chapter presents the current knowledge about the role of PGs in oviductal function with special emphasis on information related to the human fallopian tube.

Ovum Pickup

The process of ovum transport starts with the pickup of the ovum cumulus mass from the surface of the ruptured follicle, a function that is normally carried out by sweeping movements of the fimbriae over the ovarian surface. The fimbrial movements occur only at ovulation and are accompanied by an approximation of the ovary and the tubal "funnel," the infundibulum, brought about by muscular elements in the ovarian ligament and the mesosalpinx. The mechanisms controlling this series of movements are unknown but it has been speculated that a substance in the follicular fluid released at ovulation could act as a mediator. In fact, crude follicular fluid may stimulate muscular activity in isolated human tubo-ovarian ligaments and fimbriae.[1] Since the preovulatory follicle may produce considerable amounts of prostaglandins,[2] it may be conjectured that PGs could be of importance to induce contractile effects of these structures. In fact, PGI_2, PGE_2, and $PGF_{2\alpha}$ have been shown to increase the contractile activity of the human tubo-ovarian ligament at ovulation whereas only $PGF_{2\alpha}$ increases the activity of the fimbriae.[1] In addition, all three prostaglandins stimulate the contractile activity of the human mesosalpinx.[3] It is thus possible that PGs in the follicular fluid are involved in a chemotactic process to se-

The Fallopian Tube: Basic Studies and Clinical Contributions, edited by Alvin M. Siegler, M.D. Mount Kisco, New York: Futura Publishing Company, Inc.

cure the pickup of the ovum from the ovarian surface.

Ciliary Activity

Ovum pickup and the subsequent transport into the midportion of the tube (i.e., the proximal part of the ampulla), take place within a few hours of follicular rupture.[4] It has been convincingly demonstrated that ciliary activity plays a central role for the ampullary transport in the rabbit's oviduct.[5–7] The superior control of ciliary activity is thought to be exerted by ovarian hormones but detailed information concerning the role of steroids in ciliary beating is still insufficient.[8] Verdugo et al.[9] studied the influence of PGF_{α}, PGE_2, and $PGF_{2\alpha}$ on the frequency of ciliary beats in cell cultures by laser light-scattering spectroscopy. The method is based on the analysis of the spectrum of the intensity fluctuations of laser light reflected by moving objects. All three PGs were found to induce a steady and reversible increase in frequency of ciliary beat. Maximal activity was obtained at 0.1–1.0 μM. At higher concentrations, a tendency to inhibit ciliary activity was observed. At equimolar concentrations the order of efficacy was $PGF_{2\alpha} > PGE_1 > PGE_2$.

The observation that women with the immotile cilia syndrome may become pregnant[10,11] casts doubt on the importance of ciliary activity in human ovum transport. However, it is not yet known whether the women in question possess normal or optimal fertility and direct motility studies in these subjects are lacking.[7] In this connection, it is important to realize that no single part of the oviduct is essential to ovum transport: a pregnancy can occur in the absence of fimbriae, the ampulla, the ampullary-isthmic junction, the uterotubal junction, and also in the absence of both oviducts.[12] Pregnancies occurring after total hysterectomy show that not even the uterus is critical in human reproduction![13]

Muscular Activity

In spite of these observations, most investigators now consider muscular activity as the primary factor controlling ovum transport in women.[14,15] Although data are contradictory concerning the influence of exogenous sex steroids on oviductal contractility,[16] endogenous estrogens do seem to stimulate tubal contractility, whereas progesterone is inhibitory.[17] Prostaglandins have potent actions on tubal motility and were put forward early as mediators of the hormonal effects.

In-vivo Studies

Coutinho and Maia[18] showed that PGE_2 decreased the intraluminal pressure in the human fallopian tube in vivo, while $PGF_{2\alpha}$ had an opposite effect. In the monkey, the oviductal response to $PGF_{2\alpha}$ was significantly increased after both spontaneous and HCG-induced ovulation. An important finding was observed in the domestic hen by Wechsung and Houvenaghel.[19] They found that intraaortic injection of the PG precursor arachidonic acid caused an abrupt pressure increase in all parts of the oviduct and that this could be blocked by pretreatment with indomethacin. The response resembled that of PGE_2 and $PGF_{2\alpha}$. Obviously, enzyme systems are available in the intact oviduct for a rapid transformation of arachidonic acid to prostaglandins. In the rabbit, the E- and F prostaglandins are mutually antagonistic: PGF overcomes the suppressive effect of PGE and PGEs abolish the increase in tubal activity caused by F prostaglandins.[20] The PGEs also inhibit spontaneous spasmodic contractions. At ovulation, there appears to be an increased response to $PGF_{2\alpha}$, whereas the increase in ovarian estradiol and progesterone secretion during the three and a half days following coitus results in decreased responsiveness to $PGF_{2\alpha}$ and increased responsiveness to PGE.[21] It is possible that these changes might cause

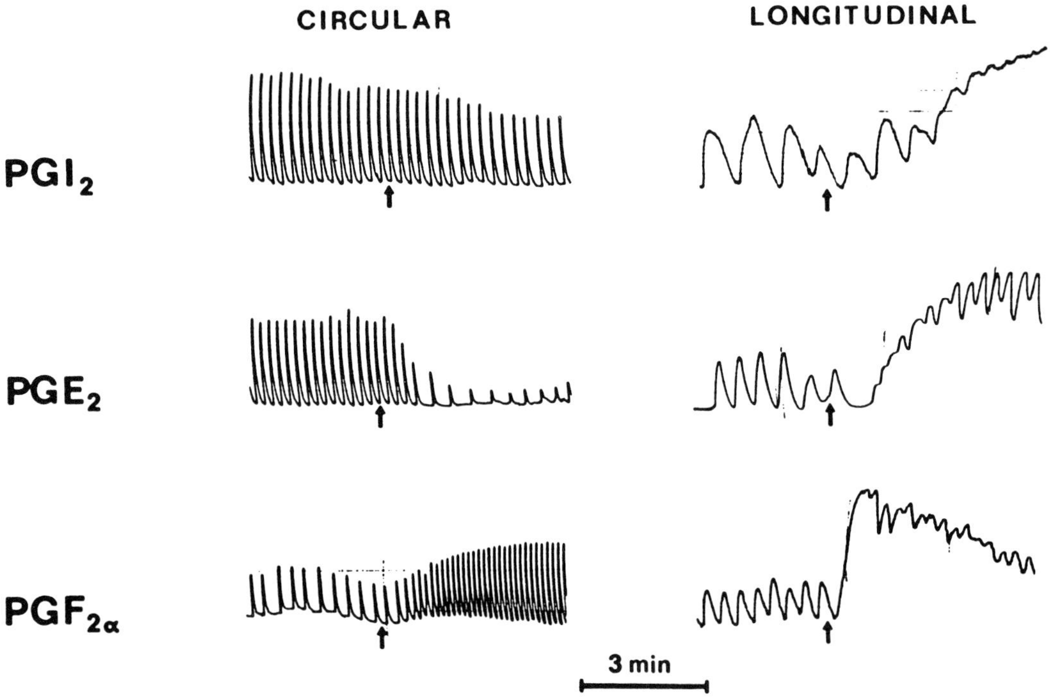

FIGURE 11:1—*The effects of PGI_2, PGE_2 and $PGF_{2\alpha}$ (10 ng/ml) on the contractile activity of muscle strips from the circular and longitudinal layers at the ampullary-isthmic junction of the human oviduct.*

relaxation of isthmic tone and allow movement of eggs through the isthmus to the uterus. Furthermore, the inhibitory effect of PGE_1 on the rabbit's oviductal response to electrofield stimulation was enhanced and the stimulatory response of $PGF_{2\alpha}$ significantly reduced 72 hours after HCG administration.[22] Using intraluminal microtransducers to record changes in diameter in unanesthetized rabbits, Blair and Beck[23] found that PGE_2 blocked spontaneous activity of both circular and longitudinal muscles, but produced little change in the internal diameter of the tube. The $PGF_{2\alpha}$, on the other hand, caused an increase in both frequency of contraction and oviductal diameter. It was thus suggested that $PGF_{2\alpha}$ accelerates egg transport in the isthmus by two mechanisms: an increase in luminal diameter causing less resistance to ovum passage and an increase in contraction frequency providing more propelling force to the egg.

In-vitro Studies

In-vitro investigations on tubal motility may provide more detailed knowledge about the interplay between different tubal segments and the various muscle layers within the tube. By microscopic dissection, pieces of circular and longitudinal muscle were isolated from the human oviduct and the contractile properties studied in organ chambers.[24] It was found that PGE_1 and PGE_2 relaxed the circular muscle layer of the isthmus at concentrations lower than 1 ng/ml, but contracted the longitudinal muscle. On the other hand, $PGF_{2\alpha}$ caused a powerful stimulation of both muscle layers (Fig. 11:1). Compared to the classic prostaglandins, PGI_2 had a comparatively weak effect.[25,26] In the ampullary portion, PGE_2 was inhibitory on the circular as well as the longitudinal layers, whereas $PGF_{2\alpha}$ was excitatory on both layers[27] (Fig. 11:2). A still more complex response was

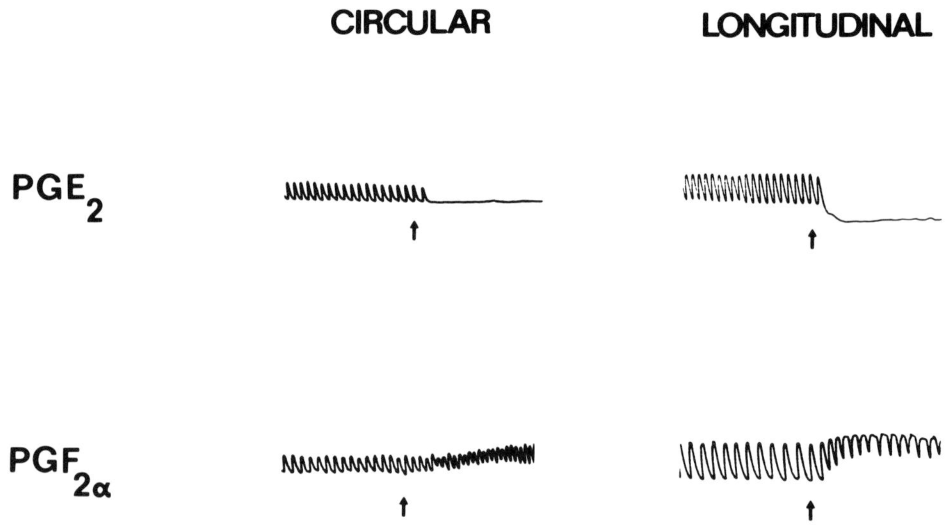

FIGURE 11:2—*Effects of PGE_2 and $PGF_{2\alpha}$ (10 ng/ml) on the contractile activity of the circular and longitudinal layers of the ampulla. PGE_2 inhibits and $PGF_{2\alpha}$ stimulates both types of strips.*

achieved at the uterotubal junction, where three different muscle layers are present. PGE_2 inhibited the activity of the innermost longitudinal layer in all phases of the menstrual cycle except in the periovulatory period, when a clearcut stimulatory response occurred.[28] Irrespective of cycle phase, the circular and outer longitudinal layers showed the same response as in the distal isthmus (Table 11:1).

Inhibitors of Prostaglandin Biosynthesis

Although the fallopian tubes thus seem to be responsive to various prostaglandins, these data do not prove that endogenous PGs play a role in the control of tubal motility. Such evidence, however, is provided by experiments using PG synthetase inhibitors. Thus, Tonpe and Lindblom[29] found that indomethacin caused a concentration dependent and reversible inhibition of tubal contractions in vitro (Fig. 11:3). Treatment with 5,8,11,14-eicosatetraynoic acid (ETYA), blocking both the cyclooxygenase and the lipooxygenase pathways in arachidonate metabolism, also causes inhibition of contractile activity of the human oviduct and normal activity can be restored in both the circular and longitudinal muscle layers of the ampullary-isthmic junction by low concentrations of $PGF_{2\alpha}$.[30] Furthermore, it was shown that arachidonic acid could induce a stimulatory response, which was blocked by ETYA. Together these data provide strong evidence that the smooth muscle of the human oviduct has the capacity to convert both endogenous and exogenous arachidonic acid to active PGs. In this context it is of interest that studies on the mechanisms responsible for the contraceptive effect of copper-bearing intrauterine devices have indicated a role for PGs in the stimulatory effect of copper on contractility of the human oviduct.[31] The response to copper ions was almost identical to the stimulatory effect of $PGF_{2\alpha}$ and the response to copper could be completely blocked by indomethacin. Furthermore, after maximal stimulation of contractility by exogenous $PGF_{2\alpha}$, copper was ineffective as a stimulant (Fig. 11:4), whereas other agents, phenylephrine, a sympathomimetic amine, may cause a further stimulation after such "loading" of the muscle with $PGF_{2\alpha}$. The

Table 11:1

Effects of PGE_2 on Different Muscle Layers within the Various Segments of the Human Fallopian Tube

	Myosalpinx		
Tubal Segment	*Inner longitudinal*	*Circular*	*Outer longitudinal*
Ampulla	Absent	Inhibition	Inhibition
Ampullary-isthmic junction	Absent	Inhibition	Stimulation
Uterotubal junction	Inhibition Stimulation	Inhibition	Stimulation

conclusion is that copper ions released from a copper intrauterine contraceptive device may increase the contractility of the oviducts by an action on endogenous synthesis of prostaglandins, predominantly of the F series. The significance of this effect in comparison with other mechanisms of action of these IUDs remains to be explored.

Modes of Action

The effector systems behind the excitatory and inhibitory effects of PGs on tubal motility are far from clear, but evidence is accumulating that $PGF_{2\alpha}$ exerts its action via different mechanisms from those of PGEs. For example, the excitatory effects of both PGs on the outer longitudinal muscle layer at the ampullary-isthmic junction (AIJ) occur with a different influence on the tissue levels of cyclic AMP.[32] In the circular muscle layer where the effects of PGE_2 and $PGF_{2\alpha}$ are opposite and antagonistic, PGE_2 abolishes the discharge of action potentials whereas $PGF_{2\alpha}$ increases the spike discharge and, hence, the contractile frequency (Fig. 11:5).[33] The high degree of conformity between the effects of PGE_2 and those of PGI_2 points to a similar mechanism of action, and perhaps a common receptor.

The interesting difference between the circular and the longitudinal muscle coat of the oviduct, both with regard to spontaneous activity and response of various drugs, has recently been further analyzed by Forman et al.[34] Using the calcium antagonist nifedipine, they found evidence that the phasic spontaneous contractions in the circular layer depend on calcium influx via potential-sensitive membrane channels, while receptor-operated calcium channels seem to be involved in the PG-induced tonic contractions observed mainly in the longitudinal smooth muscle.

Blocking of α- and β-adrenoceptors does not seem to interfere with the effects of PGs and blocking of PG biosynthesis has no effect on the excitatory action of catecholamines.[17,29] Furthermore, a maximal contraction evoked by $PGF_{2\alpha}$ can be further augmented by phenylephrine. These observations strongly suggest that catecholamines and prostaglandins, at least in part, may stimulate smooth-muscle cells within the oviduct by different mechanisms. Both kinds of stimuli, however, seem equally sensitive to removal of extracellular calcium and pharmacological blocking of calcium channels.[24,29] Furthermore, an influence of PGE_2 on noradrenaline release from adrenergic terminals has been demonstrated.[35,36]

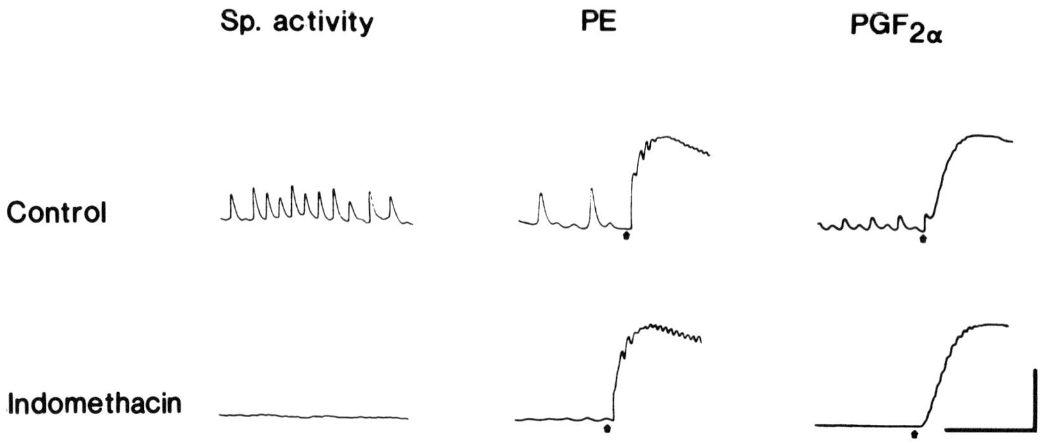

FIGURE 11:3—Left*: Spontaneous contractile activity (upper tracing) and the effect of indomethacin (40 μg/ml) (lower tracing) on the spontaneous contractile activity of longitudinal musculature from the human oviductal isthmus.* Middle*: The stimulatory effect of phenylephrine (10 μM) (upper tracing) and the effect of phenylephrine after total inhibition of spontaneous activity induced by indomethacin (40 μg/ml) (lower tracing).* Right*: The stimulatory effect of $PGF_{2\alpha}$ (0.1 μg/ml) (upper tracing) and the effect of $PGF_{2\alpha}$ after total inhibition of spontaneous activity induced by indomethacin (40 μg/ml) (lower tracing). Vertical calibration = 4 mN; horizontal calibration = 3 min.*

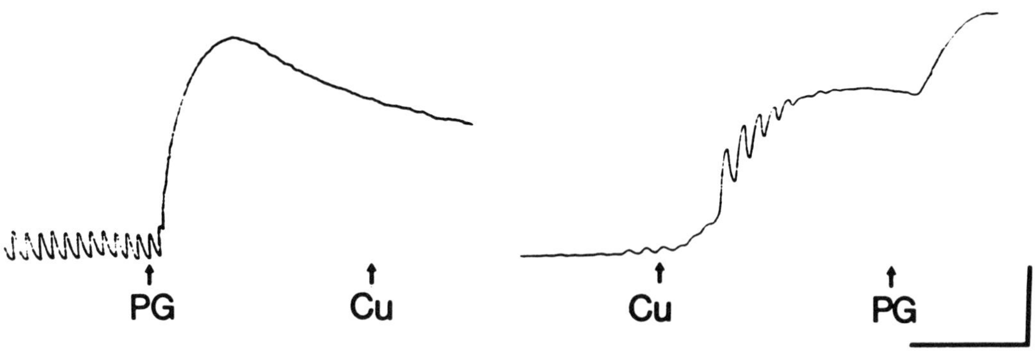

FIGURE 11:4—*After maximal response induced by $PGF_{2\alpha}$ (1 μg/ml), copper (3,000 μM) is unable to produce any further stimulation (left). After a maximal copper response, $PGF_{2\alpha}$ causes a further stimulation (right). Note the progressively developing response after administration of copper and the more acute PG response. Longitudinal muscle strips, ampullary-isthmic junction. Vertical calibration = 4 mN; horizontal calibration = 3 min.*

Prostaglandins and Ovum Transport

Despite the knowledge that has been attained with regard to the influence of endogenous and exogenous PGs on tubal motility as well as their mode of action, the involvement of PGs in human ovum transport is far from being elucidated. In 1972, Chang and Hunt[37] reported that a subcutaneous injection of $PGF_{2\alpha}$ 24 hours after insemination caused the elimination of ova from the oviducts and uteri of rabbits. Later it was shown that both PGE_1 and $PGF_{2\alpha}$ could accelerate ovum transport and reduce implantation rate appreciably if administered 13 hours after ovulation.[38] These and other findings[39] seemed promising as possibilities for using these effects of PGs for the development of a new approach for human contraception. Also, inhibitors of PG bio-

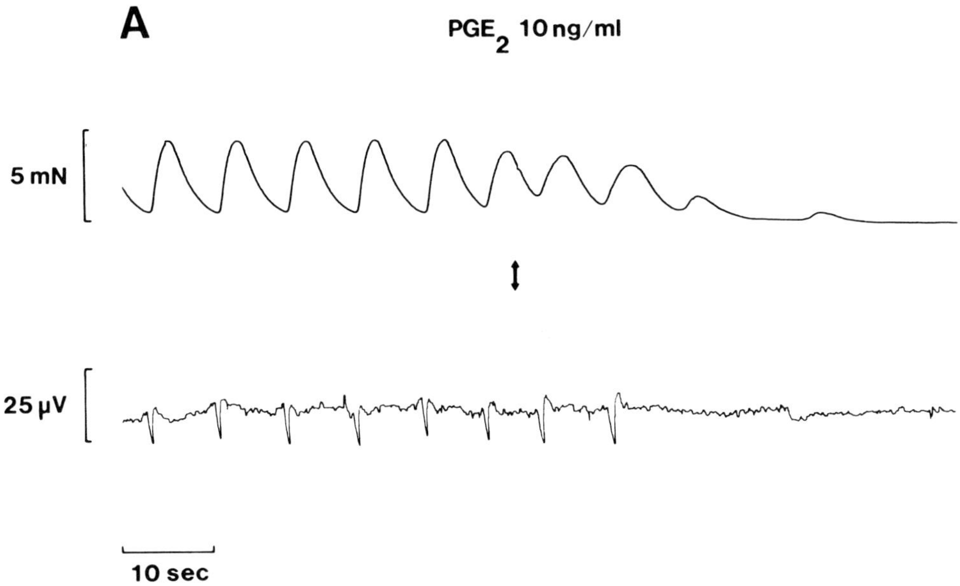

FIGURE 11:5A—*Recordings after PGE_2 treatment. PGE_2 caused no observed effect on the configuration of the action potentials during the initial phase of its inhibitory effect on contractility. After a delay of 25 to 30 sec, the action potentials suddenly disappear, concomitant with a state of complete inhibition of mechanical activity.*

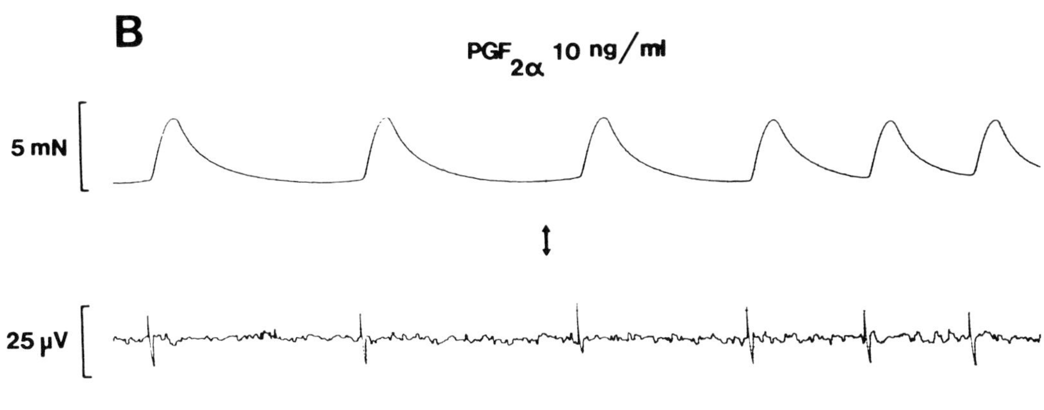

FIGURE 11:5B—*Recording of the $PGF_{2\alpha}$ effects on electrical and mechanical activity. The excitatory response is produced by an increase in the frequency of spikes.*

synthesis were shown to accelerate ovum transport in rabbits by antagonizing estrogen-induced "tube-locking." [40] However, the initial enthusiasm in this regard turned rather soon into skepticism, since clinical trials using PG analogues and other drugs were unsuccessful.[41,42]

These studies ultimately showed that compounds which stimulate tubal contractility do not necessarily accelerate ovum transport. Actually, this conclusion was not surprising in view of the fact that much of the basic knowledge derived from research in laboratory animals was applied somewhat uncritically in humans. In fact, and as mentioned previously, the details of PG action on the human oviduct are just about to emerge. The human oviducts seem to synthesize significant amounts of PGs[43] and there appears to be a correlation between the concentration of prostaglandins and egg transport in the rabbit,[44,45] but whether ovum transport can be influenced by PG compounds sufficiently to be clinically useful still remains uncertain. If a contraceptive tool acting on ovum transport is to be efficient, it probably needs to continue its attack on the uterine level, since early ovum arrival in the uterus by itself does not protect readily against pregnancy.[46]

Concluding Remarks

Prostaglandins seem to be centrally involved in a number of tubal functions. In particular, the isthmic musculature appears to be influenced by PGEs and PGFs, probably operating in a balanced system regulated by ovarian steroids. At least as regards women, knowledge about pharmacological possibilities for a contraceptive attack is still limited. It is to be hoped that the use of modern technology will lead to a deeper insight into the role of PGs in the mysteries of oviductal function and its significance in human reproduction and fertility.

Acknowledgments: Supported by grants from the Swedish Medical Research Council, (No. 2873) Magnus Bergvalls foundation and Harald Jeansson's and Harald and Greta Jeansson's foundation. Thanks are due to Mrs. Ann-Louise Dahl for expert secretarial help.

References

1. Sterin-Speziale N, Gimeno MF, Zapata C, et al: The effect of neurotransmitters, bradykinin, prostaglandins, and follicular fluid on spontaneous contractile characteristics of human fimbriae and tubo-ovarian ligaments isolated during different stages of the sexual cycle. *Int J Fertil*, 23:1, 1978.
3. Hoppen HO, Calabrese R, Voss S, et al: Prostaglandins in human follicular fluid. *Acta Endocrinol* (Suppl.), 205:135, 1983.
4. Gimeno MF, Gimeno AL, Borda E, et al: Physiological and pharmacological aspects of tubal motility. Implications of the contractile activity of the mesosalpinx. In Muldoon TG, Mahesh VB, Ballester BP (Eds): *Recent Advantages in Fertility Research, Part B, Developments in the Managements of Reproductive Disorders.* New York: Alan R Liss, Inc., 1982:77.
5. Croxatto HB, Ortiz ME, Diaz S, et al: Studies on the duration of egg transport by the human oviduct. II. Ovum location at various intervals following luteinizing hormone peak. *Am J Obstet Gynecol*, 132:629, 1978.
6. Halbert SA, Tam PY, Blandau RJ: Egg transport in the rabbit oviduct. The roles of cilia and muscle. *Science*, 191:1052, 1978.
7. Verhage et al, 1976.
8. Eddy CA: The role of cilia in tubal function. In Muldoon TG, Mahesh VB, Ballester BP (Eds): *Recent Advances in Fertility Research, Part B, Developments in the Management of Reproductive Disorders.* New York: Alan R. Liss, Inc., 1982:91.
9. Weström L, Mardh PA, von Mecklenburg C, et al: Studies on ciliated epithelia of the human genital tract. II. The mucociliary wave pattern of fallopian tube epithelium. *Fertil Steril*, 28:955, 1977.
10. Verdugo P, Rumery RE, Tam PY: Hormonal control of oviductal ciliary activity: Effects of prostaglandins. *Fertil Steril*, 33:193, 1980.
11. Afzelius BA, Camner P, Mossberg B: On the function of cilia in the female reproductive tract. *Fertil Steril*, 29:72, 1978.
12. Jean Y, Langlais J, Roberts KD, et al: Fertility of a woman with nonfunctional ciliated cells in the fallopian tubes. *Fertil Steril*, 31:349, 1979.
13. Pauerstein CJ, Carlton AE: The role of the oviduct in reproduction; Our knowledge and our ignorance. *J Reprod Fertil*, 55:223, 1979.
14. Meizner I, Glezerman M, Harroch DB, et al: Abdominal pregnancy following hysterectomy. *Obstet Gynecol*, 39:145, 1984.

14. Anand S, Guha SK: Mechanisms of transport of the ovum in the oviduct. *Med Biol Eng Comput*, 16:256, 1978.
15. Blandau RJ: Comparative aspects of tubal anatomy and physiology as they relate to reconstructive procedures. *J Reprod Med*, 21:7, 1978.
16. Aref I, Hafez ESE: Utero-oviductal motility with emphasis on ova transport. *Obstet Gynecol Surv*, 28:680, 1973.
17. Lindblom B: Hormonal and neuronal control of human oviductal contractility. Thesis, University of Göteborg, 1979.
18. Coutinho EM, Maia HS: The contractile response of the human uterus, fallopian tubes, and ovary to prostaglandins in vivo. *Fertil Steril*, 22:539, 1971.
19. Wechsung E, Houvenaghel A: Effect of arachidonic acid on oviductal pressure in the domestic hen. *Biol Reprod*, 24:519, 1981.
20. Spilman CH, Harper MJK: Effect of prostaglandin on oviduct motility in estrous rabbits. *Biol Reprod*, 9:36, 1973.
21. Spilman CH: Oviduct response to prostaglandins: Influence of estradiol and progesterone. *Prostaglandins*, 25:465, 1974.
22. Maia J, Barbosa I, Harper MJK, et al: Effect of ovulation and hormonal treatment on the in vitro response of rabbit oviducts to prostaglandins E_1 and $F_{2\alpha}$. *Fertil Steril*, 28:91, 1977.
23. Blair WD, Beck LR: In vivo effects of prostaglandin $F_{2\alpha}$ and E_2 on contractility and diameter of the rabbit oviduct using intraluminal transducers. *Biol Reprod*, 16:122, 1977.
24. Lindblom B, Hamberger L, Wiqvist N: Differentiated contractile effects of prostaglandins E and F on the isolated circular and longitudinal smooth muscle of the human oviduct. *Fertil Steril*, 30:553, 1978.
25. Omini C, Pasargiklian R, Folco GC, et al: Pharmacological activity of PGI_2 and its metabolite 6-oxo-$PGF_{1\alpha}$ on human uterus and fallopian tubes. *Prostaglandins*, 15:1045, 1978.
26. Lindblom B, Wilhelmsson L, Wiqvist N: The action of prostacyclin (PGI_2) on the contractility of the isolated circular and longitudinal muscle layers of the human oviduct. *Prostaglandins*, 17:99, 1979.
27. Cashetto S, Lindblom B, Wiqvist N, et al: Prostaglandins and contractile function of the human oviductal ampulla. *Gynecol Obstet Invest*, 10:212, 1979.
28. Wilhelmsson L, Lindblom B, Wiqvist N: The human utero-tubal junction: Contractile patterns of different smooth muscle layers and the influence of prostaglandin E_2, prostaglandin $F_{2\alpha}$, and prostaglandin I_2 in vitro. *Fertil Steril*, 32:303, 1979.
29. Tonpe N, Lindblom B: The influence of prostaglandin synthetase inhibition on the spontaneous contractile activity and induced responses of the human oviduct. *Acta Physiol Scand*, 107:181, 1979.
30. Lindblom B, Andersson A: The influence of cyclooxygenase inhibitors and arachidonic acid on contractile activity of the human fallopian tube. *Biol Reprod*, 32:475, 1985.
31. Lindblom B, Hamberger L: Copper and contractility of the human fallopian tube. *Am J Obstet Gynecol*, 141:398, 1981.
32. Lindblom B, Hamberger L, Ljung B: Contractile patterns of isolated oviductal smooth muscle under different hormonal conditions. *Fertil Steril*, 33:283, 1980.
33. Lindblom B, Wikland M: Simultaneous recording of electrical and mechanical activity in isolated smooth muscle of the human oviduct. *Biol Reprod*, 27:393, 1982.
34. Forman A, Andersson KE, Ulmsten U: Effects of calcium and nifedipine on noradrenaline- and $PGF_{2\alpha}$-induced activity of the ampullary-isthmic junction of the human oviduct in vitro. *J Reprod Fertil*, 67:343, 1983.
35. Paton DM, Johns A: Effects of prostaglandin E_2 and indomethacin on responses of the isthmus of rabbit oviduct to norepinephrine and transmural stimulation. *Chem Pathol Pharmacol*, 11:15, 1975.
36. Moawad AH, Hedqvist P, Kim MH: Correlation of plasma estrogens and progesterone levels with the in vitro adrenergic response in the isthmus of the human oviduct. In Harper MJK, Pauerstein CJ, Adams CE, et al (Eds): *Ovum Transport and Fertility Regulation*. Copenhagen: Scriptor, 1976: 276.
37. Chang MC, Hunt DM: Effect of prostaglandin $F_{2\alpha}$ on the early pregnancy of rabbits. *Nature*, 226:120, 1972.

38. Ellinger JV, Kirton KT: Ovum transport in rabbits injected with prostaglandin E_1 and $F_{2\alpha}$. *Fertil Steril*, 29:456, 1978.
39. Takeda T, Tsutsumi Y, Hara S, et al: Effects of prostaglandin $F_{2\alpha}$ on egg transport and in vivo egg recovery from the vaginas of rabbits. *Fertil Steril*, 30:79, 1978.
40. Valenzuela G, Ross HD, Hodgson BJ, et al: Effect of inhibitors of prostaglandin synthesis and metabolism on ovum transport in the rabbit. *Fertil Steril*, 28:992, 1977.
41. Croxatto HB, Ortiz ME, Guiloff E, et al: Effects of 15(s)-15-methyl prostaglandin $F_{2\alpha}$ on human oviductal motility and ovum transport. *Fertil Steril*, 30:408, 1978.
42. Croxatto HB, Ortiz ME, Hess R: Attempts to modify ovum transport in women. *J Reprod Fertil*, 55:231, 1979.
43. Ogra SS, Kirton KT, Tomasi TB, et al: Prostaglandins in the human fallopian tube. *Fertil Steril*, 25:250, 1974.
44. Saksena SK, Harper MJK: Relationship between concentration of prostaglandin F(PGF) in the oviduct and egg transport in rabbits. *Biol Reprod*, 13:68, 1975.
45. Rajkumar K, Garg SK, Sharma PL: Possible role of prostaglandins in the regulation of ovum transport in rabbits. *Indian J Med Res*, 70:636, 1979.
46. Adams CE: Consequences of accelerated ovum transport, including a re-evalution of Estes' operation. *J Reprod Fertil*, 55:239, 1979.

12

Biochemistry and Immunology of Oviductal Fluid

Gene Oliphant

Collection of Oviductal Fluid

To analyze the components in the oviductal environment effectively, an efficient means of collecting oviductal fluid is required. This problem has been addressed by simply flushing the lumen; while such a method has the advantage of no previous surgical trauma to the oviduct, the amount of fluid that can be thus collected is small and it remains possible for the fluid to be contaminated by blood. A means of increasing the amount of collectible fluid is by ligation of the distal and proximal ends. Bishop[1] demonstrated that oviductal fluid would continue to accumulate up to a pressure of 77 mmHg. However, the extent to which the increased pressure affects transudation from plasma or secretion by the oviductal epithelium has not been ascertained. Cannulation of the fimbriated ends with concurrent ligation of the uterotubal junction and exteriorization of the cannula allows intermittent aspiration. This method minimizes the buildup of pressure and allows larger amounts of fluid to be collected over extended periods of time.[2,3] The disadvantage of direct cannulation is that aspiration requires the use of negative pressure on the oviduct, which may induce artificial movement of plasma across the epithelium. Further, preventing bacterial infection and contamination of the fluid during long-term collections are major problems.

Continuous flow collections have circumvented some of the problems of previous methods. Mastroianni's laboratory[4,5] has established a continuous collection technique whereby the oviductal fluid is refrigerated, thus providing better storage conditions. However, the fluid must transverse a long cannula whose capacity may represent many hours of secretion and the experimental animal must be restrained or fitted with an extensive apparatus during the period of collection. Bacterial contamination of the oviduct and oviductal fluid are potential problems. The intra-abdominal flask collection method developed by Hamner and Williams[6] attempts to limit bacterial contamination by inclusion of a "Pasteur loop" within the flask

The Fallopian Tube: Basic Studies and Clinical Contributions, edited by Alvin M. Siegler, M.D. Mount Kisco, New York: Futura Publishing Company, Inc. © 1986.

design. The design of the intraabdominal flask allows filtered air to enter the flask during fluid aspiration, eliminating the problem of negative pressure within the oviduct affecting movement of material from plasma to the oviductal lumen. The method has the advantage of long-term collection of oviductal fluid with no need to restrain the experimental animal. The intraabdominal flask method does not have the advantage of the refrigerated storage associated with the method developed by Mastroianni. If at all feasible during the use of any of the cannulation methods, time should be provided to assure recovery from minor bleeding and initial inflammatory reactions caused by cannulization.

None of the present techniques provides the perfect method for collection of oviductal fluid. However, despite the shortcoming of the collection techniques, significant advances have been made in evaluating the oviductal environment.

Oviductal Fluid Volume

The amount of oviductal fluid produced in the species investigated is mostly dependent on the animal's hormonal state. In general, high circulating concentrations of estrogen result in maximal production of oviductal fluid. In the rabbit the maximal amount of fluid produced during estrogen dominance ranges from 2.2 to 1.3 ml/day, with a mean of 1.6 ml/day.[3,7–9] The maximal amounts of oviductal fluid in rabbits is not much different from that produced by sheep in estrus, ranging from 1.0 to 1.4 ml/day,[10,11] or from monkeys just prior to ovulation, which produce 2.8 to 0.8 ml/day.[12,13] Lippes et al.[14] have reported large variations in human oviductal fluid volumes, ranging from 0.1 to 20 ml/day; however, if the first postoperative day is eliminated from collection, the average fluid volume is 1.3 ml/day which favorably compares to the results of 0.9 ml/day found by Moghissi.[15] Oviductal fluid collected from patients likely to be under estrogen domination indicated an average daily production of 1.7 ml.[14]

Either high progesterone or depressed estrogen concentrations may result in a large decrease in the daily production of oviductal fluid. Hamner[16] demonstrated that when progesterone and estrogen were administered concurrently to an ovariectomized rabbit, oviductal fluid volume decreased relative to that with estrogen treatment alone. On the other hand, the same investigator showed that ovariectomy without hormone replacement resulted in a 75 percent decrease in rabbits' oviductal fluid production.[7] Thus, maintenance of maximal fluid volumes is likely the result of positive effects of estrogen and the absence of progesterone's negative effects. In the normal intact animal, the minimal oviductal fluid volumes should therefore occur in the postovulatory period. This has been found to be the case in the species carefully examined. The average minimal volumes from many investigations of several species indicate that a 45 to 75 percent decrease occurs in the daily fluid production. Consequently, the mininal average volumes for rabbits, sheep, monkeys, and humans are 0.7, 0.4, 0.3, and 1.0 ml, respectively.[3,8–13,16,17]

Oviductal Fluid, Inorganic Compounds, and Small Metabolites

Electrolytes

Table 12:1 provides a compilation of data from many laboratories that have evaluated the inorganic constituents of oviductal fluid from women, monkeys, sheep, and rabbits. In producing this table, all values for the components have been averaged and therefore reflect a forced consensus. Also, where data were available, oviductal fluid values are compared to serum concentrations by giving a percentage of serum concentration.

Several laboratories have indicated that the osmolality of oviductal fluid is somewhat higher than that of serum.[8,16,22] In the species extensively

Table 12:1

*Electrolytes and Small Metabolites in Oviductal Fluid during Estrogen (E) or Progesterone (P) Domination**

	Units	*Human*	*Monkey*	*Sheep*	*Rabbit*
Sodium (E)	meq/1	137 (.97)†	150 (1.0)	137 (0.9)	139 (1.0)
Sodium (P)	meq/1	143 (1.01)	143 (0.9)	140 (0.9)	141 (1.0)
Potassium (E)	meq/1	13 (2.8)	4.7 (1.0)	9.1 (1.5)	6.4 (1.2)
Potassium (P)	meq/1	7 (1.6)	4.6 (1.0)	8.3 (1.4)	5.8 (1.1)
Chloride (E)	meq/1	126 (1.2)	122 (1.1)	122 (1.1)	111 (1.1)
Chloride (P)	meq/1	114 (1.1)	118 (1.0)	130 (1.1)	115 (1.1)
Calcium (E)	meq/1	1.5 (0.6)	3.1 (1.2)	2.9 (1.1)	4.8 (1.2)
Calcium (P)	meq/1	2.4 (1.0)	4.3 (1.6)	3.1 (1.2)	5.4 (1.4)
Magnesium (E)	meq/1	1.0 (1.0)		.63	.3 (1.2)
Magnesium (P)	meq/1			.96	
Bicarbonate (E)	meq/1	20 (.7)		22	37 (1.0)
Bicarbonate (P)	meq/1			22	31 (0.8)
Glucose (E)	mg%	54 (.4)	7.3	28	24 (.2)
Glucose (P)	mg%	43 (.3)	8.3		24 (.2)
Lactate (E)	mg%		1.3	2.1	24 (.5)
Lactate (P)	mg%		1.3	4.2	28 (.5)
Pyruvate (E)	mg%		1.28	6.2	1.6 (.3)
Pyruvate (P)	mg%				2.2 (.4)

*Riddick,[3] Holmdahl and Mastroianni,[4] Iritani et al.,[8] Lippes et al.,[14] David et al.,[18] Borland et al.,[19] Mastroianni et al.,[20] Restall and Wales,[21] Iritani et al.,[22] Brunton and Brusilow,[23] David et al.[24]
†Values in parentheses are percentages of serum concentrations.

studied it appears that the increased osmolality may be attributed to somewhat elevated potassium, chloride, and calcium concentrations. Sodium seems not to exceed serum concentrations and is essentially equal to serum in rabbits, sheep, and women, while the monkey appears to have somewhat decreased sodium concentration relative to serum. These concentrations are consistent with the physiological studies that concluded that sodium flux is the result of simple diffusion based on no net flux of sodium across the isolated, short-circuited rabbits' oviductal ampulla.[25] In contrast, chloride, which is consistently elevated above serum concentrations in all oviductal fluid, is actively transported, as demonstrated by the net chloride flux and short-circuit measurements.[25] Active transport of chloride was further substantiated by the reduction or abolition of the short-circuit current by cyanide, dinitrophenol, ouabain, and anoxia. The authors point out that the short-circuit current can be totally accounted for by chloride flux, although other ions could be actively transported and concealed either by being coupled to an oppositely charged ion crossing in the same direction (such as potassium, which is often found in oviductal fluid in concentrations greater than serum [Table 12:1]), or by being exchanged across the membrane for an ion of the same charge. In addition, transport of ions may differ in different regions of the oviduct, as suggested by the results of David et al.,[24] who showed that isthmic concentrations of bicarbonate were significantly higher than those found in the ampulla when fluids were analyzed after collection from ligated segments of the rabbit oviduct.

Many laboratories have evaluated the

changes that may take place when the hormonal state of the animal switches from estrogen domination to progesterone influence (two or more days postovulatory) (Table 12:1). The increase in the concentration of calcium in oviductal fluid appears to be the most consistent change in the inorganic constituents as a function of increased circulating progesterone concentrations.

Specific functions for the inorganic constitutents of oviductal fluid have been suggested by wide-ranging studies of oocyte maturation, fertilization, and embryonic development. Bicarbonate has been suggested as a facilitator of sperm motility[26] and as functioning to remove the corona radiata cells after fertilization.[27] Calcium is required for the sperm acrosomal reaction[28] and therefore the relatively high concentration of calcium in oviductal fluid may play a role in that process. Elevated potassium might, as described by Douglas,[29] facilitate a steady base line secretion from the secretory cells of the epithelium.

Glucose, lactate, pyruvate and amino acids

Glucose in the oviductal fluid has been found in low concentrations, typically 20 to 40 percent of serum concentrations (Table 12:1). That appears to be the case for many species, including humans, and it has been reported that glucose gains access to the oviductal fluid by facilitated diffusion.[30] However, recent results from our laboratory, using coperfusion of the oviductal lumen and ovarian artery with labeled 3-0-methyl-glucose or L-glucose, suggest that glucose entry may be by simple diffusion.[31] To what extent glucose is important in the function of the oviductal fluid might be questioned because, at least for mouse and rabbit, glucose is not used by oocytes or early preimplantation embryos.[32] In addition, high concentrations of glucose block the hamster acrosomal reaction[33] and thus the low levels found in the oviduct may aid fertilization.

All of the 20 common amino acids are present in oviductal fluid.[6,8,22,34–37] The concentrations of amino acids that reach the oviductal lumen during a four-hour period of recycled perfusion ranges from 53 percent of plasma concentrations for glycine to 2 percent for cysteine. Under the same conditions, urea gains 100 percent access.[37] Those investigators have also found that the oviductal fluid-to-plasma ratios for alanine, valine, isoleucine, leucine, and tyrosine significantly increased after ovulation. Active transport of amino acids was not observed in their study nor did they demonstrate whether simple or facilitated diffusion was the mechanism for amino acid entry into the rabbit oviduct.

Oocytes of the mouse and rabbit readily take up and metabolize lactate and pyruvate and these energy sources will allow normal development.[32,38–40] Thus, the presence of the substrates in oviductal fluid can provide the exogenous energy requirements of the developing embryos. Analysis of oviductal fluid for lactate and pyruvate has demonstrated that it is present in mouse, rabbit, sheep and monkey,[4,6,8,20–22,41,42] but typically at concentrations lower than are found in serum (Table 12:1). Leese and Aldridge[41] report the linear accumulation of both lactate and pyruvate over a four-hour period of recycled perfusion of the oviduct. During this period both lactate and pyruvate reached only 10 percent of serum concentrations while urea was at 100 percent of serum levels. This investigation does not indicate the mechanism of accumulation of these substrates. A more recent report[43] indicates that propionate stimulates accumulation of pyruvate in oviductal fluid and is converted to pyruvate by oviductal tissue, which suggests that metabolism of the oviduct could be a major contributing source of this substrate to oviductal fluid.

The observation that lactate and pyruvate increase in rabbit oviductal fluid after ovulation[4,8] has been supported and extended by quantitative histochemical measurements in the mouse oviduct.[42,44] They have shown a significant elevation in ampullar pyruvate and lactate concentrations by 12 hours after mating but no change in isthmic pyruvate. Isthmic lactate concentrations increase until 12 hours after ovulation and remain elevated for at least 72 hours after ovulation in pregnant animals. That is in contrast to the return to preovulatory concentrations occurring by 48 hours after ovulation in pseudopregnant mice. Nieder and Corder[44] conclude that the maintenance of lactate only in pregnant animals appears to be a direct response of the oviduct to viable embryos, which thus provides optimal conditions for embryonic growth.

Steroids

Steroid hormone concentrations have been evaluated in oviductal fluid from monkeys and rabbits.[13–15] Estradiol, while decreasing in serum after ovulation, increases significantly in rabbit's oviductal fluid. The oviductal fluid-to-serum ratio goes from 1.2 during estrus to 4.0 at midpseudopregnancy (10 days after ovulation). However, this only reflects an increase in oviductal fluid estradiol from 63 pg/ml at estrus to 93 pg/ml 10 days after ovulation. In the monkey, the estradiol concentrations of oviductal fluid also become greater (approximately double) than serum concentrations after ovulation. However, there is a significant decrease in total estradiol concentration in the oviductal fluid during this period. Progesterone concentrations of rabbits' oviductal fluid are approximately equal to serum concentrations during estrus, but after ovulation when serum concentrations increase more than 30-fold, oviductal fluid progesterone concentrations only increase 3- to 5-fold. This results in low oviductal fluid-to-serum ratios for progesterone. In the oviductal fluid of monkeys, progesterone is approximately one-quarter of the serum concentration just prior to ovulation. Concentrations of progesterone in oviductal fluid do not keep pace with increases of progesterone in serum after ovulation such that three days after the ovulating doses of HCG, oviductal fluid progesterone is roughly only 15 percent of serum concentration. This provides a hormonal environment for the developing embryos that does not differ much from preovulatory serum concentrations.

Macromolecular Components of Oviductal Fluid

Total protein and general serum protein constituents

The protein concentration of oviductal fluid is typically much lower than that of plasma. Protein present in estrogen-dominated rabbit's oviductal fluid has been reported to range in concentration from 2.2 to 8 mg/ml, while in the mouse, sheep, monkey, and human, protein concentrations are 5.2, 9.3 to 30.0, 3.0 to 4.8, 1.0 to 18.0 mg/ml, respectively.[4,8,9,14,17,18,20–22,46–48] These measurements represent the protein from the entire oviduct, which may not reflect the microenvironment within separate regions. That possibility is supported by the protein concentration in the rabbit's oviductal ampulla being approximately 50 percent less than the concentration in the isthmus.[24] It should be pointed out that in this same study, the total volume in the fluids obtained from the ampulla and the isthmus differed by a ratio of 3.6:1 (ampulla:isthmus), indicating that the ampulla transfers more protein from plasma than the isthmus does.

The effect of ovulation and subsequent increase in progesterone on total protein in the oviductal fluid is not clear. In the rabbit, for instance, there are two reports of no increase in protein concentration,[4,9] a report of a decrease of 50 percent,[36] and one of a 3.5-fold increase.[8] The reasons for the differences are obscure since the techniques of collection were similar. It is possible that the different methods used for protein quantitation played a role but it would seem that the

Table 12:2

Amino Acid Composition: Family of Sulfated Glycoprotein and Oviductal Fluid (Residues/1,000 Amino Acids)

Amino Acid	*Peak A*	*Peak B*	*Peak C*	*Ratio to others' data**
Asp	93.7 ± 6.9	83.3 ± 11.2	88.8 ± 19.6	.9
Thr	40.3 ± 1.8	37.9 ± 0.4	34.9 ± 1.4	2.1
Ser	111.6 ± 4.9	120.5 ± 13.5	109.8 ± 2.9	.7
Glu	129.8 ± 1.5	141.0 ± 13.3	126.3 ± 4.1	.6
Pro	34.8 ± 6.8	31.7 ± 1.0	40.6 ± 7.8	1.8
Gly	169.1 ± 8.0	153.3 ± 21.2	169.3 ± 29.6	.4
Ala	58.6 ± 1.7	63.8 ± 3.5	63.2 ± 1.8	1.2
Val	69.5 ± 14.2	58.9 ± 8.5	54.4 ± 2.1	.8
Met	8.2 ± 1.2	8.0 ± 1.6	8.0 ± 0.7	1.2
Ile	28.0 ± 4.3	31.1 ± 1.9	32.0 ± 0.8	1.3
Leu	47.6 ± 5.5	54.4 ± 5.5	58.9 ± 0.9	2.0
Tyr	36.7 ± 0.3	35.2 ± 4.8	36.2 ± 1.5	.6
Phe	35.9 ± 2.1	35.8 ± 6.6	36.2 ± 2.7	1.2
His	27.3 ± 0.7	32.6 ± 4.2	27.7 ± 1.1	1.0
Lys	68.7 ± 7.2	69.7 ± 8.9	68.2 ± 7.0	.9
Arg	30.3 ± 3.0	35.1 ± 5.6	36.6 ± 3.6	1.4

*Amino acid concentrations from peak A were converted into units used by Shapiro et al.[50] and used to obtain the ratio between values reported by Shapiro and peak A.

relative amounts of protein before and after ovulation should have been consistent within the studies. The total protein in oviductal fluid of other species after ovulation suggests no common characteristic. The mouse's oviductal fluid decreases to 1.6 mg/ml.[21,22,35] In the cow there was no apparent cyclic variation of protein concentration of oviductal fluid, which averaged 32 mg/ml.[49] However, the authors did report considerable variation from one cow to another, with average concentrations for some as low as 3.1 mg/ml. The protein in oviductal fluids of monkeys and women increases to 5.5 to 7.0 mg/ml for the monkey[20] and 12 to 70 mg/ml in women.[17,18]

Even though there is considerably lower concentration of protein in oviductal fluid relative to serum, many of the typical serum proteins are present in all oviductal fluid (Table 12:2). The need for the many diverse serum proteins in oviductal fluid is unclear; Glass,[51] however, has demonstrated that serum proteins injected into the circulation of mice are transferred into the oviductal lumen and can be taken up by developing embryos at specific stages of development. Trypsin inhibitors might also be transferred from the plasma to protect against release of sperm enzymes in the oviductal fluid.[52]

The ability of several serum proteins to gain access to the rabbit's oviductal fluid was evaluated by quantitative measurement of plasma proteins present in the oviductal fluid. After infusing radiolabeled proteins into the circulation, the average amounts present in the serum and in oviductal fluid over a 24-hour period were compared.[9] Figure 12:1 shows that the apparent ability to enter the oviductal fluid is dependent on the macromolecular size. While this is the case for these macromolecules, examples of LDH attaining 50 percent of serum concentrations[41] and complement component C3 occurring at 17 percent of serum concentrations[9]

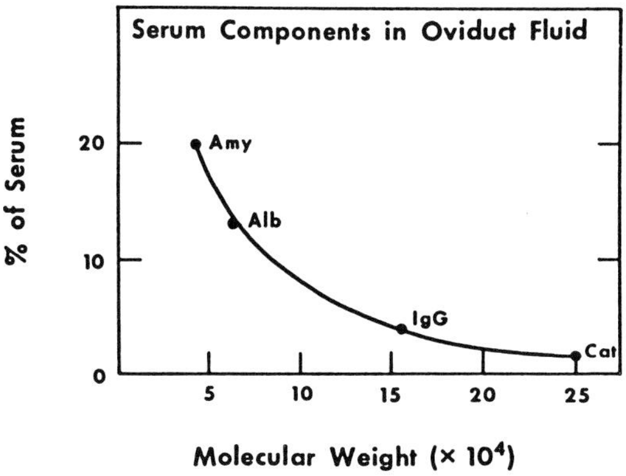

FIGURE 12:1—*The percentage concentrations of serum proteins present in oviductal fluid plotted against their molecular weights. These specific components are: amylase (Amy), Albumin (Alb), Immunoglobulin G (IgG), and Catalase (Cat). The concentrations present in the oviductal fluid were measured both by quantitative evaluation of the normal concentrations of each component in serum and oviductal fluid and by the evaluation of the relative concentrations of these components present at equilibrium 24 hours after injecting the radioactive labeled components (from Oliphant et al.[9]).*

would suggest that molecular size is not the only factor affecting serum protein entry into the oviductal fluid.

Components of the Humoral Immune System in Oviductal Fluid

Components of oviductal fluid of all species investigated have protein bands that migrate electrophoretically to regions typical for immunoglobulins (Table 12:2). Immunoglobulins have subsequently been quantitated in oviductal fluid from several species. In rabbits, three separate reports indicate that IgG is present at 4 to 11 percent of serum concentration or 0.4 mg/ml.[53–55] The same investigations demonstrated different IgA values with two reports of relatively high concentrations, 0.35 to 0.58 mg/ml,[53,54] and a very low concentration of 0.02 mg/ml.[55] On the one hand, the high levels would suggest local secretion of IgA while the low value would reject this possibility. One point that is clear from the reports is that circulating IgG can and does enter the oviduct; thus, systemic immunization to sperm or embryonic antigens is reflected in the oviductal luminal environment. Electrophoretic analysis of the monkey's oviductal fluid led also to the conclusion that immunoglobulins were present in low concentration.[56] Monkeys' oviductal fluid has recently been carefully evaluated for immunological components[57,58] and as in the rabbit, IgG is approximately 10 percent of serum concentration. Interestingly, animals that were immunized against T4 coliphages showed depressed titers for the T4 in apparent response to induction of ovulation, such that titers of 10 percent of serum levels dropped an additional 50 to 67 percent in response to HCG injections.[58] Quantitation of immunoglobulins in human oviductal fluid showed IgG in a range from 8 to 62 percent of serum concentrations and an average of 31 percent.[14] The same investigators reported an average of 49 percent of serum concentration of IgA in the human oviductal fluid. The IgA concentration added to the earlier report[59] that the secretory piece can be observed by immunohistologic localization within the oviduct suggests that local synthesis and secretion of IgA may occur in the human oviduct. The variability of these concentrations likely reflects the problems associated with collection of fluid from human oviducts and the inability to allow the woman the typical two- to three-week recovery period before oviductal fluid collection, as is generally used with experimental animals. Although IgM is not found in oviductal fluid of other species, there are conflicting reports for human oviductal fluid suggesting either none[15] or low to moderate concentration.[14]

The cytotoxic characteristic of the humoral immune system is facilitated by immunological complement. Using the classic hemolytic assay for total complement activity, none could be observed in oviductal fluids of the rabbit or monkey.[53,58] Immunological complement is, however, composed of many components.

When the most abundant component, C_3, was quantitated, it was found at 17 percent of serum concentrations in the oviductal fluid of rabbits.[53] This suggests that the complement system is not necessarily inactive because it is not present in the oviductal fluid; indeed, our laboratory has demonstrated the presence of an inhibitor to complement activity in rabbits' oviductal fluid.[60,61]

Specific Macromolecules Secreted by the Oviduct

The classic histology of the oviduct shows that the oviductal epithelium is composed mainly of two kinds of cells: ciliated and nonciliated (secretory).[62,63] Electron microscopic observations of oviducts of the mouse, rabbit, sheep, and human show similar characteristics of the nonciliated cells.[64–69] Typically, the secretory cells are covered with microvilli and contain secretory granules of varying electron densities. In the ampulla the luminal surface of the cells has pedunculated protrusions containing most of the secretory granules. Isthmic cells seem to lack these protrusions but have many more secretory granules within the cell. The secretory cells are most abundant in the isthmus and it was early assumed that they may contribute oviduct-specific components to the luminal fluid.

Electrophoretic and immunological evaluation of human oviductal fluid demonstrated many of the typical serum proteins.[15] In addition, use of antiserum against human oviductal fluid in conjunction with immunoelectrophoresis showed an extra component not present in serum, which was designated the X-glycoprotein. Very recently, further electrophoretic and immunological analyses indicate that a specific component of human oviductal fluid has a molecular weight of 60 to 100 K daltons and electrophoretically it migrates close to serum albumin.[17,70] If this component represents the mucoid material reported to be secreted by the human isthmus,[69] a study of this component may provide a good biochemical marker to evaluate oviductal function.

Specific protein components for other species include a protein in the monkey that appears after ovulation and migrates electrophoretically close to transferrin under conditions that maintain the native state of the molecule.[5] Small, oviduct-specific proteins that migrate toward the cathode during electrophoresis have been indicated as being present in oviductal fluid from the cow and sheep.[49,71]

The most extensively studied oviductal fluid is that from rabbits because it is produced in sufficient amounts for analysis and the experimental animal can be comfortably housed for easy access. Bacsich and Hamilton[72] reported from histologic staining that the "albuminous coat of tubal eggs" (mucin layer) was composed of sulfated mucopolysaccharide of oviductal epithelial origin. Although Urzua et al.[73] reported electrophoretic differences between oviductal fluid and serum proteins, the differences were not described and are unclear. Shapiro et al.[74] reported extensive similarities between serum and oviductal fluid but also pointed out two different components in oviductal fluid as well as an enrichment in the area associated with the albumin band. The presence of specific components was confirmed and better defined by Feigelson and Kay[2] who reported two to four proteins in rabbit oviductal fluid that are not detectable in serum. These components were a glycoprotein (PAS staining) which migrated at a relative mobility (Rm) of approximately 0.1, and proteins at relative mobilities of about 0.25 and 0.5.

The band at Rm = 0.5 (a postalbumin) was examined further and demonstrated to have a subunit molecular weight of 16 K daltons. The concentration of this protein diminishes to undetectable levels following ovariectomy and is restored with estrogen administration.[75] That component of oviductal fluid was subsequently identified as uteroglobin[76] and its presence in the oviductal fluid has been corroborated by several reports.[77,78] The most recent evaluation of the number of specific com-

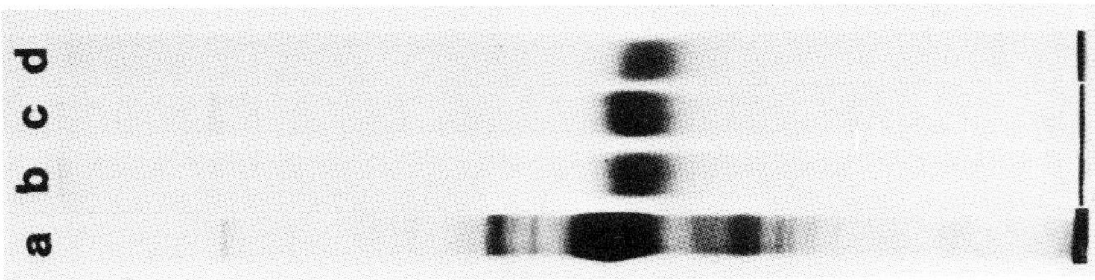

FIGURE 12:2—*SDS electrophoresis of oviductal specific glycoproteins.* (a) *Whole oviduct fluid and fractions A* (b), *B* (c), *and C* (d) *representing three components of the family of glycoproteins secreted by the oviductal epithelium. Gel demonstrates that under reducing conditions, the three components have a subunit molecular weight of 71,000 daltons. Some material remained in an aggregated state at the top of the gel.*

ponents in rabbit oviductal fluid again reported two or three components.[78] That report also equated two of these components with uteroglobin and the uteroglobin dimer. The third component was more than 200 K daltons and increased twofold in concentration in oviductal fluid after ovulation.

Some evaluation of the species similarity of these oviductal fluid components has been made by evaluating antigenic cross-reactivity. The antibodies specific to the three components of oviductal fluid[78] showed two cross-reacting bands with rabbits' uterine fluid, likely uteroglobin, and no cross-reaction with the oviductal fluids of the monkey or cat. Six oviductal tissue antigens were reported by Sacco and Shivers.[79] Of these antigens, two cross-reacted with extracts of oviduct tissue of mice and one with oviductal tissue of the rat. No cross-reaction occurred with tissue extracts of the oviducts of guinea pigs or hamsters.[80] While comparisons between the tissue antigens observed by Sacco and Shivers and the specific oviductal fluid components[2,74,78] have not been made, it seems likely that some of the tissue antigens may represent the oviductal fluid components. Whether these are the species' cross-reactive components remains unanswered.

Using only gel filtration techniques, Shapiro et al.[50] reported the isolation of an acidic glycoprotein from rabbit oviductal fluid. The glycoprotein has a subunit molecular weight of 73 K daltons and was demonstrated to be a component of the mucin surrounding the oocyte recovered from the oviduct. The investigators did not establish whether the glycoprotein was specific to the oviduct and the purity of their preparation was not well defined. Our laboratory isolated a family of sulfated glycoproteins from oviductal fluid of rabbits and demonstrated that they are synthesized in culture by the oviductal epithelium.[81,82] This family of glycoproteins has three components that can be distinguished by electrophoresis under native conditions on an agarose matrix[83] and have been separated by ion exchange chromatography.[82] The three components are immunologically similar, producing only one continuous band when antiserum produced against each specific component is diffused against whole oviductal fluid. When extensively reduced with dithiothreotol and electrophoresed in the presence of sodium dodecyl sulfate (SDS), each of these componets has a major component migrating with a molecular weight of 71 K daltons (Fig. 12:2). While the estimation of molecular weight is totally consistent with what Shapiro et al.[50] observed, a comparison of the amino acid analysis for each of these three sulfated glycoproteins and the component isolated by Shapiro et al. indicates significant differences (Table 12:2). These differences might be attributed to a somewhat impure preparation as a result of the investigators' use of only gel filtration for purification. It is interesting that the three components isolated by our laboratory are extremely similar in amino acid content. Aside from providing an internal consistency which supports the purity of these components,the result supports the preliminary evi-dence that these glycoproteins differ mainly by the extent of their sulfation.[84]

Hormonal Control of Synthesis and Secretion of Macromolecular Components of Oviductal Fluid

Electrophoretic analysis of oviductal fluids of monkeys and women indicates the presence of specific oviductal fluid components only during and after ovulation and not immediately pre- or postmenstruation.[5,17] Cytologic evaluation of the oviducts indicates a similar transitory secretion of a mucoid material from the human oviductal isthmus,[69] which corresponds with the period when Lippes et al.[17] observed oviduct-specific proteins.

Electron and light microscopic evaluations of rabbits' oviduct also suggest that maximal secretion takes place after ovulation.[66,67,85,86] This is supported by the amount of mucin deposited on ovulated oocytes or glass beads injected into the oviduct.[87] Greenwald[87] has suggested that progesterone induces secretion of oviductal mucin in the rabbit. Some mucin, however, is deposited on embryos by the oviducts of rabbits that have been ovariectomized for two weeks and then hormonally stimulated only with estradiol.[88] Further, Stone et al.[78] showed that a component of high molecular weight specific to the oviduct, likely mucin, is present at a baseline concentration during estrus but increased twofold after ovulation.

Our laboratory has used light and electron microscopic immunocytochemical techniques to localize a family of sulfated glycoproteins to the secretory granules of the oviductal epithelium (Fig. 12:3). After ovariectomy, the granules disappear and injection of estradiol induces reappearance. The synthesis of the glycoproteins was evaluated by incorporation of tritiated amino acid and S-35 sulfate into the glycoproteins. Synthesis does not occur after ovariectomy unless estradiol is administered.[61] Solid-phase radioimmunoassay indicated that the sulfated glycoproteins were present in oviductal fluid of the estrous rabbit at concentrations of approximately 0.5 mg/ml, which increased two- to threefold after ovulation. When this quantitative information is superimposed on the progesterone profile (Fig. 12:4), it becomes obvious that either initial secretion is stimulated by very small increases in progesterone or something else is inducing secretion. Neither the radioimmunoassay nor the immunocytochemical techniques differentiate between the different forms of the sulfated glycoproteins. However, with present information, reinterpretation of the data of Hanscom and Oliphant[83] would suggest that the most sulfated form of these glycoproteins is secreted during estradiol administration (Fig. 12:5). As the result of hormonal withdrawal or progesterone administration, less sulfated forms are secreted.

Biological Function of Oviductal Fluid

The oviductal fluid is the fluid environment for oocytic maturation, maintenance of sperm during transport, fertilization, and early embryonic development. Attempts to evaluate each of these functions have been made in different species; however, clear functions for specific components of oviductal fluid remain for the most part speculative.

The sperm of rabbits and rams have increased respiration in oviductal fluid from either species.[89,90] This was attributed to bicarbonate ion in rabbit oviductal fluid.[26] However, a nondialyzable, heat-labile factor in rabbits' oviductal fluid was indicated as providing some of the increase in respiration.[90] Whether these factors also contribute to changes in motility of sperm observed in the oviducts of the hamster and rabbit[91,92] is unclear. However, it is clear that oviductal fluid affects sperm and it is well documented that sperm capacitation can be induced in the oviduct, regardless of the hormonal state of the animal.[93]

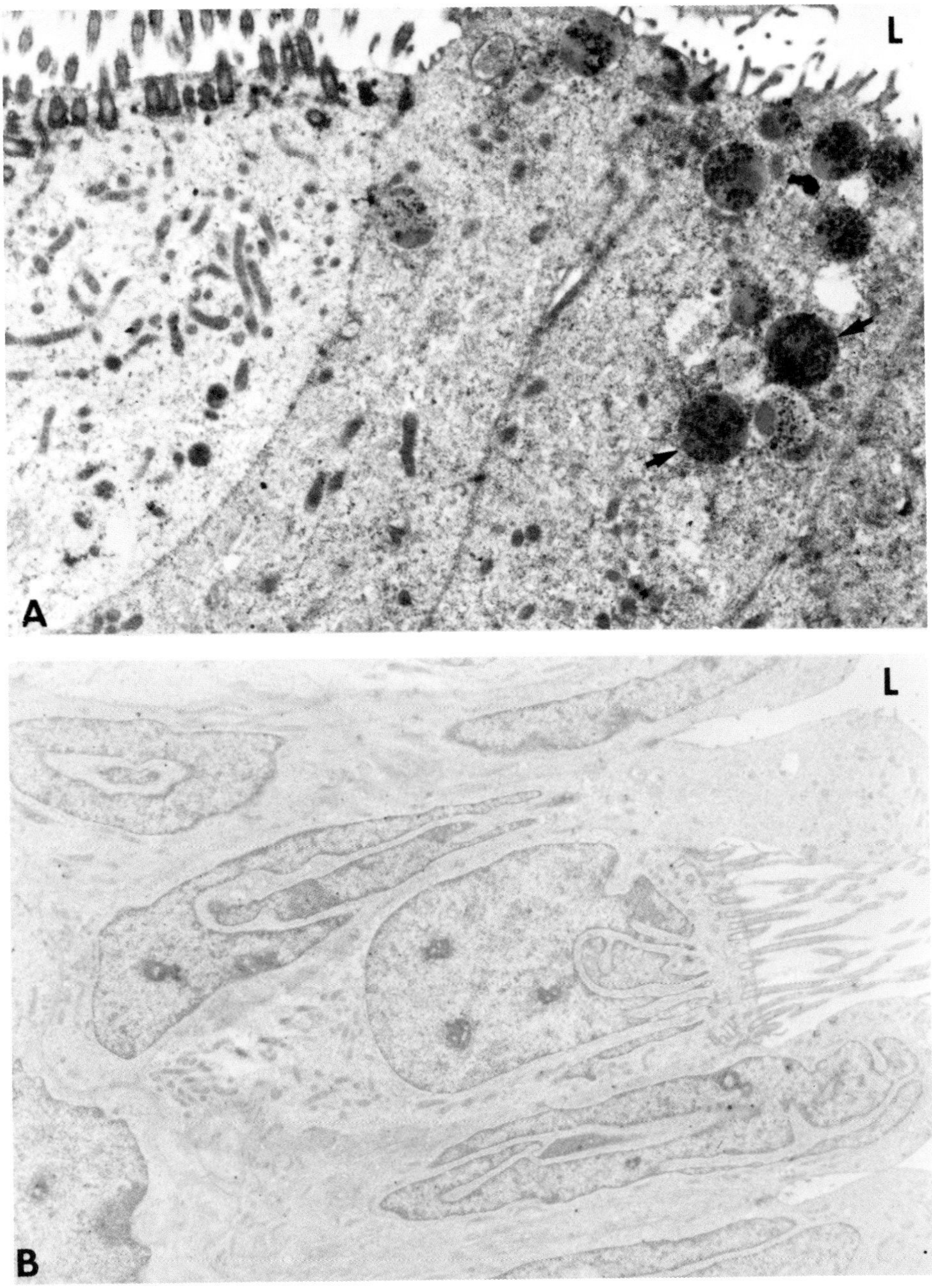

FIGURE 12:3—*Electron microscopic immunocytochemical localization of the family of sulfated glycoproteins of oviductal fluid. Sections were stained with antiserum to sulfated oviduct-specific glycoproteins and peroxidase-antiperoxidase complex; counter-staining was with uranyl acetate and lead citrate. Substrate for the peroxidase was 4-chloro-1-naphthol, which gives a granular reaction product at the site of localization.* (A) *Portions of the proximal isthmus under the influence of estrogen. Reaction product is concentrated over the secretory vesicles in the secretory cells and none is found in the ciliated cells.* (B) *In a similar region of the isthmus obtained ten days after ovariectomy, secretory cells are greatly reduced in height and contain no immunoreactive material.*

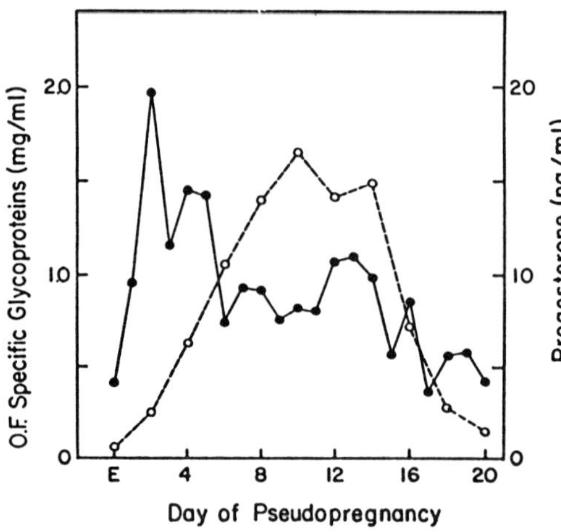

FIGURE 12:4—*Progesterone concentration versus secretion from the oviductal epithelium. (-●-) shows the concentration of sulfated oviduct-specific glycoproteins present in oviductal fluid. Measurements were made by a solid-phase RIA for the sulfated oviduct-specific glycoproteins. (-○-) shows serum progesterone concentrations as determined by an RIA. Secretion precedes the progesterone peak, thus secretion is either stimulated by small increases in progesterone or by some other factor.*

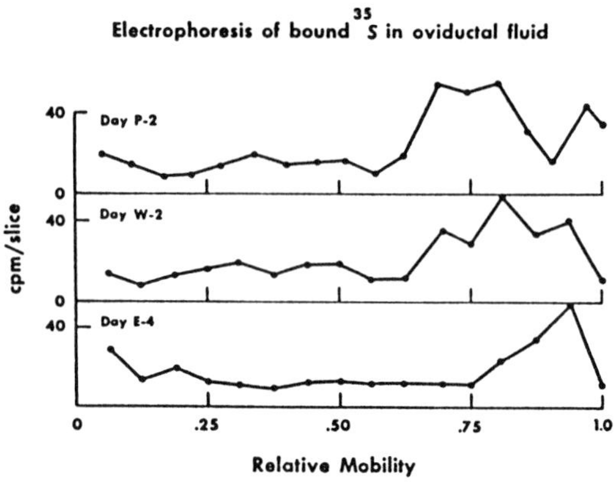

FIGURE 12:5—^{35}S *cpm per 2 mm slice (less background) after agarose-disc electrophoresis of dialyzed oviductal fluid collected after ovariectomy on day 4 of estrogen treatment (E-4), day 2 of estrogen withdrawal (W-2), and day 2 of progesterone treatment (P-2). Typical results of at least six measurements and peaks were statistically different at the* $p < 0.001$ *confidence level. (From Hanscom and Oliphant.[83]) With recent results, these data suggest that different forms of the components of the family of sulfated oviduct-specific glycoproteins may be secreted under different hormonal conditions.*

The function of oviductal fluid in embryonic development has been evaluated by several methods. Embryos have been transferred to ligated oviducts and evaluated for normal development. Adams[94] demonstrated that rabbit embryos cannot develop beyond the early blastocyst stage irrespective of the endocrine environment of the oviduct and that four-cell embryos developed best when the endocrine stimulation of the oviduct was in the early luteal phases. When pronuclear rabbit embryos were transferred to the ampulla of ovariectomized rabbits, abnormal embryonic development occurred under estrogen supplementation but not when embryos were transferred during the progesterone phase of a sequential regimen of estrogen followed by progesterone.[88] Thus, both of these studies suggest that the estrogenic phase does not provide optimal environment within the oviduct for embryonic development. That has been supported by culture of embryos in vitro in oviductal fluid collected under varying hormonal regimens. Embryos of rabbits and mice do not develop well in oviductal fluid from animals in estrus, or ovariectomized and estrogen-supplemented. In contrast, apparently normal development occurs in oviductal fluid from either pseudopregnant animals or those ovariectomized and supplemented with estrogen followed by progesterone.[46,95–97] The negative effects on development are not the direct effect of estrogen[46,96] and may be attributed to a peptide inhibitor of embryonic development.[98] The peptide nature of this inhibitor was suggested by experiments that demonstrated that the inhibitor is dialyzable, yet elutes at the void volume of a G-25 column and may be destroyed by protease but not by heating.[98] The source of the inhibitor may be by transudation from serum.[96] Thus, the mechanism for eliminating the inhibition during normal development could be by exclusion from the oviductal lumen or by production of specific secretions within the oviduct to block the effects of the inhibitor. Why such an inhibitor should exist in oviductal fluid is unclear but that it exists in at least rabbits and mice is well documented and the effect might be used as a method for birth control.

The role of the mucin secreted from the oviductal epithelial cells and readily observed around rabbit oocytes or within the human oviductal lumen[69,99] has been under investigation for at least three decades. Both Adams[100] and Greenwald[101] carried out experiments that suggested that rabbit ova had decreased ability to develop and implant when they were coated with reduced amounts of mucin. However, the ability of some embryos to complete development with the reduced amounts of mucin, along with numerous reports of in-vitro fertilization, culture, and embryo transfer, makes it highly improbable that the developing embryo directly requires specific secretions of the oviduct. On the other hand, it is likely that the oviductal secretions function in vivo to facilitate those developmental processes in an indirect manner. For example, the secretions may act to inactivate the embryonic inhibiting peptide which appears to enter the oviductal lumen from blood.[96] Such protection from serum components by oviductal secretions is also represented by the ability of the oviductal fluid to protect developing embryos and sperm from the maternal humoral immune system. Our laboratory has recently purified material inhibiting immunological complement from rabbit oviductal fluid.[102] Further analysis of this isolated complement inhibitor has shown it is the sulfated glycoproteins that are synthesized and secreted by the oviductal epithelium.[61,82] Thus, recent analysis of oviductal fluid has resulted in isolation of specific components from the oviductal fluid that can be attributed directly to the secretory cells of the oviduct. Subsequently, these sulfated glycoproteins have been found to function to protect sperm and embryos from the maternal humoral immune system.

References

1. Bishop DW: Active secretion in the rabbit oviduct. *Am J Physiol*, 187:347, 1956.
2. Feigelson M, Kay E: Protein patterns of rabbit oviductal fluid. *Biol Reprod*, 6:244, 1972.
3. Riddick DH: The composition of rabbit oviductal fluid collected continuously throughout gestation. *J Reprod Fertil*, 43:563, 1975.
4. Holmdahl TH, Mastroianni L: Continuous collection of rabbit oviduct secretions at low temperature. *Fertil Steril*, 16:587, 1965.
5. Mastroianni L, Urzua M, Stambaugh R: Protein patterns of monkey oviductal fluid before and after ovulation. *Fertil Steril*, 21:817, 1970.
6. Hamner CE, Williams WL: Composition of rabbit oviductal secretions. *Fertil Steril*, 16:170, 1965.
7. Hamner CE: Oviductal fluid—composition and physiology. In Greep RO (Ed): *Handbook of Physiology*. Washington, D.C.: American Physiological Society, 1973: p 141, Sect. 7, Part 2.
8. Iritani A, Nishikawa Y, Gomes WR, et al: Secretion rates and chemical composition of oviduct and uterine fluids in rabbits. *J Anim Sci*, 33:829, 1971.
9. Oliphant G, Bowling A, Eng LA, et al: The permeability of the rabbit oviduct to proteins present in the serum. *Biol Reprod*, 18:516, 1978.
10. Black DL, Druby RT, Riesen J: Apparatus for the continuous collection of sheep oviduct fluid. *J Reprod Fertil*, 6:257, 1963.
11. Belve AR, McDonald MF: Directional flow of fallopian tube secretion in the Romney ewe. *J Reprod Fertil*, 15:357, 1968.
12. Mastroianni L, Wallach RC: Effects of ovulation and early gestation on oviduct secretions in the rabbit. *Am J Physiol*, 200:815, 1961.
13. Wu CH, Mastroianni L, Mikhail G: Steroid hormones in monkey oviductal fluid. *Fertil Steril*, 28:1250, 1977.
14. Lippes J, Enders RG, Pragay DA, et al: The collection and analysis of human fallopian tube fluid. *Contraception*, 5:85, 1972.
15. Moghissi KS: Human fallopian tube

fluid. I. Protein composition. *Fertil Steril*, 21:821, 1970.
16. Hamner CE: Biochemistry of oviductal secretions. In Hafez ESE, Blandau RJ (Eds): *The Mammalian Oviduct*. Chicago: University of Chicago Press, 1969: p. 333.
17. Lippes J, Krasner J, Alfonso LA, et al: Human oviductal fluid proteins. *Fertil Steril*, 36:623, 1981.
18. David A, Serr DM, Czernobilsky B: Chemical composition of human oviduct fluid. *Fertil Steril*, 24:435, 1973.
19. Borland RM, Biggers JD, Lechene CP, et al: Elemental composition of fluid in the human fallopian tube. *J Reprod Fertil*, 58:479, 1980.
20. Mastroianni L, Urzua M, Stambaugh R: The internal environmental fluids of the oviduct. In Segal SJ, Crozier R, Corfman PA, et al (Eds): *The Regulation of Mammalian Reproduction*, Springfield, IL: CC Thomas, 1973: p. 376.
21. Restall BJ, Wales RG: The fallopian tube of the sheep. III. The chemical composition of the fluid from the fallopian tube. *Austral J Biol Sci*, 19:687, 1966.
22. Iritani A, Gomes WR, Vandemark NL: Secretion rates and chemical composition of oviduct and uterine fluids in ewes. *Biol Reprod*, 1:72, 1969.
23. Brunton WJ, Brusilow S: In Johnson AD, Foley CW (Eds): *Oviduct and Its Functions*. New York: Academic Press, 1974: p. 138.
24. David A, Brackett BG, Garcia CR, et al: Composition of rabbit oviduct fluid in ligated segments of the fallopian tube. *J Reprod Fertil*, 19:285, 1969.
25. Brunton WJ, Brinster RL: Active chloride transport in the isolated rabbit oviduct. *Am J Physiol*, 221:658, 1971.
26. Hamner CE, Williams WL: Identification of sperm stimulation factor of rabbit oviduct fluid. *Proc Soc Exper Biol Med*, 117:240, 1964.
27. Stambaugh R, Noriega C, Mastroianni L, Jr: Bicarbonation; the corona cell dispersing factor of rabbit tubal fluid. *J Reprod Fertil*, 18:51, 1969.
28. Yanagamachi R, Usui N: Calcium dependence of the acrosome reaction and activation of guinea pig spermatozoa. *Exper Cell Res*, 89:161, 1974.
29. Douglas WW: Stimulus-secretion coupling: The concept and clues from chromaffin and other cells. *Br J Pharmacol*, 34:451, 1968.
30. Leese HJ, Jeffries KS: Evidence for the facilitated diffusion of glucose into rabbit oviductal fluid. *J Reprod Fertil*, 51:93, 1977.
31. Burman S, Oliphant G: Unpublished data.
32. Brinster RL: In vitro cultivation of mammalian ova. *Biosciences*, 4:199, 1969.
33. Rogers BJ, Yanagamachi R: Retardation of guinea pig sperm acrosome reaction by glucose: The possible importance of pyruvate and lactate metabolism in capacitation and the acrosome reaction. *Biol Reprod*, 13:568, 1975.
34. Gregoire AT, Gongsakdi R, Rakogg AE: The free amino acid content of the female rabbit gential tract. *Fertil Steril*, 12:322, 1961.
35. Perkins JL, Goode L: Effects of stage of the estrous cycle and exogenous hormones upon the volume and composition of oviduct fluid in ewes. *J Anim Sci*, 25:465, 1966.
36. Foley CW, Engle CC, Plotka ED, et al: Influence of early pregnancy on proteins and amino acids of uterine tubal fluids in rabbits. *Am J Vet Res*, 33:2059, 1972.
37. Leese HJ, Aldridge S, Jeffries KS: The movement of amino acids into rabbit oviductal fluid. *J Reprod Fertil*, 56:623, 1979.
38. Brinster RL: Studies on the development of mouse embryos in vitro. IV. Interaction of energy sources. *J Reprod Fertil*, 10:227, 1965.
39. Brinster RL: Studies on the development of mouse embryos in vitro. III. The effect of fixed-nitrogen source. *J Exper Zool*, 158:59, 1965.
40. Brinster RL: Studies on the development of mouse embryos in vitro. II. The effect of energy source. *J Exper Zool*, 158:59, 1965.
41. Leese HJ, Aldridge S: The movement of pyruvate, lactate, and lactate dehydrogenase into rabbit oviductal fluid. *J Reprod Fertil*, 56:619, 1979.
42. Nieder GL, Corder CN: Quantitative histochemical measurement of pyruvate and lactate in mouse oviduct during the estrous cycle. *J Histochem Cytochem*, 30:1051, 1982.
43. Leese HJ: The stimulation of pyruvate

appearance in the rabbit oviduct lumen by sodium proprionate. *J Reprod Fertil*, 59:421, 1980.
44. Nieder GL, Corder CN: Pyruvate and lactate levels in oviducts of cycling, pregnant, and pseudopregnant mice. *Biol Reprod*, 28:566, 1983.
45. Richardson LL, Oliphant G: Steroid concentrations in rabbit oviductal fluid during oestrus and pseudopregnancy. *J Reprod Fertil*, 62:427, 1981.
46. Cline EM, Randall RA, Oliphant G: Hormone-mediated oviductal influence on mouse embryo development. *Fertil Steril*, 28:756, 1977.
47. Carlson D, Black DL, Howe GR: Oviduct secretion in the cow. *J Reprod Fertil*, 22:549, 1970.
48. Stone SL: Personal communication.
49. Roberts GP, Parker JM, Symonds HW: Proteins in the luminal fluid from the bovine oviduct. *J Reprod Fertil*, 45:301, 1975.
50. Shapiro SS, Brown NE, Yard AS: Isolation of an acidic glycoprotein from rabbit oviductal fluid and its association with the egg coating. *J Reprod Fertil*, 40:281, 1974.
51. Glass LE: Immunocytological studies of the mouse oviduct. In Hafez ESE, Blandau RJ (Eds): *The Mammalian Oviduct*. Chicago: University of Chicago Press, 1969: p. 459.
52. McLaughlin KC, Hamner CE: Preliminary characterization of rabbit oviduct fluid trypsin inhibitors. *Biol Reprod*, 12:556, 1975.
53. Oliphant G, Randall P, Cabot CL: Immunological components of rabbit fallopian tube fluid. *Biol Reprod*, 16:463, 1977.
54. Collins S, Menge AC, Archie JT, et al: Immunologic response of the rabbit oviduct. *Int J Fertil*, 24:149, 1979.
55. Kille JW, Goldberg E: Female reproductive tract immunoglobulin responses to a purified sperm specific antigen. *Biol Reprod*, 20:863, 1979.
56. Marcus SL, Saravis CA: Oviduct fluid in the rhesus monkey: A study of its protein components and its origin. *Fertil Steril*, 16:785, 1965.
57. Schumacher GFB: Humoral immune factors in the female reproductive tract and their changes during the cycle. In Dhindsa D, Schumacher GFB (Eds): *Immunological Aspects of Infertility and Fertility Regulation*. New York: Elsevier Press, 1980: p. 93.
58. Yaung SL, Schumacher GFB, Broer KA, et al: Specific antibodies and immunoglobulin in the oviductal fluid of the rhesus monkey. *Fertil Steril*, 39:359, 1983.
59. Lippes J, Swtantarta O, Tomasi TB, et al: Immunohistological localization of IgG, IgA, IgM, secretory piece and lactoferrin in the human female genital tract. *Contraception*, 1:163, 1970.
60. Oliphant G, Cabot C: Control of humoral immune cytotoxic activity in the oviduct. Presented at the Society for the Study of Reproduction, Corvallis, Oregon, Abstract 184, 1981.
61. Oliphant G, Reynolds AB, Smith PF, et al: Immunocytochemical localization and determination of hormone-induced synthesis of the sulfated oviductal glycoproteins. *Biol Reprod*, 31:165, 1984.
62. Novak E, Everett HS: Cyclical and other variations in the tubal epithelium. *Am J Obstet Gynecol*, 16:499, 1928.
63. Guerriero C: Étude morphologique de l'épithélium de la trompe utérine au repos sexual chez la lapine adulte, impubère, et castre. *Compt Rend Soc Biol*, 102:1972, 1929.
64. Nilsson O, Reinius S: Light and electron microscopic structure of the oviduct. In Hafez ESE, Blandau RJ (Eds): *The Mammalian Oviduct*. Chicago: University of Chicago Press, 1969: p. 57.
65. Hadek R: The secretory process in the sheep's oviduct. *Anat Rec*, 121:187, 1955.
66. Brower LK, Anderson E: Cytological events associated with the secretory process in the rabbit oviduct. *Biol Reprod*, 1:130, 1969.
67. Jansen RPS, Bajpai VK: Oviduct acid mucus glycoproteins in the estrous rabbit: Ultrastructure and histochemistry. *Biol Reprod*, 26:155, 1982.
68. Fredricsson B, Bjorkman N: Studies on the ultrastructure of the human oviduct epithelium in different functional stages. *Ztschs Zellforsch*, 58:387, 1962.
69. Habseb RS: Cyclic changes in the human fallopian tube isthmus and their functional importance. *Am J Obstet Gynecol*, 136:292, 1986.

70. Lippes J, Van Oss CJ, Bronson PM, et al: Human oviductal fluid proteins. II. Preparation of an antiserum to a human oviductal fluid protein: Existence of autoantibodies against it in some sera. *Fertil Steril,* 39:824, 1983.
71. Roberts GJ, Parker JM, Symonds HW: Macromolecular components of genital tract fluids from the sheep. *J Reprod Fertil,* 48:99, 1976.
72. Bacsich P, Hamilton WJ: Some observations on vitally stained rabbit ova with special reference to their albuminous coat. *J Embryol Exper Morphol,* 2:81, 1954.
73. Urzua MA, Stambaugh R, Flickinger G, et al: Uterine and oviduct fluid protein patterns in the rabbit before and after ovulation. *Fertil Steril,* 21:860, 1970.
74. Shapiro SS, Jestsch JR, Yard AS: Protein composition of rabbit oviduct fluid. *J Reprod Fertil,* 24:403, 1971.
75. Kay E, Feigelson M: An estrogen modulated protein in rabbit oviductal fluid. *Biochem Biophy Acta,* 271:436, 1972.
76. Feigelson M, Noske IG, Goswami AK, Reproductive tract fluid proteins and their hormonal control. *Ann NY Acad Sci,* 286:273, 1977.
77. Tucker EB, Schultz A: Temporal changes in proteins of oviduct and uterine fluids during preimplantation period in the rabbit. *Biol Reprod,* 17:749, 1974.
78. Stone SL, Huckle WR, Oliphant G: Identification and hormonal control of reproductive-tract-specific antigens present in the rabbit oviductal fluid. *Gamete Res,* 3:169, 1980.
79. Sacco AG, Shivers CA: Antigens of the rabbit ovary, oviduct and uterus. *J Reprod Fertil,* 32:403, 1973.
80. Sacco AG, Shivers CA: Comparison of antigens in the ovary, oviduct and uterus of the rabbit and other mammalian species. *J Reprod Fertil,* 32:421, 1973.
81. Barr SH, Oliphant G: Sulfate incorporation into macromolecules produced by cultured oviductal epithelium. *Biol Reprod,* 24:952, 1981.
82. Oliphant G, Ross PR: Demonstration of production and isolation of three sulfated glycoproteins from the rabbit oviduct. *Biol Reprod,* 26:537, 1982.
83. Hanscom DR, Oliphant G: Hormonal regulation of incorporation of 35-sulfate into macromolecules of oviduct fluid. *Biol Reprod,* 14:599, 1976.
84. Oliphant G, Ross PR: Unpublished data.
85. Wislocki GB, Bunting H, Dempsey EW: Metachromasia in mammalian tissues and its relationship to mucopolysaccharides in the rabbit uterus, oviducts, and vagina. *Acta Endocrinol* (Copenh), 29:18, 1947.
86. Jansen RPS: Fallopian tube isthmic mucus and ovum transport. *Science,* 201:349, 1978.
87. Greenwald GS: Endocrinology of oviductal secretions. In Hafez ESE, Blandau RJ (Eds): *The Mammalian Oviduct.* Chicago: University of Chicago Press, 1969: p. 183.
88. Stone SL, Hamner CE: Hormonal and regional influences of the oviduct on the development of rabbit embryos. *Biol Reprod,* 16:638, 1977.
89. Hamner CE, Williams WL: Effect of the female reproductive tract on sperm metabolism in the rabbit and fowl. *J Reprod Fertil,* 5:143, 1963.
90. Iritani A, Gomes WR, Vandemark NL: The effect of whole, dialyzed and heated female genital tract fluids on respiration of rabbit and ram spermatozoa. *Biol Reprod,* 1:77, 1969.
91. Katz DF, Yanagimachi R: Movement characteristics of hamster spermatozoa within the oviduct. *Biol Reprod,* 22:759, 1980.
92. Suarez SS, Katz DF, Overstreet JW: Movement characteristics and acrosomal status of rabbit spermatozoa recovered at the site and time of fertilization. *Biol Reprod,* 29:1277, 1983.
93. Hamner CE, Jones JP, Sojka NJ: Influence of the hormonal state of the female on the fertilizing capacity of rabbit spermatozoa. *Fertil Steril,* 19:137, 1968.
94. Adams CE: The development of rabbit eggs in the ligated oviduct and their viability after re-transfer to recipient rabbits. *J Embryol Exper Morphol,* 29:133, 1973.
95. Kille JW, Hamner CE: The influence of oviductal fluid on the development of one-cell rabbit embryos in vitro. *J Reprod Fertil,* 35:415, 1973.
96. Stone SL, Richardson LL, Hamner CE, et al: Partial characterization of hormone-mediated inhibition of em-

bryo development in rabbit oviduct fluid. *Biol Reprod,* 16:647, 1977.
97. Touigny M, Lambert RD, Guilbert-Blanchette L: Influence des milieux tubaire ou utérin sur le developpement des embryons de lapins. *L'union Med Canada,* 106:300, 1977.
98. Richardson LL, Hamner CE, Oliphant G: Some characteristics of an inhibitor of embryonic development from rabbit oviductal fluid. *Biol Reprod,* 22:553, 1980.
99. Adams CE: Egg development in the rabbit: The influence of post-coital ligation of the uterine tube and of ovariectomy. *J Endocrinol,* 16:283, 1958.
100. Adams CE: Development of rabbit eggs with special reference to the mucin layer. *Acta Endocrinol,* 51:687, 1960.
101. Greenwald GS: The role of the mucin layer in development of the rabbit blastocyst. *Anat Rec,* 142:407, 1962.
102. Oliphant G, Cabot C, Ross PR, et al: Control of the humoral immune system within the rabbit oviduct. *Biol Reprod,* 31:202, 1984.

13

Ovum Pickup

Yoram Beyth and
Shlomo Mor-Yosef

History and Theories

The problem of ovum transit from the ovary to the distal end of the fallopian tube has been the subject of numerous investigations. Although various theories have been brought forward, no final conclusion has yet been reached. According to a review of the history, the anatomy and course of the fallopian tube were described by Andreas Vesalius in 1538 and by his student, the Italian anatomist Gabriele Fallopio in 1561. About a hundred years later Reijnier de Graaf published explanatory notes on the fimbriae and fimbria ovarica. The mechanism of ovum pickup, however, has remained an enigma throughout the centuries. The earliest speculation on ovum migration we were able to trace was published by de Graaf in 1672.[1] He was apparently also the first to look at the fimbriae through a microscope; he realized the importance of the fimbriae in ovum pickup stating that "the expansions at the end of the tube embrace the 'testicle' from all sides."

Some of the initial investigations carried out by Walter (1776) and Halber (1788) on human cadavers, led them to speculate that "hyperaemia in the tubal tissues during coitus causes the tube to become stiff and the fimbriae to embrace the ruptured follicle." Another theory, advanced by Leukhart in 1853 stated that "The Graafian follicles act as a projective apparatus that forcibly discharges the ovum into the open tubal funnel." Rouget in 1858 emphasized the importance of the smooth-muscle fibers in the various ovarian and tubal ligaments, stating that "The tube and mesosalpinx on ovulation sweep round the ovary. The infundibulum is dragged down over the surface of the ovary. Thus the ova are prevented from getting lost in the peritoneal cavity." Pend in 1862 suggested the membrane theory, that is, "the tube and ovary are united by pseudomembranes being formed at the time of ovulation, later to disappear." Fischel (1914) advocated the suction theory: "The ova are brought down to the pouch of Douglas, and suspended in fluid. Later they are sucked up by the tube from the floor of the pouch of Douglas." Fraenkel believed that two factors were involved in

The Fallopian Tube: Basic Studies and Clinical Contributions, edited by Alvin M. Siegler, M.D. Mount Kisco, New York: Futura Publishing Company, Inc. © 1986.

ovum pickup; the ovum is shot out from the dense follicle, and the suction action of the infundibulum.

Westman[2] investigated the transit of ova and suggested that: (1) the tube and ovary come in intimate contact by the tube's own movements; (2) rotatory movements of the ovary caused by smooth muscle in the ovarian ligament; (3) these movements enable the fimbriae to come into contact with all aspects of the ovarian surface, thus affording direct ovum pickup from the site of ovulation. According to Blandau,[3] the mechanism by which freshly ovulated eggs are transported into the oviduct depends on three factors: (1) the anatomic configuration of the fimbriae of the infundibulum and its relationship to the surface of the ovary at the time of ovulation; (2) the manner in which the cumulus oophorus and its contained egg are expressed from the follicle at the time of ovulation; and (3) the physical characteristics of the antral fluid and that of the fluid of the matrix of the cumulus oophorus. In spite of all these theories and speculations, the physiology of ovum pickup is far from clear and many questions are still awaiting their answers. To name but a few:

1. How many factors are involved in ovum pickup and how does each factor contribute to this particular phase of ovum transport?
2. Is normal function of all these factors mandatory for fertility, or can ovum capture also occur in the absence or dysfunction of one or more of them?
3. In cases where one factor is neutralized, do the others fulfill a compensatory role by functioning more efficiently?
4. Are the factors involved in ovum pickup identical in all species, and is it at all possible to extrapolate conclusions drawn from animal experiments to ovum capture in women?

Anatomy

The human fallopian tube is an intraperitoneal cylindrical organ measuring 12 cm in length. It extends from the uterus in a transverse direction toward the pelvic wall as far as the uterine pole of the ovary, at which point it changes direction backward and upward along the lateral border of the ovary to bend itself finally around the tubal pole of the ovary. This looped course of the tube, together with the fossa ovarica (the depression on the lateral pelvis in which the ovary is nestled), causes the ovary to be located in a semi-isolated compartment in the abdominal cavity. The fimbriated end, which opens into the peritoneal cavity, enables ova, sperm, foreign bodies (starch, oil droplets, carbon particles, talc, china ink), and under certain circumstances, also bacteria to be transferred from the vagina through the uterus and tube into the peritoneal cavity or in reverse direction.[4–9]

Careful observations of the various anatomical and histologic details of the female genital tract may help elucidate the method of ovum pickup.

Ligaments and mesenteries of the ovary and tube

Various tubal and ovarian ligaments and mesenteries are responsible for keeping the tube and ovary in place and in proximity to one another, thus shortening the distance between the tubal ostium and ovulation sites on the ovarian surface.

The mesosalpinx is attached to the tube along its entire length, thereby stabilizing it. The peritoneal serosa, which forms the outer layer of the tubal wall, encloses the tube except for the site of insertion of the mesosalpinx. At this point the serosa divides into two thin layers which cover the mesosalpinx and extend toward the pelvic walls, forming the broad ligament. The tube is often much longer than the distance between the uterus and ovary, and this disparity in length causes the tube to bend in the shape of a loop.

The mesotubarium ovarica (MTO), the distal part of the mesosalpinx, extends from the fimbrial end to the ovary where it is attached to the tubal pole. The fimbria ovarica (FO) is an elongated fimbria of variable length which adheres to the MTO; in a considerable number of women, its length enables it to reach as far as the tubal pole of the ovary at the insertion site of the MTO. The elongated FO was already depicted by de Graaf in *On the Human Reproductive Organs* (1672). These two structures, the MTO and FO, contribute to fimbrial-gonadal approximation.

The ovarian ligament, stretching from the uterine pole of the ovary toward the uterine corner, and the infundibulopelvic ligament connecting the tubal pole of the ovary to the pelvic wall, are both responsible for stabilizing the ovary and holding it close to the tube.

The presence of smooth-muscle fibers in all the ligaments has been reported. Already in 1858, Rouget[10] mentioned a complex muscular network as well as smooth musculature in the ovarian ligaments. He also depicted muscle fibers radiating from the uterine horn to the ovarian ligament, some of them continuing across the ovarian hilus, finally reaching the tubal pole of the ovary whence they spread into the mesotubarium ovarica. Okamura et al.[11] demonstrated the existence of typical smooth-muscle cells in the human MTO with both thin and thick myofilaments. The bundles of smooth-muscle cells are described as running from the ovarian stroma to the fimbrial wall. This morphological feature suggests a possible role of ovarian follicular wall contractility in determining the fimbrial movement toward the ovary. Mahran et al.[12] studied in vitro the structure of the ovarian ligaments of 11 women who had undergone hysterectomy. They discovered that the ligaments consist mainly of nonstriated muscle fibers arranged in a central longitudinal core. It is interesting that large amounts of nonstriated muscular fibers were also found embedded in the mesotubarium of the adult rabbit and of other animals[4] and that excision or dissection of the rabbit mesotubarium may decrease the animal's fertility.[12–14]

The length of the ligaments may influence fertility. In the presence of a very long MTO (more than 2 cm), fertility may be impaired because of the enlarged distance between the tubal ostium and ovary.[15]

Tubal-ovarian relation: Comparative anatomy

Observations on the morphology of the periovarial sac and its relation to the fimbria and ovary in 41 mammalian species may shed light on ovum pickup mechanisms in different anatomical structures. Beck[16] discriminates between eight morphological types that are distinguished by the extent to which the ovary is enclosed by the oviductal mesenteries and the positional relationship of the oviduct to the ovary. The variations are extreme, ranging from species that lack a definite periovarian sac (such as women) to species that exhibit a periovarian sac that completely encloses the ovary (such as the rat). The closed sac may have evolved to provide safe conduction of the ova from the ovary to the oviduct. The mode of transportation of the eggs from the site of ovulation on the ovarian surface varies greatly in different species. There seems to be a functional relationship between the anatomical configuration and the manner in which the eggs are caught by the fimbriae.

Histological Features of the Fallopian Tube

Certain characteristics of histologic structure of the tube enable it to participate actively in ovum pickup. The tubal mucosa is composed mainly of two cell types: ciliary and secretory cells. The former play an important role in propagating the egg along the tube, especially in the ampulla.[17] The fimbriae, as part of the tube, are also lined with ciliated cells, whose cilia beat actively in the direction of the tubal ostium.[18] The percentage of ciliated cells in the fimbriae is very high,[19] and their participation in mammal ovum pickup has been established. The "ciliation index" (percentage of ciliated cells) in human tubal mucosa is in direct correlation to fertility. Fredericsson reported a decrease in glycogen content in cilia following ovulation.[20] Critoph and Dennis[21] examined human fallopian tubes in vitro and demonstrated increased ciliary activity in both ampullary and isthmic regions, but not in the fimbriae, following ovulation.

From an anatomical point of view, it would seem that the transit of ova from the ovarian surface to the tube is ensured by the above-mentioned structures which tend to isolate the ovary from the rest of the abdominal cavity. In animals in which such isolation is either lacking or incomplete, the fimbrial apparatus is well developed and is able to reach almost any point on the ovarian surface. The various anatomical descriptions and results of the investigations have permitted several theoretical interpretations as to the problem of ovum transit from the ovary to oviduct. Direct observation of these organs during ovulation has provided additional information.

Direct Observations on the Tube and Ovary During Ovulation

Studies in women

It is commonly assumed that for ovum capture the fimbriae have to be positioned such that the mucosa is able to make physical contact with the cumulus mass and the ovum it contains.[22] At the time of ovulation, muscular contractions displace the fimbriae of the oviduct, causing them to surround almost completely the ovary. Mikulicz-Radecki studied the relative positions of the ovary and the fallopian tubes at different stages of the menstrual cycle during abdominal operations.[23] He observed that at ovulation the fimbriae became hyperemic and enlarged. Their increased weight caused them to descend along the medial surface of the ovary and come into contact with its lower pole. The contractions of the ligaments and the tubes drew the isthmus, ampulla, and mesosalpinx across the ovary like a curtain, thus segregating it in a peritoneal pocket.

Caffier[24] observed the pelvic anatomy while operating during ovulation, and found the tube curving around the ovary with the fimbriae spreading over it. In one patient he observed one tube extending across the peritoneal cavity to the contralateral ovary, enfolding the latter with its infundibulum. Stimulated by the fact that the two ligaments which stabilized the ovary contained muscle fibers, Westman studied the intrinsic movement of the ovary during ovulation.[2] He assumed that the position of the ovary depended on fluctuations in tension of the ovarian ligaments. While operating on three patients, Westman deposited two drops of lipiodol in the uterine pole of one ovary at a distance of one centimeter from each other. Serial x-ray exposures three weeks after surgery showed wave-like motion of the lipiodol drops. He further described two positional changes of the ovary: upward displacement and to-and-fro rotation on the long axis.

Doyle observed the ovary and tube at ovulation during colpotomy with the patients in horizontal lithotomy position.[25,26] He found the tube lying in the cul-de-sac and described watching the egg falling into the pouch of Douglas, from which it was probably sucked up by the fimbria. When the tubal fimbriae were firmly placed against the ovary, the tube promptly fell away from the ovary. He also looked at the pelvic organs for 90 minutes during laparotomy and discerned the fimbriae attached to the ovarian surface which, however, remained immobile during his entire observation. Changing the position of the patient had a much greater effect on tubal displacement than the contractions of the mesosalpinx. It may well be, however, that muscular contractions had been suppressed by the general anesthesia.

Decker performed culdoscopies in the knee-chest position during ovulation and observed contractions of the ovarian ligament, causing the ovary to move toward the uterus into the fossa ovarica, thus approximating it to the tube and ensuring contact between the fimbriae and the ovarian surface.[27]

There are a number of clinical observations with respect to the contribution of cilia to ovum pickup. Blandau[18] and others[28] showed that the fimbrial ciliated cells beat synchronously in the direction of the tubal ostium. The sticky cumulus mass surrounding the egg is caught by these cilia and propagated into the tube.[29] Eliasson et al. described the immotile cilia syndrome.[30] This rare syndrome provides a unique opportunity to study the role of the cilia in ovum pickup. Despite the speculation that fertility is impaired in women with this syndrome, six out of eight women became pregnant.[31,32] These and additional data[33,34] strongly suggest that in the absence of other gential tract abnormalities, ciliary motility is not mandatory for female fertility. An alternative explanation is that in this syndrome, while the cilia in the upper and lower respiratory tract and elswhere in the body are immotile, those in the fallopian tubes are motile. However, it is not likely that there are two different types of cilia in one organism. More conclusive proof could be obtained if the affected women were subjected to an ultrastructural investigation of the oviductal cilia, and the lack of dynein arms demonstrated.[35] Affected men are infertile since their spermatozoa are usually immotile.[31]

Observations in animals

The use of the "abdominal window" technique, first proposed by Katsch and Borchers,[36] enabled Westman[4] to scrutinize living organs and to follow the movements of the tube and ovary at ovulation in the rabbit. To facilitate direct viewing of the organs that are attached to the posterior abdominal wall, the part of the peritoneal cavity containing the adnexa was exposed. To this end, the bowel was displaced to the upper abdomen and the cecum was fixed to the lateral abdominal wall. Westman observed that during the estrous period, strong contractions of the ovarian ligament caused rotatory movements of the ovary.[4] The musculature of the mesotubarium drew the tube toward the ovary and expanded the fimbriae. These two activities, which occur concomitantly, enabled the fimbriae to come into close contact with all aspects of the ovarian surface.

Laparoscopic observations by Westman in the rhesus monkey revealed that the tube was strongly twisted during the entire estrual period so that the infundibulum partly encircled the ovarian surface.[4] Only minor movements which constantly dragged the fimbriae to and fro over the ovarian surface were discerned. The ovary itself was also seen to move, causing its displacement cranially and caudally, while at the same time it rotated along its long axis. Blandau reported that in rabbits and guinea pigs, too, the fimbriae of the oviduct almost completely embraced the ovaries at ovulation.[18] When the animals were not in heat, the fimbriae appeared shrunken and only partially covered the ovaries; they expanded at ovulation, almost entirely enclosing the ovary and forming a distinct ovarian bursa. In rats, hamsters, and mice the periovarial space filled with fluid within which the eggs move about freely. When approaching the area of the infundibulum, ciliary currents directed the eggs to the ostium of the oviduct. The bursa formed by the periovarial sac prevented the eggs from escaping into the peritoneal cavity, thus ensuring their entry into the oviduct.

Animal Experiments Designed to Evaluate the Contribution of Various Factors to Ovum Pickup

Direct viewing of the tube and ovary during ovulation has obvious limitations: (1) Observations are carried out while the patient or animal is anesthetized, a condition which may affect tubal motility. The relaxation of the abdominal wall musculature, as a result of anesthesia, combined with the fact that the subject is quiescent and immobilized (almost paralyzed) may have an impact on the motility of other pelvic organs, such as the bowel, which eventually may affect ovum pickup. (2) Laparotomy obviously alters intraabdominal pressures. (3) Precise timing of ovulation must be established. All these drawbacks stimulated investigators to go one step further, that is, not to limit themselves to passive observations but to design experiments that would enable one to test the tube's ability to capture eggs under altered anatomical and physiological circumstances. In almost all these investigations animals were used as models. These studies can be divided into three major groups, encompassing experiments evaluating the role (1) of the ligaments, (2) of the fimbriae, and (3) of the tubal mucosal cilia in ovum pickup.

Experiments designed to evaluate the role of the ligaments and of the tubo-ovarian approximation in fertility

In women fimbrial-gonadal approximation is important, since ovum pickup is most commonly achieved by direct contact of the fimbrial cilia with the surface of the ovary at the site of ovulation.[18,37,38] This is achieved by coordinated movements of the ligaments supporting the tube and ovary. Morikawa et al. described the spontaneous contractile activity of the human mesotubarium ovarica (MTO) in vitro during the various phases of the menstrual cycle.[22] Tissue strips of the MTO, which is known to contain bundles of smooth-muscle cells,[11] were obtained at laparotomy. This experimental evidence demonstrated that the MTO contracts spontaneously and that it responds to norepinephrine (NE), acetylcholine (Ach) and prostaglandins $F_{2\alpha}$ ($PGF_{2\alpha}$) in vitro. The endocrine status of the women from whom the strips were taken influenced the spontaneous in-vitro contractile activity of the MTO: the strips obtained during the ovulatory phase showed the highest spontaneous contractile activity as well as the greatest contractile response to NE, Ach, and $PGF_{2\alpha}$. The authors concluded that the increased activity of the MTO during the ovulatory phase may play a role in ovum pickup by the tubal fimbriae.

Cohen has documented, in sheep, the importance of correct apposition of the fimbria ovarica and ovarian ligaments in ensuring a significantly higher yield of pregnancies following contralateral vascularized autotransplantation of the fallopian tubes.[39] These findings do not correlate with experiments performed on rabbits by Beyth and Winston, who showed that fertility following fimbriectomy did not depend on reconstruction of the fimbria ovarica.[40] Eddy and Laufe, examining the functional importance of an intact fimbrial-ovarian relationship for ovum pickup in rhesus monkeys, also obtained contradictory data.[41] They transected bilaterally the fimbria ovarica and mesotubarium superius (MTS) in 20 adult female monkeys; 12 conceived following a mean 2.8 mated menstrual cycles.

In the rabbit, the MTS, which is attached to the oviduct along the entire course of the oviduct, has a free margin extending from the uterotubal junction to the infundibulum. In-vitro observations in the rabbit have shown that vigorous intermittent contractions of the MTS draw the mouth of the oviduct, together with its fimbriae, over the ovary. It was therefore suggested that the rabbit MTS plays a role in the process of ovum pickup.[4,42] In-vitro mechanical and electrical activity of the MTS recorded for a few hours following ovulation also revealed a significant increase in the muscular activity at the estrual stage.[43–45] This enhanced activity may contribute to ovum pickup by moving the fimbriae and approximating the tubal ostium to the ovary.

Westman studied the problem of transit of the ovum from ovary to uterus in rabbits.[4] He extirpated the MTS and excised small, thin, transparent portions of the mesotubarium inferius, thus creating direct and free communication between the bursa ovarica and the rest of the abdominal cavity. Of the six rabbits exposed to this operation, five conceived. On the basis of these results, he concluded that the presence of a bursa enclosing the ovary is not obligatory for transit of ovum. However, since these experiments were performed on a relatively small number of animals, and since no data are available concerning the nidation index (the ratio between the numbers of embryonic sacs and corpora lutea), it is not possible to evaluate fully the precise impact of this anatomical alteration on fertility. To fill this gap in information, the following experiment was designed[13]: In 14 rabbits, the MTS of one oviduct was excised and the contralateral side of the genital tract was left intact to serve as control. All 14 rabbits conceived. Embryonic sacs were present in the uterine horn of all control sides, while in the operated sides, these sacs were found in only 12 rabbits. Although this difference between the results was not statistically significant, when the nidation index of the operated side (0.57) was compared with that of the control side (0.73) the difference proved significant ($p < 0.01$). These findings are a clear indication as to the contribution of an intact MTS to fertility. Partial damage to the MTS and to the utero-ovarian ligament by means of transection of the ligaments (but without removal) did not affect fertility in rabbits.[14]

Kelly studied the effect of an open ovarian bursa on fecundity in albino rats.[46] He cut the ovarian bursa at one side, with the intact contralateral genital tract serving as control. Of the 18 animals that conceived, complete regeneration of the bursa had occurred in 13, partial regeneration in one, and absence of regeneration was noted in only four animals. In 8 of the 18 animals, no fetuses were found on the operated side, whereas all animals had embryonic sacs on the control side. The total number of fetuses on the operated side in animals with completely regenerated bursa was 33 percent of that on the control side, and in animals with partial or no regeneration, this number was not higher than 13 percent. These results constitute clear evidence as to the role played by the intact bursa ovarica in ovum pickup in the rat, most probably in retaining the periovarian fluid accumulating during ovulation. Although the anatomical distance between the tubal ostium and the ovarian surface had not been increased in these experiments, the surgical manipulations had influenced the conception rate.

It was speculated that fertility is reduced in rabbits following extirpation of the MTS because of increased distance between the fimbriae and the ovary and, possibly, the absence of to-and-fro movements of the fimbriae over the ovary during ovulation. In a study of 11 rabbits (Pappo and Beyth, unpublished data), the MTS was removed and the fimbria ovarica separated from the ovary, thus disconnecting the infundibulum from the ovary and allowing the distal end of the tube to move freely (Table 13:1) (group A).[47] Another group of eight rabbits underwent the same surgical procedure, but here the distal end of the ampulla was fixed to the lateral abdominal wall (Table 13:2) (group B). In each animal the contralateral genital tract remained intact and served as control. Fertility was evaluated following mating by counting the embryonic sacs and corpora lutea at each side of the genital tract and calculating the nidation index. The results in group A (Table 13:1) showed that fertility was not reduced in the presence of a disconnected, free distal fallopian tube. In group B, however, in which the distance between the distal ampulla and ovary was increased and no approximation was possible, fertility was impaired as manifested by the significant difference in nidation index between operated and control sides (Table 13:2). It is of interest that in several experiments (no. 7 in group A and nos. 5, 6, and 7 in group B), the number of embryonic sacs in the uterine horn of the control side was higher than that of corpora lutea in its adjacent ovary. This finding would be difficult to explain but for the assumption that ova transmigrated through the peritoneal cavity from the site of ovulation on the ovary of the operated side to the fimbriated end of the contralateral intact tube. As early as 1894 Lode already mentioned this

Table 13:1

*Fertility Following Removal of Mesotubarium Superius and Separation of Fimbria Ovarica from the Ovary in Rabbits (Group A)**

	Operated side			Control side		
Rabbit no.	*CL*	*ES*	*NI*	*CL*	*ES*	*NI*
1	8	4	4/8	5	4	4/5
2	5	4	4/5	6	4	4/6
3	10	3	3/10	4	1	1/4
4	3	3	3/3	7	5	5/7
5	5	1	1/5	6	3	3/6
6	7	4	4/7	5	4	4/5
7	8	1	1/8	4	5	5/4
8	6	3	3/6	7	4	4/7
9	8	1	1/8	6	1	1/6
10	9	7	7/9	6	4	4/6
11	4	2	2/4	8	5	5/8
Total			33/78			40/64
Mean ± SD			0.45 ± 0.29			0.63 ± 0.29

CL = Corpora lutea; ES = embryonic sac; NI = nidation index.
*From Pappo and Beyth.[47]

Table 13:2

*Fertility Following Removal of Mesotubarium Superius Separation of Fimbria Ovarica and Fixation of the Distal End of the Ampulla to the Lateral Pelvic Wall in Rabbits (Group B)**

	Operated side			Control side		
Rabbit no.	*CL*	*ES*	*NI*	*CL*	*ES*	*NI*
1	5	3	3/5	3	0	0/3
2	4	1	1/4	6	5	5/6
3	4	1	1/4	7	7	7/7
4	5	1	1/5	7	6	6/7
5	6	0	0/6	4	6	6/4
6	8	2	2/8	2	4	4/2
7	6	1	1/6	4	7	7/4
8	6	4	4/6	3	1	1/3
Total			13/44			36/36
Mean ± SD			0.30 ± 0.22 †			1.00 ± 0.69†

CL = Corpora lutea; ES = embryonic sacs; NI = nidation index.
†$0.005 < p < 0.01$.
*From Pappo and Beyth.[47]

Table 13:3

*Ovum Transmigration in Rabbits**

	I II	No OF EXP.	No. OF ANIMALS CONCEIVED, SIDE II / No. OF ANIMALS OPERATED	No. OF EMBRIONIC-SACS SIDE II / No. OF CORPORA-LUTEA SIDE I
A	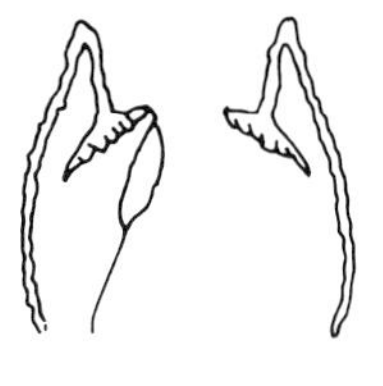	18	$\frac{0}{18}$ = 0%	$\frac{0}{169}$ = 0%
B	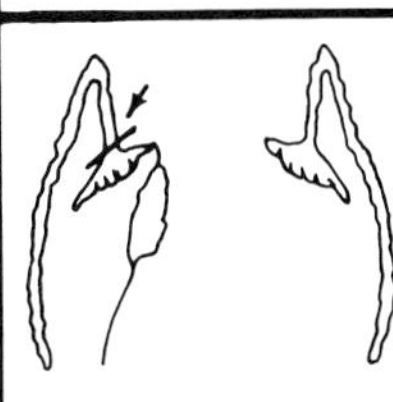	19	$\frac{7}{19}$ = 36.8%	$\frac{11}{164}$ = 6.7%
C	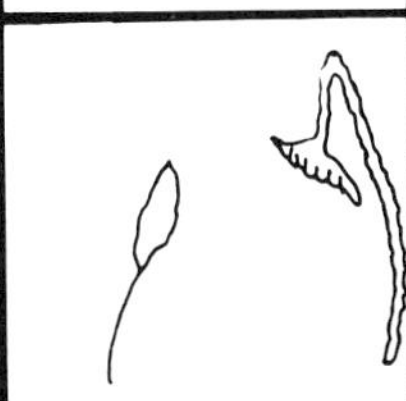	18	$\frac{15}{18}$ = 83.3%	$\frac{37}{136}$ = 27.2%
			A-B P=0.005 A-C P=0.001 B-C P=0.01	A-B P=0.05 A-C P=0.001 B-C P=0.01

*From Beyth et al.[48]

phenomenon of transmigration[48] and Westman[4] reported transperitoneal ovum transit in three rabbits. Beyth et al. investigated ovum transperitoneal migration in 55 rabbits after unilateral oophorectomy.[49] The animals were divided into three groups (Table 13:3). In group A (18 animals), the contralateral genital tract was left intact. All animals in this group conceived; and while all had embryonic sacs on the intact side, none was found in the uterine horn of the contralateral oophorectomized side. In group B (19 rabbits), distal ampullary occlusion was performed in the contralateral side, using a single clip. In seven of these rabbits, embryonic sacs were present in the uterine horn of the oophorectomized side. In all 19 animals, a total of 164 corpora lutea were counted, and as many as 11 (6.7 percent) embryonic sacs were found in the contralateral uterine horn. In group C (18 animals), contralateral salpingectomy was performed; 15 of the animals conceived with an ovum trans migration rate of 27 percent. Statistical evaluation of the results revealed the differences between the three groups to be significant.

Experiments evaluating the role of the fimbriae and of tubal patency in ovum pickup

It was generally accepted that the fimbriae play an indispensable role in ovum capture. In fimbriectomized rabbits and cats, the cumulus mass was found to adhere to the site of rupture for many hours during ovulation.[3,50] Dubreuil examined the morphology of the lymphatics of the fimbriae and infundibulum and suggested that the rapid absorption of luminal fluid into the lymphatic system causes currents within the tube that aid in ovum pickup.[51] Maia and Coutinho demonstrated negative pressures following contractions recorded by means of intraluminal catheters placed in the fallopian tubes.[52] Clewe and Mastroianni evaluated the importance of this postulated tubal suction mechanism in ovum capture.[53] In order to study the fimbrial function without any possible tubal suction interference, they placed a ligature around one tube at the base of the infundibulum in 11 rabbits. Ovulation was then induced and 14 hours later the animals were sacrificed. The ova were flushed from the control tube and removed from the fimbriae of the ligated side and counted. The number of ova recovered from each side was calculated as percentage of the number of ovulation sites on the associated ovary. There was no statistical difference between the percentages of ova recovered from either side. Since these results indicate that ova are quite efficiently captured by ligated tubes, suction does not seem to be an essential factor in ovum pickup in the rabbit. These findings correlate with those of the ovum transperitoneal migration study cited earlier[49] in which intact fimbriae, with or without distal ampullary occlusion close to the solitary ovary, reduced ovum transmigration to the contralateral tube (Table 13:3, groups A and B). The reduction in the percentage of transmigrated ova may be attibuted to their capture by the adjacent fimbriae. The development of delicate microsurgical techniques in gynecology[54–56] has afforded new perspectives in fertility research and, in particular, with respect to the study of ovum pickup and tubal transport of ova. Furthermore, these techniques also allow fimbriectomy, as well as various other surgical procedures to be performed without damage to the surrounding organs (adhesions, anatomical distortions, etc.), thus excluding additional factors that may interfere with fertility. Unilateral fimbriectomy, with removal of the fimbria ovarica, was performed in 16 rabbits.[40] The intact contralateral tube served as control. The rabbits were divided into two groups: In one, no attempt was made to construct a fimbria ovarica-like structure. In the second group, the new ostium was fixed to the ovarian capsule at the site where the fimbria ovarica would normally be attached. Of the 16 rabbits with patent tubes, 15 became pregnant in both the operated and control uterine horns (Table 13:4). The mean nidation index on the fimbriectomized side was 0.70 ± 0.28 SD and of the controls 0.87 ± 0.13 SD, a difference which was not statistically significant. In seven animals, the nidation index was 100 percent on the operated side. Ovum capture efficacy did not appear to be lessened when the neostomy was left lying free in the peritoneal cavity. On the basis of this evidence it was concluded that fimbriectomy, even without reconstruction of a fimbria ovarica does not prevent conception. This observation is supported by a number of works: Metz and Mastroianni, after performing fimbriectomy on a small number of rabbits, were able to recover a few ova from the tubes of two animals of the four with patent tubes.[57] Halbert and Patton recovered ova in the ampullae of all four oviducts that had remained patent following fimbriectomy with infundibular reconstruction in experiments carried out in rabbits.[58] The ovum capture rate

Table 13:4

*Fertility Following Fimbriectomy in the Rabbit**

	Operated side				Control side		
Rabbit no.	*CL*	*ES*	*NI*	*Distance†*	*CL*	*ES*	*NI*
1	3	3	3/3	0	5	4	4/5
2	6	5	5/6	0	5	4	4/5
3	4	2	2/4	0	5	4	4/5
4	2	1	1/2	0	4	3	3/4
5	3	3	3/3	0	9	8	8/9
6	5	5	5/5	0	9	7	7/9
7	7	4	4/7	0	7	7	7/7
8	6	4	4/6	1	3	2	2/3
9	2	2	2/2	3	7	7	7/7
10	4	2	2/4	3	7	7	7/7
11	2	2	2/2	3	6	6	6/6
12	2	1	1/2	6	6	6	6/6
13	6	0	0/6	7	7	7	7/7
14	5	5	5/5	7	6	6	6/6
15	6	6	6/6	10	10	6	6/10
16	5	3	3/5	11	4	3	3/4
Total			48/68				87/100
Mean ± SD			0.70 ± 0.28				0.87 ± 0.13

CL = corpora lutea; ES = embryonic sac; NI = nidation index.
*From Beyth and Winston.[40]
†The distance in mm between the neostomy and the nearest part of the ovary.

was 63 percent on the operated side and 80 percent in the control oviducts. Perez et al. performed unilateral fimbriectomy in 14 rabbits and created a distal ampullary flap that was oversewn to the exposed ovarian surface.[59] Ten of the 14 uterine horns on the operated side and 13 on the control sides became pregnant. The nidation indices on the operated and control sides were 0.38 and 0.73, respectively. The lower index on the manipulated side may have been merely the result of the neostomy flap technique, and its value may correlate with that portion of the ovarian surface which was covered by the flap. Since ovum pickup in the rabbit may take place quite efficiently without fimbriae, even when the distal end of the tube is not in close proximity to the ovary, it is not surprising that pregnancy occurred subsequent to the neostomy flap technique. This indicates again the role of the cilia in the propagation of ova, surrounded by their cumulus mass, from the ovarian surface into the oviduct.

Experiments evaluating the role of the cilia of the fimbrial mucosa in ovum pickup

It is believed that the ciliary activity of the mucosal cells of the fimbriae have a crucial task in transporting the ovulated eggs in their cumuli from the ovary, over the surface of the fimbriae, into the tubal ostium and down the ampulla.[17,19,28,60] In all species examined by Blandau et al. (rat, guinea pig, rabbit, pig, sheep, cow, monkey, and human), the programmed beat of the cilia plays the primary role in egg transport from the ovarian surface into the oviduct, irrespective of the anatomical configuration of the fimbriae.[19] Blandau showed that when the fimbriae of a cat having just ovulated, were lifted gently from the ovarian surface long, streamers of cumulus and matrix became evident.[3] They were attached to each ovulation site and extended into the tubal ostium. The fimbrial cilia swept the sticky, ovulated material from the ovarian surface. The ovum adhered to the epithelial surface because the tips of the cilia physically interacted with elements in the cumulus. The strength of adhesion appeared as a function of the number of cilia. Norwood and Andersen administered a polycation (poly-L-lysine) to intact rabbit oviduct.[61] This polycation is known to inhibit cilia-mediated ovum transport totally in the rabbit oviduct in vitro[62] through interaction with the high-density negative charges located in the cilia.[63] When poly-L-lysine was administered in vivo, it inhibited the ability of the tube to pick up freshly ovulated ova in cumuli. Inhibition of ovum transport amounted to 94 percent: only 4 percent of the ova entered the inhibited oviduct, as compared with 65 percent in the contralateral control side.

Contractions of smooth muscle in the oviductal wall may also contribute to ovum transport. Halbert et al. inhibited this muscle activity by administering acepromazine to anesthetized rabbits, upon which the contractions of the ampullary muscles ceased.[29] All cumulus eggs placed on the fimbriae before and after acepromazine administration moved slowly and smoothly across the fimbria into the tubal ostium. This experiment underlines the ability of the cilia to propagate and direct the egg into the tube without any contributory physical factors such as peristaltic muscular activity or suction.

Clinical Observations on Ovum Pickup in Women

Fertility in the presence of abnormal fimbrial-ovarian relationship

It was believed that direct contact of the fimbrial cilia with the surface of the ovary is mandatory for ovum pickup in women,[23,24,64–66] and that coordinated movements of the ligaments supporting the ovaries and the fallopian tubes are responsbile for the organs' proximity.[67] Cohen and Katz[68] measured the length of the fimbria ovarica and the ovarian ligament in fertile women and found that they were considerably shorter than in some infertile patients. On the basis of this evidence, Cohen instituted a method to restore normal fimbrial-gonadal relationship by plication of the fimbria ovarica (FO).[15] He observed prospectively seven infertile patients in whom the only abnormality diagnosed was deranged fimbrial-gonadal relationship caused by elongation of the FO. During the 12 months of observation, one of the women conceived; the remaining six patients underwent plication of the FO and five of them conceived. Cohen suggested that in the course of a fertility operation, the FO should be evaluated and, if appropriate, the plication procedure should be carried out to facilitate fimbrial-ovarian approximation during ovulation.

In the normal process of ovum capture, the fimbriae and tubal ostium come into contact with the ovary. The fimbriae move across the surface of the ovary in a to-and-fro motion, thus lying over and touching the site of ovulation. However, there are quite a few clinical observations that point out that this direct contact is not a critical factor for conception. Burckhard[69] in 1904, and later Westman[4] and Caffier[70] discussed in detail the possibility of ovum capture by the fimbria contralateral to the ovulatory ovary. Transperitoneal migration of ova from one ovary to the opposing oviduct has been reported,[71] and pregnancies have occurred in women with one ovary and one contralateral tube.[72–74] A reasonable explanation for ovum capture in these cases may be pickup of the ovum by the fimbriae from a pool of fluid in the cul-de-sac. However, ovum capture may also occur in women in whom the fimbriae do not reach the pouch of Douglas. Such a phenomenon is usually associated with a congenital malformation of the genital tract in which the anatomical location of the fimbriae allows neither contact with the ovary nor their descent into the pouch of Douglas. Ectopic pregnancy was reported in a heterotopic tube in the left upper quadrant of the peritoneal cavity.[75] Eggs can also be picked up by accessory tubes, which are small, nonpatent cylindrical structures attached to the ampulla of a normal-sized tube. At their distal end there is a fimbria-like small structure which is lined with ciliated epithelium.[76] These "fimbriae" do not reach the ovarian surface or the pouch of Douglas. Nevertheless, ectopic pregnancies in accessory tubes, probably as a result of peritoneal migration of ovum and spermatozoa, have been reported by Hensok[77] in 1888, and later by Ekler.[78] One is therefore justified in speculating that in certain circumstances, the ovum together with its cumulus following its detachment from the ovarian surface is carried by the fluid in the peritoneal cavity and, when passing close to the fimbriae, is captured by them.

Ovum capture in the absence of fimbriae

Intact fimbriae apparently play an important part in ovum capture. Yet, there are clinical conditions where fertility is preserved even in the absence of fimbriae. Since the fimbriae were considered indispensable for ovum pickup, bilateral fimbriectomy, as suggested by Kroener, seemed an obvious and efficient sterilization procedure.[79] The eventual and potential reversibility of sterilization by fimbriectomy was also discussed, and Kroener stated that "turning back the cuff would be a simple surgical procedure, though whether it would be an efficient method of producing fertility, I do not know." Since microsurgical reversal of female sterilization has become a successful technique, with a pregnancy rate of over 70 percent,[56,80–82] and in view of the accumulated clinical and experimental evidence that fimbrial resection per se does not prevent pregnancy, it was suggested that surgical reversal might be attempted in selected fimbriectomized patients. Novy created a new ostium by transverse salpingostomy and a cuff eversion technique, achieving a tubal patency rate of 83 percent and an intrauterine pregnancy rate of 44 percent.[83,84]

Fimbriectomy as a sterilization procedure was considered very safe since it involved removal of the infundibulum of the tube and interruption of the fimbrial-ovarian relationship. This, presumably, would seriously impair egg capture, even when the closure of the ampulla by ligation became incomplete because of fistula formation. Nevertheless, Metz reported ten conceptions in 388 patients (2.6 percent) who underwent fimbriectomy,[85,86] and several other publications[87,88] also document fimbriectomy failures.

Pelvic inflammatory disease is known to cause a wide spectrum of damages to the fallopian tubes. The extent of the damage to the fimbriae can be estimated and graded according to the classification of Rock et al.[89] The outcome of reconstructive surgery in such patients depends on the degree of tubal and fimbrial abnormality. In patients with agglutinated fimbriae (classified as "slight fimbrial damage"), microsurgical fimbrioplasty should result in a high incidence of postoperative pregnancy. Where excellent fimbriae were encountered following fimbrioplasty, a highly satisfactory pregnancy rate was achieved.[89,90] However, if tubal infection persists or remains untreated, permanent destruction of the normal tubal architecture, including that of the fimbria, may ensue. Such patients require cuff salpingostomy in an attempt to regain fertility. Even patients with destroyed fimbriae, in whom, supposedly, the tubal mucosa including the ciliated cells, were also damaged, did conceive following surgery. The success rate of salpingostomy in these patients displays extreme variations but proves to correlate well with the extent of tubal damage. The absence of fimbriae does not prevent conception, and intrauterine pregnancies have been reported in up to 44 percent of women who were subjected to terminal salpingostomy.[91–95]

Fistula formation, a possible complication of any kind of tubal sterilization procedure, may appear on either side of the ligation. A fistula on that tubal segment which is in continuity with the uterus may capture an ovum, despite both its distance from the ovulation site and its lack of fimbria, with resultant intrauterine or ectopic pregnancies.[74,88]

From the foregoing it is inferred that although neither intact fimbria nor normal fimbrial-ovarian anatomical relations are prerequisites for ovum pickup, both are conducive to efficient ovum capture. In the above-presented clinical pathological conditions, there are usually additional factors, such as shortened tubes, damage to tubal mucosa and musculature, and/or periovarian and peritubal adhesions, which by themselves may impair fertility. Because of these frequent abnormalities, we are unable to evaluate the effect of fimbriectomy per se on fertility in women.

The role of ciliary activity in fertility

In the intact female genital tract, the ciliated cells in the fimbriae are assumed to play a role in ovum pickup. At ovulation, when the fimbriae are drawn across the ovarian surface, the cilia come into contact with the sticky cumulus mass that envelops the ovum, and the cumulus mass is then conducted into the ostium, primarily by action of the cilia.

Critoph and Dennis, who investigated the ciliary activity in the human oviduct in vitro, were unable to establish any differences in the rate of ciliary beat in the fimbriae at different times of the menstrual cycle.[21] Afzelius et al[31] and Eliasson et al.[30] depicted the absence of dynein arms in cilia obtained from bronchial and nasal mucosa of two women with complete Kartagener's triad, and in the sperm tail of four subjects who produced immotile spermatozoa.[35] Bleau et al. presented the same findings in cilia of endocervical cells of a patient with Kartagener's triad.[32] The data in the literature[31,32,34] concerning fertility in women suffering from immotile cilia syndrome strongly suggest that ciliary motility in the genital tract is not imperative for female fertility and, furthermore, that motile cilia are not critical for ovum pickup in women.

Concluding Remarks

The transfer of the ovum from the ovulation site on the ovarian surface to the fimbriae is the first step of a much longer journey during which the egg is transported through the tube into the uterine cavity to the implantation site. Theoretically, there are three possible ways by which the egg reaches the fimbriae:

1. intrinsic motion of the ovulated egg leading it toward the fimbria;
2. movements of the tube, causing the fimbriae to embrace the ovarian surface at the ovulation site during ovulation; or
3. extrinsic forces that propagate the egg in the pelvic peritoneal cavity, eventually bringing it into close proximity with the fimbriae.

Obviously, simultaneous action of two, or even all three of these mechanisms is also conceivable.

By itself, the ovum in its cumulus does not have the ability to move, since it lacks the appropriate mechanisms (i.e., muscle fibers or cilia). The first speculation is therefore unfeasible, nor is chemotaxic attraction of the ovum by ciliated cells of the fimbriae, requiring intrinsic movement, plausible. There exists sufficient evidence and data as to the role of the muscle fibers of the ovarian and tubal ligaments and mesenteries in approximating the fimbriae and ovary to one another during ovulation in certain mammalian species, including the human female. The close relation between intact fimbrial ciliated cells and the site of ovulation probably accounts for optimal efficiency in ovum pickup in these species. However, since ovum capture by the fimbriae also occurs without direct contact between fimbria and ovary (admittedly less efficiently), there must be an alternative way to conduct the egg from the ovary to the tubal ostium.

This brings us to the third possible mechanism, i.e., extrinsic forces propelling the egg. In cases where the distance between the fimbriae and ovary prohibit direct contact between these organs, streams of intraperitoneal fluid (the amount of which increases in the human female toward ovulation) may carry the egg around in the peritoneal cavity. When it incidentally approaches the fimbria, the cumulus mass sticks to its cilia, which then propagates it toward the tubal ostium.

It seems that the efficacy of ovum capture by the fimbriae depends on several factors; when all function normally, optimal efficiency is achieved. However, even in the presence of dysfunction of one or more factors (compromised ciliary activity with absence of fimbriae in patients with cuff salpingostomy following pelvic inflammatory disease) or with total nonfunctioning of one factor (absence of fimbriae in reversed Kroener sterilization or immobile cilia in Kartagener's syndrome), ovum capture is still possible.

In apparently all mammalian species, once the egg in its cumulus reaches the fimbriae, it sticks to the cilia of the ciliated cells that propagate it toward the tubal ostium. However, the mechanisms by which the egg reaches the fimbriae varies in different species; hence, it is difficult to transpose the findings on animal ovum capture to that which occurs in women.

References

1. Jocelyn HD, Setchell BP: On the human reproductive organs: De mulierum organis generationi in servientibus tractatus novus. *J Reprod Fertil* 28 (Suppl 70): 1, 1972.
2. Westman A: Investigations into the transit of ova in man. *J Obstet Gynaecol Br Emp*, 44:821, 1937.
3. Blandau RJ: Gamete transport in the female mammal. In Greep RO (Ed): *Handbook of Physiology*. Washington, D.C.: American Physiological Society, 1973; p. 153, Sect. 7, Part 2.
4. Westman A: Transit of ovum from ovary to uterus in rabbits. *Acta Obstet Gynecol Scand*, 5:7, 1926.
5. Anderes E: Zur Frage des Eitransportes durch die Tube. *Schweiz Med Wochnschr*, 71:364, 1941.
6. Wimsatt WA, Waldo CM: The normal occurrence of a peritoneal opening in the bursa ovarii of the mouse. *Anat Rec*, 93:47, 1945.
7. Decker A, Decker WH: A tubal function test. *Obstet Gynecol*, 4:35, 1954.
8. Scheffery JB: A method for determining tubal patency and tubal ciliary activity. *N Y State J Med*, 54:3092, 1954.
9. Yaffe H, Beyth Y, Reinhartz T, et al: Foreign body granulomata in peritubal and periovarian adhesions, a possible cause for unsuccessful reconstructive surgery in infertility. *Fertil Steril*, 33:277, 1980.
10. Rouget C: Recherches sur les organs erectile de la femme et sur l'appareil musculaire tubo-ovarien. *J Physiol l'Homme Anim*, 1: 320, 1858.
11. Okamura H, Morikawa H, Oshima M, et al: A morphologic study of mesotubarium ovarica in human. *Obstet Gynecol*, 49:197, 1977.
12. Mahran M, Fadel HE, Saleh A: Human ovarian ligaments: Structure and possible function. *Obstet Gynecol*, 37:711, 1971.
13. Beyth Y, Meini U: Fertility following excision of the mesotuberium superius in the rabbit. *Israel J Med Sci*, 18:519, 1982.
14. Fredericks CM, Anderson WR: The ef-

fect of transection of the accessory ligaments of reproduction in the rabbit. *Fertil Steril*, 32:219, 1979.

15. Cohen BM: Surgical repair of abnormal fimbrial gonadal relationship in the human female. *J Reprod Med*, 25:33, 1980.
16. Beck LR: Comparative observations on the morphology of the mammalian periovarial sac. *J Morphol*, 136:247, 1972.
17. Gaddum-Rosse P, Blandau RJ: Comparative observations on ciliary currents in mammalian oviducts. *Biol Reprod*, 14:605, 1976.
18. Blandau RJ: Gamete transport, comparative aspects. In Hafez ESE, Blandau RJ (Eds): *The Mammalian Oviduct*, Chicago: University of Chicago Press, 1969: p. 129.
19. Blandau RJ, Bracket B, Brenner RM, et al: The oviduct. In Greep RO (Ed): *Frontiers in Reproduction and Fertility Control*, Cambridge, MA: The MIT Press, 1977: p. 137.
20. Fredericsson B: Studies on the morphology and histochemistry of the fallopian tube epithelium. *Acta Anat*, 37 (Suppl):38, 1959.
21. Critoph FN, Dennis KJ: Ciliary activity in the human oviduct. *Br J Obstet Gynaecol*, 84:216, 1977.
22. Morikawa H, Okamura H, Takenaka A, et al: Physiological study of the human mesotubarium ovarica. *Obstet Gynecol*, 55:493, 1980.
23. Mikulicz-Radecki V: Der Eiauffangsmechanismus bei der Frau und die sich daraus ergebenden Schlussfolgerungen für die operative Behandlung der Sterilität. *Arch Gynäkol*, 161:128, 1936.
24. Caffier P: Studien zum Eitransport beim Menschen. I. Mitteilung: Der Eiabnahmemechanismus. *Zentralb Gynäkol*, 60:1873, 1936.
25. Doyle JB: Exploratory culdotomy for observation of tubo-ovarian physiology at ovulation time. *Fertil Steril*, 2:475, 1951.
26. Doyle JB: Tubo-ovarian mechanism: Observations at laparotomy. *Obstet Gynecol*, 8:686, 1956.
27. Decker A: Culdoscopic observations on the tubo-ovarian mechanism of ovum reception. *Fertil Steril*, 2:253, 1951.
28. Gaddum-Rosse P, Blandau RJ, Thiersch JB: Ciliary activity in the human and Macaco nemestrina oviduct. *Am J Anat*, 138:269, 1973.
29. Halbert SA, Tam PY, Adams RJ, et al: An analysis of the mechanisms of egg transport in the ampulla of the rabbit oviduct. *Gynecol Invest*, 7:306, 1976.
30. Eliasson R, Mossberg B, Camner P, et al: The immobile cilia syndrome. *N Engl J Med*, 297:1, 1977.
31. Afzelius BA, Camner P, Mossbery B: On the function of cilia in the female reproductive tract. *Fertil Steril*, 29:72, 1978.
32. Bleau G, Richer CL, Bousquet D: Absence of dynein arms in cilia of endocervical cells in a fertile woman. *Fertil Steril*, 30:362, 1978.
33. Arge E: Transposition of the viscera and sterility in men. *Lancet*, 1:412, 1960.
34. Katsuhara K, Kawamoto S, Wakabayashi T, et al: Situs inversus totalis and Kartagener's syndrome in a Japanese population. *Chest*, 61:56, 1972.
35. Afzelius BA: A human syndrome caused by immobile cilia. *Science*, 193:317, 1976.
36. Katsch G, Borchers E: Beiträge zum Studium der Darmbewegungen. *Ztschr Pathol Therap*, 12:225, 1913.
37. Pauerstein CJ: Gamete transport in the mammalian oviduct. In Brosens I, Gognat M, Constantin A, et al (Eds): *Oviducte et Fertilite*. Paris: Masson, 1979: p. 127.
38. Kistner RW: Management of endometriosis in infertile patients. *Fertil Steril*, 26:1151, 1975.
39. Cohen BM: A modified microsurgical method of transplanting the fallopian tube. In Phillips JM (Ed): *Microsurgery in Gynecology*. Downey: American Association of Gynecologic Laparoscopists, 1977: p. 176.
40. Beyth Y, Winston RML: Ovum capture and fertility following microsurgical fimbriectomy in the rabbit. *Fertil Steril*, 35:464, 1981.
41. Eddy CA, Laufe LE: Fertility following microsurgical dissociation of the ovary and fimbriae in the rhesus monkey. *Fertil Steril*, 39:566, 1983.
42. Boling JL, Blandau, RJ: Egg transport through the ampullae of the oviduct of rabbits under various experimental conditions. *Biol Reprod*, 4:174, 1971.
43. Halbert SA, Conrad JT: In vitro con-

tractile activity of the mesotubarium superius from the rabbit oviduct in various endocrine states. *Fertil Steril*, 26:248, 1975.
44. Conrad JT: Bioelectrical and contractile behavior of rabbit mesotubarium superius: estrogen withdrawal. *Am J Physiol*, 233:180, 1977.
45. Meiri U, Meiri H, Marshall JM: Effects of ovarium steroids on spontaneous and nerve induced electrical activity of the oviduct and its attached membranes in the rabbit. *Biol Reprod*, 19:183, 1978.
46. Kelly GL: Effects of opening the ovarian bursa on fecundity in the albino rat. *Anat Rec*, 73:401, 1939.
47. Pappo I, Beyth Y: Unpublished data, 1981.
48. Lode A: Experimentelle Beiträge zur Lehre der Wanderung des Eies vom Ovarium zur Tube. *Arch Gynäkol*, 45:293, 1894.
49. Beyth Y, Margara R, Winston RML: Transperitoneal migration of ova. III World Congress of Human Reproduction, Berlin, 1981.
50. Clewe TH: The attachment of the cumulus oophorus to the follicle after ovulation in the absence of the fimbria in rabbits. *Anat Rec*, 139:217, 1961.
51. Dubreuil G: Le réseau lymphatique fonctionnel des franges et des plis de la trompe, son rôle dans la captation et le cheminement de l'oeuf chez la femme. *Gynécol Obstét*, 44:397, 1944.
52. Maia H, Coutinho EM: Peristalsis and antiperistalsis of the human fallopian tube during the menstrual cycle. *Biol Reprod*, 2:305, 1970.
53. Clewe TH, Mastroianni L Jr: Mechanisms of ovum pick up. 1. Functional capacity of rabbit oviducts ligated near the fimbria. *Fertil Steril*, 9:13, 1968.
54. Swolin K: Electromicrosurgery and salpingostomy: Long term results. *Am J Obstet Gynecol*, 121:418, 1975.
55. Winston RML: Microsurgical tubocornual anastomosis for reversal of sterilisation. *Lancet*, 1:284, 1977.
56. Gomel V: Tubal reanastomosis by microsurgery. *Fertil Steril*, 28:59, 1977.
57. Metz KGP, Mastroianni L Jr: Dispensability of fimbriae: Ovum pickup by tubal fistulas in rabbit. *Fertil Steril*, 32:329, 1979.
58. Halbert SA, Patton DL: Ovum pick-up following fimbriectomy and infundibular salpingostomy in rabbits. *J Reprod Med*, 26:199, 1981.
59. Perez LE, Flores JJ, Bajpal VK, et al: Fertility following fimbriectomy and tubo-ovarian microsurgery in the rabbit. *Fertil Steril*, 35:573, 1981.
60. Gaddum-Rosse P, Blandau RJ: In vitro studies of ciliary activity within the oviducts of the rabbit and pig. *Am J Anat*, 136:91, 1973.
61. Norwood JT, Anderson RG: Evidence that adhesive sites on the tips of oviduct cilia membranes are required for ovum pick up in situ. *Biol Reprod*, 23:788, 1980.
62. Norwood JT, Heim CE, Halbert SA, et al: Polycationic macromolecules inhibit cilia-mediated ovum transport in the rabbit oviduct. *Proc Natl Acad Sci*, 75:4413, 1978.
63. Anderson RGW, Hein CE: Distribution of anionic sites on the oviduct ciliary membrane. *J Cell Biol*, 72:482, 1971.
64. Elert R: Der Mechanismus der Eiabnahme im Laparskop. *Zentralbl Gynäkol*, 69:38, 1947.
65. Gomel V: An odyssey through the oviduct. *Fertil Steril*, 39:144, 1983.
66. Speroff L, Glass RH, Kase NG: *Clinical Gynecologic Endocrinology and Infertility*, 3 ed. Baltimore: Williams and Wilkins, 1984: p. 453.
67. Hafez ESE: Gamete transport. In Hafez ESE, Evans TN (Eds): *Human Reproduction: Conception and Contraception*. Hagerstown, MD: Harper and Row, 1973: p. 106.
68. Cohen BM, Katz M: The significance of the convoluted oviduct in the infertile woman. *J Reprod Med*, 21:31, 1978.
69. Burckhard G: Ist eine innere und aussere Ueberwanderung des Eies möglich? *Ztschr Geburtsh Gynäkol*, 52:471, 1904.
70. Caffier P: Studien zum Eitransport beim Menschen. II. Mitteilung: Zur Frage der ausseren Ueberwanderung des Eies. *Zentralb Gynäkol*, 60:2466, 1936.
71. Doyle LL, Lippes J, Winters HS, et al: Human ova in the fallopian tube. *Am J Obstet Gynecol*, 95:115, 1966.
72. First A: Transperitoneal migration of ovum or spermatozoon. *Obstet Gynecol*, 4:431, 1954.
73. Kamrava M, Seibel MM, Thompson IE, et al: Intrauterine pregnancy following

transperitoneal migration of the ovum. *Obstet Gynecol*, 60:391, 1982.

74. Mastroianni L Jr, Metz KGP: Tubal pregnancy subsequent to transperitoneal migration of spermatozoa. *Obstet Gynecol Surv*, 34:554, 1979.
75. Granat M, Evron S, Navot D: Pregnancy in heterotopic fallopian tube and unilateral ovarian hyperstimulation. *Acta Obstet Gynecol Scand*, 60:215, 1981.
76. Beyth Y, Kopolovic J: Accessory tubes: A possible contribution factor in fertility. *Fertil Steril*, 38:382, 1982.
77. Hensock H: Cited by Ekler,[78] 1888.
78. Ekler R: Gravidität in einer Nebentube. *Arch Gynäkol*, 113:605, 1920.
79. Kroener WF Jr: Surgical sterilization by fimbriectomy. *Am J Obstet Gynecol*, 104:247, 1969.
80. Siegler AM, Perez RJ: Reconstruction of fallopian tubes in previously sterilized patients. *Fertil Steril*, 26:383, 1975.
81. Brosens I, Winston R: *Reversibility of Female Sterilization*. London: Academic Press, 1978.
82. Eddy CA: Tubal physiology and microsurgery. *Aust NZ J Obstet Gynaecol*, 21:129, 1981.
83. Novy MJ: Reversal of Kroener fimbriectomy sterilization. *Fertil Steril*, 32:498, 1979.
84. Novy MJ: Reversal of Kroener fimbriectomy sterilization. *Am J Obstet Gynecol*, 137:198, 1980.
85. Metz KGP: Failures following fimbriectomy. *Fertil Steril*, 28:66, 1977.
86. Metz KGP: Failures following fimbriectomy: A further report. *Fertil Steril*, 30:269, 1978.
87. Editorial comment (re: Kroener WF Jr: Surgical sterilization by fimbriectomy). *Obstet Gynecol Surv*, 24:1400, 1969.
88. Hughes GJ: Sterilisation failure. *Br Med J*, 2:1337, 1977.
89. Rock JA, Katayama P, Martin EJ, et al: Factors influencing the success of salpingostomy techniques for distal fimbrial obstruction. *Obstet Gynecol*, 52:591, 1978.
90. Patton GW: Pregnancy outcome following microsurgical fimbrioplasty. *Fertil Steril*, 37:150, 1982.
91. Winston RML: Is microsurgery necessary for salpingostomy? The evaluation of results. *Aust NZ J Obstet Gynaecol*, 21:143, 1981.
92. DeCherney AH, Kase N: A comparison of treatment for bilateral fimbrial occlusion. *Fertil Steril*, 35:162, 1981.
93. Frantzen C, Schlösser HW: Microsurgery and post-infectious tubal infertility. *Fertil Steril*, 38:397, 1982.
94. Cholst IN: Surgery on the fimbrial portion of the fallopian tube. *Semin Reprod Endocrinol*, 2:160, 1984.
95. Wallach EE, Manara LR, Eisenberg E: Experience with 143 cases of tubal surgery. *Fertil Steril*, 39:609, 1983.

II

Tubal Pathology

Editorial Comments

The Effect of Exposure to DES in Utero

Newbold and McLachlan describe and illustrate the significant alterations in oviductal development as a consequence of prenatal exposure to diethylstilbestrol (DES) in animals. Significant changes are seen both grossly and microscopically, especially proliferative lesions within the oviduct, evidence of its teratogenic effect.

The concern for the neoplastic consequences of prenatal DES exposure has receded but genital tract abnormalities do exist. The unique characteristics seen on hysterosalpingography are the small endometrial cavity, the concavities beneath the uterine cornua, and the T-shaped uterine configuration (Fig. II:1). On hysteroscopic examination, these radiological changes can be explained by structural alterations within the myometrium that resemble submucous myomas. To date, there is no method of surgical correction for this uterine abnormality.

Although radiological configuration of the fallopian tubes is not characteristic of prenatal DES exposure, Newbold and McLachlan show significant proliferative changes within the endosalpinx, quite similar to those seen in salpingitis isthmica nodosa or tubal diverticulosis. Such morphological alterations cause a characteristic honeycomb appearance on the hysterosalpingogram. However, such changes were described long before DES was used. There is no evidence of any increase in proximal tubal obstruction or alteration in the intramural portion of the oviduct in women exposed prenatally to DES. These women seem to have some predisposition to tubal pregnancy so that the mechanism of ovum transport may be abnormal. Whether prenatal DES exposure is associated with an increased frequency of infertility remains controversial.

Pelvic Inflammatory Disease

Much has been written about *Chlamydia trachomatis* as a possible cause of pelvic inflammatory disease. Several articles in the Scandinavian literature suggest a concurrent chlamydial infection in 30 to 60 percent of patients with gonococcal cervicitis. Chlamydia grow intracellularly and may be identified as

The Fallopian Tube: Basic Studies and Clinical Contributions, edited by Alvin M. Siegler, M.D. Mount Kisco, New York: Futura Publishing Company, Inc. © 1986.

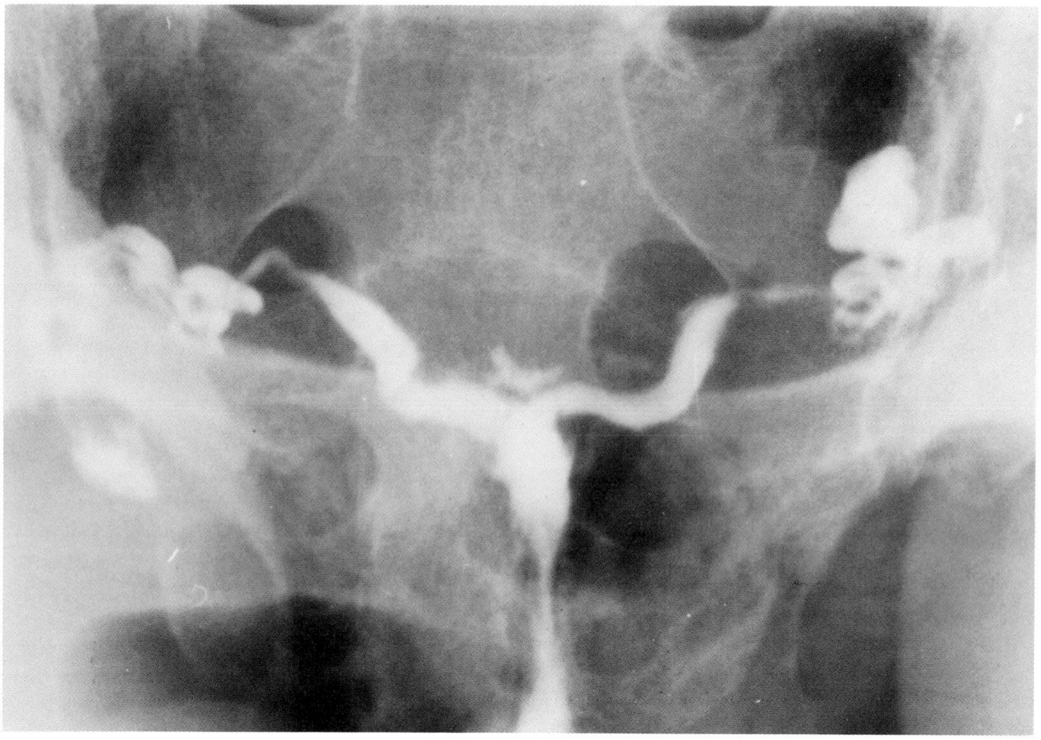

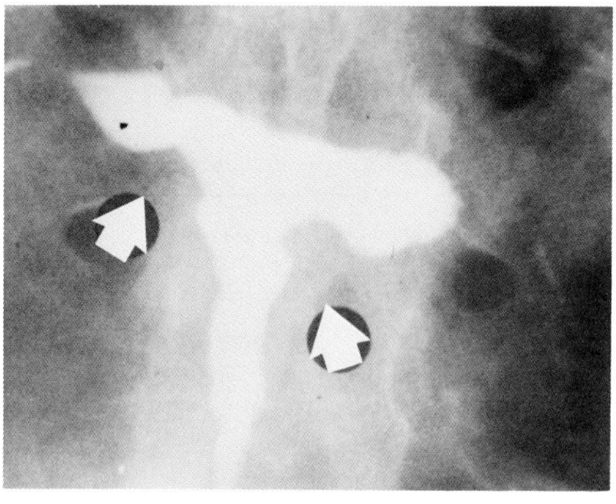

FIGURE II:1—a (above). *Odd-shaped uterine cavity resembles steer horns.* b (left). *More characteristic uterine deformity with lateral concavities (arrows) is seen.*

inclusion bodies with special staining techniques. Culture is the most reliable method of identification; the specimen sent for culture or staining must include cellular material to yield meaningful results.

The tetracyclines are the drugs of choice for many sexually transmitted diseases caused by selective organisms such as chlamydia and mycoplasma. These drugs act to inhibit protein synthesis by binding to 30 S ribosomes. Since only a small portion is irreversibly bound, the tetracyclines are bacteriostatic. Ultimate destruction of the bacterium depends on host defense mechanisms. If not phagocytized, the bacterium may subsequently renew its replication when the tetracycline is eliminated from the cell. The recent renaissance of the tetracyclines has resulted from the development of two analogues, doxycycline (Vibramycin, Pfizer) and minocycline (Minocin, Lederle). Doxycycline is given orally, 100 mg b.i.d., with a minimum dose of 100 mg. Its serum half-life is 15 hours, it has high patient compliance, and gastrointestinal absorption is virtually complete.

The augmented protein binding enables the antibiotic levels in the serum to be sustained for a prolonged amount of time, thus decreasing the frequency of antibiotic administration. This new generation of tetracycline permits the use of one-fifth to one-tenth the dose required with the older generation of tetracyclines. Food does not appear to alter gastrointestinal absorption significantly so that blood levels for doxycycline, with or without meals, are comparable. Both Hager and DeCherney emphasize the need for the early, accurate diagnosis and prompt treatment of salpingitis to prevent serious tubal damage resulting in infertility.

Nodular formation in the tubal isthmus caused by diverticulosis is associated with acute and chronic salpingitis in most patients. However, endometriosis, tubal polyps or, less frequently, tuberculosis, are other possibilities, as pointed out by Badaway, Beller, and Ansari.

Descriptions of the roentgenological appearance of tubal diverticulosis were reported in the early 20th century. Nodular isthmic disease should be suspected whenever interruption in the clear, linear continuity of the luminal shadow is associated with flecks of contrast agent above or below the main canal. The honeycombed appearance is characteristic of tubal diverticulosis and this condition has been confirmed at laparotomy or laparoscopy in many instances. (Fig. II:2).

The honeycombed roentgenographic appearance of salpingitis isthmica nodosa, endometriosis, and tuberculosis can be difficult to differentiate from each other so that other features of these diseases should be sought. With tubal tuberculosis, the tubes appear rigid, with pipe stem configurations and sometimes calcifications appear in the tubes, ovaries or in regional lymph nodes (Fig. II:3). With salpingitis, distal tubal obstruction and hydrosalpinges are associated with isthmic disease.

Tubal Endometriosis

Laparoscopic examination that shows evidence of endometriosis in the cul-de-sac and ovaries, associated with a nodular tubal isthmus, should make one suspicious of tubal endometriosis as the cause of the problem. Although biopsy is not feasible, a course of hormonal therapy with ovulation suppression for six months and either a repeat hysterosalpingogram or laparoscopy could furnish valuable additional information.

Tubal endometriosis has been seen in the proximal segment of previously sterilized patients in whom the sterilization was done by tubal coagulation, ligation, or the application of rings. The tubal serosal surface can become involved with endometrial implants and associated adhesions may be dense or filmy. The most severe forms of endometriosis cause distal tubal occlusion with extensive adhesions and almost always involve the ipsilateral ovary. The cause of infertility in instances cited above, in which the tubes are involved significantly, is obvious, but the presence of minimal or mild endome-

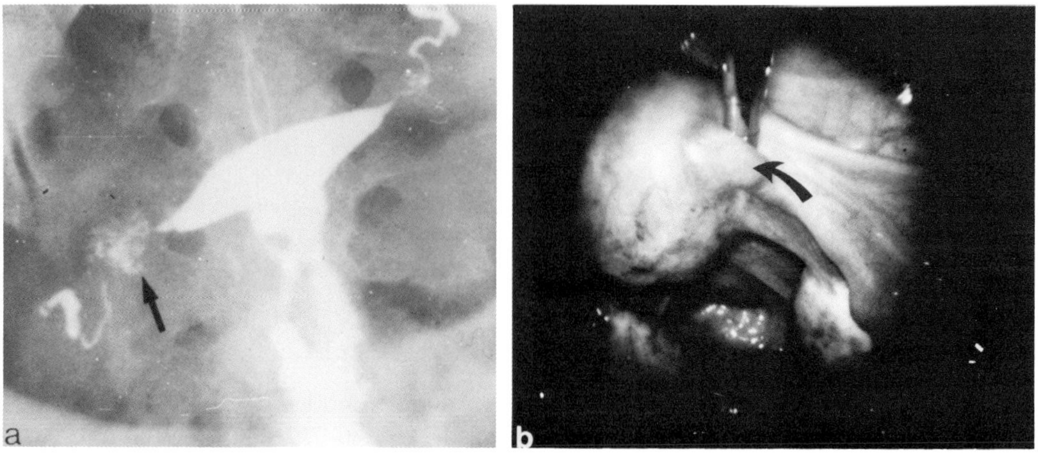

FIGURE II:2—a. *Hysterosalpingogram shows characteristic appearance of salpingitis isthmica nodosa (arrow).* b. *At laparoscopy isthmic nodularity (arrow) is present under the probe.*

triosis can also create an unsuitable pelvic environment. Badaway discusses some recent data on peritoneal reactions and hormonal content of cul-de-sac fluid as they pertain to endometriosis.

The IUD

The reports of an increased risk of tubal infertility because of the use of inert intrauterine devices (IUDs) especially in nulliparous women and those with multiple sexual partners make the comprehensive contributions by Eibshitz and coworkers quite timely. Indeed, manufacturers have made additions to the professional labeling and to patient information leaflets. The IUD remains a safe and effective method of contraception for parous women, especially when no more children are desired and neither partner wants to be sterilized. It is particularly useful in women over 35 and especially women who smoke, in whom the risks of oral contraceptives are increased.

Actinomyces appears to have the same incidence in the vagina regardless of whether or not an intrauterine device is present, about 3 to 4 percent. In a recent study by Persson and Holmberg (*Acta Obstet Gynecol Scand,* 63:207, 1984), it was found that *A. israelii* was part of the natural flora of the lower genital tract. Heretofore the general impression was that this organism thrived only when a foreign body was present. The type of IUD and the length of its use appear to influence the positivity of the culture. Most positive cases appear in women wearing plastic devices rather than copper ones, and in those users whose devices have been in place for over two years.

When the only finding is cytologic evidence of actinomyces, patients should not be treated for pelvic inflammatory disease (PID). The colonization cannot be ignored because, while rarely serious, IUD-associated actinomycoses can be fatal. *A. israelii* is susceptible to penicillin, tetracyclines, and clindomycin; however, attempts to eradicate this organism from the genital tract have been unsuccessful when the IUD has been left in place. The finding of actinomyces on Papanicolaou smear will disappear gradually if the IUD is removed. Accepted current practice is to remove the IUD and repeat the smear in four to six weeks. If the smear is negative and the patient is asymptomatic, the IUD can be reinserted. If the patient is symptomatic, the IUD should be removed and the patient treated with adequate amounts of an appropriate antibiotic for two weeks.

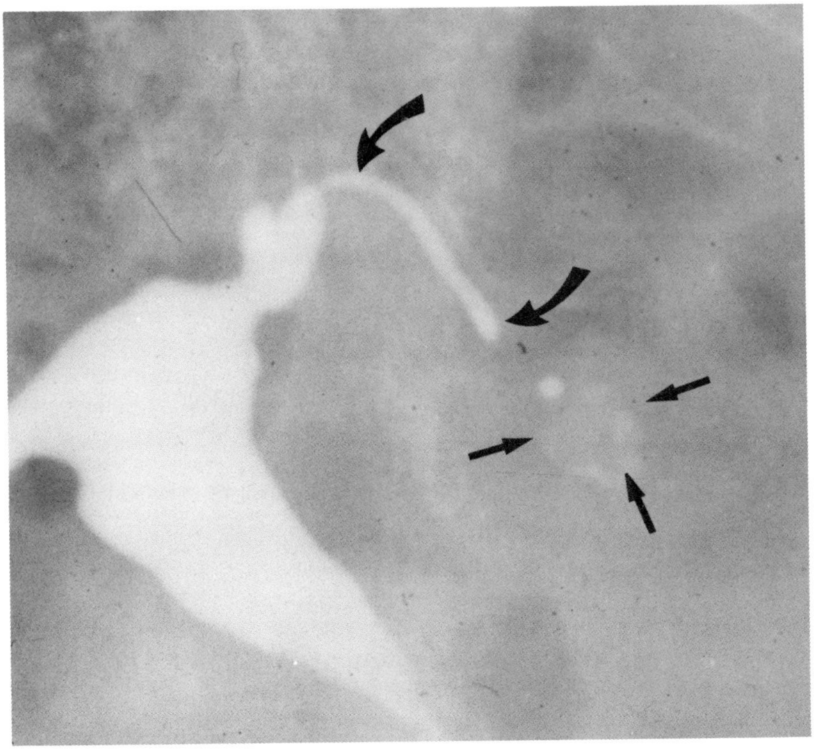

FIGURE II:3—*Pipe stem configuration and rigid appearance tube (curved arrow) and ovarian calcification (straight arrow) indicate tuberculosis.*

From 9 to 17 percent of all pregnancies with the IUD in place are ectopic. The IUD reduces the risk of intrauterine pregnancy by 99.5 percent, the risk of tubal pregnancy by 95 percent, and that of ovarian pregnancy not at all; hence, the relevant increase in tubal and ovarian pregnancies in IUD users. In a well-designed case control study analyzing 615 women with previous ectopic pregnancies and 3,453 control subjects matched by several variables including risk factors for ectopic pregnancies, Ory et al. (*Obstet Gynecol*, 51:137, 1981) concluded that an IUD user had the same risk as a nonuser for an ectopic pregnancy. Incorporation of a progestogen into the IUD appears to increase the incidence of ectopic pregnancy over that seen with the unmedicated device.

Struthers and her colleagues have collected data from many investigators and conclude that copper and inert IUDs do not seem to be risk factors for tubal pregnancy and indeed confer some degree of protection against ectopic gestations.

Tubal Pregnancy

Tubal pregnancy still presents the gynecologist with difficult problems in diagnosis and therapy. It remains a potentially fatal condition and currently accounts for 6 to 8 percent of all maternal deaths in the United States.[1]

Many concerns persist about the management of this condition, including its apparently rising incidence, the identification of the high-risk patient, the need for prompt and early diagnosis before tubal rupture, the selection of the proper operative procedure, the subsequent infertility of most patients, and an incidence of repeat ectopic gestation of nearly 15 percent. The principal case against tubal conservation has always been the predisposition to recurrence of pregnancy in the repaired tube.

Instances of unruptured tubal pregnancy were occasionally found and reported as early as the 17th century.[2] However, the diagnosis was rarely suspected before severe bleeding ensued. Rogers, in 1867,[3] described quite clearly the symptoms and signs of this entity, and he even suggested the use of a trocar to search for blood in the peritoneal cavity. Although he and Harbert indicated the need for surgical intervention to arrest the bleeding, it was not until 1884 that Tait performed laparotomies on five women.[5] Four of these patients had salpingectomies and all survived. One woman who had a conservative operation, closing of the tubal rent and removing the products of conception, succumbed. Before the end of the 19th century, other reports appeared in the literature on the management of tubal abortion and successful conservative tubotomy.[6–8] Until this time, nonoperative management had included starvation, purgation, ergot, and electrocution of the tubal gestation.[9] Colpotomy, with vaginal drainage and removal of the products of conception, was described by Kelly et al.[10] in 1896 and Ford[11] in 1906. Exciting discussions followed both of these historic presentations with commendation and condemnation of the technique.

To gather some idea concerning the prospects of a repeat tubal gestation or normal pregnancy post-operatively, Schumann,[12] in 1921, collected the reports of 280 patients in whom pregnancy was possible following salpingectomy/or salpingo-oophorectomy for a tubal pregnancy. He noted that 35 (12.5 percent) had a repeated ectopic gestation and 134 (47.8 percent) had an intrauterine pregnancy. This ratio of 1:4 has not changed significantly until the present time. Rubin,[13] in 1934, hoping to improve the postoperative fertility of his patients, suggested concurrent salpingostomy or lysis of adhesions of the contralateral tube if it appeared obstructed. He also alluded to the possibility of partial salpingectomy or removal of the products of conception by simple tubal incision, with or without curettement, followed by tubal suture to conserve the tube in selected patients. It seemed logical that the early diagnosis of unruptured tubal gestation would make conservative operations on the pregnant tube safer and more feasible. In 1941, Caffier[14] described ten conservative operations on the pregnant tubes of women whose contralateral adnexa had been previously removed for ectopic gestations. Only one of them reported a repeat ectopic, and four women had a total of six intrauterine pregnancies. In the English literature, it appears that Stromme[15] was the first physician to describe precisely a successful salpingotomy for an unruptured tubal gestation.

Management of patients suspected of having an extrauterine pregnancy includes a good history and proper physical examination. Abdominal pain is the most consistent symptom of ectopic pregnancy and the most common predisposing factor is previous pelvic inflammatory disease. A history of infertility, the use of an IUD, a previous tubal pregnancy, or tubal ligation also increase the risk. The classic symptoms of pregnancy are inconsistent but abnormal vaginal bleeding associated with pain and a history of PID should arouse suspicion. However, a pelvic mass is not present in at least 50 percent of the patients and this is one of the reasons why an examination under anesthesia can be misleading. In addition, this type of examination could rupture a tubal pregnancy. Finally, the degree of abdominal pain and pelvic tenderness are masked by the anesthesia.

Culdocentesis is occasionally used to detect hemoperitoneum. With the decrease in frequency of tubal rupture, the incidence of hemoperitoneum may be expected to decline, and the value of culdocentesis may change. A positive test with nonclotting blood in association with a positive serum HCG is almost always pathognomonic of an extrauterine pregnancy. In these situations, laparoscopy may be avoided unless the surgeon believes it is possible to remove the pregnancy endoscopically. It must be remembered that a positive culdocentesis does not necessarily indicate tubal rupture and hemoperitoneum can exist in the absence of signs of peritoneal irritation. This procedure is inexpensive, rapid, and easily performed with a 20 ml syringe, a 19 gauge needle, and perhaps a needle extender. Ultrasound, laparoscopy, and blood tests are extremely helpful, but there are situations in which culdocentesis can corroborate the diagnosis, avoid the need for laparoscopy, and in some instances, influence the decision to wait for further results of beta-HCG titers.

Although reliable sonographic identification of an extrauterine pregnancy is not always possible, the technique is helpful for the diagnosis of an intrauterine pregnancy so that an unnecessary operation can be avoided. In some instances, a definitive diagnosis cannot be made with the use of laparoscopy. However, the combination of a beta-HCG pregnancy titer of greater than 6,000 mIU and a sonogram that does not show an intrauterine pregnancy indicates the extrauterine position of the fetus. Holtz and Hosseinian have devised a workable screening procedure for the patient suspected of having a tubal pregnancy in which they have clearly incorporated the diagnostic tests described above.

Surgical management

Conservative operations are designed principally for nulliparous patients and for those with a poor reproductive performance or infertility who wish to preserve their potential for fertility.

Tubal resection by laparoscopy

Specific techniques for removal of some unruptured tubal pregnancies with the use of laparoscopy have been described by several authors. One prerequisite is a 2 to 3 cm gestational mass in a freely movable, intact, middle or outer tubal segment. Given this gross appearance, a linear salpingostomy can be done. The pathological area is incised by electrocautery. The products of conception are removed through an accessory puncture and bleeding is controlled with bipolar forceps. The operative site is copiously irrigated with lactated Ringer's solution and scrutinized to ensure proper hemostasis. The products of conception should not be removed by squeezing the affected tubal segment or "milking it" out.

Bruhat[16] and co-workers reported on 60 extrauterine pregnancies removed by using a triple-puncture technique that included an 11 mm fiberoptic laparoscope inserted subumbilically and two operating trocars, 5 to 6 mm, placed in the lower quadrants for insertion of atraumatic laparoscopic forceps, a monopolar electrode, or a device for aspiration. In 17 instances, the conceptus was squeezed out of the distal third of the tube toward the fimbria, and the contents were then aspirated. Although this technique appeared easiest, it was most dangerous because of the uncertainty of complete evacuation of the products of conception. It is essential to filter the aspirated material or to look for a villous configuration, since there were three instances in which patients subsequently required a laparotomy for tubal bleeding. In 43 other women who had isthmic or midampullary gestations, the tube was incised 1 to 2 cm with electrocautery, the contents evacuated with aspiration, and hemostasis obtained by compression or bipolar cautery.

These laparoscopic procedures decrease the length of postoperative hospitalization. Morbidity appears to be minimal, and the subsequent tubal patency and intrauterine pregnancy rates compare favorably with conservative management by laparotomy. Laparoscopic treatment for extrauterine pregnancy is possible only if the surgeon has had previous experiences with pelvic dissection under laparoscopic control using special forceps, scissors, and cautery; the patient should be in excellent condition with evidence of minimal bleeding from the tube. Gonadotropin markers must be used to identify patients who have residual trophoblastic disease following a conservative operation. Such surveillance is recommended prior to discharge from the hospital, and if positive, sequential HCG radioreceptor assay or beta subunit HCG determinations must follow. If persistently positive, reoperation is probably indicated to avoid serious delayed hemorrhage.

Laparotomy

Once the physician has ascertained that the tube can be salvaged, and the patient has a desire to retain her fertility, several options are possible.

Partial salpingectomy

When the gestation is in the isthmus, effective removal of the products of conception by partial salpingectomy is preferable. It is also possible to carry out this procedure for a ruptured tubal pregnancy, providing the remaining tubal segments are not severely disorganized. The resected ends of the remaining tubal segments are closed with an absorbable suture and tubal repair should be postponed to a subsequent operation. Taylor and Cumming[17] performed partial salpingectomy through a minilaparotomy after having made the diagnosis by laparoscopy. In six patients, clamps were placed proximal and distal to the gestational sac through a minilaparotomy, the tips of the clamps entering into the mesosalpinx, and the tube divided and transfixed.

Once an isthmic pregnancy is removed, either an immediate or delayed anastomosis is possible. Both techniques have been reported with good results. Whether or not such women should be placed on contraception until the anastomosis is done is controversial.

Salpingotomy

When the conceptus is implanted in the ampulla (90 percent), a linear incision is made in the tube parallel to its long axis along the antimesenteric border either with a fine microunipolar electrode needle or a scalpel. Microsurgical principles using fine sutures, irrigation, and selected careful use of electrosurgery are important. The operating microscope is of no value in these patients. The products of conception are removed with forceps and hemostasis is achieved with bipolar cautery. The placental bed is irrigated and the incised tubal edges can be sutured with a synthetic absorbable fine suture (5-O) with a running stitch. Another option is to close the incision with a few interrupted fine sutures. In these cases, the fimbriae, although edematous and identifiable, are in otherwise good condition. Overzealous cauterization or debridement of the placental bed or probing the tube to detect patency of the proximal segment are all to be avoided. Linear salpingotomy is the operation of choice for ampullary pregnancies.

Salpingostomy

When the pregnancy is almost at the infundibulum or fimbriated end, it is possible to open the tube by inserting a blade of a scissors into the tubal orifice and the opposite blade on the antimesenteric border. The tube is then cut to the level of the pregnancy. Again the products of con-ception are removed and hemostasis is achieved. Irrigation and selective use of electrocautery should reduce the incidence of postoperative peritubal adhesions.

Manual expression (milking)

The technique of squeezing out the products of conception in situations in which the gestation seems close to the end of the tube has not given good postoperative results. It would appear from several series that these tubes are more predisposed to occlusion or become the sites of recurrent extrauterine pregnancy. Uncontrollable manual pressure may cause more endosalpingeal damage than incisional techniques and direct observation of the placental site.

When is salpingectomy conservative?

On opening the abdomen, the surgeon may encounter large amounts of fluid or clotted blood. Initially no attempt is made to remove this material, but the uterus and adnexa are lifted out of the pelvis and the site of tubal pregnancy is identified. Bleeding is controlled by clamps applied to the affected tube close to the uterus and along the mesosalpinx. The clamps are replaced by ligatures. Cornual wedge resection is not recommended; the tube is severed close to the uterine serosal surface. Raw areas are peritonealized with a loop of round ligament. Cornual resection is no guarantee against a subsequent ipsilateral interstitial pregnancy; it increases the duration of the operative procedure over simple salpingectomy and predisposes the patient to the risk of a ruptured uterus in a future pregnancy.

Ipsilateral oophorectomy

A different approach to improve fertility in selected patients has been proposed in the form of a "paradoxical oophorectomy." It is argued that if the contralateral tube and ovary appear normal, the performance of a salpingo-oophorectomy on the involved side will assure all subsequent ovulations from the remaining ovary and eliminate transmigration as a factor predisposing to recurrent tubal pregnancy. Salpingectomy might compromise the blood supply to the ipsilateral ovary.

However, several series have not substantiated any reduction of tubal pregnancy following salpingectomy when compared with patients having salpingo-oophorectomy. In addition, no significant increase in viable pregnancies has been shown to occur from this policy. Although a tube may appear grossly normal, it is not possible to test tubal patency safely during the operative management of a tubal pregnancy. Thus, it would appear that preserving the ipsilateral ovary is warranted because normal ovarian tissue is important for young women who might require a unilateral oophorectomy later in their reproductive lives for adnexal disease. In addition, the possibility of in-vitro fertilization and embryo transfer could become the only chance for fertility in some of these patients.

Medical management

Tanaka and colleagues[18] found an interstitial pregnancy at laparotomy and treated the patient with three subsequent courses of methotrexate. They followed the patient with serial HCG levels to observe the effect of the medication and the gestation was apparently destroyed. A subsequent HSG revealed bilateral tubal patency. Nonsurgical management without the use of antimetabolites has also been reported. Falling titres of beta HCG indicated resorption of the pregnancy previously identified as having been within the fallopian tube.

Results

Jarvinen and co-workers[19] performed conservative operations on 43 patients with tubal pregnancy in the middle or distal third of the tube, followed by daily hydrotubation for nine to ten days. Hysterosalpingography performed an average of five months postoperatively showed the affected tube completely open in 24 of 32 patients examined. In patients with only a treated residual tube, term pregnancies resulted but there were repeated ectopic pregnancies and two miscarriages.

Sherman, Langer, and colleagues[20] followed 154 patients from 3 months to 11 years. One hundred and twenty-five (81 percent) subsequently became pregnant and 113 had an intrauterine pregnancy. The incidence of repeat tubal pregnancy was 6.5 percent. These results are quite remarkable. Subsequent fertility was influenced by the presence of periadnexal adhesions, associated tubal disease, a history of infertility before conception, the degree of damage to the pregnant tube, and the patient's age at operation. Only 26 percent of their operations conserved the affected tube. The only statistically significant difference in subsequent reproductive performance between the salpingectomy (radical) and salpingotomy (conservative) patients was found among women with coexistent fertility factors.

The real measure of successful conservative surgery occurs in those patients who have only one remaining tube, the site of the extrauterine pregnancy. DeCherney and his co-workers[21] had 15 such women on whom they performed linear salpingostomy and 50 percent of these women eventually had a viable pregnancy. Twenty percent had repeat tubal pregnancies. All of the tubes were patent postoperatively. Conservation of the tube preserves and probably prolongs reproductive potential.

A patient who has had two tubal pregnancies has a slim chance of having a subsequent intrauterine pregnancy. She must be counseled in this regard so that choices can be made that include contraception, in-vitro fertilization and embryo transfer (IVF/ET), or another attempt at pregnancy. An HSG showing tubal patency or a laparoscopy with a positive chromopertubation do not eliminate the possibility of another extrauterine pregnancy. Tubal function and endosalpingeal damage are difficult to assess.

Most studies report a subsequent viable pregnancy rate of about 40 percent; an additional 10 percent of repeat extrauterine pregnancies and the remainder of the women do not become pregnant. The conservative operation or retaining the tube is theoretically attractive but difficult to support with good data. The most persuasive arguments are those few series with conservative operations on the single residual tube followed by subsequent viable pregnancies.

Summary

Conservative operations in selected instances of tubal pregnancy are feasible, safe, and do not further impair tubal function. It logically follows that the involved tube should be salvaged whenever fertility is desired, such as in the nulliparous patient or one who has a history of poor reproductive performances. It has been shown that satisfactory function can remain in a repaired tube so that a normal pregnancy can occur in patients having only a solitary tube that has been treated conservatively. On the other hand, there is no compelling evidence to show an increase in postoperative intrauterine pregnancies in patients whose opposite tube is normal.

Laparoscopy

Chronic recurrent pelvic pain is a common gynecologic complaint. Although patients with this problem may or may not have a positive history or documented evidence of sexually transmitted disease, pelvic inflammatory disease is often used to explain the symptoms. When there is no evidence of active infection, pelvic adhesions are presumed to be the cause of the pain.

Pittaway and Fayez emphasize that therapy should not be instituted before an accurate diagnosis is made. Nonspecific symptomatic treatment, heat, analgesics, and repetitive use of antibiotics are the most common errors in emergency room management.

Laparoscopy is used very frequently for diagnosis and therapy of the infertile woman. Although its benefits are numerous, it remains an operative procedure and should be performed for precise indications. The basic infertiity evaluation should not be circumvented. Laparoscopy is reserved for selected patients depending on the preoperative findings: the history, the physical examination, the results of the postcoital test, the endometrial biopsy, the hysterosalpingogram, and semen analysis.

The basic techniques for laparoscopy are well known and need not be repeated here. Infertility studies do require a double-puncture technique and an apparatus for instilling the colored solution into the uterine cavity. Inhalation anesthesia with cuffed intubation and assisted ventilation are best for a comprehensive laparoscopic exploration of the pelvis. The time in the cycle for the operation depends on the indication for the study. For example, the proliferative phase is best in patients who have associated hysteroscopy because it is easier to observe the uterine cavity, the cornua and uterotubal ostia. When unexplained infertility exists and a properly timed endometrial biopsy specimen is required, laparoscopy is performed during the secretory phase. In women selected for follicular aspiration, laparoscopy is timed in accordance with the endocrinologic and sonographic findings that indicate a mature, ripening ovum.

An organized, routine method for inspection of the internal genitalia is essential. One should begin with the uterus and proceed in a clockwise fashion to inspect the fallopian tubes, the ovaries, and the round, uterosacral and infundibulopelvic ligaments. These structures are manipulated, mobilized, and measured with a tactile, calibrated probe. One must remember and record the size, shape, surface, color, consistency, and mobility of each organ, and proceed with chromopertubation. After completing the operation, the result is noted on an appropriate form. The promptly written record is most valuable, whereas those dictated at the end of the operative schedule are almost worthless. It is not possible to remember the details of each laparoscopic examination at the conclusion of three or four operations. The need to inform the patient postoperatively and for subsequent comparison mandates that the physician have available an illustration of the significant findings.

The five basic tubal conditions are normal patency, proximal obstruction, distal occlusion, hydrosalpinges with or without minimal patency, and phimotic ostia. A presumptive diagnosis of proximal occlusion can be made if the uterus becomes visibly distended during the injection, the cornual areas become pale, and resistance to further injection rises. Occasionally, venous intravasation is seen in association with proximal tubal obstruction, the fluid passing easily into the uterine cavity but the tubes do not fill. The patency and position of the cannula must be checked. Has its end slipped too far into the uterine cavity? Is it still in the cervical canal? Is there extensive leakage at the cervical os?

Salpingitis isthmica nodosa has a characteristic nodularity, readily observed and palpated. Dye is occasionally seen to intravasate into the hypertrophied myosalpinx. The isthmic extent of the disease can be surmised from these findings but not the intramural involvement. The condition is usually bilateral. Tubal endometriosis presents a similar gross appearance; the physician should therefore search for other sites of pelvic endometriosis.

In distal tubal disease, the tubes fill and become distended but sometimes spill of dye is seen into the cul-de-sac or behind occlusive adhesions. The least diseased club-shaped, distally occluded tubes appear pink and soft, and the blue dye is seen almost at the characteristic "spoke-wheel" tip. The size of the hydrosalpinx is not related to the chance of conception following repair. A firm or nodular enlarged tube suggests infiltration of the myosalpinx with fibrosis and scarring, and these lumens do not show rugal markings. The phimotic ostium causes the tube to distend with the instilled dye, the fimbria being observed, with minimal passage of fluid into the peritoneal cavity. The impediment to its free flow could be endosalpingeal adhesions or thick fibrous bands. A cul-de-sac free of adhesions and ovaries that are easily mobilized improve the chance for a successful tubal repair.

Biochemical and bacteriological studies on fluids obtained from a hydrosalpinx, and hematoxylin and eosin stains have not revealed any significant information. Tubal biopsy under laparoscopic control has been done to study the distribution of ciliated and secretory cells. It has been suggested that a certain percentage of ciliated cells must be present in the ampulla to expect success from tuboplasty.

Laparoscopy is essential in women

who have demonstrable proximal tubal occlusion on hysterosalpingography so that the tube distal to the point of obstruction can be evaluated. Bipolar disease and associated periovarian adhesions contraindicate an attempt at reconstructive surgery because the prognosis is so poor. Occasionally, proximal obstruction detected radiographically turns out to be caused by spasm and chromopertubation during laparoscopy shows the tubes to fill and spill.

Patients sterilized by the application of clips or Falope rings, or by excision of 1 to 2 cm of tube in a Pomeroy ligation do not require a laparoscopic "peek" to assure the physician that reversal is feasible. However, laparoscopy is essential in instances of sterilization with either bipolar or unipolar electrocoagulation because the extent of vascular damage and subsequent tubal atrophy are unpredictable with these techniques.

The findings on the endoscopic examination in certain instances can detect patients having minimal tubal disease or irreparable tubal damage. In the former instance, thereapeutic laparoscopic procedures such as salpingolysis or dilatation of phimotic ostia are feasible. In women with severe pelvic adhesions and tubal obstructions, the condition and accessibility of the ovaries can be evaluated for the eventual possibility of follicular aspiration, should such a patient elect to undergo in-vitro fertilization and embryo transfer.

Finally, a diagnostic laparoscopic examination for unexplained infertility will occasionally reveal unsuspected endometriosis or significant pelvic adhesions. Both of these conditions often can be treated under laparoscopic control with the use of accessory instruments and additional punctures in the lower quadrants.

In this section on Tubal Pathology, Sedlis has succinctly described significant benign and malignant tumors of the fallopian tube, their diagnosis and management. The nonobstructing tubal polyp does not require excision.

References

1. Breen J: A 21-year survey of 654 ectopic pregnancies. *Am J Obstet Gynecol*, 106:1004, 1970.
2. Ricci JV: *The Genealogy of Gynaecology*. Philadelphia: The Blakiston Company, 1943: p. 374.
3. Rogers S: *Extrauterine Foetation and Gestation, and the Early Signs which Characterize It*. Philadelphia: Collins, 1867.
4. Harbert WW: A case of extrauterine pregnancy. *West J Med Surg*, 3:110, 1849.
5. Tait RL: Five cases of extrauterine pregnancy operated upon at the time of rupture. *Br Med J*, 1:1250, 1884.
6. Kelly HA: The treatment of extrauterine pregnancy, ruptured in the early months by vaginal puncture and drainage. *Trans Am Gynecol Soc*, 21:180, 1896.
7. Martin A: Zur Kenntniss der Tubarschwangerschaft. *Geburtsh Gynäkol*, 5:1244, 1897.
8. Prochownick L: Ein Beitrag zur Mechanik des Tuben. *Geburtsh Gynäkol*, 2:266, 1894.
9. Woodruff, JD, Pauerstein CJ: *The Fallopian Tube*. Baltimore: Williams and Wilkins, 1969: p. 220.
10. Kelly MT, Santos-Ramos R, Duenhoelter JH: The value of sonography in suspected ectopic pregnancy. *Obstet Gynecol*, 53:703, 1979.
11. Ford WE: Results of vaginal secretion and drainage in early cases of ectopic gestation. *Trans Am Gynecol Soc*, 31:157, 1906.
12. Schumann EA: *Extrauterine Pregnancy*. New York: D. Appleton, 1921: p. 161.
13. Rubin IC: The status of the residual tube following ectopic pregnancy in relation to sterility and further pregnancy. *Am J Obstet Gynecol*, 28:698, 1934.
14. Caffier P: Die konservativ Operation des schwangeren Eileiters. (Ein Beitrag zur Sterilitätsverhutung). *Arch Gynäkol* 173:261, 1941.
15. Stromme WB: Salpingotomy for tubal pregnancy. *Obstet Gynecol*, 1:472, 1953.
16. Bruhat MA, Manhes H, Mage G, et al: Treatment of ectopic pregnancy by means of laparoscopy. *Fertil Steril*, 33:411, 1980.

17. Taylor PJ, Cumming DC: Combined laparoscopy and minilaparotomy in the management of unruptured tubal pregnancy; A preliminary report. *Fertil Steril*, 32:521, 1979.
18. Tanaka T, Hayashi H, Kutsuzawa T, et al: Treatment of interstitial ectopic pregnancy with methotrexate: Report of a successful case. *Fertil Steril*, 37:851, 1982.
19. Jarvinen PA, Nummi S, Pietila N: Conservative operative treatment of tubal pregnancy with postoperative daily hydrotubations. *Acta Obstet Gynecol Scand*, 51:169, 1972.
20. Sherman D, Langer R, Sadovsky G, et al: Improved fertility ectopic pregnancy. *Fertil Steril*, 37:497, 1982.
21. DeCherney AH, Romero R, Naftolin F: Surgical management of unruptured tubal pregnancy *Fertil Steril*, 35:21, 1981.

14

Effects of Perinatal Exposure to Diethylstilbestrol on Oviductal Development

Retha R. Newbold
and John A. McLachlan

Exposure of pregnant women to drugs or chemicals has been associated with teratogenic and carcinogenic effects on their offspring. The dramatic and known toxic effect of maternal treatment with diethylstilbestrol (DES) has illustrated this problem.

For almost three decades, DES, a synthetic estrogen, had been used as a therapeutic agent for threatened abortion. In 1971, an association between the use of DES during pregnancy and an increased incidence of vaginal and cervical adenocarcinoma in the offspring was reported.[1] While the full extent of DES use is unknown, it is estimated that at least two to three million pregnant women may have been treated with the drug. Although DES is no longer used clinically to prevent threatened abortion, the number of progeny at risk will peak in this decade.

Since the initial observation of DES-induced adenosis and adenocarcinoma,[2] the incidence of the malignant lesion has been reported to be low.[2,3] However, other benign changes throughout the female reproductive tract appear quite commonly in exposed offspring. Changes of uterine contour and morphological features resulting in "T-shaped" uteri, malformed cervices, and vaginal abnormalities have been described.[4–7] These DES-associated anatomical changes in reproductive tract tissues may be associated with reduced reproductive capacity.

Altered reproductive tract development caused by treating rodents with DES or other estrogenic substances during fetal life has been of special interest in our laboratory and has led to the development of a useful experimental model to investigate the anomalies associated with intrauterine exposure to DES. Studies from our laboratory showed that prenatal

The Fallopian Tube: Basic Studies and Clinical Contributions, edited by Alvin M. Siegler, M.D. Mount Kisco, New York: Futura Publishing Company, Inc. © 1986.

DES treatment of mice resulted in a dose-related decrease in reproductive capacity.[8] Abnormalities, including adenocarcinoma in the cranial vagina, cervix, and uterus have been observed in mice exposed to DES in utero.[9,10] In addition, these studies demonstrated that the oviduct may be another target for DES-induced dysmorphology.[9,11,12] The increased incidence of tubal pregnancies in prenatally DES-exposed women[4,6,13,14] and the reduced fertility in animals[8] and women[4] exposed to DES are consistent with the oviduct being a target for DES action. Since oviductal dysmorphogenesis is an apparently rare finding,[15] and morphological alterations of this organ have received little attention, oviductal abnormalities found in mice exposed perinatally to DES will be presented and compared to preliminary observations reported for women.

Comparative Morphogenesis of the Oviduct

The murine and human oviducts are highly specialized structures that are derived embryonically from the cranial regions of the fetal müllerian (paramesonephric) ducts.[16] Prenatal development of the oviductal segment of the müllerian duct has received far less attention than that of the uterus and upper vagina. Descriptive studies of oviductal development have been reported for a few species,[16] but hormonal influence on oviductal development has not been well studied.

During fetal development, after the formation of the ostium, the müllerian duct is closely applied to the wolffian (mesonephric) duct; it then grows caudally to the urogenital sinus in close association with the preexisting mesonephric duct. It has been suggested that the müllerian duct depends on the wolffian duct for directional cues. Some investigators have reported an actual contribution of cells from the wolffian duct to the growing müllerian duct.[17,18] The cranial portion of the müllerian duct continues to differentiate into the definitive oviduct through a series of morphogenetic and histogenetic changes. It becomes distinguishable from the uterus. The epithelium differentiates, the muscle layer develops, mucosal folds are defined, fimbriae form, and the segments (fimbriae, ampulla, isthmus, intramural) are identifiable. Timing of this differentiation process differs in mice and humans, but the order of the various developmental cues is similar.

There are, however, easily recognized differences between mice and humans with regard to the degree of development of the ovarian bursa, the complexity of the uterotubal junction, and the structural details of the oviductal segments.[19] For example, the human fimbriae form a fringed open funnel which encircles the ovary; in mice the fimbriae form a sac around the ovary (ovarian bursa). There are also differences in the uterotubal junction. The mouse's oviduct enters the uterus at an angle and is always protected by a polyp-like projection or mucosal fold which prevents fluid from passing from the uterus to the oviduct.[20] The presence of this polyp-like projection makes tubal insufflation impossible because the uterus will rupture before fluid can enter the oviduct. In women, the oviductal opening has no polyp-like projections but rather a "sphincter" at the uterotubal junction which permits passage of either gases or liquids from the uterus to the oviduct. The structural details of the oviductal segments also vary between mice and women, especially in the isthmic region. The mouse's oviduct is characterized by tortuous coils in the isthmic region, while in women this segment is relatively straight.

In summary, while the function and developmental events surrounding oviductal development and differentiation are generally similar in mice and women, there are specialized features that distinguish the species.

DES-induced Alterations in the Embryogenesis of the Mouse's Oviduct

To study the latent expression of abnormal structure and function of the gen-

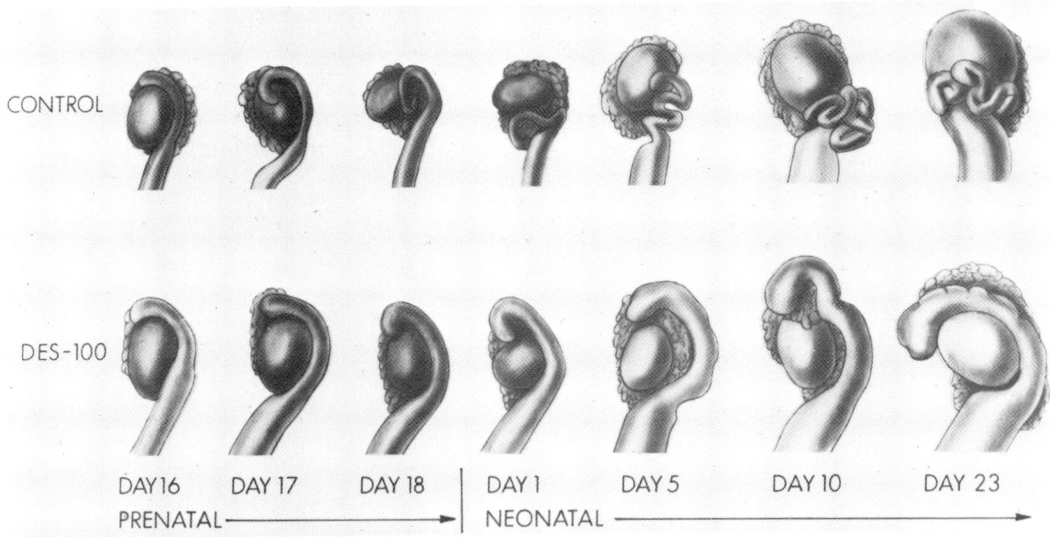

FIGURE 14:1—*Schematic drawing of oviductal development. Composite drawing from control female mice (upper panel) and mice exposed to DES (100 μg/kg) on 9 to 16 days of gestation (lower panel) demonstrate oviductal morphogenesis. Each drawing represents three to five females examined at each age. Prenatal DES treatment retards oviductal development; the oviduct fails to lengthen or coil and it retains a "fetal-like" appearance. The retention of this fetal anatomical relationship between ovary, oviduct, and uterus suggests the term "developmentally arrested oviduct." This malformation persists throughout the animal's life.*[11]

ital tract of female mice exposed transplacentally to DES, outbred CD-1 mice were treated subcutaneously with 100 μg/kg of DES on days 9 through 16 of gestation. This period of gestation encompasses the major events of genital tract organogenesis in the female mouse and should provide useful information that can be extrapolated to women.

Significant differences were observed when oviductal development in DES-exposed animals was compared to untreated animals (Fig. 14:1). The oviductal segment appears initially late on gestational day 16 with a narrowing of the cranial portion of the müllerian duct (Fig. 14:1, upper panel). On day 17, the oviduct starts to coil and the müllerian duct develops slight undulations in the oviductal region, then a series of loose wavy folds, followed by deep coils. By day 1 of neonatal life, the oviduct is identifiable as a discrete region and its caudal limits are demarcated from the uterus. By postnatal day 10, the ovary rotates into the position it has in adult life, and the loosely coiled oviduct enters the uterus at an angle.

In contrast, DES treatment retards oviductal development in mice exposed in utero (Fig. 14:1, lower panel). Differences are evident by neonatal day 1 when normal müllerian duct coiling is absent in DES female offspring. Differences become more obvious during postnatal development because the oviduct in DES mice fails to lengthen or coil and retains a fetal-like appearance. These differences persist throughout the animal's life (Fig. 14:2) and distort the anatomical relationships among uterus, tube, and ovary. In the DES-treated animals, the ovary does not rotate and there is little or no demarcation between the oviduct and the uterus. Also, the oviduct's angle of entry into the uterus is altered. The oviduct appears to join the uterus at its apex and forms a straight tube. This oviduct malformation is observed in all females treated prenatally with this dosage

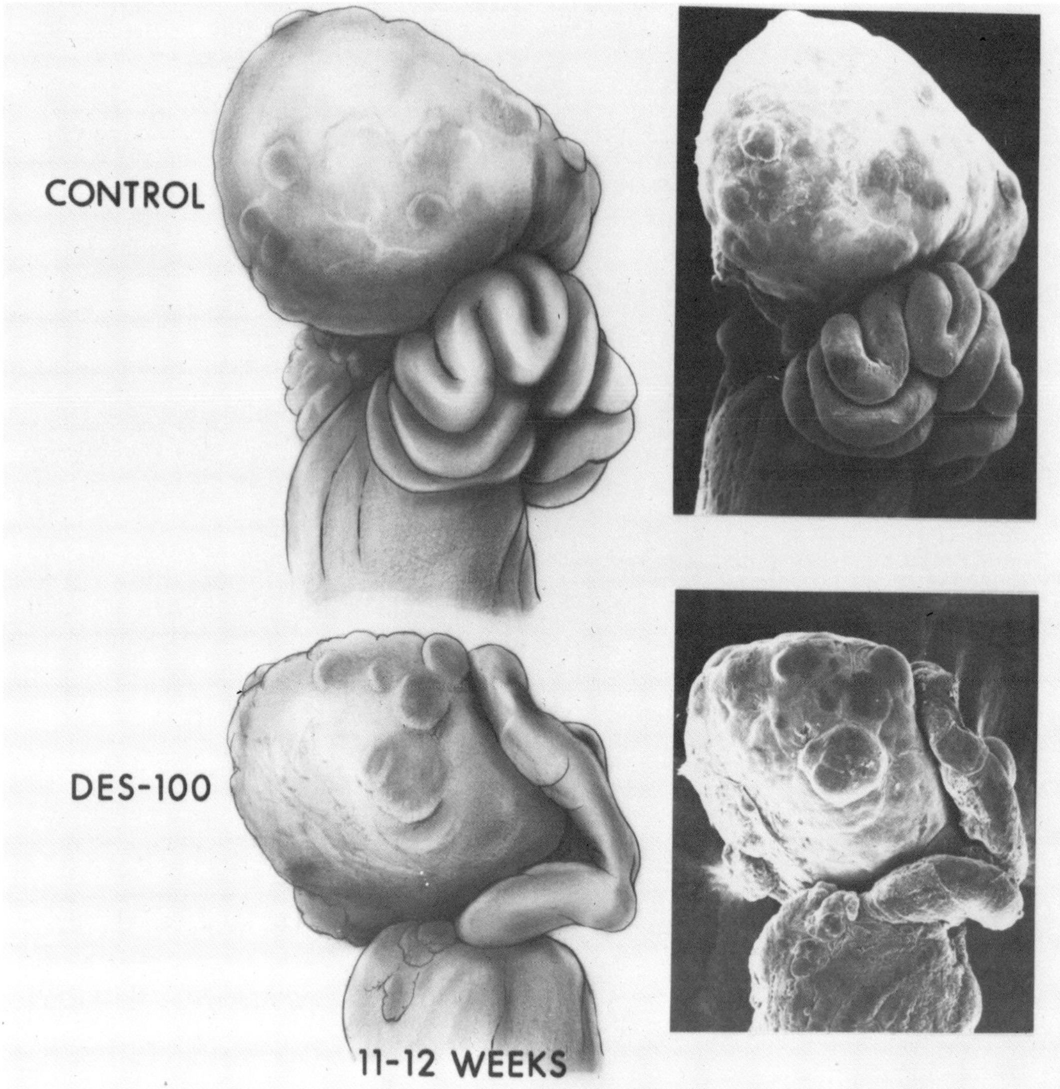

FIGURE 14:2—*A drawing and a scanning electron micrograph (SEM) from a 12-week-old control female offspring and an offspring exposed to 100 μg/kg/day of DES on days 9 to 16 of gestation. Note the relationship of the ovary, oviduct, and uterus in the control as compared to the DES-exposed structures. The oviductal coils in the control offspring form regular loops that are uniform in diameter whereas the DES-exposed oviduct is closely adherent and wrapped around the ovary.*[11]

of DES but is not seen in any control animals.

The retention of a fetal anatomical relationship among ovary, oviduct, and uterus suggests the term "developmentally arrested oviduct" to describe the phenomenon.[12] This is supported by the relative lack of growth of the oviductal segment. Although the body weights of DES-treated and control offspring are similar (38 g versus 36 g, respectively), the average length of the oviducts of the treated females is only about half that of the controls (8 mm versus 16 mm).

Microscopic alterations accompany the teratogenicity associated with prenatal DES treatment.[21] In the control animals, the histologic differentiation coincides with the morphogenetic development. The epithelium shows an increase in cell height, pseudostratification, and evidence of secretory activity. In contrast, the oviductal differentiation is halted in DES mice and the fimbriae develop minimally. In the ampulla of both control and treated animals, there are ciliated and secretory cells. However, the arrangement of the columnar cells lining the lumen and the mucosal folds is irregular in DES animals. In addition, gland formation was observed in the DES animals which extended through the muscularis, a feature never observed in control mice. Epithelial hyperplasia was also noted and inflammatory changes were more prevalent in all segments of the oviduct of DES animals as compared to controls.

Prenatal exposure to DES was also associated with functional alterations of the oviduct.[11] Dye injected into the uterine lumen of DES females passed readily into the oviduct and ovarian bursa, indicating that the uterotubal junction did not function normally to retain the dye in the uterus. In only one of 17 control animals could dye be forced into the lumen of the oviduct following injection into the uterus. In light of the extensive malformation of the oviduct and uterus in DES animals, this result is not surprising. In fact, scanning electron microscopy (SEM) of the area of the uterotubal junction of control animals demonstrated a papillary projection where the oviduct enters the uterus (Fig. 14:3A). This papillary structure is present in fewer than half of the DES animals (Fig. 14:3B). For example, there is no papillary structure, and the oviductal opening in the DES animal illustrated in Figure 14:3C resembles uterine epithelial foldings.

Alteration in Proliferative Properties of Oviductal Epithelium in Mice Treated Neonatally with DES

To study the developmental alterations induced by DES further, the exposure period was extended into neonatal life, a time when cellular morphogenesis continues. Neonatal female mice were each treated by subcutaneous injection of 2 μg of DES in corn oil on days 1 to 5 of age. Animals were sacrificed at various times following treatment and their oviducts examined (Table 14:1). Altogether, 70 neonatally DES-treated females and 47 age-matched controls were evaluated.

At the ages indicated in Table 14:1, mice were sacrificed and the oviducts removed and fixed in 10 percent neutral buffered formalin. Tissues were dehydrated, embedded in paraffin, and serially sectioned at 6 μ. Microscopic evaluation resulted in a staging analysis to describe the oviductal lesion: *Stage 1:* focal epithelial hyperplasia with a single epithelial fold extended into the muscle wall; *Stage 2:* general epithelial hyperplasia with several mucosal folds extended through the muscularis; some folds split the muscle wall and sent another layer of connective tissue around the epithelial elements; "gland-like structures" connected with lumen; *Stage 3:* irregular oviductal serosal surface with marked adenomatous proliferation through the muscularis; no apparent connection of some glandular structures with lumen; *Stage 4:* cellular changes and degree of severity of folds increased to resemble adenocarcinoma. Glands were never seen in groups of 10 to 15 untreated mice evaluated at corresponding ages at various stages of the estrous cycle (Fig. 14:4A).[21]

Within one month after treatment, changes were noticeable in 89 percent of the treated mice (Fig. 14:4B) and by six months, changes (Stage 3, Fig. 14:4C) were noted in 100 percent of the animals. One year after treatment, 34 percent of the mice had Stage 3 and 66 percent had severe Stage 4 growth disturbances in

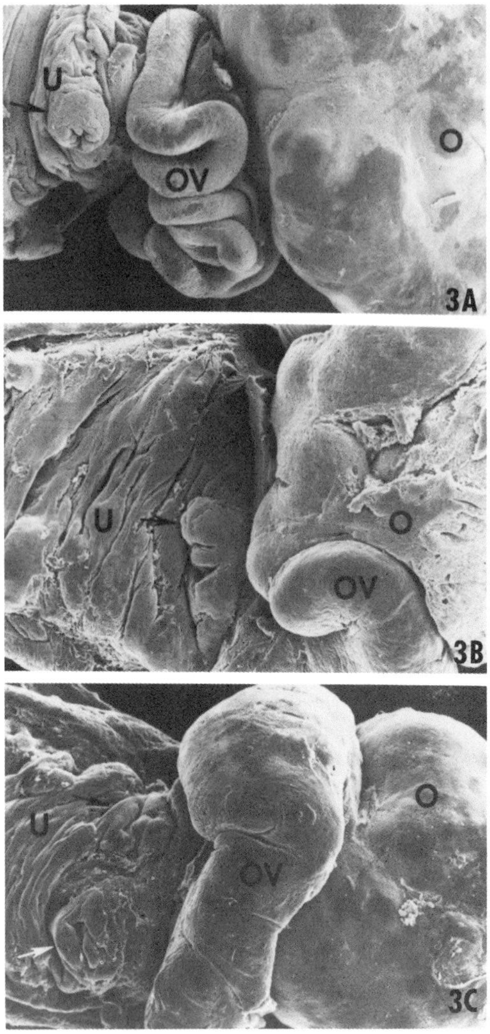

FIGURE 14:3—*(A) Scanning electron micrograph (SEM) of the ovary (o), oviduct (ov), and uterine lumen (u) of a control (10 to 15 week) animal shows the entry of the oviduct into the uterus forming a papillary projection (black arrow). (B) Scanning electron micrograph (SEM) of the ovary (o), oviduct (ov), and uterine lumen (u) of an offspring (10 to 15 weeks) exposed prenatally to DES (100 μg/kg). Entry of the oviduct into the uterus forms a papillary protrusion (black arrow); however, the oviduct is not coiled and is closely adherent to and wrapped around the ovary. (C) Scanning electron micrograph (SEM) of the ovary (o), oviduct (ov), and uterine lumen (u) of an offspring (10 to 15 weeks) exposed prenatally to DES (100 μg/kg). There is no papillary structure at the entry of the oviduct into the uterus and the oviductal opening (black arrow) resembles uterine epithelial folds (white arrow).[11] (Original magnification ×36)*

terms of proliferation and altered differentiation (Fig. 14:4C). In DES mice at one month of age, focal epithelial folds extended into the muscle wall. These mucosal folds had an adenomatous (gland-like) appearance but maintained connection with the oviductal lumen. By four months, the entire epithelium was hyperplastic while the muscle wall and stroma were thinner than in corresponding controls. The number of adenomatous mucosal folds and the degree of extension through the muscle wall increased with age, splitting the muscle wall and extending to the serosal surface. Connection of these "gland-like" structures with the lumen was demonstrated with tissues sectioned serially (Table 14:1: Stage 2). At six months of age, one animal had a thick sclerotic muscle wall with epithelial components isolated in sclerotic connective tissue while other animals had a severe form of adenomatous proliferation through a thin muscle wall (Table 14:1: Stage 3). The serosal surface at this age was irregular with areas resembling polyps which appeared to be pinched off rather than connecting to the oviductal lumen (Table 14:1: Stage 3). When treated animals were one year old, (Table 14:1: Stage 4), this proliferative lesion, which was first observed in only the ampulla, had progressed to include the entire tube. The epithelium was severely hyperplastic and the cells were irregular (Fig. 14:4D). Epithelial proliferation in the wall of the oviductal muscularis resembled adenocarcinoma although this lesion did not spread along the serosal surface and no metastases were observed. Figure 14:5 schematically represents the progressive proliferation of this oviductal lesion.

Biological and Clinical Significance

Subfertility has been described in mice treated in utero with DES,[8,22] and in

Table 14:1

Progressive Proliferative Lesion of the Oviduct

Age after DES treatment (months)	*Number of animals*	*Mice with oviductal lesions*				
		No lesion	*Stage 1*	*Stage 2*	*Stage 3*	*Stage 4*
1	18	2 (11%)	16 (89%)	0	0	0
4	10	1 (10%)	0	9 (90%)	0	0
6	12	0	0	0	12 (100%)	0
12	30	0	0	0	10 (34%)	20 (66%)

DES-exposed women.[4,6,13,14] Oviductal abnormalities may play a role in the reduced reproductive capacity seen in both species.

The experimental animal model clearly establishes the oviduct as a target for the teratogenic effect of DES. Moreover, the arrested development resulting from prenatal exposure to DES suggests a role for estrogens in the normal morphogenesis of the mouse oviduct. It is possible that an increase in estrogen levels during oviductal development may play a role in the ultimate structural or functional integrity of this organ in women and mice. In fact, some of the salient features of the "developmentally arrested oviduct" in DES mice, such as decreased oviductal length, relative lack of fimbriae, and abnormal anatomical location, have also been described in 16 women exposed to DES during gestation.[23] This altered or arrested development of the mammalian oviduct may be a general biological consequence of prenatal exposure to DES.

In addition to the teratogenic changes in the oviduct of mice following DES exposure, microscopic changes were also observed. Histologically, the cellular changes—i.e., epithelial hyperplasia and gland formations (diverticuli) of the oviductal mucosa which extend into the muscle wall—resemble salpingitis isthmica nodosa.

Since it was described by Chiari in 1887,[24] the etiology and pathogenesis of salpingitis isthmica nodosa has been the subject of much debate. Although Chiari suggested that the lesion resulted from chronic salpingitis, more recent reports suggest that salpingitis isthmica nodosa is a primary noninflammatory process similar to adenomyosis of the uterus[25] and diverticulosis of other organs,[26] although secondary infection may be a common occurrence.[27] Clinically, this lesion has been related to tubal pregnancy[27–29] and infertility.[29–34] Although the incidence is not known, Siegler and Hellman found salpingitis isthmica nodosa in 1 to 5 percent of the general population.[35] Another study reported an occurrence of 2.86 percent in a group of patients with tubal pregnancy and 50 percent in a group of infertility patients.[29] Bundey and Williams considered this lesion to be neoplastic since no chronic inflammation was present in their material and because a tumor swelling was found.[36] Although there are few other reports in the literature to support the neoplastic potential of salpingitis isthmica nodosa, the lesion has been described as progressive and capable of involving the whole oviduct.[34] The data obtained from our experimental animal model raise the possibility that these clinically noted cases of salpingitis isthmica nodosa may be the result of altered hormonal environment during early development. A recent study describes salpingitis isthmica nodosa in the oviduct of women exposed prenatally to DES.[37]

The mechanisms for regulating epithethelial cell proliferation of the repro-

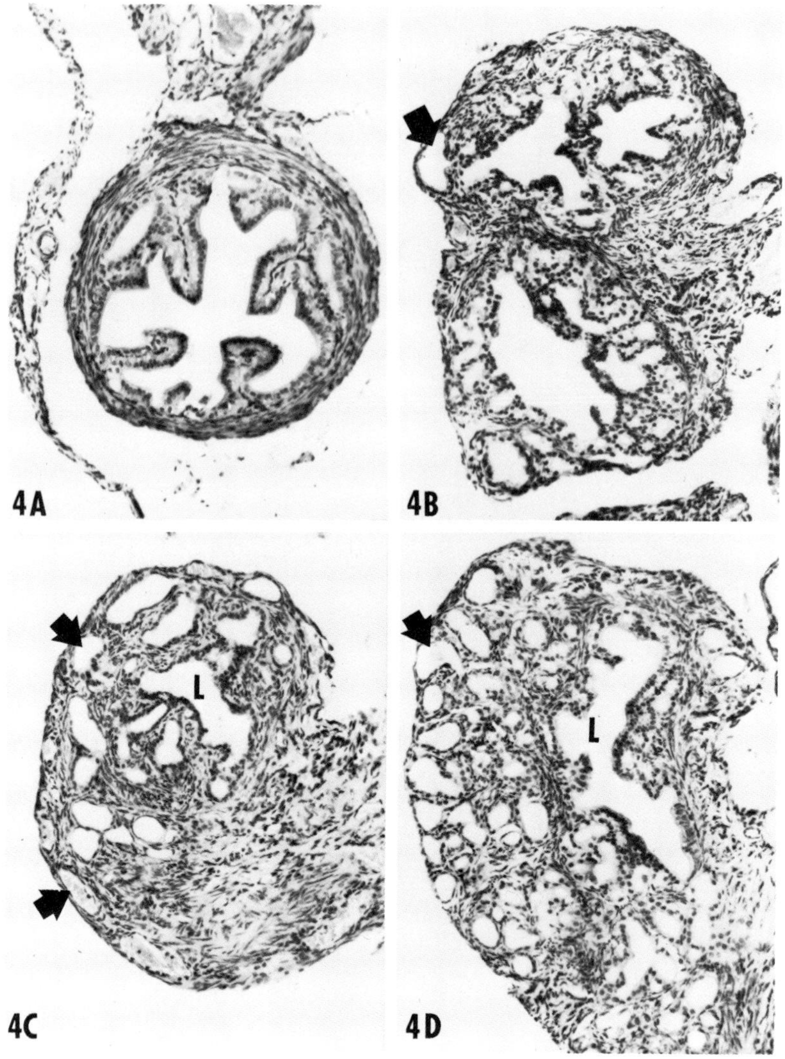

FIGURE 14:4—*Progressive proliferative change in the oviductal epithelium of neonatally DES-exposed mice. (A) Photomicrograph of the isthmic region of a control mouse oviduct. (B) Stage 1 progressive proliferative lesion; photomicrograph of the isthmic region of the oviduct from a one-month-old mouse exposed to DES (2 μg/day) on days 1 to 5 of neonatal life. There is focal epithelial hyperplasia with epithelial folds extending into the muscle wall (arrow). (C) Stage 3 progressive proliferative lesion; photomicrograph of the isthmic region of the oviduct from a six-month-old mouse exposed to DES (2 μg/day) on days 1 to 5 of neonatal life. There is general epithelial hyperplasia with mucosal folds extending through the muscularis (arrows); some folds split the muscle wall and send another layer of connective tissue around the epithelial elements; no apparent connection of some glandular structures with the oviductal lumen (L). (D) Stage 4 progressive proliferative lesion; photomicrograph of the isthmic region of the oviduct from a 12-month-old mouse exposed to DES (2 μg/day) on days 1 to 5 of neonatal life. Cellular changes and degree of severity of adenomatous folds (arrow) has increased and at this stage, involves the entire length of the oviduct. The oviductal lumen (L) is labeled for reference. (H and E, original magnification × 125)*

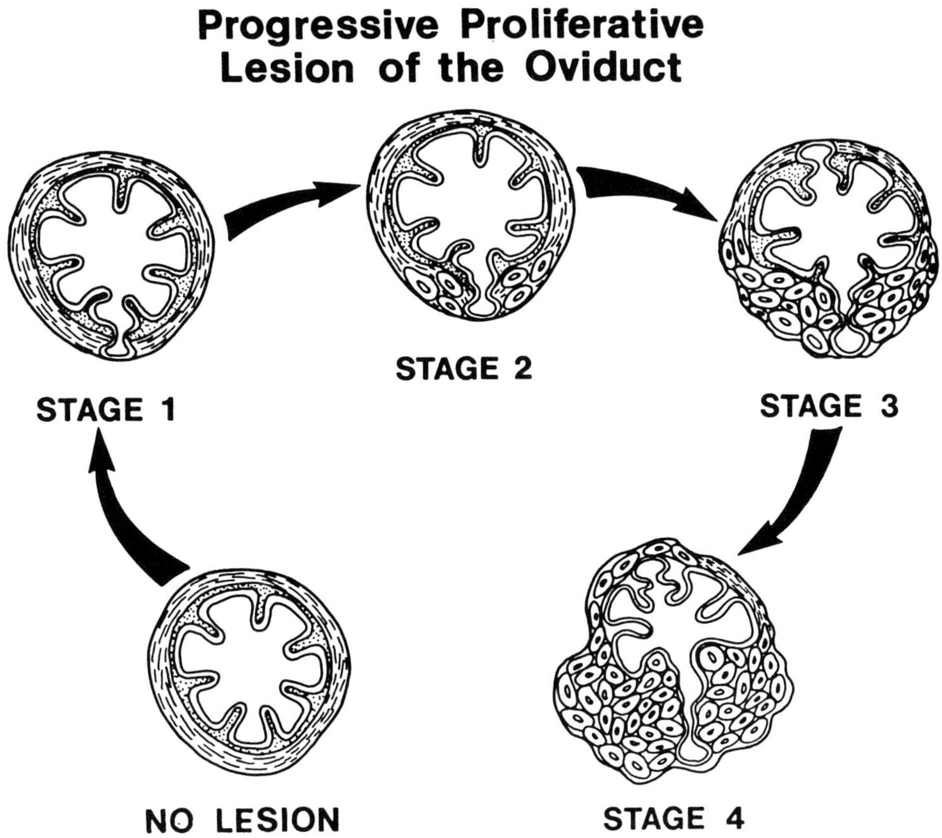

FIGURE 14:5—*Schematic representation of the progressive proliferation of the oviductal epithelium following neonatal exposure to DES.*

ductive tract are unknown; however, the observations in the oviduct following neonatal exposure to DES provide a unique model in which enhanced proliferation occurs. In addition, the oviduct has the ability to differentiate to form gland-like structures. Thus, this experimental model provides an opportunity to study the regulation and differentiation of müllerian epithelium. While the observed changes reside in the epithelium, it is not clear whether the epithelium is responding independently or in combination with factors from the underlying stroma. Since the connective tissue stroma in these DES-treated mice is relatively thin and hypoplastic, it may be a defect in this compartment that modifies the epithelial response. In view of these observations in mice, it is apparent that the proliferative capacity of the different regional epithelia in the müllerian duct (uterus, oviduct) may be affected by hormonal exposure during development. If estrogen levels are significantly elevated, as with prenatal DES treatment, the proliferative capacity may be altered. A similar situation may occur with salpingitis isthmica nodosa where oviductal epithelium possesses an increased capacity for proliferation and forms gland-like structures into the muscle wall.

Moreover, these data on abnormal oviductal epithelial proliferation in mice may be useful in examining the hypothesis that precursor cells for vaginal adenocarcinoma in women exposed prenatally to DES resemble oviductal cells (tuboendometrial cells).[38] Evidence has accumulated during the last few years to indicate that clear-cell adenocarcinoma of the vagina and cervix arises in a background of tuboendometrial cells after developmental exposure to DES.

Conclusion

Oviductal malformation and gland formation have been described in both laboratory animals and women exposed developmentally to DES. The laboratory animal studies shed light on the etiologic factors, natural history, and functional significance of DES-induced genital tract lesions, especially in the region of the oviduct, which might be relevant to similarly exposed women.

References

1. Herbst AL, Ulfelder H, and Poskanzer DC: Adenocarcinoma of the vagina. Association of maternal stilbestrol therapy with tumor appearance in young women. *N Engl J Med,* 284:878, 1971.
2. Herbst AL, Kurman RJ, Scully RE, et al: Clear-cell adenocarcinoma of the genital tract in young females. *N Engl J Med,* 287:1259, 1972.
3. Herbst AL, Cole P, Colton T, et al: Age-incidence and risk of diethylstilbestrol-related clear cell adenocarcinoma of the vagina and cervix. *Am J Obstet Gynecol,* 128:43, 1977.
4. Herbst AL, Hubby MM, Blough RR, et al: A comparison of pregnancy experience in DES-exposed and DES-unexposed daughters. *J Reprod Med,* 24:62, 1980.
5. Kaufman RH, Binder GL, Gray PM, et al: Upper genital tract changes associated with exposure in utero to diethylstilbestrol. *Am J Obstet Gynecol,* 128:51, 1977.
6. Kaufman RH, Adam E, Binder GL, et al: Upper genital tract changes and pregnancy outcome in offspring exposed in utero to diethylstilbestrol. *AM J Obstet Gynecol,* 137:299, 1980.
7. Haney AF, Hammond CB, Soules MR, et al: Diethylstilbestrol-induced upper genital tract abnormalitics. *Fertil Steril,* 31:142, 1979.
8. McLachlan JA, Newbold RR, Shah HC, et al: Fertility of female mice exposed prenatally to diethylstilbestrol. *Fertil Steril,* 38:364, 1982.
9. McLachlan JA, Newbold RR, and Bullock BC: Long-term effects on the female mouse genital tract associated with prenatal exposure to diethylstilbestrol. *Cancer Res,* 40:3988, 1980.
10. Newbold RR, and McLachlan JA: Vaginal adenosis and adenocarcinoma in mice exposed prenatally to diethylstilbestrol. *Cancer Res,* 42:2003, 1982.
11. Newbold RR, Tyrey S, Haney AF, et al: Developmentally arrested oviduct: A structural and functional defect in mice following prenatal exposure to diethylstilbestrol. *Teratology,* 27:417, 1983.
12. Newbold RR, Bullock BC, and McLachlan JA: Exposure to diethylstilbestrol during pregnancy permanently alters the ovary and oviduct. *Biol Reprod,* 28:735, 1983.
13. Rosenfeld DL, and Bronson RA: Reproductive problems in the DES-exposed female. *Obstet Gynecol,* 55:453, 1980.
14. Schmidt G, Fowler WC, Talbert LM, et al: Reproductive history of women exposed to diethylstilbestrol in utero. *Fertil Steril,* 33:21, 1980.
15. Jeffcoate TNA: Malformations and maldevelopments of the genital tract. In Jeffcoate TNA (Ed): *Principles of Gynaecology,* London:Butterworths, 1975: p. 134.
16. Price D, Zaaijer JJP, and Ortiz E: Prenatal development of the oviduct in vivo and in vitro. In Hafez ESE, and Blandau RJ (Eds): *The Mammalian Oviduct.* Chicago: University of Chicago Press, 1969: p. 29.
17. Gruenwald P: The relation of the growing müllerian duct to the wolffian duct and its importance for the genesis of malformations. *Anat Rec,* 81:1, 1941.
18. Burns RK: Urogential system. In Willier BH, Weiss PA, and Hamburger V (Eds): *Analysis of Development.* Philadelphia: WB Saunders, 1955.
19. Nalbandov AV: Comparative morphology and anatomy of the oviduct. In Hafez ESE, and Blandau RJ (Eds): *The Mammalian Oviduct.* Chicago: University of Chicago Press, 1969: p. 47.
20. Hafez ESE, and Black DL: The mammalian uterotubal junction. In Hafez

ESE, and Blandau RJ: (Eds): *The Mammalian Oviduct*. Chicago: University of Chicago Press, 1969: p. 85.
21. Newbold RR, Bullock BC, and McLachlan JA: Progressive proliferative changes in the oviduct following developmental exposure to diethylstilbestrol. *Teratogenesis, Carcinogenesis, Mutagenesis,* 5:473, 1985.
22. McLachlan JA: Prenatal exposure to diethylstilbestrol in mice: Toxicological studies. *J Toxicol Environ Health,* 2:527, 1977.
23. DeCherney AH, Cholst I, Naftolin F: Structure and function of the fallopian tubes following exposure to diethylstilbestrol (DES) during gestation. *Fertil Steril,* 36:741, 1981.
24. Chiari H: Zur pathologischen Anatomie des Eileiterkatarrhs. *Ztschr Heilk,* 8:457, 1887.
25. Benjamin CL, and Beaver DC: The pathogenesis of salpingitis isthmica nodosa. *Am J Clin Pathol,* 21:212, 1951.
26. Benirschke K: Pathologic processes of the oviduct. In Hafez ESE, and Blandau RJ (Eds): *The Mammalian Oviduct,* Chicago: University of Chicago Press, 1969.
27. Freakley G, Normal WJ, Ennis JT, et al: Diverticulosis of the fallopian tubes. *Clin Radiol,* 25:535, 1974.
28. Majmudar B, Hendeson PH III, and Semple E: Salpingitis isthmica nodosa; A high risk factor for tubal pregnancy. *Obstet Gynecol,* 62:73, 1983.
29. Honore LH: Salpingitis isthmica nodosa in female infertility and ectopic tubal pregnancy. *Fertil Steril,* 29:164, 1978.
30. Craig JM: The pathology of infertility. *Pathol Ann,* 10:299, 1975.
31. DeBrux J, Palmer R, and Monteforte C: Etude istologique et prostic des lesions tubaries dans la stérilité. *Gynécol Obstét* (Paris), 68:11, 1969.
32. Thomas ML, Rose DH: Salpingitis isthmica nodosa demonstrated by hysterosalpingography. *Acta Radiol,* 14: 295, 1973.
33. Woodruff JD, and Pauerstein CJ: *The Fallopian Tube.* Baltimore: Williams and Wilkins, 1969: p. 117.
34. Cioltei A, Tasca L, Titirga L, et al: Nodular salpingitis and tubal endometriosis. II. Diagnosis and differential diagnosis. *Acta Europ Fertil,* 10:147, 1979.
35. Siegler AM, and Hellman LM: Tubal plastic surgery: A retrospective study of 50 cases. *Am J Obstet Gynecol,* 86:448, 1963.
36. Bundey JG, and Williams JD: Salpingitis isthmica nodosa with tumor formation resembling torsion of an ovarian cyst. *J. Obstet Gynaecol Br Commonw,* 70:519, 1963.
37. Shen SC, Bansal M, Purrazzella R, et al: Benign glandular inclusions in lymph nodes, endosalpingiosis and salpingitis isthmica nodosa in a young girl with clear cell adenocarcinoma of the cervix. *Am J Surg Path,* 7:293, 1983.
38. Robboy SJ, Welch WR, Young RH, et al: Topographic relation of cervical ectropion and vaginal adenosis to clear cell adenocarcinoma in DES exposed progeny. *Obstet Gynecol,* 60:546, 1982.

15

Acute Salpingitis

W. David Hager

The term "pelvic inflammatory disease" has been used to describe infections of the female genital tract resulting from ascending spread of pathogenic bacteria. This term has not always been applied specifically to a sexually transmitted infection but has been used for many pelvic infections including those occurring after delivery, abortion, curettage, and other pelvic surgery. In this presentation the term salpingitis will be used to denote a clinical syndrome consisting of a complex combination of symptoms and signs resulting from the ascending, contiguous spread of pathogenic endocervical microorganisms along the endometrium to the endosalpinx and adjacent structures.

Since salpingitis is the most common infectious cause of tubal damage and subsequent tubal occlusion and infertility, it is essential that any text on tubal diseases should contain a discussion of this entity whose accurate and prompt diagnosis and treatment are essential.

Incidence

The exact incidence of salpingitis is difficult to ascertain because of the variation in diagnostic terminology, the inclusion of postpartum and postoperative infections within the discharge diagnosis of "pelvic inflammatory disease," and because salpingitis is not a reportable disease. Based on recent data for inpatient discharges, outpatient visits to private physicians' offices, and correlates with the incidence of gonorrhea, it is estimated that 700,000 to 850,000 cases of salpingitis will occur in the United States each year.[1] Recently the number of inpatients with salpingitis has reached a plateau, indicating that perhaps more affected patients are detected and treated effectively as outpatients (Figs. 15:1 and 15:2).

The incidence of salpingitis appears to follow the total number of cases of gonorrhea reported in the United States, even though this organism is only isolated from 30 to 60 percent of patients. Along with the plateau in incidence of reported cases of gonorrhea in the United States, there has also been a plateau in the estimated number of cases of salpingitis; however, this disease remains a major medical problem.[2]

The Fallopian Tube: Basic Studies and Clinical Contributions, edited by Alvin M. Siegler, M.D. Mount Kisco, New York: Futura Publishing Company, Inc. © 1986.

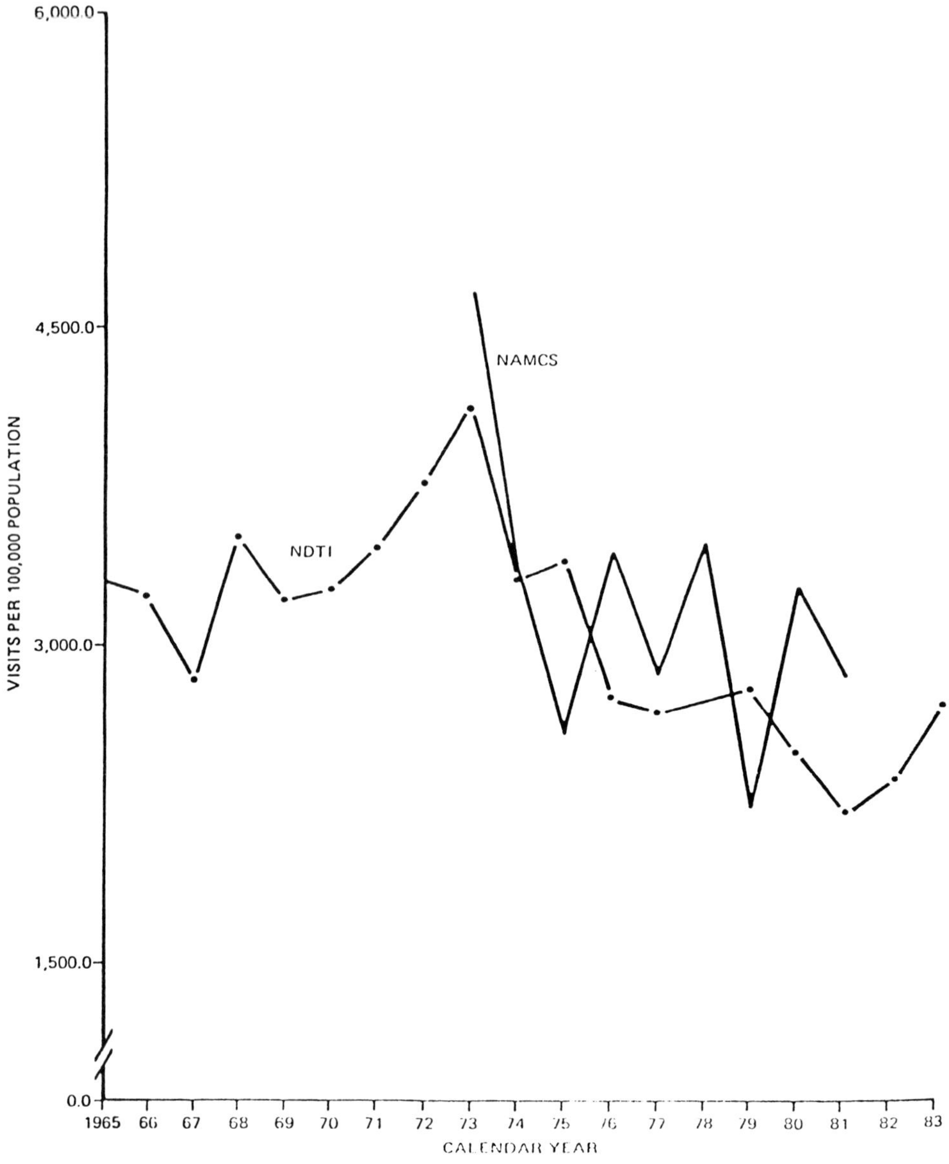

FIGURE 15:1—*Total visits for pelvic inflammatory disease; visits per 100,000 population in the United States for the calendar years 1965–1983. Rate is for female population (age group 15–50) and women with PID in age groups 15–50. NDTI = National Disease and Therapeutic Index; NAMCS = National Ambulatory Medical Care Survey.*

Predisposing Factors

A number of identifiable factors have been associated with the occurrence of salpingitis. Exposure to pathogenic bacteria is obviously a prerequisite to infection, although these bacteria may originate from the host's own vaginal flora. The combination of pathogenic bacteria and one of several predisposing factors increases the chance of developing tubal infection. Acute salpingitis is a sexually transmitted infection and is not found in

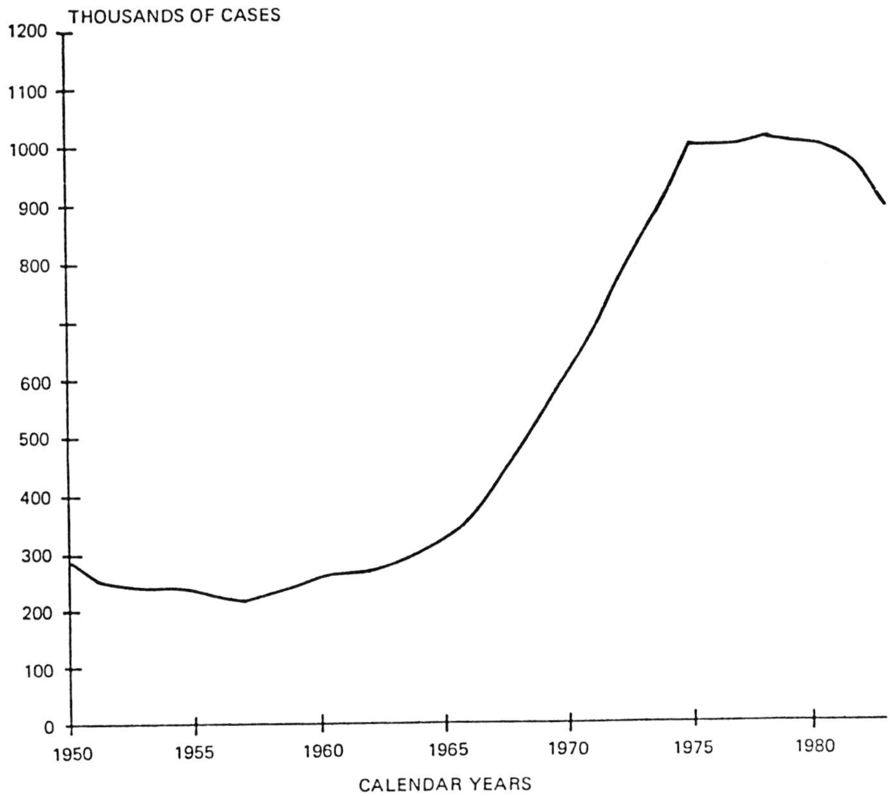

FIGURE 15:2—*Gonorrhea cases in the United States for the calendar years 1950–1983.*

sexually inactive women unless they have an intrauterine contraceptive device (IUD) in place.[3,4] Exposure to multiple sexual partners increases the risk of developing any sexually transmitted disease (STD) including salpingitis. Prior uncomplicated gonococcal infection and/or a prior episode of salpingitis predispose a woman to subsequent salpingitis because of the susceptibility to infection resulting from previous damage to the endosalpinx.

Several investigators have reported an association between the menstrual period and salpingitis. Falk[5] reported that two-thirds of all instances of salpingitis have their onset of symptoms within seven days of a previous menstrual period. This may indicate that shedding of the endometrium and patency of the endocervix allow for easier access of pathogenic bacteria to the endometrium and fallopian tubes.

Ory has reviewed the literature and reported that salpingitis occurs two to five times more frequently in women who wear IUDs compared with sexually active women using other methods of contraception.[3] Among IUD users, young, nulliparous, sexually active women are at greatest risk. Burkman, on the other hand, has reported no significant increase in salpingitis among such women in his study.[4]

Causes

For many years most investigators equated salpingitis with gonococcal infection. Most early studies on pathogenesis used endocervical and rectal culture results as the basis for concluding that 60 to 80 percent of salpingitis was caused by

Neisseria gonorrhoeae. It was not uncommon to divide reported cases into gono-coccal and nongonococcal groupings, and to base treatment on endocervical isolation alone.

Data have recently been generated that allow a more realistic evaluation of the bacterial cause of the disease. In 1975, Eschenbach[6] indicated that salpingitis was a disease caused by multiple organisms that may be present concomitantly in the same patient. Since that publication, other investigators[7–11] have reported data to support the concept of a polymicrobial cause of salpingitis. These studies compared endocervical and rectal isolates to intraperitoneal isolates, the latter obtained either by culdocentesis or by laparoscopy. They found that in patients from whom the gonococcus was isolated from the endocervix or rectum, it was simultaneously cultured from the peritoneal cavity only 30 to 40 percent of the time. In most of these patients, multiple aerobes and anaerobes were isolated from the peritoneum.

Controversy has arisen over the issue of the initial cause of the disease. Do multiple organisms simultaneously invade the endometrial cavity and fallopian tubes in a susceptible host, or does a principal pathogen (such as the gonococcus) initiate infection, cause damage to the tubal mucosa, and allow for subsequent infection by secondary invaders? Studies on bacterial attachment would indicate that *N. gonorrhoeae* attach to nonciliated cells on the endosalpinx. Subsequent damage to ciliated cells alters host resistance and then other bacteria infect and damage the tubes and adjacent structures. Results of peritoneal cultures depend, to a great extent, on when during the course of disease they are obtained. Organisms present on the peritoneal surfaces would be most readily obtained.

Data from Europe and from the United States have more recently implicated another organism in the cause of salpingitis. In separate studies, Thompson,[11] Mardh,[12,13] Sweet,[14] and Henry-Suchet[15] reported that chlamydia may be the most common cause of salpingitis. It is the most common cause of mucopurulent cervicitis and urethral syndrome in women. An important aspect in the consideration of chlamydia, as a cause of salpingitis, is the finding that patients infected with this organism develop a characteristic type of salpingitis. Frequently they have minimal symptoms, in spite of severe tubal involvement, and may not seek medical care until significant tubal damage has already occurred.

The bacterial cause of acute salpingitis cannot be assumed to be gonococcal and must include endocervical and rectal cultures for *N. gonorrhoeae* and *C. trachomatis* and properly obtained specimens for aerobes and anaerobes from the peritoneal cavity, preferably from the tubal surfaces.

Diagnosis

Symptoms

Salpingitis is frequently confused with other causes of abdominal pain. There is a tendency to suspect any young, sexually active woman who presents with lower abdominal pain as having a tubal infection. Data indicate that it is as common to miss the diagnosis of salpingitis, by assuming that another entity is present, as it is to diagnose salpingitis and find that another disease is the cause of the symptoms.

Abdominal pain is the complaint of almost all women with confirmed tubal infection but is also the most common complaint in women with many other disorders. It is important to consider another diagnosis if the patient has no abdominal pain. Other symptoms may include fever, chills, nausea, vomiting, and abnormal vaginal discharge.

Signs

On examination, patients with acute salpingitis have abdominal direct and rebound tenderness, and there is tenderness with manipulation of the cervix, uterus, and adnexa in over 90 percent of cases. Patients with salpingitis may present for care without significant temperature elevation. Data from Jacobson and Weström[16] indicated that only 41.3 percent of more than 900 patients with confirmed salpingitis had a temperature elevation greater than 38°C. Thus, temperature elevation should not be used as an absolute criterion for diagnosis. The woman with salpingitis frequently is so uncomfortable that she has difficulty relaxing sufficiently to allow adequate evaluation of the adnexa. Hours or days may pass after antibiotic therapy is begun before the adnexa may be examined satisfactorily to detect a tubo-ovarian inflammatory mass or a fluctuant pelvic abscess. Ultrasound scan may be helpful in such patients to search for adnexal enlargement which may be found in up to 50 percent of patients.[17]

Purulent cervical discharge is noted in approximately half of these women. In patients with abdominal peritonitis, ileus with hypoactive bowel sounds may be present. The clinical findings of salpingitis are classically bilateral but unilateral disease may exist, especially in patients with IUD-associated disease.

Criteria for diagnosis

To improve diagnostic capabilities and clinical competence, and to facilitate comparison of data among studies, clinical criteria have been developed from existing data. Abdominal direct tenderness, tenderness with motion of the cervix and uterus and adnexa must be present to make the diagnosis. Findings that add credibility to the diagnosis include a gram stain of the endocervix positive for *Neisseria gonorrhoeae*, temperature elevation, leucocytosis, purulent material (with white blood cells) present in the peritoneal cavity, and an adnexal mass consistent with a tubo-ovarian inflammatory mass or a tubo-ovarian abscess (Table 15:1).

The laparoscope gives us a reliable method of confirming the clinical diagnosis of salpingitis based on direct observation of the involved structures.[18,19] This examination should be performed whenever there is uncertainty about the diagnosis and to allow classification of the severity of disease. Mild disease is classified as erythema and tubal edema without spontaneous purulent exudate. Moderate disease includes more severe erythema and edema along with gross purulent exudate or observation of exudate when the tubes are manipulated. The tubes may be less mobile and occluded. Severe disease consists of a pyosalpinx, inflammatory mass, or abscess. The severity of disease indicates the prognosis for subsequent fertility, since the rate of subsequent bilateral tubal occlusion is directly related to the severity of disease at initial laparoscopy.[20]

Laboratory findings

The diagnosis of acute salpingitis is principally made from findings on physical examination and few laboratory tests are required. According to most reports, fewer than 50 percent of patients will have a white blood cell count in excess of 12,000, with a shift to the left in the neutrophil count. The erythrocyte sedimentation rate will be elevated in 75 percent of patients. Cervical gram-stained smears may be helpful if positive for gram-negative intracellular diplococci, but the false negative rate is high. Endocervical cultures for *N. gonorrhoeae* and *C. trachomatis* and other organisms and aerobic and anaerobic intraperitoneal cultures should be obtained during laparoscopy or culdocentesis.

Differential Diagnosis

The work of Jacobson and Weström[16] has demonstrated that despite careful history taking and examination by experienced physicians, the clinical diagnosis of salpingitis is in error 35 percent of the

Table 15:1

Salpingitis: Clinical Criteria for Diagnosis[18]

Criteria	
• Abdominal, direct tenderness, with or without rebound tenderness • Tenderness with motion of cervix and uterus • Adnexal tenderness	All three necessary for diagnosis
• Gram stain of endocervix—positive for gram-negative, intracellular diplococci • Fever (greater than 38° C) • Leukocytosis (greater than 10,000) • Purulent material (WBC present) from peritoneal cavity by culdocentesis or laparoscopy • Pelvic abscess or inflammatory complex on bimanual exam or by sonography	One or more necessary for diagnosis

time when laparoscopy is used to confirm the diagnosis. Other disorders were detected 12 percent of the time and in 23 percent of patients no abnormalities were seen.[21]

Other entities frequently confused with salpingitis and comprising the differential diagnosis include: acute appendicitis, ectopic pregnancy, torsion or rupture of an ovarian cyst, septic abortion, pyelonephritis, and inflammatory intestinal disease.

Clinical Response

Many patients with early acute salpingitis can be managed as outpatients with oral antibiotic regimens.[22] These women must be seen in 48 to 72 hours and again at seven to ten days after initiation of treatment to evaluate their clinical response and to insure that an abscess has not developed. Women who fail to respond should be hospitalized. Their sexual partners should be examined, have cultures obtained from their urethra, and be treated appropriately with an acceptable oral antibiotic regimen.

Hospitalization is advisable whenever there is uncertainty about diagnosis, lack of response to oral antibiotics, a pelvic mass (greater than 5 cm) present, generalized peritonitis, and another complicating medical illness. Inpatients should be followed with daily assessment of their clinical progress. A clinical method for assessing response is the severity score index of Thompson, Hager, and colleagues.[11] This index involves a daily grading of the clinical findings used for diagnosis with the measurement of a daily percentage change in severity score. (Table 15:2). The change in score at 72 hours correlates well with prognosis for response. Patients must be examined to evaluate their response to treatment.

Therapy

Treatment recommendations for acute salpingitis have been published by the Centers for Disease Control.[23] These recommendations include regimens for outpatients and inpatients. Any regimen chosen must provide coverage for *N. gonorrhoeae*, *C. trachomatis*, and anaerobic bacteria. The primary regimen for outpatients should include a form of tetracycline to be continued for 10 to 14 days. This may include an intramuscular injection of cefoxitin. Another frequently used regimen includes intramuscular aqueous procaine penicillin G and oral ampicillin, or amoxicillin to complete 10 to 14 days. Patients must be followed frequently to evaluate their clinical response.

Table 15:2

Severity Score[11]

Abdominal tenderness (direct)
Rebound tenderness
Decreased bowel sounds*
Pain on cervical motion
Adnexal tenderness—right
Adnexal tenderness—left
Adnexal enlargement—right
Adnexal enlargement—left

0 = absent, 1 = minimal, 2 = moderate, 3 = marked. Total severity score range = 0 (normal) to 24 (most ill).

*For bowel sounds, the score is reversed.

Patients who are hospitalized should be managed with bed rest, intravenous fluids, appropriate analgesia, and an appropriate combination of parenteral antibiotics to treat a polymicrobial infection. Before antibiotics are begun, endocervical cultures for *N. gonorrhoeae* and *C. trachomatis*, a rectal culture for *N. gonorrhoeae*, and intraperitoneal cultures for aerobes and anaerboes should be obtained. The latter is ideally done laparoscopically, but may be accomplished using culdocentesis, although this procedure is fraught with contamination.

Results of several antibiotic combinations in patients hospitalized with salpingitis are not available because the use of different criteria for diagnosis and clinical response to treatment often preclude adequate comparison of studies. Selection of appropriate antibiotics for inpatients might include a cephamycin and doxycycline, a penicillin or cephalosporin combined with an aminoglycoside and clindamycin, or ampicillin or a cephalosporin with metronidazole.[24] Inpatients should be evaluated by the severity score index to assess clinical response.

The laparoscope is used selectively to make the original diagnosis, to obtain cultures, for an uncertain diagnosis, to assess response to therapy, and to provide information to determine a prognosis for future fertility.

Indications for surgical intervention include failure of clinical improvement after adequate antibiotic treatment, presence of a pelvic abscess refractory to antibiotic treatment, uncertain diagnosis, and suspected rupture or leakage of a pelvic abscess. Patients must be properly hydrated and have adequate serum levels of appropriate antibiotics before the operation is begun.

Sequelae of Disease

The development of a tubo-ovarian abscess and peritonitis may be the consequence of delayed consultation, delayed diagnosis, or inappropriate treatment. Studies by Ginsburg,[25] Landers,[26] and others report frequent resolution of abscesses in patients treated with appropriate antibiotics. We have found that patients with an abscess do not respond as well to antibiotics as do those with a tubo-ovarian inflammatory mass.[27] Failure to respond with a decrease in temperature, white blood cell count and tenderness within 72 hours is an indication for operative intervention since the abscess may have ruptured. Colpotomy may be performed to drain a fluctuant midline abscess that dissects into the rectovaginal septum.

Women who develop salpingitis with an IUD in place may form a unilateral tubo-ovarian abscess[28] and a salpingo-oophorectomy may prevent involvement of the uninvolved side.

Long-term sequelae of salpingitis include chronic pain, ectopic pregnancy, and infertility.[29] Eighteen percent of patients with an episode of acute salpingitis will have chronic pelvic pain which may require a subsequent operation for relief. Retrospective data in women with tubal pregnancy indicate that 50 percent have a history of previous salpingitis. Concomitant with the increase in incidence of this disease has been a rise in tubal pregnancy.[30] Forty percent of infertility in women has been reported to be related to salpingitis.[31] This is the most tragic consequence of the disease, other than death from sepsis or ruptured ectopic pregnancy, because it results in loss of reproductive capability. Weström reported 13 percent bilateral tubal occlusion after one episode of salpingitis, after two episodes 35 percent, and 75 percent after three or more episodes.[31]

Salpingitis has a detrimental economic impact on our society.[32] Estimates indicate total direct costs of salpingitis and ectopic pregnancy in the United States to be greater than seven hundred million dollars per year. This disease continues to cause significant disability and warrants early, accurate diagnosis, adequate treatment, and careful monitoring.

References

1. Centers for Disease Control: *Morbid Mortal Weekly Rep*, 33:665, 1984.
2. St John RK, Jones OG, Blount JH, et al: Pelvic inflammatory disease in the United States: Epidemiology and trends among hospitalized women. *Sex Trans Dis*, 8:62, 1981.
3. Ory HW: A review of the association between intrauterine devices and acute pelvic inflammatory disease. *J Reprod Med*, 20:200, 1978.
4. Burkman RT: Intrauterine device use and risk of pelvic inflammatory disease. *Am J Obstet Gynecol*, 138:861, 1980.
5. Falk V: Treatment of acute non-tuberculous salpingitis with antibiotics alone and in combination with glucocorticoids. *Acta Obstet Gynecol Scand*, 44(Suppl 6): 1965.
6. Eschenbach DA, Buchanan TM, and Pollock HM: Polymicrobial etiology of acute pelvic inflammatory disease. *N Engl J Med*, 293:166, 1975.
7. Chow AW, Malkasian KL, and Marshall JR: The bacteriology of acute pelvic inflammatory disease. *Am J Obstet Gynecol*, 122:876, 1975.
8. Monif GRG, Welkos SL, and Baer H: Cul-de-sac isolates from patients with endometritis-salpingitis-peritonitis and gonococcal endocervicitis. *Am J Obstet Gynecol*, 126:158, 1976.
9. Sweet RL, Mills J, Hadley KW, et al: Use of laparoscopy to determine the microbiologic etiology of acute salpingitis. *Am J Obstet Gynecol*, 134:68, 1979.
10. Cunningham FG, Hauth JC, Gilstrap LC, et al: The bacterial pathogenesis of acute pelvic inflammatory disease. *Obstet Gynecol*, 52:161, 1978.
11. Thompson SE, Hager WD, Wong KH, et al: The microbiology and therapy of acute pelvic inflammatory disease in hospitalized patients. *Am J Obstet Gynecol*, 136:179, 1980.
12. Mardh PA, Ripa T, and Svennson L: *Chlamydia trachomatis* infection in patients with acute salpingitis. *N Engl J Med*, 296:1377, 1977.
13. Mardh PA, and Svensson L: Chlamydial salpingitis. *Scan J Infect Dis* (Suppl), 32:64, 1982.
14. Sweet RL: Pelvic inflammatory disease: Etiology, diagnosis and treatment. *Sex Trans Dis*, 8(Suppl 4):308, 1981.
15. Henry-Suchet J, Catalan F, Loffredo V, et al: *Chlamydia trachomatis* associated with chronic inflammation in abdominal specimens from women selected for tuboplasty. *Fertil Steril*, 36:599, 1981.
16. Jacobson L, and Weström L: Objectivized diagnosis of acute pelvic inflammatory disease. *Am J Obstet Gynecol*, 105: 1088, 1969.
17. Spirtos NS, Bernstine RL, Crawford WL, et al: Sonography in acute pelvic inflammatory disease. *J Reprod Med*, 27:312, 1982.
18. Hager WD, Eschenbach DA, Spence MR, et al: Criteria for diagnosis and grading of salpingitis. *Obstet Gynecol*, 61:113, 1983.
19. Monif GRG: Clinical staging of acute bacterial salpingitis and its therapeutic ramifications. *Am J Obstet Gynecol*, 143:489, 1982.
20. Chaparro MV, Ghosh S, Nashed A, et al: Laparoscopy for the confirmation and prognostic evaluation of pelvic inflammatory disease. *Int J Gynecol Obstet*, 15:307, 1978.
21. Jacobson L: Differential diagnosis of acute pelvic inflammatory disease. *Am J Obstet Gynecol*, 138:1006, 1980.
22. Cunningham FG, Hauth JC, Strong JD, et al: Evaluation of tetracycline or penicillin and ampicillin for treatment of acute pelvic inflammatory disease. *N Engl J Med*, 296:1380, 1977.
23. Centers for Disease Control: *Morbid Mortal Weekly Rep* (Suppl), 31:33, 1982.
24. Monif GRG, Welkos SL, Baer H: Clinical response of patients with gonococcal endocervicitis and endometritis-

salpingitis-peritonitis to doxycycline. *Am J Obstet Gynecol*, 129:614, 1977.
25. Ginsburg DS, Stern JL, Hamod KA, et al: Tubo-ovarian abscess: A retrospective review. *Am J Obstet Gynecol*, 138:1055, 1980.
26. Landers DV, Sweet RL: Tubo-ovarian abscess: Contemporary approach to management. *Rev Infect Dis*, 5:876, 1983.
27. Hager WD: Followup of patients with tubo-ovarian abscess(es) in association with salpingitis. *Obstet Gynecol*, 61:680, 1983.
28. Niebyl JR, Parmley TH, Spence MR, et al: Unilateral ovarian abscess associated with the intrauterine device. *Obstet Gynecol*, 52:165, 1978.
29. Adler MW, Belsey EH, and O'Conner BH: Morbidity associated with pelvic inflammatory disease. *Br J Ven Dis*, 58:151, 1982.
30. Weinstein L, Morris MB, Dotters D, et al: Ectopic pregnancy: A new surgical epidemic. *Obstet Gynecol*, 61:698, 1983.
31. Weström L: Effect of pelvic inflammatory disease on fertility. *Am J Obstet Gynecol*, 121:707, 1975.
32. Curran JW: Economic consequences of pelvic inflammatory disease in the United States. *Am J Obstet Gynecol*, 138:848, 1980.

16

Pelvic Infection and Infertility; Mechanisms of Action

Alan H. DeCherney
and Neri Laufer

Pelvic infection is a major factor in infertility because it can result in tubal damage and anatomical distortion of the adnexa.

Grossly, tubal and ovarian structures can be significantly altered, the tube being encapsulated in scar tissue and thereby preventing normal ovulation. In addition, the tubal distortion prevents normal capture and transport of the ovum (Fig. 16:1). Microscopic damage shows cellular infiltration of bacteria and white cells followed by adherent cilia. Subsequent fragmentation and destruction of cilia ensue.[1,2] The degree of destruction depends on the severity of infection, the type of organism, and the frequency of infections. Eventually, the endosalpinx becomes denuded and there is no ciliary regeneration. Fronds of tissue become adherent, forming diverticulae and bald areas in the tubal lumen (Figs. 16:2 and 16:3).The tube becomes unable to assist in ovum transport.

Tubal tuberculosis shows the extension and end stage of damage. Hypertrophy of the epithelial cells and destruction of the normal tubal structure are seen. The degree of tubal destruction can also be appreciated with light miscroscopy.

Animal models for studying the pathogenesis of salpingitis have been primarily limited to *Neisseria gonorrhoeae* and *Chlamydia trachomatis*.[3] Gram-negative bacteria have recently been described as major infecting organisms in pelvic inflammatory disease. The predominant facilitative aerobic pathogen found in tuboperitoneal fluid obtained from women with salpingitis is *Escherichia coli,* while the prominent anaerobic pathogens are in the bacteroides species.[4]

Animal experiments have substantiated and corroborated the work in humans. Gram-negative bacteria liberate endotoxins derived from the cell wall. When injected systemically into experimental animals, these endotoxins produce a syndrome of shock, vasoconstriction, and intravascular coagulation. The effects of

The Fallopian Tube: Basic Studies and Clinical Contributions, edited by Alvin M. Siegler, M.D. Mount Kisco, New York: Futura Publishing Company, Inc.

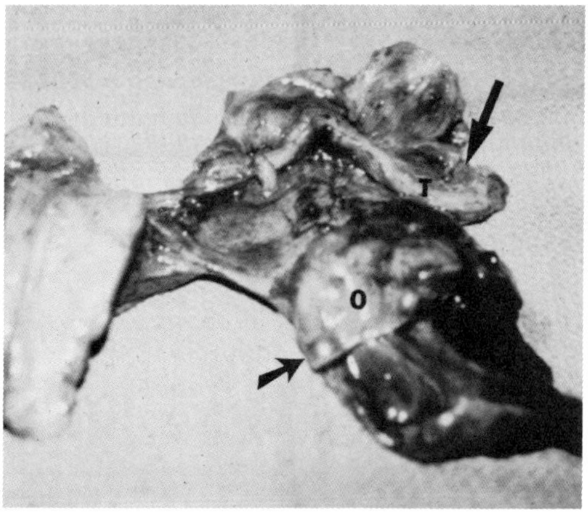

FIGURE 16:1—*Tubo-ovarian abscess shows distortion of the tube (T) and ovary (O) with dense adhesions (arrows) encapsulating the ovary. This specimen had been dissected to show the tube and ovary as separate entities.*

endotoxins and *E. coli* on the surface epithelium of the fallopian tube in the rabbit have been examined.[2] When *E. coli* endotoxin (5μg/ml) was administered into the tubal lumen in a single injection, severe ciliary damage and alterations in the surface of the secretory cells occurred. Twelve hours after the endotoxin injection, the tips of the cilia demonstrated blebs and tended to adhere to each other. At the same time, swelling of the microvilli of the secretory cells also occurred. Twenty-four hours after the injection, the cilia became shorter, swollen, and adherent to each other at the tips and appeared fused. The microvilli were shortened, giving a smooth appearance of these secretory protrusions. Light microscopy at this time revealed severe cellular swelling and edema with an infiltrate of polymorphonuclear cells and mural thrombi. Restoration of the epithelium was found after 72 hours and most of the mucosal surface appeared normal.

When *E. coli* but not endotoxin, in a concentration of 1×10^5, were injected into the lumen of the fallopian tube, the maximal endosalpingeal ciliary injury to the surface microvilli of the secretory cells occurred seven days after the initial injection. The process of regeneration began two weeks after the inoculation and it was completed eight weeks later. The pattern of injury and regeneration in response to *E. coli* was almost identical to that caused by its endotoxin alone and it was significantly different from the pattern seen from experimental endosalpingeal damage caused by *N. gonorrhoeae* and *C. trachomatis*.[3] The maximal tubal damage after endotoxin injection occurred after 24 hours, and after seven days from *E. coli* alone. The intact bacteria probably liberated their endotoxin over time, thereby delaying the peak of maximal damage. These experiments shed light on the pathogenesis of tubal surface injury from gram-negative bacteria and suggest that the major effects on tubal mucosa are mediated through endotoxin liberated from the bacterial cell wall.

The macroscopic changes parallel those seen with light and electronmicroscopy. Normal fimbria have a pink, velvety appearance and promptly spill transcervically injected dye. Macroscopically, the sequence of tubal changes secondary to infection begin, as they do microscopically, with adherence of ciliated epithelial surfaces. Fimbrial tips agglutinate, forming a meshwork (Fig. 16:4). Theoretically, this conglutination is an impediment to ovum pickup and transport. Thickening of the peritoneal band in the infundibulum follows (Fig. 16:5). This causes the fimbria to roll inward, and the overgrowth of visceral peritoneum produces phimosis. Eventually, the thickened visceral peritoneum occludes the tube. The white lines represent demarcation of peritoneal fusion (Fig. 16:6).

Once the tube is totally occluded, it becomes unable to handle the daily production of luminal fluid. Instead of flowing out of the normal fimbrial opening, the 3 to 5 ml of fluid produced daily is forced into the uterine cavity through the interstitial segment. The pressure necessary to force this fluid through a smaller opening causes hypertrophy of the muscularis (Fig. 16:7), The myosalpinx is prominent, in contrast to the nearly transparent layer seen in a normal tube. Eventually, this

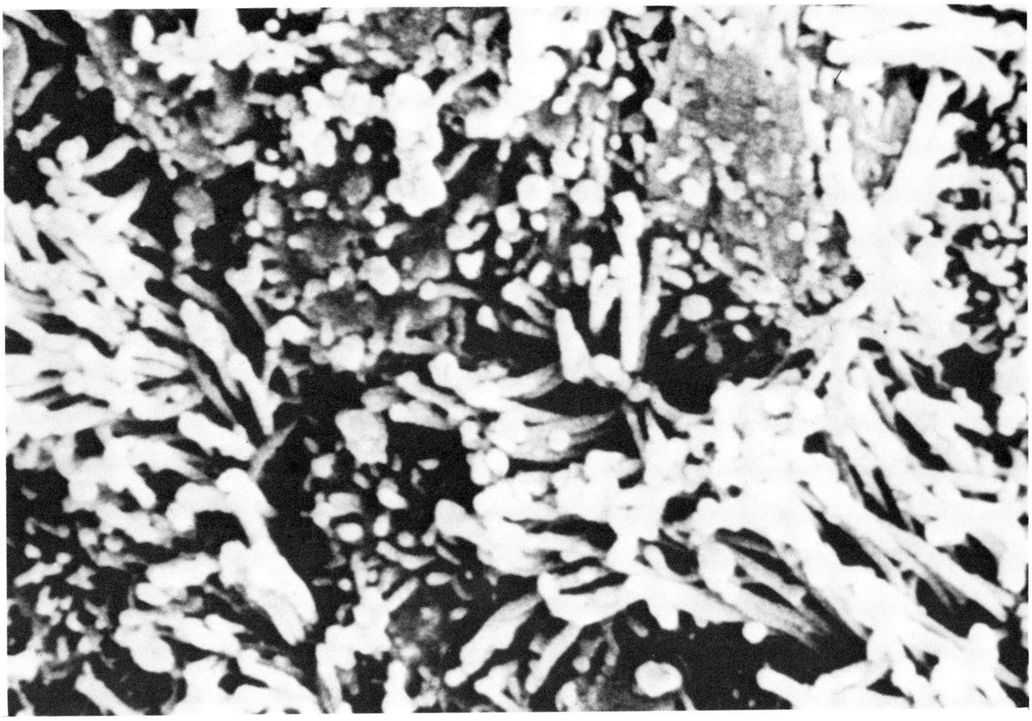

FIGURE 16:2—*Destruction of cilia occurs after an infection.*

clubbed tube is unable to overcome the resistance and dilatation occurs with the formation of a hydrosalpinx. Pressure necrosis of the ciliary lining results in a "bald" tube; such damage is not reversible. This sequence of tubal changes is descriptive of disease resulting from gonorrheal or chlamydial infections, followed by secondary invasion by gram-negative anerobes and aerobes.

Peritubal adhesions can prevent the tube from moving freely so as to capture the ovum. Even if the intraluminal architecture and transport ability remain intact, infertility results. This condition is seen following pelvic peritonitis caused by a ruptured appendix where the tubal lumen is normal.[6,7] Postoperative infections, especially those associated with peritonitis, may also result in similar periadnexal adhesions. Indeed, any pelvic surgery entails such a risk. Procedures commonly performed on young women such as ovarian cystectomy or wedge resection may cause such adhesions (Fig. 16:8).

Tubal obstruction sometimes occurs in the intramural segment (Fig. 16:9) and is caused by either a postpartum or a postabortal infection; sometimes it results from an intercurrent infection associated with an intrauterine contraceptive device (IUD). The mechanism of IUD action is to initiate a low-grade, chronic endometritis that prevents implantation. However, in approximately 5 percent of IUD users, the infection can cause tubal obstruction.[8–10] Statistically, the incidence of tubal damage and infertility per years of IUD use is not precisely known but pelvic infection is increased over the baseline rate. Chronic endometritis, whether associated with an IUD or not also results in infertility. A classic instance of chronic endometritis is seen with hemosiderin deposits along with a plasma cell

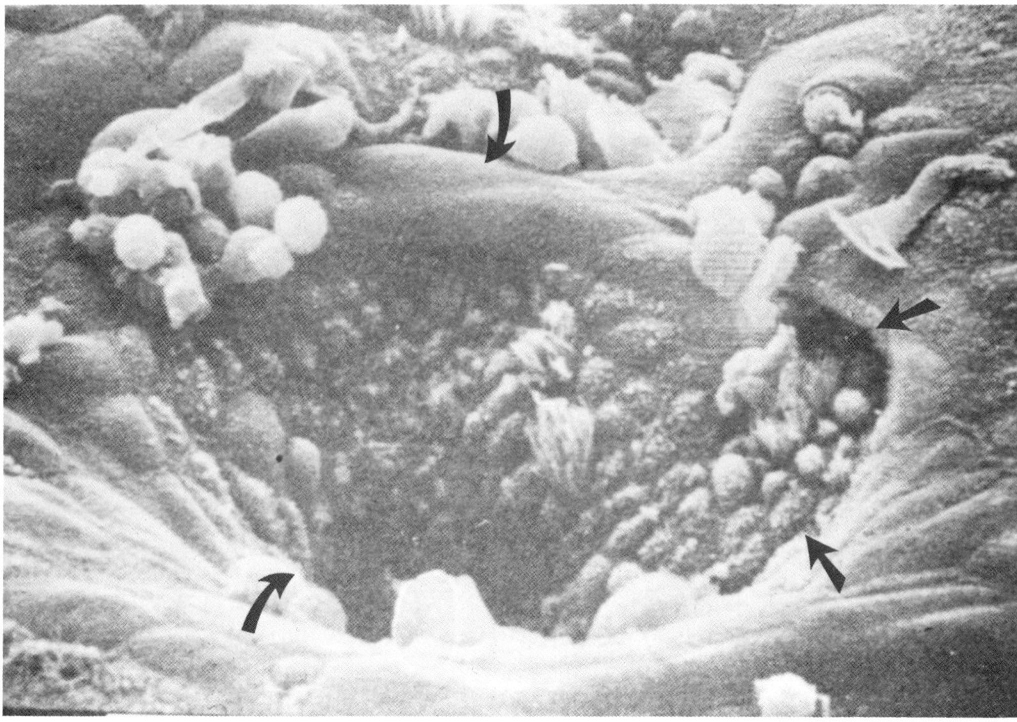

FIGURE 16:3—*Experimental microdiverticulum (arrows) follows induced infection. (Reproduced with permission from Draper et al.[3])*

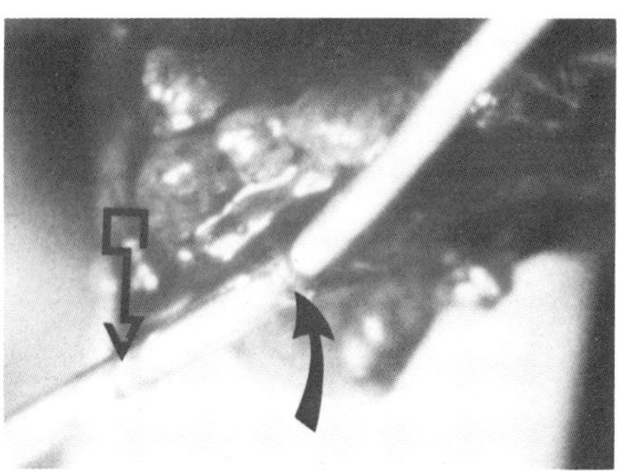

FIGURE 16:4—*Fimbrial conglutination (arrow) is present.*

and leukocytic infiltration (Fig. 16:10). This condition is detected from an endometrial biopsy specimen and should be treated with a broad-spectrum antibiotic such as a tetracycline.

Does the knowledge of the sequence of tubal changes seen after pelvic infection have any immediate bearing on clinical gynecology? As Weström[11] demonstrated in his study of over 1,000 women, the rate of tubal occlusion increased from 12.8 percent to 75 percent as the number of episodes of PID increased. Each attack carries an increased risk of sterility. Does the severity of the infection correlate with subsequent infertility? Data from Weström[11] revealed that patients with severe pelvic inflammatory disease (PID) at the time of the initial laparoscopy had a higher incidence of subsequent tubal occlusion than those who had mild PID. Thus, the extent and severity of an infection may have some prognostic value in predicting future fertility.

Chlamydia trachomatis and *N. gonorrhoeae* cause most severe reproductive damage. Gonorrhea was assumed to be the major cause of pelvic inflammatory disease, but a review of the literature showed the incidence to range from 33 percent to 81 percent.[5] Since pelvic infec-

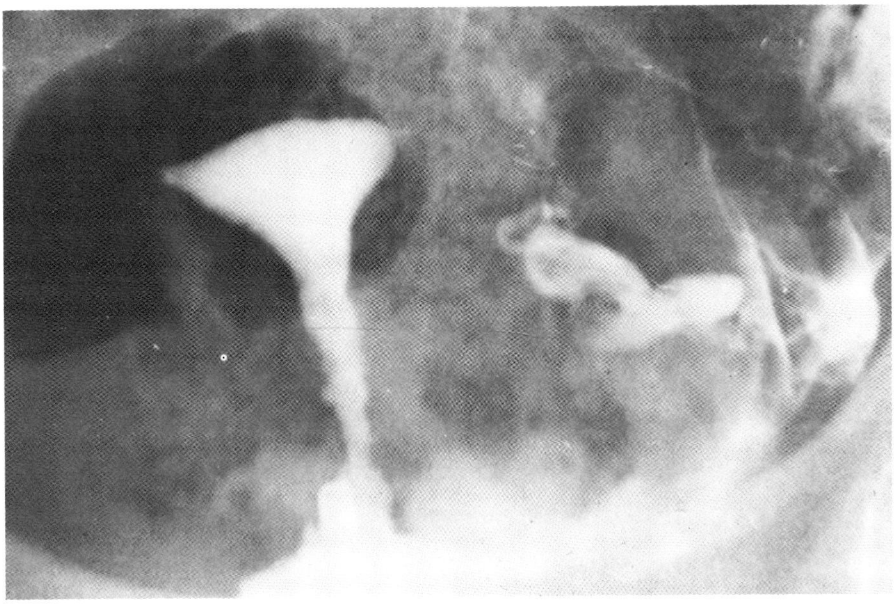

FIGURE 16:5—*Hysterosalpingogram shows fimbrial phimosis caused by thickening of the visceral peritoneum of the infundibulum.*

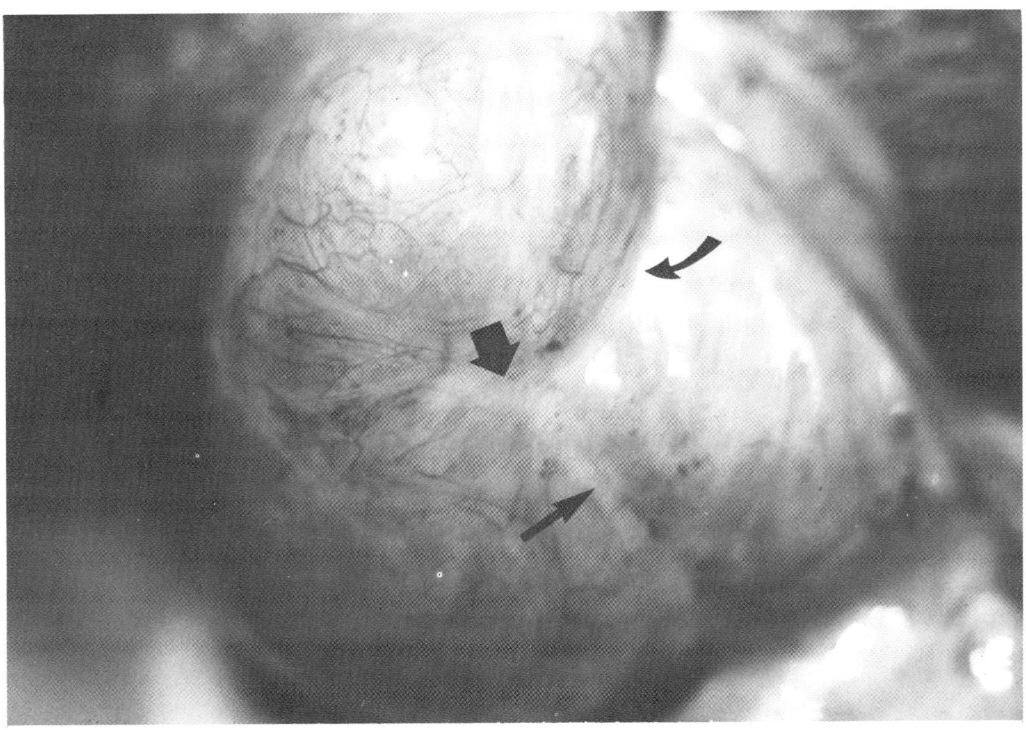

FIGURE 16:6—*Clubbed tubes showing overgrowth of the visceral peritoneum at white lines (arrows).*

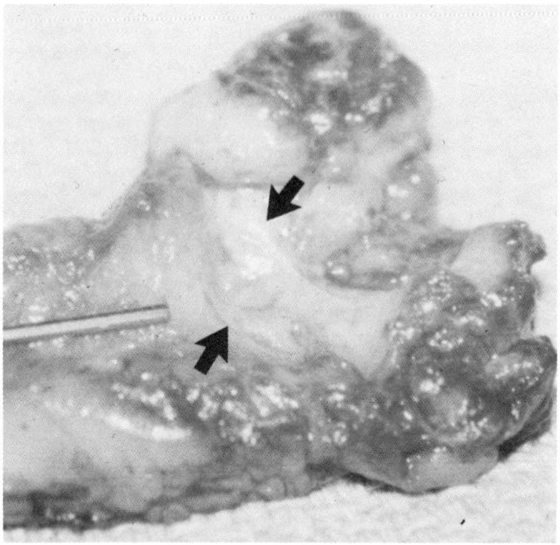

FIGURE 16:7—*Severe salpingitis causes muscular hypertrophy (arrows) and scarring at the fimbriated end.*

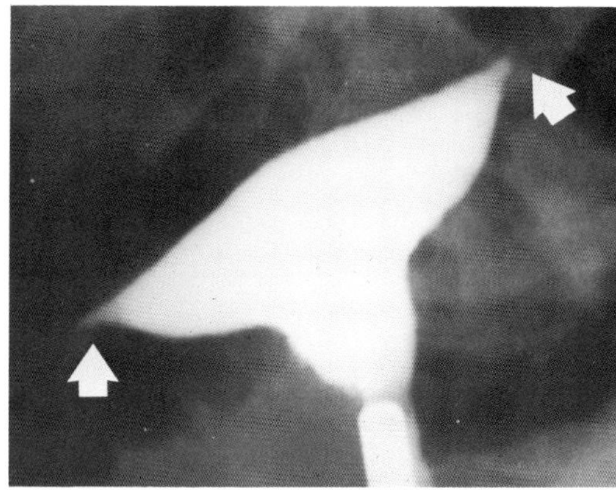

FIGURE 16:9—*Bilateral cornual obstruction (arrows) demonstrated on hysterosalpingogram.*

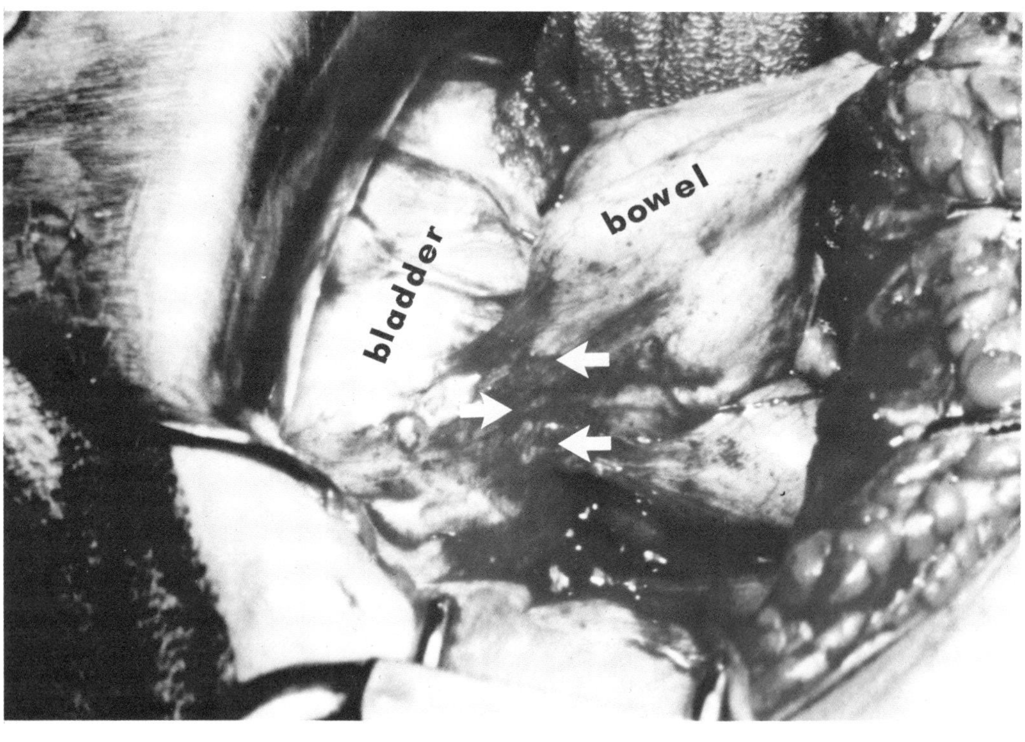

FIGURE 16:8—*Dense pelvic adhesions (arrows) formed after a ruptured appendix.*

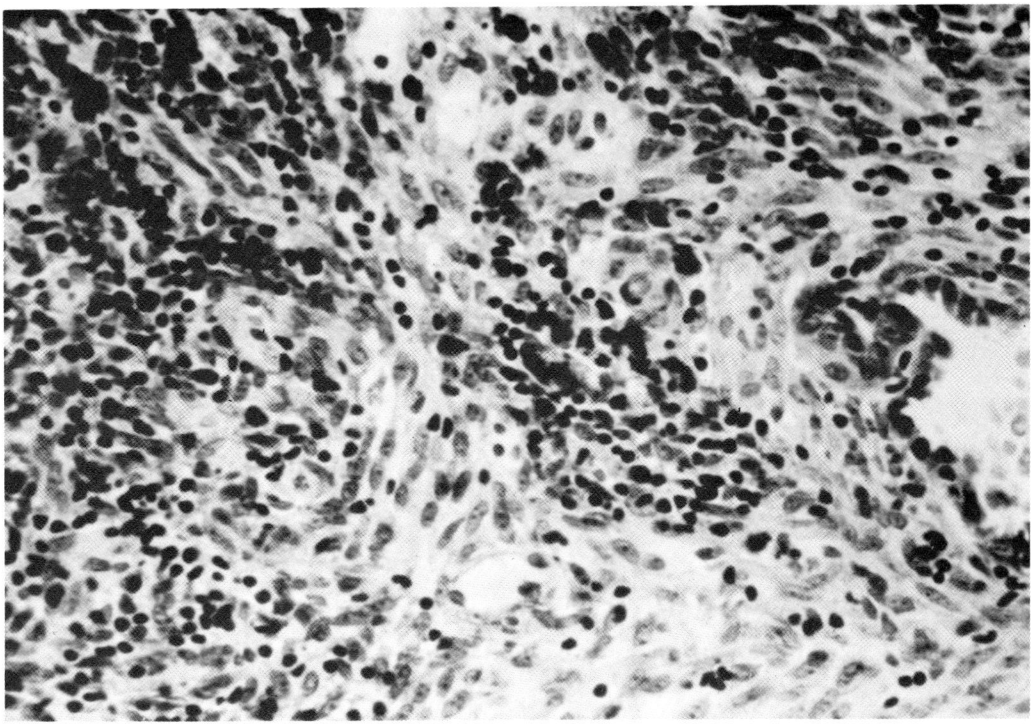

FIGURE 16:10—*Chronic endometritis showing polys, hemosiderin, and plasma cells.*

tion with other organisms also results in infertility, the gynecologist must search carefully to make an adequate diagnosis and recommend proper treatment of pelvic inflammatory disease. Perhaps all patients should have laparoscopy at the time of the diagnosis of PID.[12,13] Misdiagnosis could be minimized. In a study of over 905 patients by Weström,[13] 98 women or roughly 10 percent had a changed diagnosis based on laparoscopy. In addition, 184 patients were found to have normal pelves, indicating the significant extent of errors in diagnosis.

As the infecting organisms and concepts change, therapy also must be altered. At present, *C. trachomatis* appears to be the major infecting organism, with anerobes and mycoplasma being secondary offenders. These bacteria also cause severe damage. Penicillin or its derivatives are no longer the drugs of choice. In selected clinical situations, multiple drug therapy is required, including cephalosporins, aminoglycosides, and other anaerobicidals.

Chlamydia trachomatis is an intracellular organism, forming inclusion bodies. It must be grown in cells and is difficult and expensive to culture; the recovery rates are often low. This infection often causes small peritubal inclusion cysts giving a "frog's eggs" appearance (Fig. 16:11). Occasionally, these are mistaken for hydatids but on close inspection they appear quite different and cultures may grow chlamydia. Henry-Suchet et al[14] studied patients who presented for tubal surgery; they had significantly more women with either previously or currently active PID cultured chlamydia when compared with a control group presenting for other gynecologic surgery not related to infertility (Table 16:1).

Women who have tubal damage also are at high risk for ectopic pregnancy. Epidemiologically, there is an increased incidence of tubal pregnancy in women

Table 16:1

*Positive Abdominal Cultures: Cases of Sterility with Tubal Obstruction or Adhesions**

Positive cultures	*Group 1*	*Group 2*	*Control group*
Chlamydia trachomatis	7	5	1
Ureaplasma urealyticum	4	2	3
C. trachomatis plus *U. urealyticum*	0	1	0
Other microbiological agents	4	1	0
Total positive cultures	15	9	4
Total specimens	30	39	49
% positive cultures	50%	23%	8%

*Reproduced with permission from Henry-Suchet et al.[14]

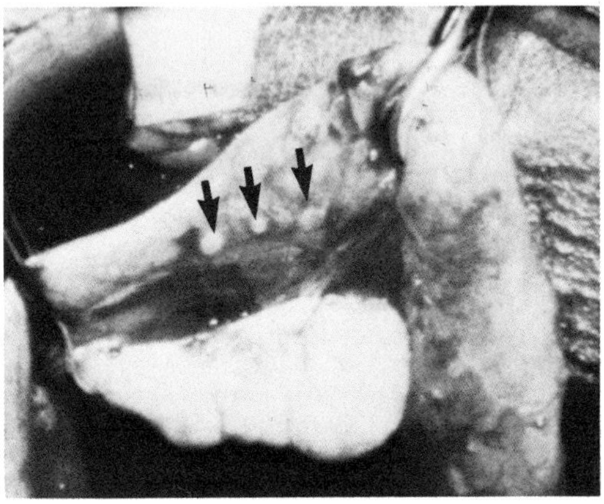

FIGURE 16:11—*Chlamydial salpingitis causes a characteristic appearance on tubal surface (arrows).*

with a history of previous pelvic inflammatory disease.[7] The micrograph from Draper et al illustrated a microdiverticulum resulting from tubal infection in an animal model (Fig. 16:3).

How can we prevent serious damage caused by pelvic inflammatory disease and its sequelae? Perhaps operative techniques have reached their limit. Such macroscopic intervention has no effect on the profound involvement in the tubal lumen and endosalpinx. Prevention of significant damage may require additional medical treatment at the time of initial infection in order to prevent anatomical changes. More effective antibiotics are necessary but adjuvant therapy with progesterone, estrogen, or prostaglandin synthetase inhibitors may have some role in preventing serious tubal damage. An epidemiological approach might also be effective. The peak incidence of pelvic inflammatory disease and tubal destruction occurs between the ages of 19 and 24.[6,7] Perhaps something happens immunologically after age 24 so that tubal damage is no longer facilitated, suggesting an early immunological treatment. Should all women with PID be treated with tetracycline to cover chlamydia? A clinical trial is under way at our institution. It involves laparoscopy whenever acute pelvic inflammatory disease is diagnosed. The extent of the disease is noted, and four months later the patient has a repeated laparoscopic examination. At the time of the initial operation, she receives either ampicillin, a third-generation cephalosporin (Claforan) and tetracycline, or tetracycline alone. The observer of both laparoscopies is not informed of the drug regimen employed.

A tantalizing question concerns the use of prompt surgery as soon as tubal damage is noted. The old concept argued that operation should be deferred until the patient desires pregnancy. Possible intervention is needed to evaluate an abnormal hysterosalpingogram. However, an operation may do nothing to stop the cascade of events and reinfection is a possibility.

We do not know the best and simplest ways to prevent or treat pelvic inflammatory disease so that future fertility will not be impaired. Perhaps antibiotic prophylaxis, immunization, immediate laparoscopy, or new hormonal or antibiotic therapy will be helpful. In the meantime, more research and clinical trials are needed to give gynecologists the ability to prevent tubal damage rather than repair it.

References

1. Ferenczy A, and Richart RM: *Female Reproductive System: Dynamics of Scan and Transmission Electron Microscopy.* New York: John Wiley, 1974.
2. Laufer N, Sekeles E, Cohen R, et al: The effects of *E. coli* endotoxin on the tubal mucosa of the rabbit. A scanning electron microscopic study. *Path Res Pract,* 170:202, 1980.
3. Draper DL, Donegan EA, James JF, et al: In vitro modeling of acute salpingitis caused by *Neisseria gonorrhoeae. Am J Obstet Gynecol,* 138:996, 1980.
4. Eschenbach DA: Acute pelvic inflammatory disease: Etiology, risk factors and pathogenesis. *Clin Obstet Gynecol,* 19:147, 1976.
5. Holmes KK, Eschenbach DA, and Knapp JD: Salpingitis: Overview of etiology and epidemiology. *Am J Obstet Gynecol,* 138:893, 1980.
6. Mardh PA: An overview of infectious agents of salpingitis, their biology, and recent advances in methods of detection. *Am J Obstet Gynecol,* 138:933, 1980.
7. Weström L: Incidence, prevalence, and trends of acute pelvic inflammatory disease and its consequences in industrialized countries. *Am J Obstet Gynecol,* 138:880, 1980.
8. Ory HW: A review of the association between intrauterine devices and acute pelvic inflammatory disease. *J Reprod Med,* 20:200, 1978.
9. Taylor ES, McMillan JH, Greer BE, et al: The intrauterine device and tubo-ovarian abscess. *Am J Obstet Gynecol,* 123:338, 1975.
10. Weström L, Bengtsson L, and Mardh PA: The risk of PID in women using IUD's as compared to non-users. *Lancet,* 2:221, 1976.
11. Weström L: Effect of acute pelvic inflammatory disease on infertility. *Am J Obstet Gynecol,* 121:707, 1975.
12. Jacobson L, and Weström L: Objectivized diagnosis of acute pelvic inflammatory disease. *Am J Obstet Gynecol,* 105:1088, 1969.
13. Sweet RL, Mills J, Hadley KW, et al: Use of laparoscopy to determine the microbiologic etiology of acute salpingitis. *Am J Obstet Gynecol,* 134:68, 1979.
14. Henry-Suchet J, Catalan F, Loffredo V, et al: *Chlamydia trachomatis* associated with chronic inflammation in abdominal specimens from women selected for tuboplasty. *Fertil Steril,* 36:599, 1981.

17

Tuberculosis of the Fallopian Tubes

Uziel Beller and
Yoram Beyth

The incidence of tuberculosis in general and of the genital tract in particular has been reduced significantly during the past four decades, especially because of the introduction of effective antimicrobial agents.[1] However, the disease is still a major medical problem causing disability and death in large areas of the world. In India, half a million people die of tuberculosis each year and even in the United States the current annual loss is 10,000.[2]

The prevalence of tuberculosis depends on factors such as country of origin, urban or rural society, and socioeconomic status. The incidence of genital tuberculosis in women is estimated by various methods: (a) postmortem studies of the general population of women; (b) postmortem studies of tuberculous patients; (c) histology of all surgically removed tubes; (d) endometrial specimens of patients with various signs and symptoms (including infertility); and (e) evaluation of female patients with extragenital tuberculosis. The reports in the literature are therefore based on selective material that is dependent on variables and thus make it difficult to draw general conclusions applicable for the entire female population.

Nevertheless, it is estimated that 1 to 5 percent of infertility in women can be attributed to tuberculosis and close to 40 percent of genital tuberculosis is detected during an infertility evaluation. Since the tubes are involved in all cases of genital tuberculosis, this disease should seriously be considered when dealing with mechanical infertility in a high-risk patient.

Pathogenesis

A thorough pathological study by Nogales-Ortiz and co-authors[3] evaluated 1,400 surgical specimens from tuberculous women collected from the Universities of Madrid and Seville. They found the following frequency of involvement of the genital organs: fallopian tubes, 100 percent; endometrium, 79 percent; cervix, 24 percent; myometrium, 20 percent; and ovaries, 10 percent.

Except for rare and poorly documented cases, the genital involvement is

The Fallopian Tube: Basic Studies and Clinical Contributions, edited by Alvin M. Siegler, M.D. Mount Kisco, New York: Futura Publishing Company, Inc. © 1986.

secondary to a pulmonary lesion and the spread is hematogenous. The tubes, and especially the submucosa, create an optimal site for bacilli to lodge and multiply. Other less common modes of spread are through lymphatic vessels from the gastrointestinal tract or direct spread from the adjacent involved bladder or rectum.[1,4]

The involvement of the genital structures is through direct extension from the primary tubal lesion and not as part of miliary spread. Therefore, the extent of involvement usually decreases from the tubes to the cervix. When ovaries are involved, they are directly involved from the tubes and present as tuberculous periophoritis. Several rare cases of hematogenous spread to the ovaries causing parenchymal hilar disease have been described.[4] The reason for selective involvement of the tubes by tubercle bacilli is unknown. Primary tubal tuberculosis is rare. Endometrial involvement exists in 50 percent of patients who have tubal involvement, indicating a preexisting tubal lesion. However, tubal occlusion resulting from tuberculous salpingitis may prevent endometrial spread. Genital involvement may also occur from the urinary tract through the lymphatic system, or as a result of ascending tubal infection following coitus with a male who has tuberculous epididymitis.

Pathology

Grossly, the disease may resemble pelvic inflammatory disease; gonorrhea or any other pyogenic organism can cause similar macroscopic findings. Rarely, a reaction to an oil-soluble contrast medium used in hysterosalpingography can be the reason for the pathological state. If tubercles and caseation are not present, a nonspecific pyosalpinx, chronic interstitial salpingitis, or salpingitis isthmica nodosa can be erroneously diagnosed from the gross appearance.[1,4] Both the tubes are usually involved, although not necessarily to the same degree, and it is the ampulla that is affected initially. In the early stages, only slight alteration of the tubal caliber is seen. Later, the fimbriated end becomes swollen although the ostia may remain open.

The initial tubal lesion is the acute exudative form, in which a pyosalpinx is present, which is relatively free of adhesions and mobile. The subsequent chronic productive-adhesive stage is characterized by tubes that are studded with tubercles, at the mesosalpingeal side, and densely adherent to surrounding organs. The tubes are thickened but less swollen and occasionally contain calcifications and fibrosis.

Histologically, typical tuberculous lesions are in the tubal wall with giant cells and caseation. In submucosal disease, ulcerations of the endosalpinx are found accompanied by hyperplastic reaction of the endosalpingeal folds creating an adenomatous pattern that can be confused with carcinoma.

The presence of Shauman bodies (crystals) can assist in diagnosis. In the absence of acid-fast bacilli, the diagnosis of a granulomatous infection is assumed. This could result from a foreign body reaction to talc or oil contrast media, sarcoidosis, Crohn's disease, leprosy, actinomycosis, bilharziasis, or *Enterobius vermiculosis*.[4,5]

Diagnosis

The presenting symptoms among gynecologic patients suffering from genital tuberculosis are sterility (45 to 55 percent), pelvic pain (50 percent), irregular bleeding (20 percent), and vaginal discharge (4 percent). Once genital tuberculosis is suspected, several investigative steps should be followed, as suggested by Schaefer[1]:

1. *Familial history*. More than 20 percent of the patients will reveal close contact with tuberculosis in childhood.

2. *History*. Close to half the patients were affected by tuberculosis in their youth, sometimes without a correct diagnosis. As stated by Ylinen[6] and Sutherland,[7] previous infection with tuberculosis as pleurisy and peritonitis has been

reported in 30 percent of women with genital tuberculosis.[8]

3. *Infertility.* Sterility is reported by 85 percent of patients with genital tuber culosis and the disease developed one year from their last delivery in half of the remaining 15 percent. Depending on the country and society, tuberculosis is seen in 0.69 percent of infertile women in Australia, 5 percent in certain areas of the United States, and 17.4 percent in India.[1]

4. *Symptoms.* Pelvic pain, a common symptom, is vague, aggravated by coitus and menses, but rarely develops to an acute abdomen because of secondary infection. General malaise, fatigue, weight loss, and low-grade fever are seen in chronic systemic diseases. Amenorrhea, usually a late manifestation of end organ failure as a result of endometrial destruction, was reported by Sutherland in less than 5 percent of his patients, over the past 30 years.[7]

5. *Physical examination.* Unless peritoneal tuberculosis is present, the pelvic findings are not specific. A tubo-ovarian abscess is sometimes palpable but the tubes can be normal in size, slightly thickened, and tender in the range of normal to mild salpingitis.

6. *Laboratory aids in diagnosis.*

a. *chest x-ray:* can detect pulmonary or pleural tuberculosis.

b. *tuberculin test:* two days after injection of purified protein derivative of tuberculosis (PPD) to the forearm, an erythematous reaction of 10 mm or more is considered positive. A negative test excludes tuberculosis but a positive one is not indicative of location of the disease or its activity.

c. *endometrial specimen:* a better chance for detecting the disease is offered by curettage rather than biopsy. The curettage should be performed several days prior to the expected menses so that the tubercles will have time to develop fully from the previous shedding of endometrium. It is therefore sometimes advised to delay the menstrual flow by progestational agents to facilitate a full histologic study. During the curettage, the cornual areas should be thoroughly explored since these are the first sites for direct spread from the tubes. Often the histologic diagnosis cannot be made and further bacteriological confirmation is required.

d. *bacteriology:* since direct staining is sometimes not positive because of a low concentration of bacilli in the material, cultures and animal inoculation are more accurate with results in six to eight weeks. Menstrual blood can also be used for culture and animal inoculation.

e. *hysterosalpingogram:* several descriptive findings of tuberculosis have been reported. Among them are calcified pelvic lymph nodes, pipe-stem (or "drumstick"-type) tubes of smaller caliber, obstructed and constricted in several points, endometrial adhesions, deformities as well as lymphatic and venous extravasation (Fig. 17:1).[8–10] These roentgenographic findings are not pathognomonic and should be confirmed by histology or bacteriology. Hysterosalpingography is contraindicated in the presence of a recent history of acute pelvic infection and it is certainly inappropriate to use as a method for the differential diagnosis of salpingitis. Nevertheless, the roentgenographic findings in some infertile women are often the first clue to the existence of latent female genital tuberculosis. Latent tubal tuberculosis frequently causes changes first in the ampulla, then in the isthmus; the intramural portion almost always remains unaffected. Tuberculosis is the presumptive diagnosis when calcified pelvic or mesenteric glands are associated with bilaterally occluded rigid tubes. Diverticula are sometimes seen extending from the sac-like tubal ends. The borders of the tubal lumen are often sawtoothed with pockets or lacunae. These finely jagged, ragged contours have multiple strictures and bulges. The occluded ampulla appears tufted, with less dilatation than other types of distal tubal obstruction. The club-shaped appearance and pipe-stem configuration of tubal tuberculosis are caused by connective tissue scars in the ampulla that constrict the lumen. Strictured tubes represent the oldest lesions. The gaps in the contrast ma-

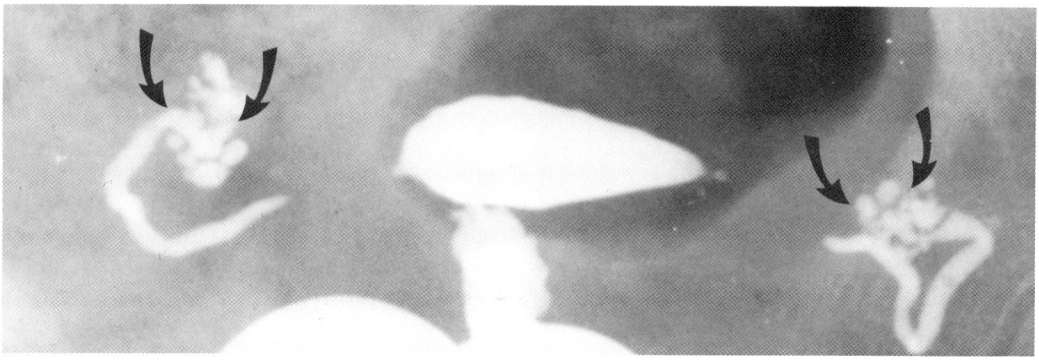

FIGURE 17:1a—*Abnormal tubes are seen with rigid ampullary segments and terminal (arrows) portions showing multiple strictures.*

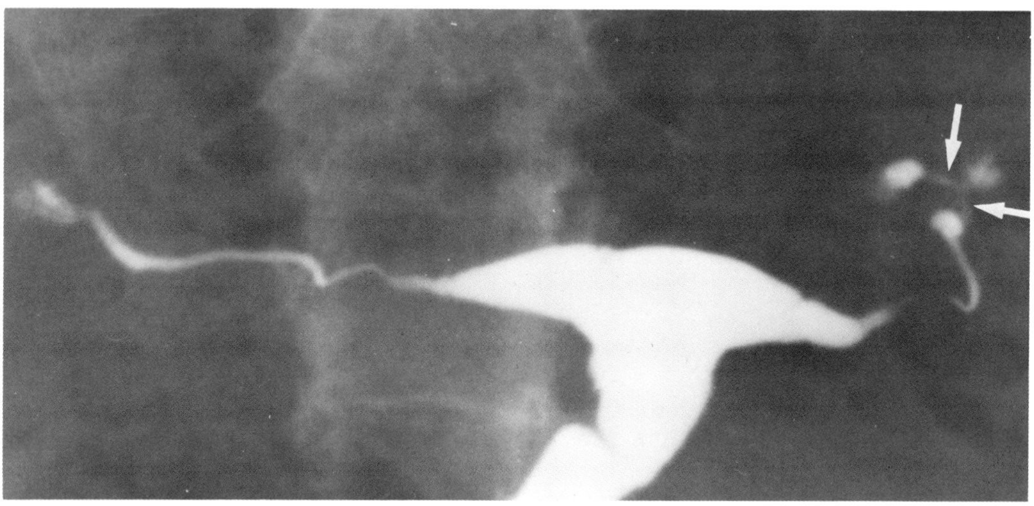

FIGURE 17:1b—*Arrows indicate strictured segment of left tube. Right tube has a tufted end.*

terial are caused by isolated groups of hypertrophic villi surrounded by areas of destroyed rugae. The ragged contours result from deep mucosal ulcerations. Proliferating tubal epithelium grows in a glandular configuration, reaching from mucosa into myosalpinx and thus accounting for extraluminal extension of the contrast medium. Tubal diverticulosis (salpingitis isthmica nodosa) presents a similar roentgenographic picture except that it is not associated with tubal, ovarian, or lymph node calcification, or uterine deformity. Genital tuberculosis is excluded by a normal hysterosalpingogram. Tubointestinal fistula often has a tuberculous cause. Although a barium enema may reveal the fistulous connection, it is more difficult to fill the sinus tract by this procedure than by hysterosalpingography. An important cause of either lymphatic or venous intravasation on hysterosalpingography is endometrial and myometrial tuberculosis. Reticular shadows surrounding the uterine cavity are caused by interstitial or lymphatic penetration of contrast material, often associated with a shrunken or deformed uterus. With lymphatic intravasation, the transfer of contrast material into reticular patterns and channels

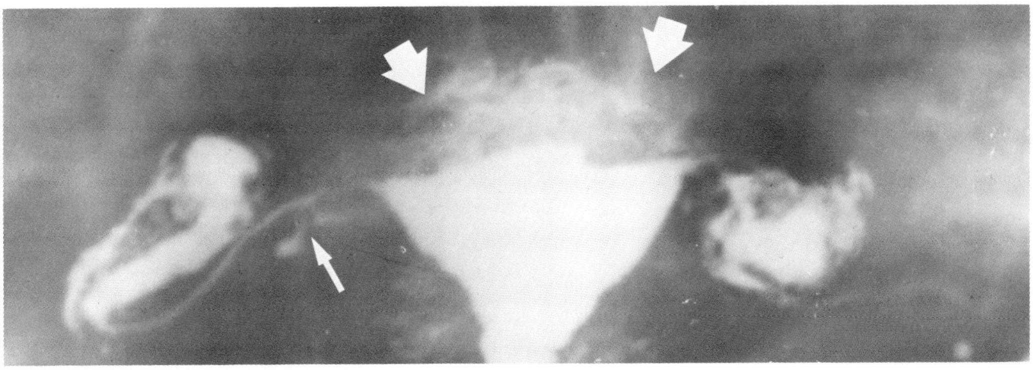

FIGURE 17:1c—*Lymphatic intravasation (large arrows) is noted surrounding the uterine shadow. Small arrow indicates isthmic diverticuli.*

persists longer than with venous penetration, and nodes are sometimes opacified.

7. *Laparoscopy.* The role of this procedure in the evaluation of genital tuberculosis is questionable.[11] We have described the phenomenon of the "blue uterus." This finding is a result of lymphatic intravasation by the intrauterine injected blue dye which colors the uterus and was seen especially in cases of genital tuberculosis.[12] Once tuberculosis is suspected and confirmed by the previously mentioned methods, the value of laparoscopy is limited. The pelvic adhesions with intestinal loops and genital organs prevent observation of the pelvic organs and may even make the procedure dangerous.

8. *Surgical specimen.* The pathologist makes the diagnosis because sectioning of the extirpated fallopian tubes may reveal the presence of caseous granulomas, the pathognomonic feature of tuberculosis. Nevertheless, without bacteriological confirmation, the possibility of foreign body reaction should be considered prior to initiation of chemotherapy.

Treatment and Prognosis

Antimicrobial therapy is recommended for minimal genital tuberculosis (that is asymptomatic, except for sterility) and confined primarily to the fallopian tubes without evidence of tubo-ovarian masses. The diagnosis must be established bacteriologically and from the endometrial curettings.

Therapy consists of isoniazid 300 mg and ethambutol 20 mg/kg daily. At six months and again at twelve months, endometrial curettings are examined bacteriologically and microscopically. If these are negative, hysterosalpingography is performed, although patency is not a guarantee for pregnancy. These two drugs are continued for two years, followed by isoniazid indefinitely. However, if abscesses develop or laboratory results turn positive during treatment, rifampin 600 mg daily is added and a laparotomy is performed.[7,13,14]

Fertility

Most investigators believe that since genital tuberculosis is detected fairly late in the course of the disease, the prognosis for fertility is hopeless.

Halbrecht[15] treated 42 patients with bilateral tubal occlusion. Treatment consisted of antituberculous drugs and prednisone. Of these, three became pregnant: two intrauterine and one tubal pregnancy. Of 12 patients who were subjected to tuboplasty, none became pregnant.

Since both tubes are not damaged to the same extent at a certain time, if one tube is patent on diagnosis, there is 5 percent chance of delivering a live infant following treatment. Schaefer[1] has re-

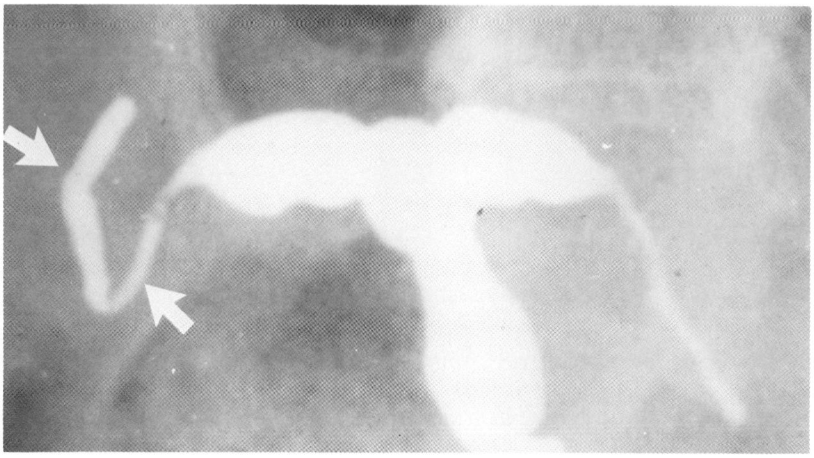

FIGURE 17:1*d*—*Rigid pipe-stem tube (arrows) are very suggestive of a tuberculous cause.*

ported a review of 7,000 cases of genital tuberculosis from the literature. There were 155 term pregnancies, 67 abortions, and 125 ectopic pregnancies. Documentation was often inadequate but when the diagnosis of tuberculosis was based on histologic and/or bacteriological evidence, the term pregnancy rate fell from 2.2 percent to 0.44 percent. Recently, Punnonen et al.[16] reported on seven cases of genital tuberculosis, all confirmed histologically during evaluation of infertility. There were two term pregnancies in two patients, one delivered two and three years after chemotherapy, the other one and two years after treatment. The role of tuboplasty in these women is minimal. Gomel[17] and Winston[18] have concluded that tuberculosis is a contraindication for tubal reconstructive surgery. It has been reported that such surgery may cause reactivation of silent tuberculosis with resultant diffuse peritoneal disease.[19]

Theoretically, the only chance for pregnancy is in-vitro fertilization and embryo transfer (IVF-ET). Following several months of treatment, with evidence of a histologically normal endometrium, this procedure could prove valuable. Although no reports have appeared in the literature thus far, we believe that as it gains popularity, the procedure will reach areas of the world where tuberculosis is still endemic.

Summary

Genital tuberculosis is suspected on the basis of a familial history of tuberculosis, past or present pulmonary tuberculosis, and infertility and amenorrhea. Tuberculous endosalpingitis may result in pyosalpinx, follicular hydrosalpinx, or pseudoadenomatous salpingitis, the latter resembling salpingitis isthmica nodosa. The ampulla is the tubal segment generally involved and the endosalpinx is most often affected.

In general, the drug regimen and duration of therapy are the same as for the management of pulmonary tuberculosis. The major change in the therapy of women with genital tuberculosis has been the diminished role of surgery and the greater use of ethambutol hydrochloride instead of PAS. Surgery is restricted to patients who have persistent adnexal masses after at least six months of therapy. Total abdominal hysterectomy and bilateral salpingoophorectomy are the procedures of choice. Postoperatively, the drugs are continued for 18 months or longer.

Attempts to reconstruct tubes occluded by tuberculous involvement are inevitably unsuccessful although postoperative patency does occur. If pregnancy results, it usually terminates in an abortion or a tubal gestation.

Tuboplasty for unsuspected tubal tuberculosis is occasionally performed inadvertently, the lesion being detected on tubal biopsy. Such patients should be treated with antimicrobial agents for at least one year. Inasmuch as a term pregnancy following either medical or conservative surgical treatment of tuberculosis is so rare and tubal gestation is more common than intrauterine pregnancy, contraception rather than tuboplasty is advisable.

References

1. Schaefer G: Tuberculosis of the female genital tract. In Sciarra JJ (Ed): *Gynecology and Obstetrics*. Philadelphia: Harper and Row, 1982.
2. Bazaz-Malik G, Makeshwari B and Lal N: Tuberculous endometritis: A clinicopathological study of 1000 cases. *Br J Obstet Gynaecol,* 90:84, 1983.
3. Nogales-Ortiz F, Tarancon I, and Nogales-Ortiz F Jr: The pathology of female genital tuberculosis. *Obstet Gynecol,* 53:422, 1973.
4. Wheeler J: Pathology of the fallopian tube. In Blaustein A (Ed): *Pathology of the Female Genital Tract*. New York: Springer-Verlag, 1982.
5. Brooks JJ, and Wheeler JE: Granulomatous salpingitis secondary to Crohn's disease. *Obstet Gynecol,* 49:315, 1977.
6. Ylinen O: Genital tuberculosis in women. *Acta Obstet Gynecol Scand,* 40(Suppl. 2); 1960.
7. Sutherland AM: The changing pattern of tuberculosis of the female genital tract. A thirty year survey. *Arch Gynecol,* 234:95, 1983.
8. Csordas SE, and Monheit BM: Gynecological tuberculosis in Victoria. A 20 year survey. *Aust N Z J Obstet Gynaecol,* 22:86, 1983.
9. Rozin S: *Uterosalpingography in Gynecology*. Springfield: Charles C. Thomas, 1965: p. 231.
10. Siegler AM, and Kontopoulos V: Female genital tuberculosis and the role of hysterosalpingography. *Semin Roent,* 14:295, 1979.
11. Palmer R, and Oliviera EM: Coelioscopy and percoelioscopy biopsies in latent genital tuberculosis. In Rippman ET, and Wenner RS (Eds): *Genital Tuberculosis*. Basel: Karger, 1966: p. 1973.
12. Beyth Y, Adoni A, and Polshuk WZ: A blue uterus, a possible sign of uterine tuberculosis. *Am J Obstet Gynecol,* 111:858, 1971.
13. Klein TA, Richmond JA, and Mishell DR: Pelvic tuberculosis. *Obstet Gynecol,* 48:99, 1976.
14. Sutherland AM: Surgical treatment of tuberculosis of the female genital tract. *Br J Obstet Gynaecol,* 87:610, 1980.
15. Halbrecht I: Cortisone in the treatment of tubal occlusion caused by healed genital tuberculosis. *Fertil Steril,* 13:371, 1962.
16. Punnonen R, Kiilholma P, and Meurman L: Female genital tuberculosis and consequent infertility. *Int J Fertil,* 28:235, 1983.
17. Gomel V: Principles of microsurgery for infertility. In Phillips JM (Ed): *Microsurgery in Gynecology*. Downey, CA: American Association of Gynecologic Laparoscopists, 1977: p. 115.
18. Winston RML: Microsurgery of the fallopian tube: From fantasy to reality. *Fertil Steril,* 34:521, 1980.
19. Ballon SC, Clewel WH, and Lamb EJ: Reactivation of silent pelvic tuberculosis by reconstructive tubal surgery. *Am J Obstet Gynecol,* 122:991, 1975.
20. Siegler AM: *Hysterosalpingography*. New York: Medcom Press, 1974: p. 159.

18

Endometriosis of the Fallopian Tube and Factors Leading to Infertility

Shawky Z. A. Badawy

Endometriosis is present in about 30 percent of infertile women.[1,2] Currently it is diagnosed more frequently because of the use of laparoscopy in the workup of those patients who may or may not have clinical evidence of the disease. The cause of infertility in patients with endometriosis is multifactorial. A tubo-ovarian dysfunction in ovum pickup is an important issue when there is advanced disease with pelvic adhesions. In the absence of adhesions, endometriosis is still associated with infertility, probably because of a pelvic reaction that leads to excess cul-de-sac fluid. This fluid, with its cellular and hormonal content, contributes to infertility in these patients. The link between endometriosis and infertility is established with the diagnosis of pelvic disease and also by the increased pregnancy rate following treatment of this problem.

Pathology

The dominant theory explaining pelvic endometriosis is that of Sampson.[3] Retrograde reflux of menstrual fluid occurs in almost every menstruating woman with patent fallopian tubes.[4] In some women, the endometrial cells either implant on the pelvic peritoneum and pelvic organs or elicit a metaplastic process leading to the development of endometriosis.[5] The factors that lead to implantation of the endometrial tissue on the celomic epithelium are not known. Some studies show that the percentage of women with endometrial cells in the peritoneal fluid is the same in patients with endometriosis as in those without endometriosis. It is suggested that lack of ovulation in patients with endometriosis leads to implantation of endometrial cells

The Fallopian Tube: Basic Studies and Clinical Contributions, edited by Alvin M. Siegler, M.D. Mount Kisco, New York: Futura Publishing Company, Inc. © 1986.

on the celomic epithelium.[6] Another theory to explain the beginning of the disease is suppression of the immune reaction in such patients. This is based on findings in the rhesus monkey, which showed significantly less lymphocytic reaction around the injected endometrial homogenate in the subcutaneous tissue of animals with endometriosis as compared to controls.[7]

Pelvic endometriosis is a disease of the reproductive age group. Its development and progress depend on the ovarian steroids. In oophorectomized monkeys, endometrial implants in the celomic cavity can survive and grow when progesterone, estrogen, or both are administered to these animals.[8] This may explain the rarity of endometriosis before puberty and after the onset of menopause.

Ovarian steroids act on cytosol receptors present in the ectopic endometrial tissue. Studies revealed that the steroid receptors in endometriosis are less than those of the normal endometrium.[9] This explains the disparity in growth between the ectopic endometrium and the normal endometrium in the same patient. The ectopic endometrium may lack such receptors and remain inactive with no evidence of progress.

The use of steroidal oral contraceptives and their effect on the incidence of endometriosis in women needs further evaluation. The current data show that the use of oral contraceptives may decrease the incidence of the disease or may lead to milder forms.[10] It is important that this issue be studied because many women do not start families until late in their reproductive age, and most depend on oral contraceptives to prevent pregnancy. Prolonged use of oral contraceptives leads to atrophy of the endometrium. The amount of flow is scantier than without the use of oral contraceptives. This may lead to less reflux of menstrual fluid through the fallopian tubes.

All the factors discussed do not explain why endometriosis occurs in some women and not in others. Endometriosis frequently affects members of the same family or women within the familial pedigree, which suggests a genetic predisposition, as some investigators have shown. Thus, a familial history of endometriosis is a significant piece of information to the clinician dealing with problems related to reproductive function in women.

Anatomical Changes in the Fallopian Tube

Although it has been stated that the fallopian tube is rarely affected by endometriosis, the disease process does affect the tube both directly and indirectly. Indirect involvement occurs as a result of a pelvic adhesive process which occurs in severe endometriosis. The adhesions may be filmy, or thick and fibrous. They lead to distortion of the normal course of the tube by fixing all or parts of it to the lateral pelvic wall or to the ovary. In addition, fixation of the ovary to the back of the broad ligament or the lateral pelvic wall is possible. The adhesions may surround the fimbriae or may directly involve them, leading to tubal occlusion and the development of hydrosalpinx. In these cases, the fimbriae are intact once the adhesions are lysed in contradistinction to distal tubal occlusion caused by pelvic inflammatory disease in which the fimbriae are destroyed.

The tube also may become directly involved by the endometriotic process. Spots of endometriosis are frequently seen on the tubal serosa. They may be superficial, involving only the serosa or the myosalpinx. In mild cases, implants are surrounded by hemosiderin and a fine vascularity. In more advanced lesions, there is some degree of fibrosis around the implants that leads to tubal contractures and distortions. In severe cases, the endometriotic process may lead to hyperplasia of the tubal wall, with extreme thickening of a tubal segment or segments resulting in complete occlusion. This condition is not usually detected during laparoscopic evaluation unless the tube is enlarged or extremely nodular. However, palpation of the tube during a laparotomy reveals these nodularities which may lead to suspicion of a tumor.

The fallopian tube may also be involved with salpingitis isthmica nodosa. This is related to endometriosis in that it results from proliferation of the endosalpinx into the myosalpinx. It is also known as endosalpingiosis, a proliferative process that can occur as a result of an inflammatory reaction. Most of these lesions have been associated with a history of IUD insertion and may or may not coexist with pelvic endometriosis. Some of them may respond to hormonal suppression therapy with resultant tubal patency.[11]

The Peritoneal Reaction

Several investigators have detected increased amounts of peritoneal fluid in the cul-de-sac of patients with endometriosis. The amount of peritoneal fluid increases during the luteal phase of the cycle.[12,13] The fluid is either straw-colored, blood-tinged, or sometimes bloody. This fluid may cover only areas of endometriosis in the pelvis. It is a good practice to aspirate this fluid to search the cul-de-sac and uterosacral ligaments for endometriosis. The source of the fluid is from the peritoneal reaction to the presence of endometriosis, follicular fluid at ovulation, and also secretions from the endosalpinx.

The macrophage population in the peritoneal fluid has been evaluated.[14–16] The findings clearly document a significant increase in the number of macrophages in the peritoneal fluid of patients with endometriosis as compared to controls. Some investigators suggest that the macrophage population occurs as a response to toxic substances in the secretory products of the endosalpinx; the macrophages are increased in patients who have patent tubes but not in women with closed tubes. The studies on the macrophage population from our unit did not document any relationship to tubal patency.[16]

The macrophages in the peritoneal fluid appear as a reaction to a foreign body (ectopic endometrium) whose purpose is to remove degradation products from the ectopic endometrium. These macrophages are biologically active and contribute secretory products such as prostaglandins, complement components, and acid phosphatase.[16]

Hormonal Content of Peritoneal Fluid

Studies in rabbits with endometrial implants revealed increased prostaglandins $F_2\alpha$ and E_2 in the peritoneal washings of these animals, as compared to controls.[17] Other investigators found increased prostaglandins in peritoneal fluid of patients with endometriosis[18] but the prostaglandin content is not increased when the examination is done during the follicular phase. The studies from our laboratories have documented a significant increase in prostaglandin E_2 and $F_2\alpha$ in the peritoneal fluid of infertile patients with endometriosis.[16,19] When the data were analyzed in relation to the stage of the cycle, it was found that the increase was significant during the periovulatory and early luteal phase. The concentrations of thromboxane B and prostacyclins were increased significantly in the peritoneal fluid of infertile patients with endometriosis.[18] The effect on reproductive function depends on the concentration of each prostaglandin. Prostaglandin $F_2\alpha$ increases the contractility of the myosalpinx. Prostaglandin E_2 decreases tubal contractility and has a relaxing effect. In addition, equal concentrations of both prostaglandins lead to a weak stimulatory effect on tubal contractility.[20] Tubal function is affected by prostaglandins in the cul-de-sac fluid and varies with the concentration of each prostaglandin. This effect may lead either to failure of ova pickup phenomena by the tubes or to rapid transfer of the ova in the tubes. Intraperitoneal injection of high doses of prostaglandin $F_2\alpha$ in golden hamsters leads to rapid disappearance of ova from the fallopian tubes and uterus, as compared to controls.[21]

Physiological concentrations of prostaglandin $F_2\alpha$ are present in the fimbriated end. The amount of this prostaglandin is increased at ovulation time in the tubal fimbriae to increase their contractility and in ovum pickup. The effect of various prostaglandin concentrations on the ciliary function of the tubal epithelium has been documented in in-vitro studies. Prostaglandins $F_2\alpha$, E_2, and E_1 have been shown to increase ciliary movement with increasing concentrations. However, when the concentrations reach 10^{-5}, the ciliary movement starts to decline. These changes in the ciliary movements may deter ovum pickup, especially if the ciliary movements are inhibited.[22]

Prostaglandins $F_2\alpha$ and E_2 also affect ovarian function. Around ovulation, the increase in their ovarian concentration is essential for ovulation under the effect of the LH surge. In-vitro ovarian perfusion studies documented the blockage of ovulation after the administration of prostaglandin synthetase inhibitors.[23] Following ovulation, the ratio of $PGE_2/PGF_2\alpha$ is increased to maintain the corpus luteum function. In the absence of pregnancy, the ratio $PGF_2/PGE_2\alpha$ is increased to cause the demise of the corpus luteum.[24] It is known that prostaglandin $F_2\alpha$ is luteolytic in animals and according to some limited studies, in women.[25] Furthermore the administration of high doses of prostaglandins to mice interferes with the process of follicular growth and the function of the corpus luteum.[26]

These data suggest that increased concentrations of prostaglandins in the peritoneal fluid affect tubo-ovarian function. The effect depends on the relative concentration of each prostaglandin, which may be additive or antagonistic.

In conclusion, endometriosis may affect the fallopian tube directly or indirectly. Both anatomical and hormonal factors contribute to infertility in endometriosis patients. Medical and/or surgical treatments depend on the classification of the disease.

References

1. McGoogan LS: Sterility and endometriosis. *Arch Surg,* 59:437, 1949.
2. Kistner RW: Endometriosis and infertility. In Behrman SJ, and Kistner RW (Eds): *Progress in Infertility,* 2d ed. Boston: Little, Brown, 1969: p. 345.
3. Sampson JA: Peritoneal endometriosis due to the menstrual dissemination of endometrial tissue into the peritoneal cavity. *Am J Obstet Gynecol,* 14:422, 1927.
4. Halme J, Hammond MG, Hulka JF, et al: Retrograde menstruation in healthy women and in patients with endometriosis. *Obstet Gynecol,* 64:151, 1984.
5. TeLinde RW, and Wharton LR: Further studies on experimental endometriosis. *Am J Obstet Gynecol,* 66:1082, 1953.
6. Koninckx PR, Ide P, Vandenbroucke W, et al: New aspects of the pathophysiology of endometriosis and associated infertility. *J. Reprod Med,* 24:257, 1980.
7. Dmowski WP, Steele RW, and Baker GF: Deficient cellular immunity in endometriosis. *Am J Obstet Gynecol,* 141:377, 1981.
8. DiZerega GS, Barber DL, and Hodgen GD: Endometriosis: Role of ovarian steroids in initiation, maintenance, and suppression. *Fertil Steril,* 33:649, 1980.
9. Tamaya T, Motoyama T, Ohono Y, et al: Steroid receptor levels and histology of endometriosis and adenomyosis. *Fertil Steril,* 31:396, 1979.
10. Buttram VC: Cyclic use of combination oral contraceptives and the severity of endometriosis. *Fertil Steril,* 31:347, 1979.
11. Ayers JWT: Hormonal therapy for tubal occlusion: Danazol and tubal endometriosis. *Fertil Steril,* 38:748, 1982.
12. Drake TS, Metz SA, Grunert GM, et al: Peritoneal fluid volume in endometriosis. *Fertil Steril,* 34:280, 1980.
13. Badawy SZA, Marshall L, and Cuenca V: Periotneal fluid prostaglandins in various stages of the menstrual cycle. Role in infertile patients with endometriosis. *Int J Fertil,* in press.
14. Haney AF, Muscato JJ, and Weinburg JB: Peritoneal fluid cell population in infertile patients. *Fertil Steril,* 35:696, 1981.
15. Halme J, Becker S, and Wing R: Accentuated cyclic activation of peritoneal macrophages with endometriosis. *Am J Obstet Gynecol,* 148:85, 1984.
16. Badawy SZA, Cuenca V, Marshall L, et

al: Cellular components in peritoneal fluid in patients with and without endometriosis. *Fertil Steril,* 42:704, 1984.
17. Schenken RS, and Asch RH: Surgical induction of endometriosis in the rabbit: Effect on fertility and concentrations of peritoneal fluid prostaglandins. *Fertil Steril,* 34:581, 1980.
18. Drake TS, O'Brien WF, Ranwell PW, et al: Peritoneal fluid thromboxane B_2 and 6 keto prostaglandins F_1 in endometriosis. *Am J Obstet Gnecol,* 140:401, 1981.
19. Badawy SZA, Marshall L, Gabal AA, et al: The concentration of 13, 14-dihydro-15-keto prostaglandin $F_2\alpha$ and prostaglandin E_2 in peritoneal fluid of infertile patients with and without endometriosis. *Fertil Steril,* 38:166, 1982.
20. Coutinho EM, and Maia HS: The contractile response of the human uterus, fallopian tubes, and ovary to prostaglandins in vivo. *Fertil Steril,* 22:529, 1971.
21. Thomas CMG, Bastiaans LA, and Rolland R: Effects of prostaglandin $F_2\alpha$, indomethacin, and estradiol on ovum transport and pregnancy in the golden hamster. *Biol Reprod,* 23:687, 1980.
22. Verdugo P, Rumery RE, and Tam PY: Hormonal control of oviductal ciliary activity: Effect of prostaglandins. *Fertil Steril,* 33:193, 1980.
23. Kobayashi Y, Santulli R, Wright KH, et al: The effect of prostaglandin synthesis inhibition by indomethacin and ovulation and ovum maturation in the in vitro perfused rabbit ovary. *Am J Obstet Gynecol,* 141:53, 1981.
24. Aksel S, Schomberg DW, and Hammond CB: Prostaglandin $F_2\alpha$ production by the human ovary. *Obstet Gynecol,* 50:347, 1977.
25. Wentz AC, and Jones GS: Transient luteolytic effect of prostaglandin $F_2\alpha$ in the human. *Obstet Gynecol,* 42:172, 1973.
26. Peluso JJ, Leiper S, and Steger RW: Effects of $PGF_2\alpha$ induced luteolysis and progesterone on follicular growth in pregnant mice. *Prostaglandins,* 19:437, 1980.

19

Salpingitis Isthmica Nodosa

Amir H. Ansari,
Steven P. Bondell,
and H. Randall Squires

Chiari[1] in 1887 was the first to describe this entity and introduced the term of salpingitis isthmica nodosa (SIN). In 1904 Meyer [2] referred to it as adenomyosalpingitis and Sampson called it endosalpingiosis.[3] Schenken and Burns[4] renamed the entity diverticulosis of the fallopian tube. Recently, McCausland[5] observed two types of mucosal proliferation (tubal and endometrial) in the proximal oviduct following tubal coagulation and introduced the term endosalpingoblastosis; he further divided these lesions into two types depending on whether the glandular component was tubal or endometrial. Epitheliomyosis is another termconsidered by Schoenholz according to Benjamin and Beaver.[6]

Various theories have been postulated as to the pathogenesis of SIN. Chiari and others believed in its inflammatory etiology, having observed a leukocytic infiltration in association with SIN.[3,4,7–9] In addition, it has been found that more than 50 percent of patients with SIN have concomitant salpingitis and pelvic inflammatory disease.[4,10] Von Recklinghausen[7] postulated that the entity was caused by wolffian duct arrest during embryonic life. Opponents of the congenital theory state that SIN is extremely rare in premenarchal children. Recently, Newbold et al.[11] experimentally produced lesions similar to those of SIN in newborn mice following exogenous administration of diethylestilbestrol (DES). Shen and associates[12] described SIN in a young girl who was prenatally exposed to DES. On the basis of these findings, the congenital concept cannot be ruled out with certainty.

Benjamin and Beaver[6] believe that SIN is adenomyosis of the tube which is acquired following menarche.

Clinical Manifestations and Diagnosis

There usually are no symptoms in patients with salpingitis isthmica nodosa other than infertility. A history of pelvic

The Fallopian Tube: Basic Studies and Clinical Contributions, edited by Alvin M. Siegler, M.D. Mount Kisco, New York: Futura Publishing Company, Inc. © 1986.

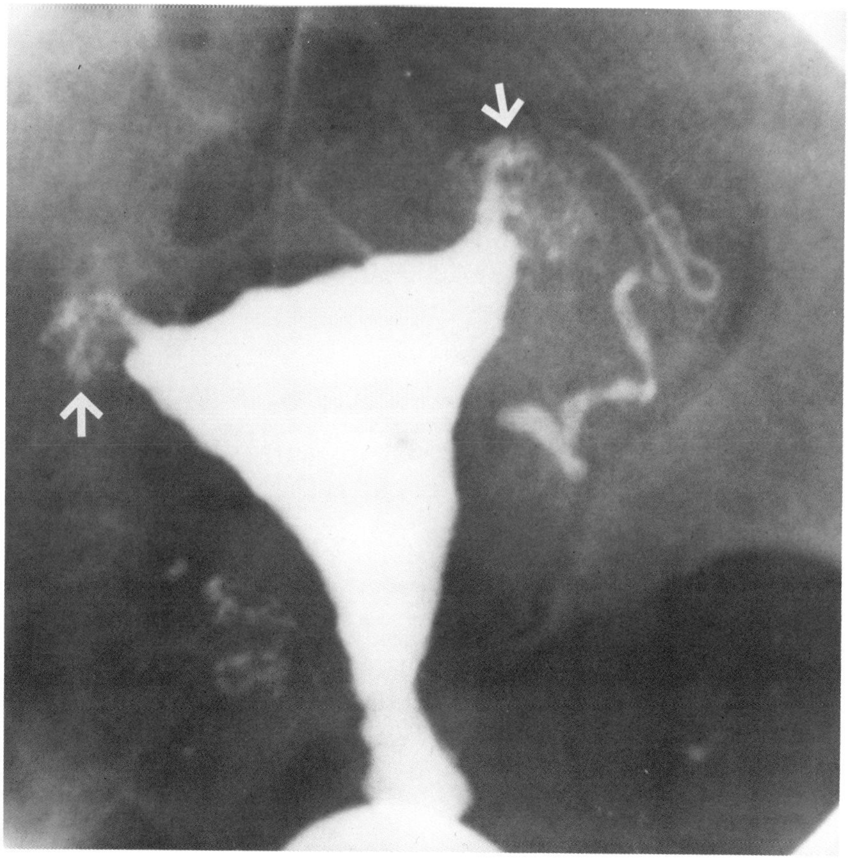

FIGURE 19:1—*Bilateral multiple diverticula (arrows) in a patient who had a partial right salpingectomy because of an ectopic gestation.*

inflammatory disease or ectopic pregnancy is also present in a majority of these cases.[4,10,13,14]

Hysterosalpingography can show a typical "honeycomb," "stippled" appearance usually in the proximal tubal segment.[15] This radiographic pattern is usually bilateral although sometimes the hysterosalpingogram may reveal the typical pattern on one side with complete occlusion of the opposite tube (Fig. 19:1). Hydrosalpinx and peritubal adhesions are frequently associated radiological findings (Figs. 19:2 and 19:3).

At laparoscopy or laparotomy, thickened or nodular proximal segments are presumptive evidence and intravasation of methylene blue into this area during chromopertubation is almost pathognomonic of SIN (Fig. 19:4).

Occasionally no gross abnormalities are seen or felt and the diagnosis is established from histologic evaluation of a resected isthmus during a tuboplasty.

Microscopic findings disclose columnar lined epithelium dispersed irregularly throughout the myosalpinx (Fig. 19:5) which is often hypertropic and hyperplastic (Fig. 19:6). These diverticular outpouches from the endosalpinx enabled Wrork and Broders[16] to propose the following classification:

Grade I. Tubal epithelium within the inner third of myosalpinx; Grade II. Tubal epithelium within the inner two

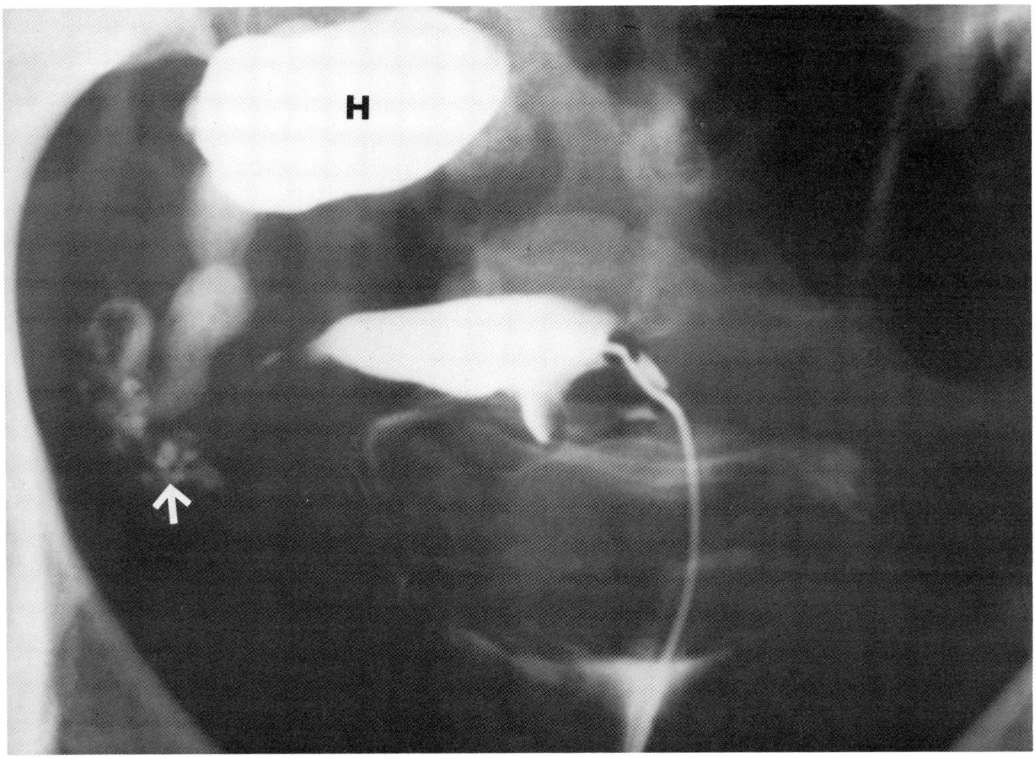

FIGURE 19:2—*Unilateral midsegmental diverticulosis (arrow) with a large hydrosalpinx (H). The opposite tube has proximal tubal obstruction.*

thirds of myosalpinx; Grade III. Extension beyond muscular layers to subserosal surface.

The presence of stromal tissue around these "glands" suggests the diagnosis of tubal endometriosis or adenomyosis.[6,9,16]

Salpingitis isthmica nodosa is often associated with ectopic pregnancy, cornual occlusion, hydrosalpinx, endometriosis, adenomyosis, and pelvic inflammatory disease.[4,6,17–21] Fortier and Haney[10] recently reported a 40 percent incidence of salpingitis in patients with uterotubal obstruction. Proximal tubal obstruction and hydrosalpinx were associated findings (28 percent and 19 percent, respectively) in another report.[16] The association of ectopic pregnancy in 50 to 57 percent of patients was also noted.[13,14] The fertilized ovum can theoretically become trapped in the channels resulting in ectopic pregnancy. However, in most cases, the ectopic gestation is in the distal tubal segment, supporting other theories; muscular hypertrophy[13] (leading to tubal stricture) and associated tubal abnormalities[14] (peritubal adhesions, salpingitis, etc.) resulting in disturbed tubal transport.

Management

On occasion, where the tubes are patent and endoscopically appear normal, except for the isthmic nodularity, surgical extirpation of the nodular isthmus may not be necessary since a normal intrauterine pregnancy may occur in these women. Treating the condition medically, perhaps with danazol for six to eight months, is recommended as an alternative to observation only. Since salpingitis isthmica

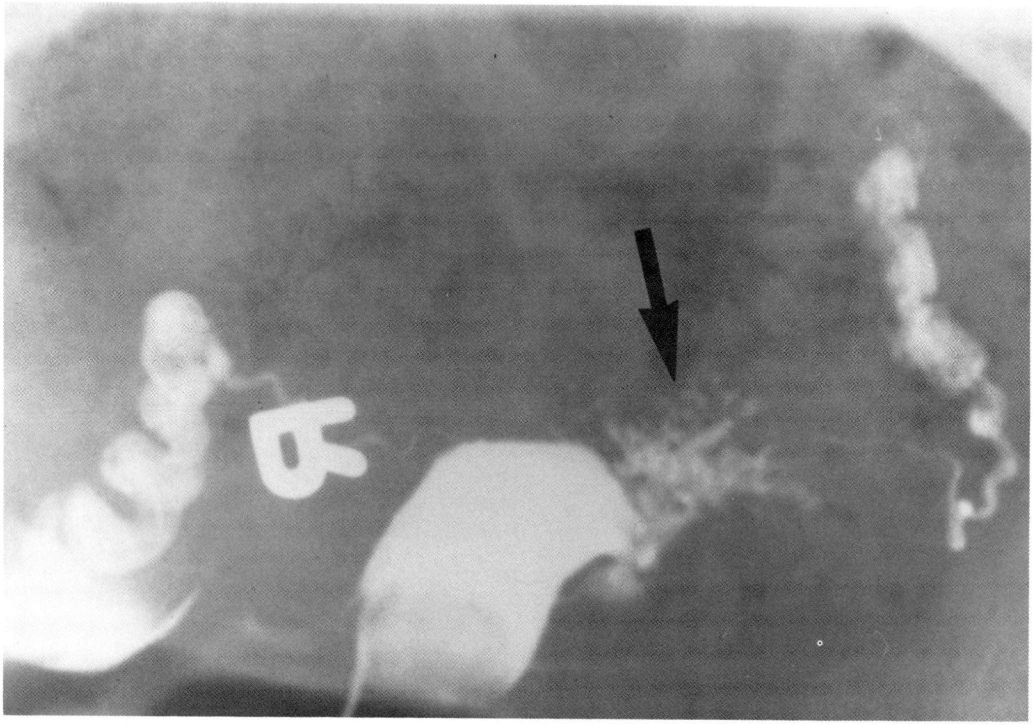

FIGURE 19:3—*Unilateral SIN is seen (arrow) with distal occlusion and right peritubal adhesions.*

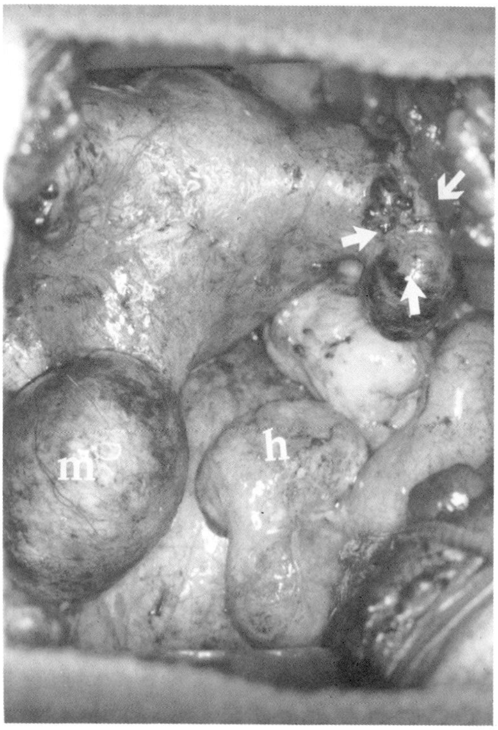

FIGURE 19:4—*Nodular isthmus is seen (arrows) with intravasation of methylene blue from chromopertubation. Associated abnormal findings are a right hydrosalpinx (h) and a myoma (m).*

nodosa is a pathological diagnosis, the value of observation and medical treatment cannot be ascertained with certainty and in most cases surgical correction is necessary. Resection with tubotubal or tubocornual anastomosis and tubal implantation may be required to remove all of the affected tissue. Examination of the operative site with high magnification is essential before deciding to allow certain tubal segments to remain. Incomplete resection of the diseased portion may be the main reason for a failed corrective procedure and recurrence.

When microscopic resection and anastomosis was performed in 15 patients, 6 became pregnant. Contraception is used for three months after surgery and a hysterosalpingography is recommended if pregnancy is not achieved within one year.

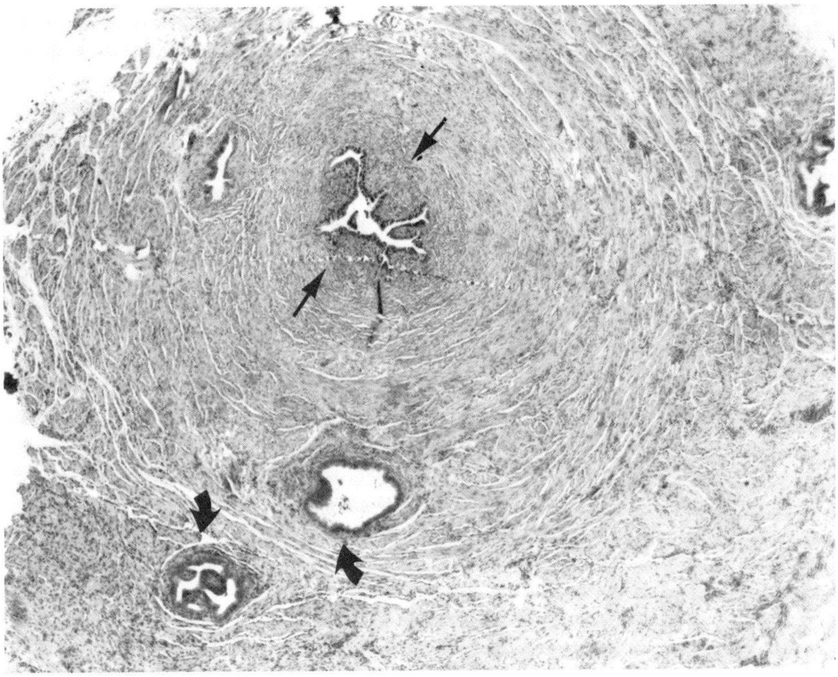

FIGURE 19:5—*Typical microscopic appearance of salpingitis isthmica nodosa showing residual salpingeal lumen (arrows) surrounded by displaced "glands" (curved arrows). (H & E, × 20)*

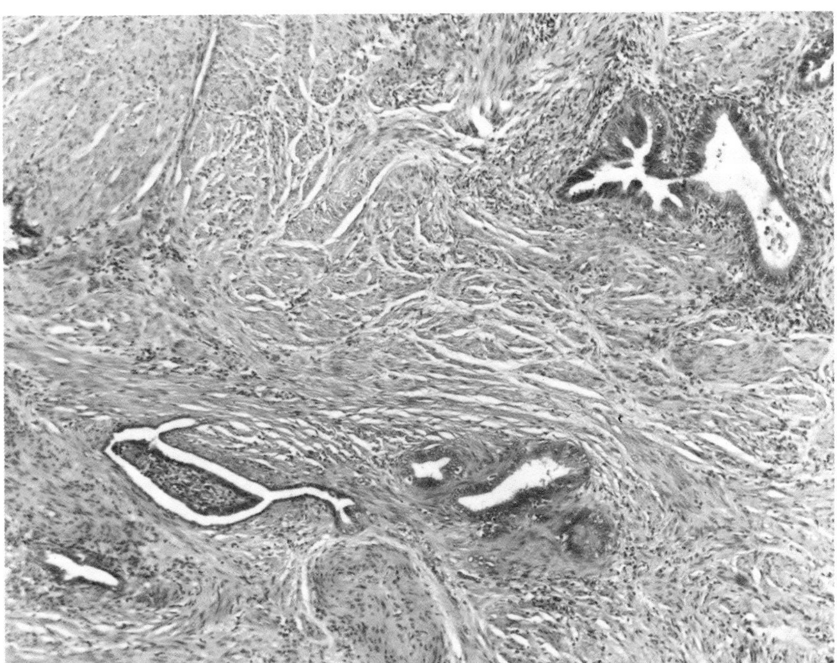

FIGURE 19:6—*Displaced "glands" are seen with irregular, muscular hypertrophy and moderate chronic inflammatory cells. (H & E, × 50)*

References

1. Chiari H: Zur pathologischen Anatomie des Eileiterkatarrhs. *Ztschr Heilk*, 8:457, 1887.
2. Meyer R: Ueber adenomatose Schleimhautwucherungen in der Uterus and Tubenwand und ihre pathologisch—anatomische Bedeutung. *Virchows Arch Pat Anat*, 172:394, 1094.
3. Sampson JA: Post-salpingectomy endometriosis (endosalpingiosis). *Am J Obstet Gynecol*, 20:443, 1930.
4. Schenken JE, and Burns EL: Study and classification of nodular lesions of the fallopian tubes. *Am J Obstet Gynecol*, 45:624, 1943.
5. McCausland A: Endosalpingiosis ("endosalpingoblastosis") following laparoscopic tubal coagulation as an etiologic factor for ectopic pregnancy. *Am J Obstet Gynecol*, 143:12, 1982.
6. Benjamin CL, and Beaver DC: The pathogenesis of salpingitis isthmica nodosa. *Am J Clin Pathol*, 21:212, 1951.
7. Von Recklinghausen F: Die Adenomyome und Cystodenome der Uterus and Tubenwand. Berlin 1896, cited by Robinovitz.[8]
8. Robinovitz M: The pathogenesis of adenomyosalpingitis (salpingitis nodosa). Report of 10 cases. *Am J Obstet Dis Wom*, 68:711, 1913.
9. Frankl O: Salpingitis isthmica nodosa und Adenomyosis tubae. *Arch Gynäkol*, 135:556, 1929.
10. Fortier KJ, and Haney AF: The pathologic spectrum of uterotubal junction obstruction. *Obstet Gynecol*, 65:93, 1985.
11. Newbold RR, Bullock BC, and McLachlan JA: Diverticulosis and salpingitis isthmica nodosa (SIN) of the fallopian tube. Estrogen-induced diverticulosis and SIN of the mouse oviduct. *Am J Pathol*, 117:333, 1984.
12. Shen SC, Bansal M, Purrazzella R, et al: Benign glandular inclusions in lymph nodes, endosalpingiosis and salpingitis isthmica nodosa in a young girl with clear cell adenocarcinoma of the cervix. *Am J Surg Pathol*, 7:293, 1983.
13. Majmudar B, Henderson PH, and Semple E: Salpingitis isthmica nodosa: A high-risk factor for tubal pregnancy. *Obstet Gynecol*, 62:73, 1983.
14. Persuad V: Etiology of tubal ectopic pregnancy. *Obstet Gynecol*, 36:257, 1970.
15. Siegler AM: *Hysterosalpingography*. New York: Harper and Row, 1967: p. 175.
16. Wrork DH, and Broders AC: Adenomyosis of the fallopian tube. *Am J Obstet Gynecol*, 44:412, 1942.
17. Freakley G, Norman WJ, Ennis JT, et al: Diverticulosis of the fallopian tubes. *Radiology*, 25:535, 1974.
18. Niles TH, and Clark JFJ: Pathogenesis of tubal pregnancy. *Am J Obstet Gynecol*, 105:1230, 1969.
19. Thomas ML, and Rose DH: Salpingitis isthmica nodosa demonstrated by hysterosalpingography. *Acta Radiol*, 14:295, 1973.
20. Honore LH: Salpingitis isthmica nodosa in female infertility and ectopic tubal pregnancy. *Fertil Steril*, 29:164, 1978.
21. Craig JM: The pathology of infertility. *Pathol Ann*, 10:299, 1975.

20

Tumors of the Fallopian Tube

Alexander Sedlis

Benign and malignant tumors of the fallopian tube are uncommon. Tubal carcinoma is the least common malignancy of the female genital tract. Data on tubal tumors derived from sporadic case reports are often sketchy. In this review, tumors will be discussed in order of their origin from the three anatomic layers: the endosalpinx, the myosalpinx, and serosa.

Tumors of the Endosalpinx

Benign tumors: polyps

Tubal polyps have been observed on hysterosalpingograms, at laparotomy, or during examination of an excised specimen. They are found in 1.8 to 2.7 percent of salpingograms.[1,2] Grossly, polyps are pedunculated structures, usually several millimeters in diameter protruding above the mucosal folds. They may be located either in the intramural or the proximal isthmic segment. The polypoid projections consist of fine fibrovascular stalks lined by epithelium (Figs. 20:1 and 20:2) containing the usual types of ciliated, mucoid, and intercalated cells. The etiology of polyps is not known but mechanical injury appears to be a likely cause since they are found in increased proportions in tubes removed after sterilization. Although 20 to 60 percent of women with tubal polyps have associated infertility, it is not known how or why these tumors contribute to infertility. Polyps suspected of causing tubal obstruction have been treated by excision using microsurgical techniques.[1]

Malignant tumors: adenocarcinoma

Since tubal carcinoma is rare, most physicians have had no experience in the diagnosis and management of this tumor. The diagnosis is often missed preoperatively and it may be difficult to make it even intraoperatively or at examination of the extirpated specimen. Tubal carcinomas vary from 0.31 to 1.11 percent of all gynecologic cancers and they are found about once in 1,000 abdominal gynecologic operations. This tumor may be encountered at any age from 19 to 80 years with a mean of 52 years.[3] It originates in the endosalpinx and expands the tubal lumen during early phases of its growth.

The Fallopian Tube: Basic Studies and Clinical Contributions, edited by Alvin M. Siegler, M.D. Mount Kisco, New York: Futura Publishing Company, Inc. © 1986.

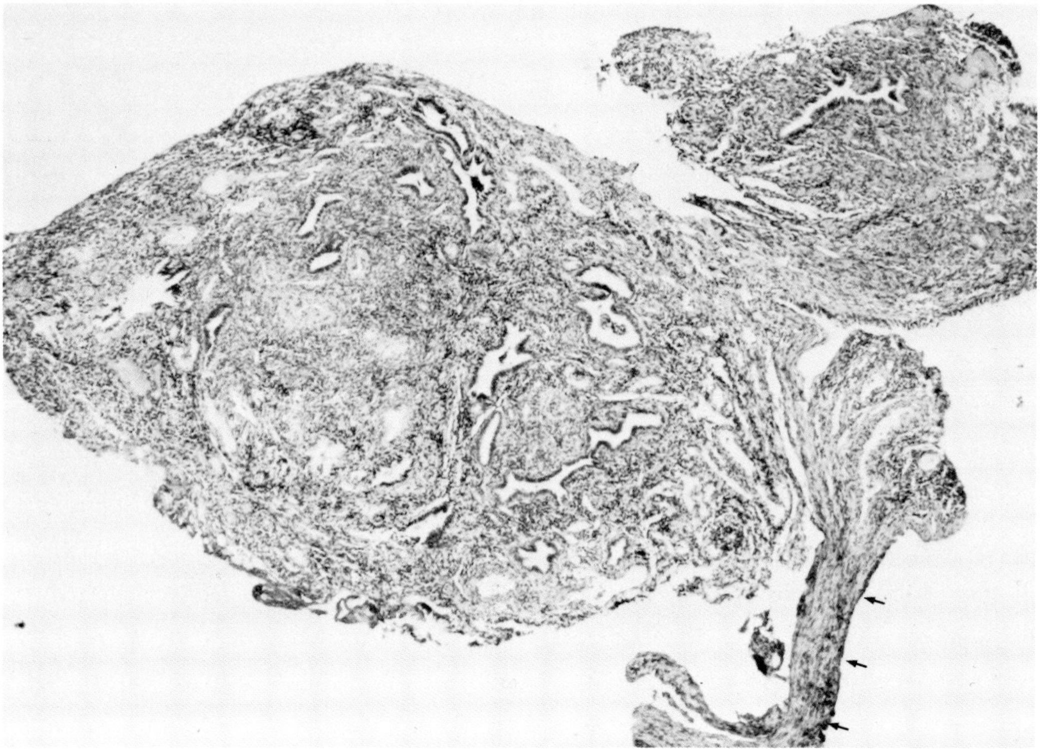

FIGURE 20:1—*Tubal polyp. Note the polypoid shape and the stalk (arrows).*

Bleeding from eroded blood vessels can cause a hematosalpinx, hemoperitoneum, or even vaginal bleeding. If the fimbrial ostium becomes occluded by tubal or preexisting inflammatory disease, a hydrosalpinx or pyosalpinx may result.

Bilateral tubal carcinoma has been reported in 26 percent of patients. Some authors believe that such involvement is caused by independent occurrence in both tubes because in most instances the size of the tumors are nearly equal in both tubes and the intervening endometrium is rarely involved by cancer.[3] The metastatic theory is supported by the observation that bilateral tubal carcinoma is found more frequently in advanced disease (30 percent of stages III and IV) than in the initial stages (7 percent of stages I and II).[4]

Grossly, the tumor appears as a polypoid growth within the tubal lumen, frequently with hemorrhagic and necrotic areas. In advanced stages, it extends to the serosal surface, the ovaries, broad ligaments, and adjacent structures; in these circumstances, it may not be properly identified as a primary tubal carcinoma. Microscopically it shows a papillary alveolar structure with intercommunicating fibrovascular stalks lined by epithelium resembling the normal endosalpinx depending on the degree of differentiation (Fig. 20:3). Stratification, cellular and nuclear pleomorphism, and increased mitotic figures are observed. Transition from a normal epithelium to a malignant type is often seen. In addition, clear-cell, endometrial and adenosquamous variants of tubal cancer have been reported.[5]

The pattern of spread is similar to ovarian cancer. It can pass through the open fimbria or erode the tubal wall and extend to other intraabdominal organs.

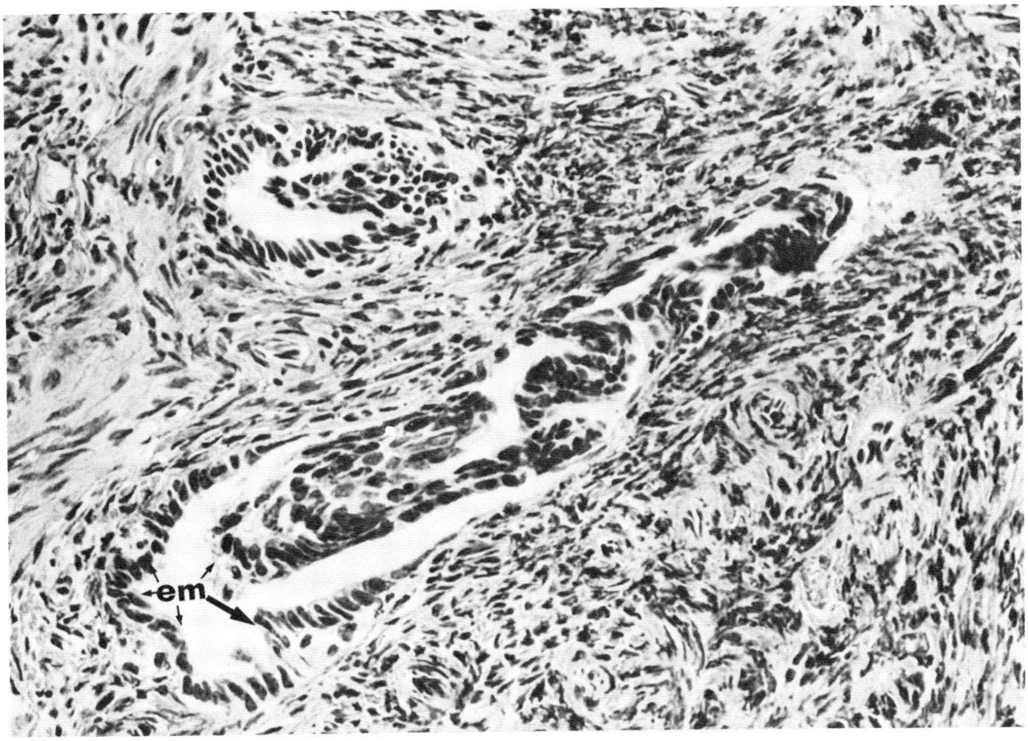

FIGURE 20:2—*Tubal polyp. High-power view with a detail of lining epithelium reproducing endosalpingeal mucosa.*

The pattern of lymphatic spread has not been studied accurately, but the preferred route appears to go into the paraaortic lymph nodes. The lymph nodes are the most common site of recurrent carcinoma (60 percent of cases).[6] The following criteria have been proposed to make a proper pathological diagnosis:

1. The tumor arises from the endosalpinx.
2. The histologic pattern produces the epithelium of the tubal mucosa.
3. Transition from benign to malignant epithelium is found.
4. The ovaries and endometrium are either normal or with tumor smaller than the tubal tumor.[3]

Most women have abdominal pain, distension, and pressure with vaginal bleeding and discharge but the symptoms are inconsistent and nonspecific. Postmenopausal or intermenstrual vaginal bleeding are the most common complaints. Abdominal pain may be intermittent and colicky, caused by tubal contraction from expansion of the tumor or a hematosalpinx. Constant pain, pressure, and heaviness may result from a large tumor mass. A vaginal discharge mixed with blood may be copious in association with abdominal pain or precipitated by compression of the tumor during an abdominal or pelvic examination. The syndrome, hydrops tubae profluens, is characterized by a copious discharge precipitated by compression and followed by relief of pain subsequent to the release of fluid from the distended tube. A palpable pelvic mass may have a characteristic sausage shape but it is difficult to distinguish it from an associated myoma.

In a recent study, malignant cells were found on cytologic preparation in 28

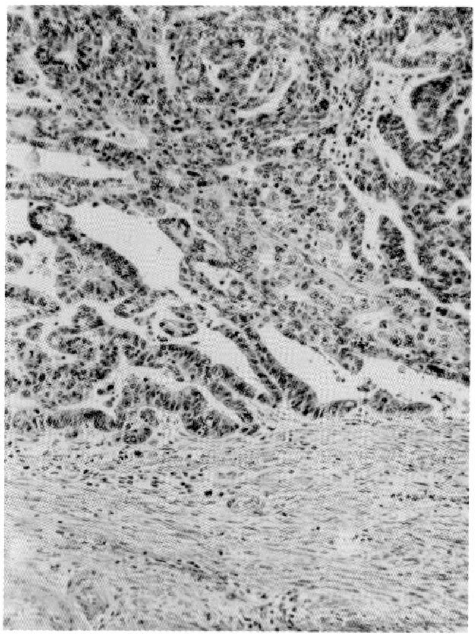

FIGURE 20:3—*Adenocarcinoma of the fallopian tube exhibiting papillary-alveolar pattern.*

out of 61 patients (45.9 percent).[7] Positive smears are found less commonly than with cervical or endometrial cancer but more frequently than with ovarian cancer. Positive cytology is especially valuable if there is no histologic proof of cervical or endometrial malignancy.

Radiological imaging techniques have been used for diagnosis and sonographic evaluation may help to detect a pelvic mass in women with unexplained vaginal bleeding or leukorrhea, or who have an unsatisfactory pelvic examination. A barium enema or gastrointestinal series may define a pelvic mass. Hysterosalpingograms also can help in the diagnosis of tubal carcinoma but there is concern for the possible dissemination of the cancer by this technique.[3]

Tubal carcinoma should be detected more frequently than an ovarian malignancy because the communication remains open between the tubal lumen and uterine cavity allowing passage of blood or malignant cells. Ovarian cancer rarely produces a positive cytology. A tubal carcinoma should be suspected in patients having a vaginal discharge in the absence of vaginitis or cervicitis, the presence of a pelvic mass, and if malignant cells are seen in the Papanicolaou smear without histologic proof of endometrial or cervical cancer.

Survival is influenced by the clinical stage. Generally the same classification has been used as the FIGO system for ovarian cancer but some systems combine the FIGO criteria with the depth of invasion of the tubal wall, as in Duke staging for intestinal cancer.[4] The survival statistics have been collected from the literature using retrospective staging with FIGO criteria.[8] Retrospective data are used because of the rarity of this disease. The recently reported actuarial three-year survival figures for stages I, II, and III are 52 percent, 50 percent, and 6 percent, respectively.[9]

At laparotomy, a tumor may be observed through the dilated fimbrial opening or eroding through the tubal wall. If a bilateral tubal malignancy causes swelling of both tubes, it may be mistaken for pelvic inflammatory disease.

Management of these patients follows the principles used for ovarian cancer. Surgery consists of hysterectomy and bilateral salpingo-oophorectomy, cytoreductive surgery (if necessary), and systematic exploration of the abdomen for evidence of distant spread, including the subdiaphragmatic region, paracolic gutters and paraaortic node dissection. Postoperatively, one chemotherapeutic protocol uses cis-platinum singly or in combination with other agents and sometimes radiotherapy is used.[6]

Malignant mixed müllerian tumor

This tumor is a rare type of sarcoma reproducing various components of the müllerian tract. In the homologous variant, the malignant tissues resemble fibrous connective tissue stroma, the glands, and the smooth muscle normally found in the müllerian tract. The heterologous type contains elements from outside of the müllerian tract, such as striated muscle, cartilage, and bone. Most mixed müllerian tumors develop in the uterine corpus and only rarely in the ovary and the fallopian tubes. Only 27 instances of primary tubal malignant mixed müllerian tumor have been reported in the literature.[10]

Grossly, these appear as fungating growths filling the endosalpinx. Microscopically, the homologous type contains bizarre spindle cells with numerous mitoses, and malignant glands featuring stratified epithelium and cellular pleomorphism. In heterologous types, one sees either malignant cartilage with bizarre nuclei or rhabdomyoblasts characterized by immature striated muscle cells with multiple nuclei and transverse striations demonstrable with phosphotungstic acid-hemotoxylin (PTH) stain.

All mixed müllerian tumors, regardless of their location, spread rapidly by direct extension and by hematogenous metastases; only 3 out of 26 reported patients with this tumor lived longer than 28 months. Aggressive therapy has been recommended even for early stages because of its rapid systemic spread.[10]

Tumors Arising from the Myosalpinx

Leiomyoma

These tumors are quite rare, unlike their counterpart in the uterus. They may originate from the myosalpinx or from the blood vessel wall. Leiomyomas cause focal thickening of the tubal wall and microscopically appear similar to the uterine leiomyoma with irregularly arranged bundles of spindle cells. Hyaline and other types of degeneration common to uterine myomas have been reported in the fallopian tube. An adenomyoma has been observed consisting of benign glands in addition to a smooth-muscle tumor.[11]

Malignant tumors: *leiomyosarcoma*

This tumor is rare. Microscopically it has spindle cells with bizarre nuclei and numerous mitotic figures. The pattern of spread is similar to the mixed malignant müllerian tumor with direct extension to the abdominal viscera and into the blood stream. The prognosis is poor.[12]

Tumors of the Tubal Serosa

Benign Tumors

Inclusion cysts

These are usually of inflammatory origin from peritubal adhesions appearing as thin-walled cystic spaces of variable size in a perisalpingeal location filled with serous fluid. Microscopically the cyst wall is thin, lined with flat cells resembling the peritoneum. Occasionally, the lining epithelium undergoes metaplastic changes resulting in stratification and formation of tuft-like excresences resembling the papillations of serous ovarian tumors.

Walthard rests

These multiple, small, grayish-yellow plaques scattered around the tubal serosa and found in large numbers may be mistaken for miliary spread of peritoneal tuberculosis. Walthard rests consist of clusters of squamous epithelium, occasionally with a cystic central space lined by cuboidal epithelium. Once considered embryonal rests, they currently are believed to develop from mesothelial metaplasia.

Adenomatoid tumor (benign mesothelioma)

These benign growths present as nodules of various sizes with indistinct borders, blending with the surrounding peritoneal surface. Adenomatoid tumors are also found on the uterus, broad ligament, and cul-de-sac. An adenomatoid tumor located at the uterotubal junction associated with an intrauterine pregnancy clinically and laparoscopically simulated a tubal gestation.[13] Microscopically, this tumor is composed of sieve-like spaces lined by a single layer of cuboidal cells with prominent nuclei and may resemble a hemangioma but the spaces do not contain blood.

These tumors, originating from mesothelium, are located subperitoneally and resemble inflammatory proliferation of the mesothelial cells lining the fallopian tube or mesosalpinx. Originally, flat mesothelial cells are cuboidal in these inflammatory lesions. Electron microscopy shows microvilli projecting from the cell surface, desmosomes present between the cells but absent over the lamina propria, and tonofilaments occasionally attached to the desmosomes.[14]

The tumor may either displace the fibromuscular stroma or diffusely infiltrate it with scattered clusters or individual cells. Although the microscopic picture of mesothelioma may suggest invasion because of lack of encapsulation and apparent infiltration, its clinical behavior is benign with only slow progression and no metastases.

Excision of the adenomatoid tumor is an adequate treatment, since they rarely recur.

Endosalpingiosis

This term has been applied to serosal implants that microscopically resemble endosalpinx and are found on serosal surfaces of tubes and the uterus, and on the mesosalpinx and omentum. Omental inclusions of endosalpingiosis were described in 25 percent of young women with salpingitis.[15] The cells lining the implant are either flat or cuboidal with tuftlike structures and glands. Laminated calcifications (psammoma bodies) may be seen occasionally with the implants. The original designation of endosalpingiosis implied an outward extension of the endosalpingeal mucosa analagous to endometriosis. Endosalpingiosis implants remain small and superficial and are asymptomatic.

The theory of the tubal origin of endosalpingiosis has not been documented. Some of the implants may represent metaplasia of mesothelium because they seem similar to the gland-like spaces and polypoid tufts observed in inflammatory adhesions of pelvic organs.

Endosalpingiosis in association with malignant or low-malignant-potential ovarian tumors may lead to a diagnostic and therapeutic dilemma. Are the implants caused by endosalpingosis or tumor extension? An accurate diagnosis is essential in deciding which type of operation to perform, especially in young women. At laparotomy the same guidelines are used as in the exploration for ovarian cancer. During microscopic examination of the specimens, attention is directed toward stratification, the lack of desmoplastic reaction, and cellular atypia to resolve the problem.

Paratubal cysts and tumors

Cystic structures found in paratubal locations may derive either from paramesonephric (müllerian), mesonephric (wolffian), or mesothelial structures. (The cysts and implants of mesothelial origin were discussed previously under the heading of adenomatoid tumor and endosalpingiosis.)

Most paratubal cystic structures arise from paramesonephric ducts.[16] According to Gendry et al.,[17] these cysts originate from accessory tubal lumina during embryogenesis by the same mechanisms as formation of the fimbria and hydatids of Morgagni. All these structures are produced by pinching off the developing oviduct between the receding pronephros and the mesonephric body. The accessory tubal lumina give rise to cystic structures that are usually located in the mesosalpinx. They are rarely symptomatic, few become larger than 5 cm, and are discovered incidentally at laparotomy. The epithelial lining closely resembles the endosalpinx, consisting of ciliated and mucinous cells with smooth muscle surrounding the lumen. The cysts occasionally contain intraluminal infoldings simulating papillations of serous ovarian tumors. Rarely does the epithelium acquire characteristics of low-malignant-potential tumors with excessive cellular proliferation and complex papillae. Since they do not spread to adjacent structures, paratubal cysts should not be placed in a low-malignant-potential category.[16] Accurate information concerning the ovary and other structures is essential to exclude the possibility of primary tumors spreading to the mesosalpinx.

Mesonephric duct (wolffian) remnants frequently are found on microscope sectioning of the mesosalpinx: these remnants appear as tubular structures with small lumens lined by uniformly sized cuboidal epithelium surrounded by a thick cuff of smooth muscle. In most recent studies, few of these cysts have been confirmed as mesonephric in origin.

Adnexal tumors of probable wolffian origin have been described as solid, encapsulated tumors from 1.3 to 12 cm in diameter.[18] Histologically, they vary from solid areas to tubular structures resembling a Sertoli cell or adenomatoid tumor. Electron microscopic features point to their origin from wolffian structures. Adrenocortical tissues may be found on careful sectioning of mesosalpinx in up to 20 percent of women and the implants look like adrenals with all three zones clearly evident. Most adrenal rests are clinically asymptomatic although instances of hypertrophy or even adenoma have been described.

Tumors of presumed displaced ovarian tissue origin

Tumors have been described in the fallopian tubes with clinical and pathological features of tumors usually seen in ovarian locations but without evidence of similar tumor in the ovary. The presumed origin of these tumors is either from displaced ovarian parenchyma, an "accessory ovary," or from a germ cell arrested during its migration from the yolk sac to the gonad during early embryogenesis.

Mature tubal teratomas may be found in the lumen, attached to the tube by a pedicle, or in an intramural or subserosal location. The sizes range from 1 to 20 cm[19] and microscopically, tissues resemble the ovarian teratoma. In one instance, a true "struma salpingitis" composed entirely of thyroid tissue produced clinical symptoms of hyperthyroidism. Other tumors in this category include dysgerminomas and granullosa cell tumors. Only one case of an immature teratoma has been reported.[20]

Trophoblastic tumors

According to Hertig and Gore, molar pregnancy occurs in one out of 5,000 ectopic gestations[21] and only one instance of tubal choriocarcinoma has been reported. The trophoblastic tissue in a tubal pregnancy may have characteristics of a hydatid mole with excessive trophoblastic proliferation and very immature appearance of the syncytiothropoblast.

Metastatic tumors

Most malignant tumors that metastasize to the tube originate from the ovary although sometimes, because of massive involvement of both structures, it becomes impossible to establish the site of the primary malignancy. Pancreatic or intestinal tumors can metastasize to the tube or ovary.

References

1. Stangel J, Chervenak F, Mouradian-Davidian M: Microsurgical resection of bilateral fallopian tube polyps. *Fertil Steril*, 35:580, 1981.
2. Fernstrom L, Lagerlof B: Polyps in the intramural part of the fallopian tubes. *J Obstet Gynaecol Br Commonw*, 71:681, 1964.
3. Sedlis A: Primary carcinoma of the fallopian tube. *Obstet Gynecol Surv*, 16:209, 1961.
4. Schiller HM, Silverberg SG: Staging and prognosis in primary carcinoma of the fallopian tube. *Cancer*, 28:389, 1971.
5. Voet RL, Lifshitz S: Primary clear cell

adenocarcinoma of the fallopian tube: Light microscopic and ultrastructural findings. *Int J Gynecol Path*, 1:292, 1982.

6. Maxson WZ, Stehman FB, Ulbright TM, et al: Primary carcinoma of the fallopian tube: Evidence for activity of cisplatin in combination therapy. *Soc Gynecol Oncol* Feb., (abstr.) 1985.
7. Takashina T, Ito E, Kudo R: Cytologic diagnosis of primary tubal cancer. *Acta Cytologica*, 29:367, 1985.
8. Sedlis A: Carcinoma of the fallopian tube. *Surg Clin North Am*, 58:121, 1978.
9. Jacobs MS, Kao E, Wolfsohn A, et al: Treatment and prognosis of fallopian tube carcinoma. *Soc Gynecol Oncol*, Feb., (Abstr.) 1985.
10. Kahanpaa KV, Laine R, Saksel E: Müllerian tumor of the fallopian tube: Report of a case with 5 year survival. *Gynecol Oncol*, 16:144, 1983.
11. Wheeler JE: Pathology of the fallopian tube. In Blaustein's *Pathology of the Female Genital Tract*, 2d ed. New York: Springer-Verlag, 1982.
12. Abrams J, Kazal HL, Hobbs RE: Primary sarcoma of the fallopian tube. *Am J Obstet Gynecol*, 75:180, 1958.
13. Grunebaum A, Sedlis A: Adenomatoid tumor of the uterus simulating interstitial pregnancy. *Obstet Gynecol*, 59:875, 1982.
14. Taxy JB, Battifora H: Female adnexal tumor of probable wolffian origin. *Cancer*, 37:2349, 1976.
15. Zinsser KR, Wheeler JE: Endosalpingiosis in the omentum: A study of autopsy and surgical material. *Am J Surg Pathol*, 6:109, 1982.
16. Samara M, Woodruff D: Paratubal cysts: Frequency, histogenesis and associated clinical features. *Obstet Gynecol*, 65:691, 1985.
17. Genadry R, Parmley T, Woodruff JD: The origin and clinical behavior of the paraovarian tumor. *Am J Obstet Gynecol*, 129:873, 1977.
18. Taxy JB, Battifora H: Female adnexal tumor of probable wolffian origin. *Cancer*, 37:2349, 1976.
19. Hertig AT, Gore H: Tumors of the ovary and fallopian tube. In Hertig AT, Gore H (Eds): *Tumors of Female Sex Organs*, part 3, *Atlas of Tumor Pathology*. Washington DC: 1961:p. 158.
20. Sweet RL, Selinger HE, McKay DG: Malignant teratoma of the uterine tube. *Obstet Gynecol*, 45:553, 1975.
21. Hertig AT, Gore H: Hydatidiform mole and choriocarcinoma. In Hertig AT, Gore H (Eds): *Tumors of Female Sex Organs*, part 1, *Atlas of Tumor Pathology*. Washington DC: 1961:p. 63.

21

The Effect of an IUD on Tubal Pathophysiology

Izu Eibschitz, Mordechai Sharf, and Karl de Vries

The IUD and Pelvic Infections

The use of the intrauterine device (IUD) has been associated with pain, bleeding, and pelvic inflammatory disease (PID). The literature dealing with the incidence of PID in IUD users should be divided into reports summarizing the decades before and after 1970. Reports before 1970 indicated that the IUD was not associated with an increased incidence of PID.[1–4] When an association of PID with IUD use was reexamined subsequently in epidemiologic studies, it was ascertained that the risk of PID secondary to an IUD in situ was increased (Table 21:1).[5–11]

These controlled studies showed that: (1) IUD use was associated with approximately a two- to tenfold increased risk of PID, evidence that the association is probably cause and effect; (2) the risk of PID in IUD users increased with more certainty of the diagnosis of PID, when a temperature of at least 38°C was required for the definition of PID[6]; (3) the risk of PID for nulligravid versus multigravid IUD users was found to be increased by some authors[7,9] while no increased risk was found for nulligravid women in the Women's Health Study[10]; (4) current IUD users were at increased risk for PID compared with users of nonpermanent contraceptive methods (i.e., pill and barrier methods) in which the risk of PID was less than one, suggesting that the latter methods provided some protection against PID[10]; (5) the risk of PID was related to insertion rather than to duration of use of the IUD: the risk was 3.8 in the first 30 days of insertion or reinsertion; otherwise, duration of use was not a significant risk factor for PID. In the first year after IUD removal, there was still an increased risk of PID but beyond 12 months the risk disappeared.[10]

The association between the IUD

The Fallopian Tube: Basic Studies and Clinical Contributions, edited by Alvin M. Siegler, M.D. Mount Kisco, New York: Futura Publishing Company, Inc. © 1986.

Table 21:1

Summary of Controlled Epidemiologic Studies of the Association between IUD Use and PID (Risk of an IUD User of Developing PID Relative to Nonuser)

Author and type of study	*No. of subjects*	*Relative Risk (95% Confidence interval)*	*Comments*
Noonan and Adams[5] (prospective)	1,706	1.8 (1.5–2.1)	In gonococcal PID, IUDs were 6.5 times more common.
Faulkner and Ory[6] (prospective)	205	5.1 (2.5–10.4)	Strict criteria for PID. With febrile PID, IUD users' risk increased.
Weström et al.[7] (prospective)	1,256	2.9 (2.1–4.0)	Cases laparoscopically confirmed PID. Nullipara at increased risk for PID at each age level.
Vessey et al.[8] (prospective)	17,032	3.5 (2.1–6.0)	Users of nonpermanent contraceptions had a significantly lower risk for PID than IUD users.
Eschenbach et al.[9] (prospective)	346	4.4 (3.0–6.9)	Nulligravida at increased risk for PID. IUD use associated with nongonococcal PID.
Burkman and the Women's Health Study[10]	1,447	1.6 (1.2–2.0)	Nulligravida not at increased risk for PID. Risk of PID for users of IUD versus oral contraceptives 4.5 and versus users of barrier methods 3.5. Increased risk of PID for 12 months after IUD removal.
Vessey et al.[11] (prospective)	17,032	10.5 (5.4–32)	Analysis limited to parous women. Acute definite PID 10.5 times commoner in current users than in nonusers, and chronic definite disease 2.5 times.

and PID was mainly caused by an ascending genital infection. Insertion of the IUD cannot be accomplished without bacterial contamination of the uterine cavity.[12] Ascending infection by neisseria is the best known cause of PID, but a wide variety of bacteria including anaerobes, actinomyces, and chlamydia as causative agents in nongonoccal PID has been identified.[13,14]

The worldwide rising incidence of gonorrhea seems to be an important factor in the increasing incidence of PID in association with IUDs.[5] Moreover, IUDs containing copper do not seem to protect the wearer against gonorrhea,[7] although copper has been demonstrated to have a gonococcicidal action in vitro.[15] After insertion of an IUD, bacteria were recovered by transfundal sampling from the uterine cavity, but one month later no bacteria were cultured.[16] Aseptic techniques are therefore recommended during IUD insertion.[17] Unilateral tubo-ovarian abscesses have been described in association with the IUD.[18–20] Not all of the symptoms of PID are related to infection; a sterile inflammatory process has been demonstrated in the tubes of IUD users, a finding possibly potentiating the susceptibility of the tubes to microbial invasion.[21,22]

Types of IUDs and Their Relationship to PID

Four groups of IUDs can be distinguished:

1. The early inert (nonmedicated) metal devices,[23]
2. Lippes loop and other inert polyethylene devices,
3. Medicated IUDs, containing copper,
4. Medicated IUDs, containing progesterone.

No evidence of PID was described in association with the early devices.[24] With the polyethylene types, the relative risk of PID was 3- to 4.4-fold greater than in nonusers.[7,9] Differences regarding the occurrence of PID are minimal between different types of polyethylene IUDs as long as the transcervical appendage is a monofilament type. The multifilament tail of IUDs, as in the Dalkon® shield, has been associated with severe ascending infections and this type of IUD has been withdrawn from sale.[25,26] A protective effect of copper-containing IUDs against gonorrheal salpingitis has not been demonstrated,[7] although copper has a toxic effect against gonococci in vitro.[27] The crude rate of PID was 1 in 445 for the Lippes loop®, 1 in 538 for Saf-T-Coil®, and for the Copper 7 (Gravigrad®) IUD it was 1 in 278 in multiparous women and 1 in 113 in nulliparous women;[28] however, a lower incidence of bacterial contamination of the uterine cavity with copper devices as compared with inert ones has been demonstrated.[29]

An association between IUD use and pelvic actinomycosis has been shown.[30] The growth of actinomyces, which is not a normal inhabitant of the vagina, may be favored in the pelvis by action of the copper as a reducing agent. In women using progesterone-medicated IUDs, the rate of PID is strongly correlated with the history of PID. The infection rate in women with a history of PID was four times greater than in those without such a history; a history of PID must therefore be viewed as a contraindication for selection of a progesterone-containing device.[31]

Progesterone-medicated IUDs have a relative risk of 2.2 for PID as compared to controls; Copper 7 and Saf-T-Coil® users had a risk of 1.9 and 1.3 for developing PID.[32]

The IUD and Ectopic Pregnancy

A number of mechanisms have been proposed to explain the association between IUDs and ectopic pregnancies:

1. IUD-induced PID as a sterile inflammation possibly leading to tubal scarring, occlusion, and changes in tubal motility.
2. IUD-induced antifertility factor, which is supposedly a humoral or chemical substance. It is maximally effective in the uterine cavity, reducing intrauterine implantations by 99.5 percent, less effective in the tubes, reducing tubal implantations by 95.5 percent, but the rate of ovarian pregnancies is unchanged in the presence of an IUD.[33]
3. Tubal motility is changed by progesterone-containing IUDs.[34]
4. A possibly IUD-related mechanism is the local release of prostaglandins.[35] According to different authors, from 4 to 8.9 percent of pregnancies occurring with an IUD in situ are extrauterine.[4,36] An index rate of ectopic pregnancy in women not using IUDs of 0.2 to 0.5 per 100 pregnancies can be expected.[37] Combining this statement with the finding of 4 to 9 percent ectopic pregnancies among IUD users, the relative risk of ectopic pregnancy for women becoming pregnant with an IUD in situ seems to be 8 to 45 times greater than for the general population of women. This increased risk cannot be explained completely by the risk of PID in IUD users (1.6 to 10.5 times greater than in women using other forms of contraception or no contraception at all). In addition to the increased incidence of PID in IUD us-

ers, these devices predispose women to ectopic pregnancies.

Reports from England and Wales[38] and from the United States have indicated an increased incidence of ectopic pregnancies, with the number from 1965 through 1977 going from 15,000 to 41,000 per year.[39] Mortality statistics show that the number of deaths from ectopic pregnancy, as a percentage of all maternal deaths, increased from 5.6 percent to 10 percent and was the largest single cause of maternal death in nonwhite women.[40] The steadily increasing number of ectopic pregnancies in young women between 1966 and 1972 in England and Wales could be associated with increasing IUD use.[38] In England and Wales, in 1967–1968, 1.3 percent of married women aged 15 to 44 years used the IUD, whereas by 1970, 4 percent of them used the device.[38] Since the introduction of copper IUDs and smaller sizes, IUD use has been extended to younger patients and to nulliparous women. Copper IUDs are efficient in preventing intrauterine implantation but less efficient than other devices in preventing ectopic pregnancies. After release of this IUD in England and Wales in 1971, the tubal pregnancy rates in 1971–1972 showed the greatest percentage increase over regional rates of the preceding three years. With progesterone-containing IUDs, the risk that a pregnancy will be ectopic is 16.3 percent.[40] Of 711 ectopic pregnancies occurring between 1966 and 1975, 70 were associated with IUDs.[41] In Finland, from 1970 to 1971, 2 percent of ectopic pregnancies were associated with an IUD, whereas from 1971 to 1975, 39 percent of ectopic pregnancies were associated with an IUD.[42] The IUD has a time-dependent protective effect against ectopic pregnancies, being most protective in the first two years of use.[38] Subsequently, the risk is the same as for patients not using contraception, and remains unchanged until the IUD is removed.

In another study of 101 unplanned pregnancies occurring in parous women using IUDs, 2 percent were ectopic among pregnancies occurring up to 24 months after insertion of the device, while 13 percent of pregnancies occurring 49 months or more after insertion were ectopic.[43] When location of pregnancies in women using a Copper-T IUD was examined, 3.4 percent of the 918 pregnancies that occurred were ectopic; the risk of the pregnancy being ectopic was increased after the Copper-T had been used for more than two years.[44]

A multicenter case control study evaluated complications related to IUD use in the United States between 1976 and 1978, among them ectopic pregnancies.[39] Women who had never used an IUD were as likely to have an ectopic pregnancy as women who had worn one. Current IUD users had 0.8 times the risk of an ectopic pregnancy as those who had never used an IUD. IUD users were three times as likely to have an ectopic pregnancy as oral contraceptive users. IUD users who had worn the device for 25 months or more had 2.6 times the risk of ectopic pregnancy as those who had the IUD for a shorter time. If a woman changed from oral contraceptives to an IUD, the increased risk of having an ectopic pregnancy is not caused by the IUD but by the absence of the oral contraceptives. The risk of an ectopic pregnancy is increased three times after the IUD is used more than two years and thereafter remains constant. After two years, histologic changes induced by the IUD become established in the tubes. Until one year after IUD removal, this foreign body reaction remains at a level sufficient to alter tubal function but not implantation. Therefore, pregnancy should be avoided in the first three months after IUD removal because of the increased risk of ectopic pregnancy. The evidence that an IUD predisposes a patient to an extrauterine pregnancy remains to be resolved.

Removal of an IUD

Fertility seemed to be decreased in parous women for the first year after contraception was stopped, but within two

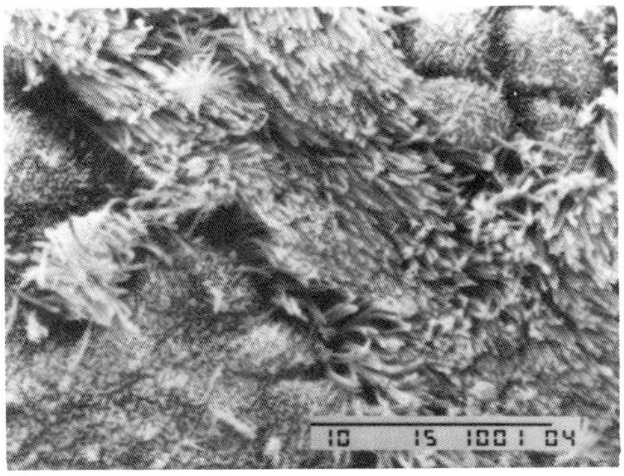

FIGURE 21:1—*Normal ciliary and secretory cells in ampulla of a patient who wore a copper IUD one year.* (× *5,000)*

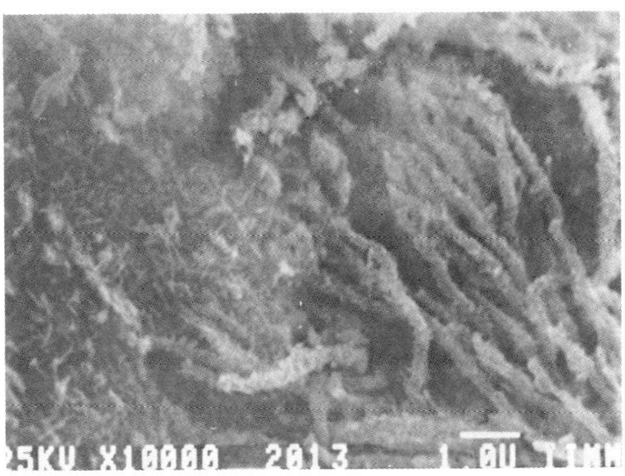

FIGURE 21:2—*Deciliated area in ampulla of women who wore a copper IUD three years. (Original magnification,* × *1,000)*

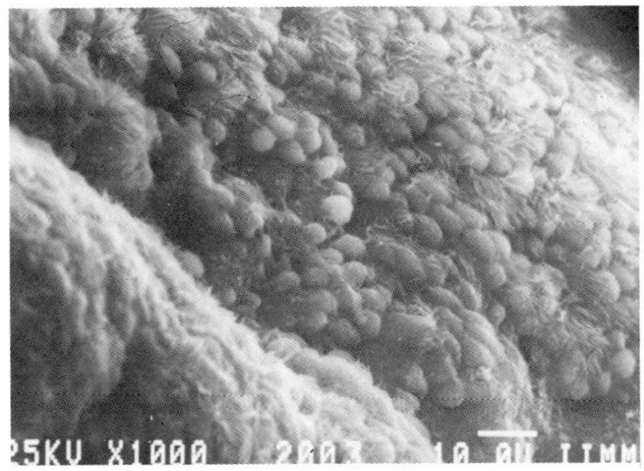

FIGURE 21:3—*The cilia appear irregular and tortuous ("worm-like") in tubes of women who wore a copper IUD three years. (Original magnification,* × *10,000)*

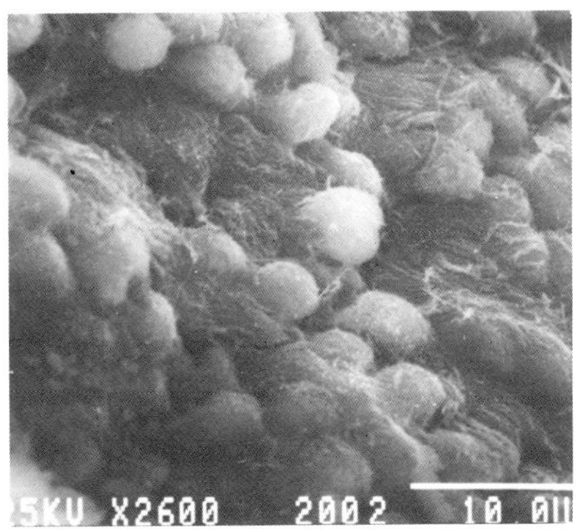

FIGURE 21:4—*A patch of secretory cells ballooning. Cilia appear to adhere to cell surface.* (× *2,600)*

years the differences in fertility were minimal.[45] Even when the IUD was removed for medical reasons such as pain or bleeding, about 86 percent of women desiring pregnancy conceived within 24 months of removal of the IUD.

The Effect of Copper IUDs on the Ultrastructure of Human Endosalpinx as Observed by Scanning Electron Microscopy

The ultrastructural changes in the endometrium induced by the presence of the IUD have been studied in the past[46,47] but no reports were found in the literature on the ultrastructure of the human endosalpinx in the presence of an IUD.

The fallopian tubes of women who had a copper IUD in situ (multiload Cu250, Copper 7 or Gyne-T 380) for at least six months were examined by scanning electron microscopy after hysterectomy performed for uterine myomata or prolapse. The women were between 30 and 40 years of age, parous, and had no history of PID or tubal disease. The operations were performed during the secretory phase. Specimens were prepared by immediate wash-

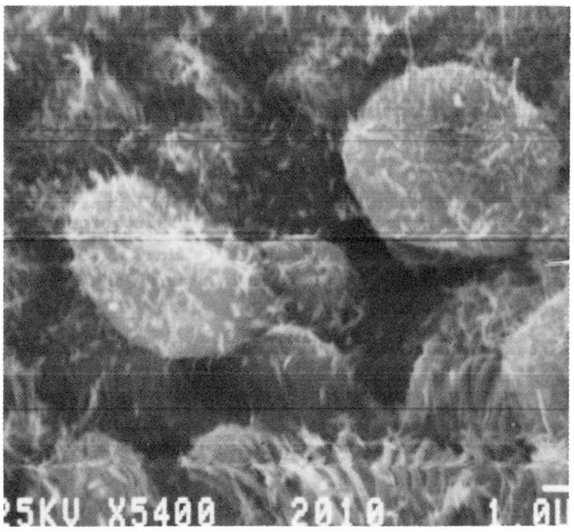

FIGURE 21:5—*Secretory cell surfaces exhibit protruding apices and abnormal microvilli.* (× *5,400*)

ing with isotonic saline, followed by fixation in 2.5 percent phosphate-buffered gluteraldehyde (pH 7.3), dehydrated in ethanol and amyl acetate, critical point dried, and coated with gold palladium. Observations were made on a JSM-U3 scanning electron microscope.

The ampullas obtained from IUD users and controls had ciliated and secretory cells. When the IUD had been in use for only one to two years, the ultrastructure appeared normal (Fig. 21:1). After more than two years of copper IUD use, areas of deciliation were consistently found (Fig. 21:2) and morphometric studies revealed a decreased ciliary cell count. In some instances, the number of cilia per ciliary cell was reduced and cilia appeared to have an uneven irregular surface (Fig. 21:3). Occasionally the cilia adhered to the apical surfaces of the cells and the secretory cells showed typical secretory phase apical protrusions ("ballooning") (Fig. 21:4). Microvilli on secretory cell surfaces were relatively sparse and uneven (Fig. 21:5).

On the basis of these findings, it appears that copper IUDs influence the ultrastructure of the epithelial lining of the fallopian tube. The IUD causes deciliation especially when the IUD has been worn three years or longer. This deciliation can predispose patients to an increased incidence of ectopic pregnancy because this loss of cilia impairs transport of the cleaving eggs.

References

1. Zipper J, Garcia ML, Pastene LL: Intrauterine contraception with the use of flexible nylon ring: Experience in Santiago de Chile. In *Proceedings of the Second International Conference on Intrauterine Contraception*. Amsterdam: Excerpta Medica, 1964: p. 88.
2. Lippes J: Contraception with intrauterine plastic loops. *Am J Obstet Gynecol*, 93:1024, 1965.
3. Tietze C: Contraception with intrauterine devices. *Am J Obstet Gynecol*, 96:1043, 1966.
4. Tatum HJ, Schmidt FH: Contraceptive and sterilization practices and extrauterine pregnancy: A realistic perspective. *Fertil Steril*, 28:407, 1977.
5. Noonen AS, Adams JB: Gonorrhea screening in an urban hospital family planning program. *Am J Public Health*, 69:701, 1974.
6. Faulkner WL, Ory HW: Intrauterine devices and acute pelvic inflammatory disease. *JAMA*, 235:1851, 1976.
7. Weström L, Bengtsson LP, Mardh PA: The risk of pelvic inflammatory disease in women using intrauterine contraceptive devices as compared to non-users. *Lancet*, 2:221, 1976.
8. Vessey MP, Doll R, Peto R, et al: A long term follow-up study of women using different methods of contraception. An interim report. *J Biosoc Sci*, 8:373, 1976.
9. Eschenbach DA, Harnisch JP, Holmes KK: Pathogenesis of acute pelvic inflammatory disease: Role of contraception and other risk factors. *Am J Obstet Gynecol*, 128:838, 1977.
10. Burkman RT: Association between intrauterine device and pelvic inflammatory disease. *Obstet Gynecol*, 57:269, 1981.
11. Vessey MP, Yeates D, Flavel R, et al: Pelvic inflammatory disease and the intrauterine device: Findings in a large cohort study. *Br Med J*, 282:855, 1981.
12. Advisory Committee on Obstetrics and Gynecology, U. S. Food and Drug Ad-

ministration: Report on Intrauterine Contraceptive Devices, 1968.
13. Schiffer MA, Elguezabal A, Sultana M, et al: Actinomycosis infections associated with intrauterine contraceptive devices. *Obstet Gynecol*, 45:67, 1975.
14. Gibson M, Gump D, Ashikaga T, et al: Patterns of adnexal inflammatory damage: Chlamydia, the intrauterine device, and history of pelvic inflammatory disease. *Fertil Steril*, 41:47, 1984.
15. Fiscina B, Oster GK, Oster G, et al: Gonococcicidal action of copper in vitro. *Am J Obstet Gynecol*, 116:86, 1973.
16. Mishell DR, Bell JH, Good RJ, et al: The intrauterine device: A bacteriological study of the endometrial cavity. *Am J Obstet Gynecol*, 96:116, 1966.
17. Mishell DR, Moyer DL: Association of pelvic inflammatory disease and the intrauterine device. *Clin Obstet Gynecol*, 12:179, 1969.
18. Dawood MJ, Birnbaum SJ: Unilateral tuboovarian abscess and intrauterine contraceptive device. *Obstet Gynecol*, 46:429, 1975.
19. Taylor ES, McMillan JH, Greer BE, et al: The intrauterine device and tuboovarian abscess. *Am J Obstet Gynecol*, 123:338, 1975.
20. Gold SH, Israel R, Ledger WJ: Unilateral tubo-ovarian abscess: A distinct entity. *Am J Obstet Gynecol*, 127:807, 1977.
21. Smith MR, Soderstrom R: Salpingitis: A frequent response to intrauterine contraception. *J Reprod Med*, 16:159, 1976.
22. Poma PA: Intrauterine contraception and tubal pathology. *Int J Fertil*, 25:287, 1980.
23. Graefenberg E: An intrauterine contraceptive method. In Sanger M, Stone H (Eds): *Proceedings of Seventh International Birth Control Conference. The Practice of Contraception.* Baltimore: Williams and Wilkins, 1931: p. 33.
24. Oppenheimer W: Prevention of pregnancy by the Graefenberg ring method. *Am J Obstet Gynecol*, 78:446, 1959.
25. Tatum HJ, Schmidt FH, Phillips DM: Morphological studies of Dalkon shield tails removed from patients. *Contraception*, 11:165, 1975.
26. Cates W, Ory HW, Rochat RW, et al: The intrauterine device and deaths from spontaneous abortion. *N Engl J Med*, 295:1155, 1976.
27. Ory HW: A review of association between intrauterine devices and acute pelvic inflammatory disease. *J Reprod Med*, 20:200, 1978.
28. Snowden R: Pelvic inflammation, perforation, pregnancy outcome associated with the use of IUDs. In Hefnawi F, Segal SJ (Eds): *Analysis of Intrauterine Contraceptions*. Amsterdam: North Holland Publishing Company, 1975: p. 139.
29. Buckingham MS, Sparks RA, Watt PJ, et al: Pelvic infection and intrauterine devices. *Br Med J*, 2:942, 1976.
30. Dische EE, Burt JM, Davidson NJH: Tubo-ovarian actinomycosis associated with intrauterine contraceptive devices. *Am J Obstet Gynecol*, 122:535, 1975.
31. Pharriss BB: Clinical experience with the intrauterine progesterone contraceptive system. J Reprod Med, 20:155, 1978.
32. Lee NC, Rubin GL, Ory HW, et al: Type of intrauterine device and the risk of pelvic inflammatory disease. *Obstet Gynecol*, 62:1, 1983.
33. Lehfeldt H, Tietze C, Gorstein F: Ovarian pregnancy and the intrauterine device. *Am J Obstet Gynecol*, 108:1005, 1970.
34. Snowden R: The Progestasert and ectopic pregnancy. *Br Med J*, 2:1600, 1977.
35. Cates W Jr, Ory HW: IUD complications: infection, death and ectopic pregnancy. In Moghissi K (Ed): *Controversies in Contraception*, Baltimore: Williams and Wilkins, 1979: p. 187.
36. Vessey MP, Johnson B, Doll R, et al: Outcome of pregnancy in women using an intrauterine device. *Lancet*, 1:495, 1974.
37. Kohl S: Data from Obstetrical Statistical Cooperative, Personal communication, 1976.
38. Beral V: An epidemiological study of recent trends in ectopic pregnancy. *Br J Obstet Gynaecol*, 82:775, 1975.
39. Ory HW: Ectopic pregnancy and intrauterine contraceptive devices: New perspectives. *Obstet Gynecol*, 57:137, 1981.
40. National Center for Health Statistics: Final natality statistics, 1977. *Monthly Vital Statistics Reports*, 27 (Suppl): 1979.
41. Hallat JG: Ectopic pregnancy associated with intrauterine device: A study of

seventy cases. *Am J Obstet Gynecol*, 125:754, 1976.
42. Erkkola R, Liukko P: Intrauterine device and ectopic pregnancy. *Contraception*, 16:569, 1977.
43. Vessey MP, Yeates D, Flavel R: Risk of ectopic pregnancy and duration of use of an intrauterine device. *Lancet*, 2:501, 1979.
44. Tatum HJ, Schmidt FH, Jain AK: Management and outcome of pregnancies associated with the Copper T intrauterine device. *Am J Obstet Gynecol*, 126:869, 1976.
45. Vessey MP, Lawless M, McPherson K, et al: Fertility after stopping use of intrauterine contraceptive device. *Br Med J*, 286:183, 1983.
46. Gonzalez-Angulo A, Aznar-Ramos R: Ultrastructural studies on the endometrium of women wearing TCu-200 intrauterine devices by means of transmission and scanning electron microscopy and X-ray dispersive analysis. *Am J Obstet Gynecol*, 125:170, 1976.
47. Verma V: Some ultrastructural observations on the endometrium of IUD users. *Gynecol Obstet Invest*, 12:220, 1981.

22

Ectopic Pregnancy in Women Using IUDs*

Barbara J. Struthers, William C. Stewart, and Francis B. O'Brien

Beral[1] was the first investigator to establish that the incidence of ectopic pregnancy (EP) had been rising in the general population since the late 1950s. Both the absolute numbers of EPs and the incidence have been shown to be increased in those western countries in which appropriate statistics are available. Using vital statistics from England and Wales, Beral reported that IUD users experienced a sixfold increase in EPs, and also reported an increase of EP with increasing age, with use of progestogen-only contraceptives, tubal surgery, and abortion. She found no correlation between pelvic inflammatory disease (PID) and EP with respect to time trend or regional distributional trend; an incidence of 2.5 EPs per 1,000 births was reported.

Hallatt,[2] in a retrospective study of 70 women who experienced EPs, found that the ratio of EPs to births was 1/54 in women not using contraception. This ratio increased to 1/18 ectopic pregnancy/intrauterine pregnancy (EP/IUP), in IUD users. He concluded that IUDs do not appear to prevent extrauterine pregnancies in predisposed patients. Erkkola and Liukko[3] studied 345 women with EP, recording history of PID, previous surgery, and IUD use. In their study, 17 percent of non-IUD users had a history of PID compared to only 5 percent of IUD users—i.e., fewer IUD users had this pre-

*It is difficult to compare the various studies of ectopic pregnancy directly, because various investigators use different bases for frequency calculation. Some studies report ectopic pregnancy as a percentage of all pregnancies, or as a percentage of all births or of live births. Other studies report a Pearl Index (frequency/100 woman-years) or frequency/100,000 women ages 15–44, or some variation of one of these. We have converted figures in this chapter, wherever possible, to either frequency/10,000 women or to frequency/thousand woman-years, for the sake of consistency.

The Fallopian Tube: Basic Studies and Clinical Contributions, edited by Alvin M. Siegler, M.D. Mount Kisco, New York: Futura Publishing Company, Inc. © 1986.

Table 22:1

*Summary of Ectopic Pregnancy/IUD Use Literature**

Reference	*Study type*	*No. of subjects*	*Findings*
Beral[1] 1975	Retrospective (vital stats.)	All women England and Wales	1. Rate of EP increases with age of women 2. 2.5 EP/1,000 births 3. Incidence of EP increased from late 1950s to 1972. 4. No relationship between time trend for PID and EP; no regional distribution trend. 5. 6× increase in EP rate in IUD users. 6. Increase in EP with progestogen-only contraceptives. 7. Tubal surgery, abortion are risk factors for EP.
Hallatt[2] 1976	Retrospective	70 cases	1. EP/births, 1:54; EP/IUP IUD in place, 1:18. 2. IUD probably doesn't prevent extrauterine pregnancies in predisposed patients. 3. Delay in diagnosis of EP with IUD in place.
Erkkola and Liukko[3] 1977	Retrospective	345 cases (59 with IUDs)	1. Frequency: 1966–70, 0.6% of deliveries; 1971–75, 1.08%. 2. PID recorded in history of 17% of patients with no IUD, 5% with IUD. 3. IUDs may play a major role in increased EP. (Protective effect of OCs not considered.)
Savolainen and Saksela[4] 1978	Retrospective case/control, + prospective uncontrolled	163 cases 351 controls 585 IUD wearers	1. EP as percent of deliveries has increased: 1968—1.3%; 1976—2.5% 2. EP occurred 12 times as often in women with EP history as in women having normal delivery only. 3. Prospective part of study: EP incidence, 2/1,000 WY 4. Estimates a twofold increase in RR of EP with IUD. 5. In IUD wearers, IUP decreased by 99.5%, EP by 93.6%. IUD does not induce abnormal implantation, but does not prevent EP very effectively.
Vessey, Yeates, Flavel[5] 1979	Prospective (1978–74)	117,032 (21 EPs)	1. Risk of EP is unrelated to duration of IUD use; incidence = 1.22/1,000 WY. 2. About 1/10 pregnancies with IUD in place may be ectopic. 3. No increase in EP incidence with age in women over 25.
Urquhart[6] 1979	Retrospective: statistics and calculations	U.S. population	1. Base: vital statistics of U.S., and estimate of incidence of PID in U.S. 2. Estimates approx. a 10× increase of EP/IUP in post-PID patients. 3. 11 EP/1,000 WY expected with IUD, taking into account percent of women with past PID. ≤1.5 EP/1,000 WY observed in IUD users. Conclusion: IUDs offer some protection against EP, and do not increase rate of EP.
Sivin[7] 1979	Prospective clinical	35,496 (Cu-T)	1. Higher risk of EP/IUP in years 3–4 compared to years 1–2 of IUD use. 2. Annual U.S. EP rate, 1965: 0.38/1,000 WY (age 15–44). 1977: 0.88/1,000 WY. IUD can't be responsible for >26% of increase in EP during this period. 3. After subtracting OC users, sterilized, sexually inactive women, and IUD users, U.S. EP rates were: 1965: 0.68—0.72/1,000 WY 1973: 1.15—1.25/1,000 WY 1976: 1.53—4.63/1,000 WY Rate didn't change when IUD users were added back.
Ambe et al.[8] 1980	Retrospective	426 EP 26 repeat EP	1. 26/426—repeat EP. (66.1% of EP). 2. Risk factors for EP: 73%—previous PID 15%—Arias-Stella reaction 12%—History of sterility 12%—History of endometriosis

Table 22:1 *Continued*

Reference	*Study type*	*No. of subjects*	*Findings*
Meirik and Nygren[9] 1980	Retrospective case-control (IUD vs. no IUD)	203 women: 142, no OC, no IUD 55, IUD	1. Prevalence of EP: 1.1/1,000 women. For copper IUD users: 1.5/1,000 WY based on *sales* of IUDs; no data on actual insertions, removals, and discontinuations. 2. IUD capacity to prevent EP may be less than usually reported. 3. IUD users had fewer other risk factors for EP than non-OC, non-IUD users.
Sandvei and Ulstein[10] 1980	Retrospective 1965–1978	450 cases (105—IUD) 345—controls	1. Absolute rate of EP in the Finnish population increased from 1965 to 1978. 2. PID, abdominal operations, adhesions, previous EP, and legal abortions were higher in non-IUD than IUD group. 3. Ovarian pregnancy more common in IUD group. 4. Evidence of PID found in 34.2% of patients with EP.
Brenner, Roy, Mishell[11] 1980	Retrospective	300	1. IUD users have significantly fewer risk factors for EP than OC users, nonusers, or ex-IUD users. 2. Of 23 women with previous EP, 20 occurred in contralateral oviduct. 3. Risk factors present in patients: 26.0%—history or evidence of PID 15.0%—history of pelvic surgery 11.0%—history of PID and surgery 14.0%—past or present IUD use 11.0%—present IUD use 4. Percent of EPs in women with history of PID lower in IUD users than in noncontraceptors. No connection between IUD use and PID seen. 5. By Tietze's method, number of EPs with years of IUD use was less than expected.
Ory and The Women's Health Study[12] 1981	Retrospective	615 EP 3,453 controls	1. Known risk factors for EP (black race, PID, prior EP) more common in cases than controls. 2. Current IUD users: 0.8 × EP RR of never users (0.6–1.0), NS. Past IUD users: 1.4 × RR of EP. 3. Women with recent past use of IUD (within 1 yr) had higher risk of EP than never-users. Women who had used IUDs more than 1 year before showed *no* increased risk. 4. No significant effect of IUD use history was seen in women with history of either PID or EP. 5. IUD use does not increase risk of EP. 6. Reevaluation of data, *Am. J. Epidemiol.*, 112:434, 1980: All current contraceptors, including IUD users, are less likely to have EP than women not using contraception.

Recalculation: Unadjusted est. RR, using noncontraceptors as controls, rather than non-IUD users:

	EP	*Control*	*RR*	*95% CL*
Current IUD	42	360	0.39	(0.28, 0.55)
Recent-past IUD	18	67	0.91	(0.53, 1.55)
Remote Past IUD	51	253	0.68	(0.49, 0.94)
Noncontraceptors	319	1078	1.00	Referent

Reference	*Study type*	*No. of subjects*	*Findings*
Weström, Bengtsson, Mårdh[13] 1981	Retrospective	All women in Lund, Sweden	1. EP/1,000 pregnancies: 1960–64, 5.8; 1975–79, 11.1 2. Risk of EP increases with age. 3. EP rate in noncontracepting women without past PID, 3/1,000 WY; EP in IUD users without past PID, 4/1,000 WY. 4. PID increases RR of EP approx. sevenfold. Without PID, incidence was 3/1,000 WY; with PID, 19/1,000 WY.

Table 22:1 *Continued*

Reference	*Study type*	*No. of subjects*	*Findings*
Pagano[14] 1981	Retrospective	3,200 controls 287 EP	1. Chronic PID found in 100/287 (35%) with EP. 2. 18 pts. had history of appendicitis compared to 25% of controls. 3. 15% of EP patients had history of infertility; PID history was similar to PID history in control women. 4. 9% of women with EP had history of EP, compared to 0.5% of controls. 5. High percent of spontaneous abortions in patients compared to controls. 6. IUD in situ in 14% of patients; only in 0.5% of controls.
Punnonen and Lauren[15] 1982		41 ovarian pregnancies	1. Incidence of ovarian pregnancy has increased: 1964–70, 1.2% of EPs were ovarian; 1971–80, 5.4% of EPs were ovarian. 2. 61% of ovarian pregnancy patients had history of legal abortion, D&C for spontaneous abortion, or EP. In 1970s, 61% of patients had IUD in situ. 3. Conclusion: both surgery and IUDs increase ovarian pregnancy.
Sivin[16] 1983	Vital statistics and review		1. Comparison of EP rate for IUDs with rates based largely on women using OCs, sterilized women, or sexually inactive women is incorrect since those methods protect against EP and IUDs do not. Noncontraceptors are the appropriate comparison group. 2. Using Ory's figures, calculated risk of past IUD use to be 0.7. 3. Concluded that Ory's evidence for a past users' effect was weak. 4. Concluded that copper and inert IUDs do not contribute to EP rate, but that Progestasert may enhance EP rate.
Vasquez et al.[17] 1983	Retrospective case/control	37 cases 20 controls	1. Ciliation of cells in tubes of normal or pregnant women is greater than in women with EP. 2. Although tubes may appear grossly normal, deciliation is present in women with hydrosalpinx or in women with EP. Contralateral fimbriae were also deciliated. 3. In women with previous EP, tubes always showed significant deciliation.
Grimes et al.[18] 1983	Retrospective 148,734 deliveries	24 cases ovarian preg.	1. Ovarian pregnancy occurs approximately 1/7,000 deliveries. 5.3% of EPs in this series were ovarian. 2. IUD use is not associated with an absolute increase in ovarian pregnancy; IUDs have no effect on ovarian pregnancy. 3. >50% of ovarian pregnancies occurred in women with previous infertility or reproductive pathology.
Majmudar et al.[19] 1983	Retrospective case-control	200 cases 100 controls	1. Salpingitis isthmica nodosa present in 57/100 tubes with EP, 5/100 in controls.
Weinstein et al.[20] 1983	Retrospective uncontrolled	154 cases	1. Tabulation of risk factors in this group showed the following: 4.5%—Prior EP 1.97—Average parity (range, 0–7) 22.7%—Prev. abortion (therapeutic) 45.5%—No live births 56.5%—No contraceptive 9.7%—IUD 6.5%—Diaphragm 19.5%—No contraceptive information 14.9%—History of PID 22.7%—Past IUD use 13.6%—Prev. infertility 44.5%—History or evidence of PID 2. Past or present IUD use not correlated with PID.
Rubin et al.[21] 1983	Vital stats	All women U.S.A. 1970–78	1. EP frequency in the U.S. rose from 4.5/1,000 preg nancies in 1970 to 9.4/1,000 in 1978. 2. Rate of EP higher in older women. 3. Rate of EP higher in nonwhite than white women.

*Abbreviations: EP = ectopic pregnancy; IUP = intrauterine pregnancy; PID = pelvic inflammatory disease; Stats = statistics; IUD = intrauterine contraceptive device; OC = oral contraceptive; RR = estimated relative risk.

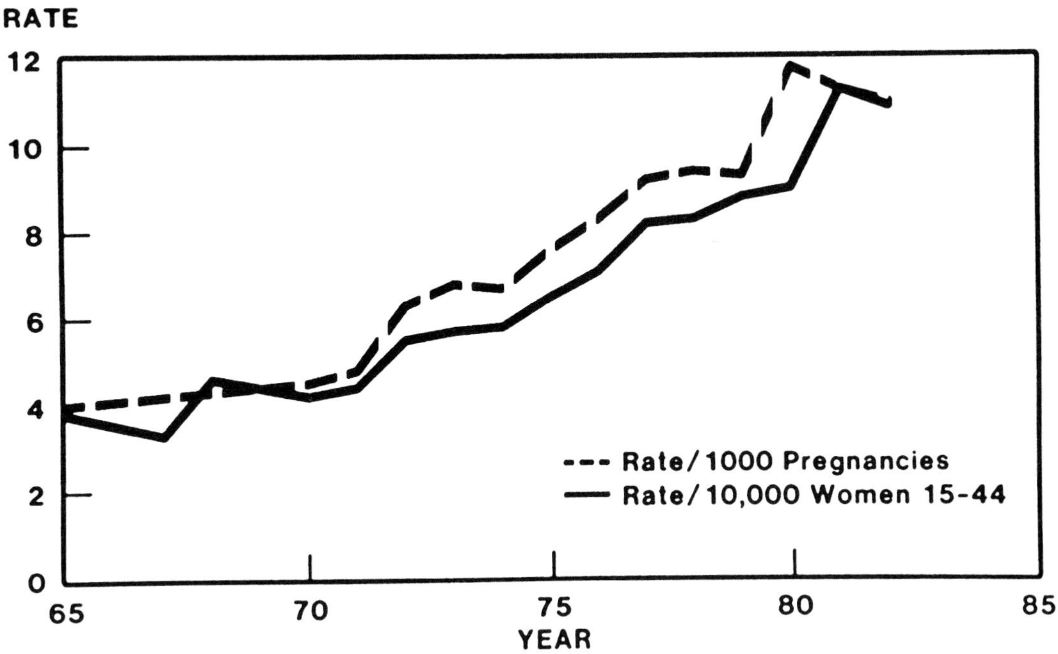

FIGURE 22:1—*Ectopic pregnancy in U.S. population, 1965–1982. (Reproduced by permission from Sivin.[16])*

disposing factor for EP. They concluded that IUDs may play a role in increased incidence of EP, although they failed to consider any protective effect of oral contraceptives against EP. Other authors have reached varying conclusions relative to the contribution of IUDs and other factors to the incidence of EP; these are summarized in Table 22:1.[1–21]

Increased Rate of Ectopic Pregnancy

Sivin[16,22] calculated the EP rate in the United States (Fig. 22:1). It can be seen that whether EP incidence is calculated per 1,000 pregnancies (live births, spontaneous and induced abortions) (Figure 22:2) or per 10,000 women of childbearing age per annum, there has been a real increase in the incidence of EP. (Because not all births are reported, these incidence figures may be about 10 percent too high.) Although these are U.S. data, increases have also been calculated for other countries. In England and Wales, during the period 1965–1969, the annual incidence of EP was 2.9/10,000 women; this rate was 3.3/10,000 women ten years later.[1,23] In Sweden, the 1960–1964 rate was 4.2, similar to U.S. figures. By 1975–1979, the Swedish incidence was 11.2/10,000 women ages 15 to 44, slightly higher than the U.S. incidence during the same period.[13] In Helsinki, Finland, there was[13] an increase in EP/IUP of 1.9/1,000 pregnancies from 1968 to 1976[4]; in Prague, Czechoslovakia, there was an increase of 1.7/1,000 from 1955 to 1966.[24]

The reason for the increase in EP incidence is uncertain; multiple factors may be involved. Several authors have reported an increase in EP incidence with increasing age.[1,12,21] At least in the United States, many women are waiting to have children until they are in their thirties. Data from Rubin[21] show the influence of age as a factor in the rising EP rate (Table 22:2). Although the EP rate per

1,000 pregnancies increased with advancing age from 4.5 (ages 15 to 24) to 15.2 (ages 35 to 44) the incidence per 10,000 women and the percentage of total EPs experienced in each age group indicate that the number of EPs is greatest in the group that experiences the majority of pregnancies, namely, 25- to 34-year-old-women.

Rubin et al.[21] have published data indicating that in the United States, race, independently of age, alters the risk of EP. In each age group, the rate was lower among white than among nonwhite women. Overall, the EP rate among nonwhite women was 1.6 times higher than among white women during the period 1970–1976 (Fig. 22:2)..

Ectopic Pregnancy and Salpingitis

Certainly one of the major recognized risk factors influencing EP is salpingitis. Kelly[25] listed this as one of several factors causing EP, and Novak[26] reported that chronic salpingitis was the primary cause of EP. Weström et al.[13] reported data indicating that women with a history of salpingitis had approximately a seven fold increased estimated relative risk (RR) of EP compared with women without such a history. These authors compared EP incidence in women using IUDs, oral and barrier contraceptives with women using no contraceptives. The results are presented in Table 22:3. Their data showed a protective effect for both oral and barrier contraceptives, but no increase in IUD users compared to noncontraceptors, using the incidence of EP/1,000 woman-years as a basis for comparing these groups.

Ambe et al.[8] noted that 73 percent of their EP patients had had previous PID. Sandvei and Ulstein[10] found evidence of PID in 34.2 percent of EP patients; a similar percentage was reported by Pagano.[14] Weinstein et al.[20] found histologic evidence of PID in 44.5 percent of their EP patients, although only 14.9 percent had a history of PID. According to data from the National Ambulatory Medical Care Survey,[27] there were nearly 1.9 million patient visits for PID per year to office-based private practicing physicians during the years 1973 to 1977. Curran[28] has estimated that if the present trend of sexually transmitted disease and PID continues unabated, for the cohort of women who reached reproductive age in 1970, by the year 2000 there will have been one case of PID for every two women in this cohort, 10 percent of these women will be infertile because of PID alone, and 3 percent of these women will have experienced EP.

Previous Ectopic Pregnancy and Infertility

Previous EP has also been found by several authors to be a risk factor for a subsequent EP[4,8,10,11,15] and a history of infertility has been reported in EP patients by some authors.[8,14,20] Vasquez et al.[17] have studied ciliation of fallopian tubes via scanning electron microscopy in normal women and in women with hydrosalpinx or a history of EP. They have shown that although the tube may appear grossly normal, deciliation is present in women who have had either of these pathological conditions. In cases of EP, the contralateral tubes always showed significant deciliation as well. Peretz et al.[29] have recently reported similar results.

IUDs and Incidence of EP

The incidence in women using IUDs depends on the method of reporting and the comparison groups used (see Table 22:1). The actual number of EPs occurring in IUD users in the population is not known. An estimate of the expected incidence of EP in women using IUDs was made by Tietze et al. in 1967.[30] Using a fertility rate of 300/TWY (thousand woman-years), and 13 ovulations/woman/year, the expected rate was calculated as 13 ovulations/year × 300 fertilizations/TWY = 3,900, or about 4,000 expected fertilizations/TWY. In 1970, the U.S. EP rate was 5/1,000 pregnancies or 20/4,000 fer-

Table 22:2

Ectopic Pregnancy Rate by Age Group, 1970 to 1978[21]

	Age group		
Tubal pregnancy	*15–24*	*25–34*	*35–44*
Rate/1,000 pregnancies	4.5	9.7	15.2
Incidence/10^4 women	5.3	10.3	2.9
Number	92,400	138,700	30,600
Percentage in age group	35	53	12

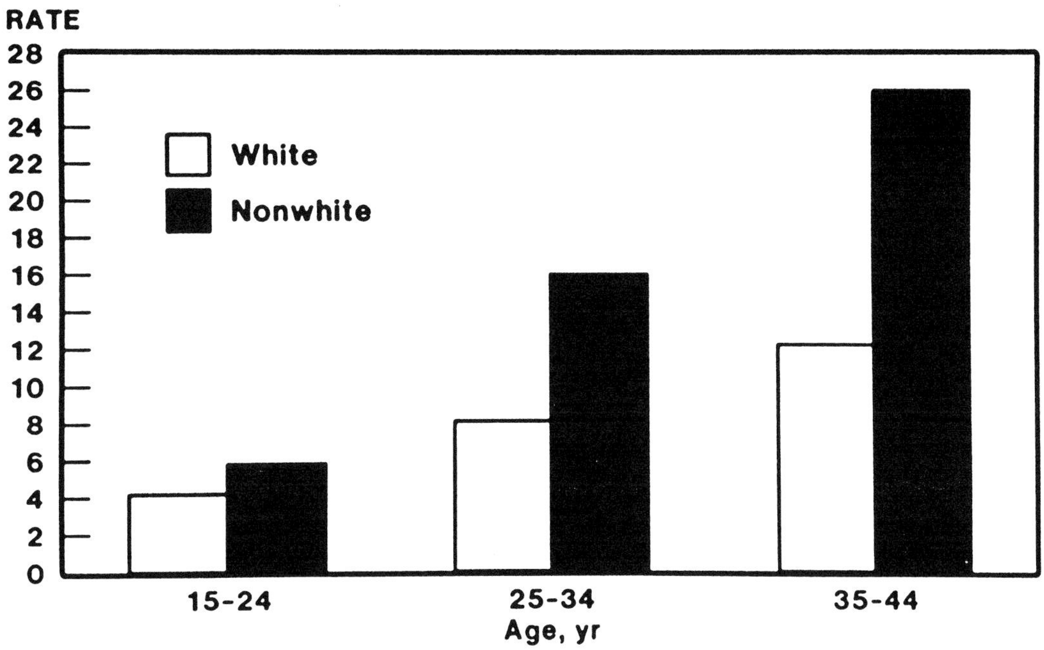

FIGURE 22:2—*Ectopic pregnancy rates per 1,000 reported pregnancies (including live births, legal induced abortions, and ectopic pregnancies) by age and race, United States, 1970 through 1978.*[21]

tilizations = 20/TWY. Thus, one would expect 20 EPs/TWY of IUD use based on 1970 EP rates (Sivin[22] has calculated the incidence of 5 EPs/1,000 pregnancies to be equivalent to 4.2 EPs/TWY). In 1981, the U.S. EP rate had increased to 11.3/TWY. These figures are both lower than the 20/TWY expected in IUD users.

It has been suggested that Tietze's estimate of 20 EPs/TWY in IUD users overestimates the actual expected rate. If, as a basis for estimating the incidence of EP in normal women, one begins with a figure of 1 EP/250 IUP (intrauterine pregnancies), which was the approximate U.S. rate of EP in 1965, the following calculation may be made:

U.S. EP/IUP (1965): 1/250 (=4/1000).
Assume: 80 percent fertility in normal noncontracepting women
(800 conceptions/TWY).

Table 22:3

*Incidence of Ectopic Pregnancy/1,000 Woman-Years, 1970 to 1974**

Contraceptive	*Woman-years*	*EP/TWY*
IUD	2,940	4.1
Oral contraceptives	16,311	0
Barrier contraceptive	7,044	0.9
No contraceptive	5,032	5.4

*Calculated from data of Weström et al.[13]

Table 22:4

Searle Cu-7® Clinical Studies, Ectopic Pregnancy/Thousand Woman-Years (TWY)

Months	*No. EP*	WY	EP/TWY
	Nulliparas (n = 4771)		
1–12	2	3,691	0.8
1–24	5	6,432	0.8
1–36	5	8,045	0.6
	Multiparas (n = 11,673)		
1–12	3	9,444	0.3
1–24	13	16,560	0.8
1–36	15	20,914	0.7
	Combined (n = 16,444)		
1–12	5	13,105	0.4
1–24	18	22,992	0.8
1–36	20	28,858	0.7
1–108	22	31,162	0.7

800/2500 = 3.2 EP/TWY.
In postsalpingitis women, there is a six-fold increase in RR of EP, plus an additional 20 percent decrease in fertility.[13]
(3.2) (6) (0.80) = 15.4 EP/TWY.

Thus, one should expect between 3.2 EP/TWY and 15.4 EP/TWY of IUD use. The actual rate in the population will vary with the number of women who have had PID, or who have other predisposing conditions (tuboplasty, congenital anomalies, and high parity are also considered by many clinicians to fall in this category, although these authors found little evidence for the inclusion of high parity as an independent risk factor).

The contribution of IUDs to the population rate of EP appears to be low. In Searle's clinical studies with the Cu-7,® EP/TWY was 0.70 during 28,858 WY (Table 22:4). Twenty of the 561 pregnancies recorded in this period, or 3.6 percent were ectopic. This included 4,771 nulliparous women during 8,045 woman-years of use over 36 months, and 11,673 multiparous women during 20,914 woman-years of use over 36 months (first insertions only) (Table 22:5). Criteria for inclusion in the clinical study have been previously reported by O'Brien et al.[31] The incidence at the completion of the study, which was conducted between 1970 and 1980, and included 16,444 women over 31,162 woman years of Cu-7® use, was 0.7/TWY. A total of 22 of the 679 pregnancies (3.2 percent) reported during this nine-year period of Cu-7® use was extrauterine.

Table 22:5

Searle Cu-7® Clinical Studies, Ectopic/Intrauterine Pregnancies

Months	*Nulliparas*	*Multiparas*	*Combined*
1–12	2/079 (2.5%)	3/218 (1.4%)	5/297 (1.7%)
1–24	2/124 (4.0%)	13/343 (3.8%)	18/467 (3.9%)
1–36	5/161 (3.1%)	15/400 (3.7%)	20/561 (3.6%)
1–108			22/679 (3.2%)

Table 22:6

IUD Device-Specific Ectopic Pregnancy Rates, 1974 to 1983[31]

IUD	*Woman-years*	*Rate/TWY*
T Cu 200	4,836	1.4
Cu-7	5,490	0.9
Nova T	1,668	0.7
T Cu 220	11,931	0.8
MLCu 250	8,207	0.2
Lippes C&D	12,621	1.1
Saf-T-Coil	4,712	0.8
Progestasert	10,128	5.2
Levonorgestrel, 20 μg	893	1.1

Table 22:7

IUDs and Ectopic Pregnancies

Weighted Average, all nonhormonal IUDs: 0.81/TWY (calculated from Table 22:6)
Woman-years: 49,465

Actual EPs:

0.81/1,000 WY × 49,465 WY = *40* EP experienced

Expected:

From Tietze, 300 fertilizations/1,000 WY

300 × 49.465 TWY = 14,840 pregnancies expected in unprotected women

Expected EP @ 1965 rate, 1/250: 59
Expected EP @ 1975 rate, 1/132: 112
Expected EP @ 1982 rate, 1/91: 163

World Health Organization studies (Table 22:6) of several IUDs (1974–1983) indicate EP rates from 0 to 1.4/TWY for several plastic and copper IUDs and one levonorgestrel-releasing IUD. All of these rates are lower than the 3.2/TWY just calculated for normal women. The progesterone-releasing device has an EP rate of 5.2/TWY, almost four times higher than any of the other IUDs tested, but similar to Weström's estimate of 5.4 for noncontracepting women[13] and substantially less than Tietze's estimate of 20/TWY of IUD use.[30] A weighted average of 0.81/TWY may be calculated from Table 22:6 (see Table 22:7 for calculation) for all nonhormonal IUDs, over 49,465 woman-years. Forty EPs were experienced by this cohort. If Tietze's figure of 300 fertilizations per TWY is used to calculate the expected pregnancies in unprotected women,[30] one would expect 14,840 fertilizations or pregnancies, including 59 EPs at the 1965 rate of 1 EP/250 IUP. The expected number increases to 112 at the 1975 rate of 1 EP/132 IUP, and 163 at the 1982 rate of 1 EP/91 IUP. When these figures are compared to the 40 actual EPs, it is apparent that copper and inert IUDs do not appear to be risk factors for EP.

Although IUDs do not prevent EP as efficiently as they prevent intrauterine pregnancy, there does seem to be some degree of protection against EP conferred by plastic and copper IUDs to the women who wear them.

Acknowledgments: The authors wish to express appreciation to Diane Fallon and Dorrel Edstrand for their assistance in preparing the manuscript, and to Dr. F.M. Sturtevant for his helpful comments.

References

1. Beral V: An epidemiological study of recent trends in ectopic pregnancy. *Br J Obstet Gynaecol*, 82:775, 1975
2. Hallatt JG: Ectopic pregnancy associated with the intrauterine device: A study of seventy cases. *Am J Obstet Gynecol*, 123:754, 1976.
3. Erkkola R, Liukko P: Intrauterine device and ectopic pregnancy. *Contraception*, 16:569, 1977.
4. Savolainen E, Saksela E: Ectopic pregnancy, relationship to the preceding

contraception. *Ann Clin Gynaecol,* 67:198, 1978.
5. Vessey MP, Yeates D, Flavel R: Pelvic inflammatory disease and the intrauterine device: Findings in a large cohort study. *Lancet,* 2:501, 1979.
6. Urqhuart J: Effect of the venereal disease epidemic in the incidence of ectopic pregnancy. Implications for the evaluations of contraceptives. *Contraception,* 19:455, 1979.
7. Sivin I: Copper T IUD use and ectopic pregnancy rates in the United States. *Obstet Gynecol Surv,* 34:693, 1979.
8. Ambe AK, Sosa TB, Luna Y, et al: Embarazo ectopice repeticion. *Ginecol Obstet Mex,* 48:95, 1980.
9. Meirik O, Nygren K: Ectopic pregnancy and IUDs: Incidence, risk rate and predisposing factors. *Acta Obstet Gynecol Scand,* 59:425, 1980.
10. Sandvei R, Ulstein M: History and findings in ectopic pregnancies in women with and without an IUD. *Contracept Deliv Syst,* 1:131, 1980.
11. Brenner PF, Roy S, Mishell DR: Ectopic pregnancy: A study of 33 consecutive surgically treated cases. *JAMA,* 243:673, 1980.
12. Ory H: Ectopic pregnancy and intrauterine contraceptive devices: New perspectives. *Am J Epidemiol,* 112:434, 1980.
13. Weström L, Bengtsson L, Mardh P: Incidence, trends, and risk of ectopic pregnancy in a population of women. *Br Med J,* 282:15, 1981.
14. Pagano R: Ectopic pregnancy: A seven-year study. *Obstet Gynecol Surg,* 37:526, 1982.
15. Punnonen R, Lauren P: Increased occurrence of ovarian pregnancy. *Eur J Obstet Gynecol Reprod Biol,* 13:139, 1982.
16. Sivin I: IUDs and ectopic pregnancy. *Stud Fam Plann,* 14:57, 1983.
17. Vasquez G, Winston RM, Brosens LA: Tubal mucosa and ectopic pregnancy. *Br J Obstet Gynecol,* 90:468, 1983.
18. Grimes HG, Nosal RA, Gallagher JC: Ovarian pregnancy: A series of 24 cases. *Obstet Gynecol,* 61:174, 1983.
19. Majmudar B, Henderson PH, Semple E: Salpingitis isthmica nodosa: A high-risk factor for tubal pregnancy. *Obstet Gynecol,* 62:73, 1983.
20. Weinstein L, Morris MB, Dotters D, et al: Ectopic pregnancy. A new surgical epidemic. *Obstet Gynecol,* 61:698, 1983.
21. Rubin GL, Peterson HB, Dorfman SF, et al: Ectopic pregnancy in the United States 1970 through 1978. *JAMA,* 249:1725, 1983.
22. Sivin I: IUD-associated ectopic pregnancies. In Zatuchni GI, Goldsmith A, Sciarra JJ (Eds): *Intrauterine Contraception.* Philadelphia: Harper and Row, 1985: p. 340.
23. Robinson N, Veral V: Risk of ectopic pregnancy. *Lancet,* 2:1247, 1979.
24. Cernoch VA: Kunstliche Schwangerschaftsunterbrechung und extrauterin Schwangerschaft. *Zentralbl Gynäkol,* 93:1784, 1971.
25. Kelly H: *Operative Gynecology,* New York: Appleton, 1898.
26. Novak E: *Textbook of Gynecology,* 3d ed. Baltimore: Williams & Wilkins, 1948.
27. St John RK, Blount J, Jones O: Pelvic inflammatory disease in the United States: Incidence and trends in private practice. *Sex Trans Dis,* 8:56, 1981.
28. Curran JW: Economic consequences of pelvic inflammatory disease in the United States. *Am J Obstet Gynecol,* 138:848, 1980.
29. Peretz BA, Lindenbaum ES, Beach D: Ectopic pregnancy effects. *Eur J Obstet Gynec Reprod Biol,* 17:19, 1984.
30. Tietze C, Lewit S: Statistical evaluation of intrauterine devices. *Advan Plann Parenth,* 3:85, 1967.
31. O'Brien FB, Stewart WC, Sturtevant FM: Incidence of pelvic inflammatory disease in clinical trials with Cu-7 (intrauterine contraceptive device): A statistical analysis. *Contraception,* 27:111, 1983.

23

Diagnosis of Tubal Pregnancy

Gary Holtz and
Abdol H. Hosseinian

A dramatic increase has been reported in the number of patients being evaluated and treated for tubal pregnancy. In 1980, over 52,000 women suffered from this condition in the United States.[1] Early diagnosis and proper management can reduce maternal morbidity and mortality secondary to acute blood loss,[2] and enable a more conservative operation that enhances subsequent fertility in some cases.[3] The present chapter describes recent advances in human chorionic gonadotropin (HCG) assay techniques, ultrasonography, and endoscopy, which facilitate early and accurate diagnosis.

Clinical Diagnosis

Tubal pregnancy must be differentiated from pelvic inflammatory disease, rupture or torsion of functional ovarian cysts, anovulatory bleeding, threatened or incomplete abortion, endometriosis, appendicitis, gastroenteritis, urinary tract abnormalities, and pain of undetermined cause. Symptoms and signs are often nonspecific, as reflected in the high frequency of diagnostic errors (36 to 53 percent) reported in recent series of patients with ectopic pregnancies[4–6] and in the large percentage of patients with this tentative diagnosis, in whom it subsequently was not found. Only 20 percent of patients evaluated for tubal pregnancy in a contemporary study[7] had this diagnosis confirmed.

Knowledge of predisposing risk factors involved in the pathogenesis of tubal gestations can often be helpful in evaluating patients (Table 23:1). The increasing incidence of pelvic inflammatory disease clearly correlates with the rise in ectopic pregnancy.[8] Such disease has been estimated to increase the risk six- to tenfold.[9] Also frequently associated is a history of pelvic surgery; approximately 25 percent of patients with a tubal pregnancy had undergone previous pelvic operations.[5] Tubal reconstructive surgery is a significant risk factor, but other operations such as appendectomy and ovarian cystectomy are also predisposing factors.

Tubal sterilization more effectively prevents intrauterine pregnancy than ec-

The Fallopian Tube: Basic Studies and Clinical Contributions, edited by Alvin M. Siegler, M.D. Mount Kisco, New York: Futura Publishing Company, Inc. © 1986.

Table 23:1

Risk Factors for Tubal Pregnancy

Risk factor
Previous PID/endometritis
Previous pelvic surgery
IUD in situ
Previous ectopic pregnancy
Progestin-only oral contraceptive
Estrogen for introception
HMG-induced ovulation
Endometriosis
Advanced maternal age
Abortion
Infertility
Intrauterine DES exposure

Table 23:2

Presenting Symptoms and Signs of Tubal Pregnancy

Symptom	*Frequency (%)*
Abdominal pain	87–99
Abnormal uterine bleeding	48–86
Amenorrhea	61–79
Symptoms of pregnancy	23
Faintness/syncopy	6–37
Shoulder pain	5–22
Passage of tissue	6–7
Physical finding	
Abdominal tenderness	97–99
Adnexal tenderness	87–99
Peritoneal signs	71–76
Adnexal mass	33–53
Enlarged uterus	6–30
Shock	2–17

topic gestations and 12 percent of patients with tubal pregnancies have previously been sterilized.[10] The risk appears to be greatest within the first three years after sterilization and it is particularly high for those who have had tubal cauterization.[11] Patients who have previously had a tubal pregnancy have an increased risk of suffering another one.[12] Indeed, all conceptions achieved by individuals with such previous histories should be considered ectopically located until proven otherwise. Since IUDs prevent intrauterine gestations more effectively than extrauterine ones, tubal conceptions occur proportionately more often in patients with IUDs in situ. Progestin-containing IUDs actually increase the incidence of tubal pregnancy,[13] as do "progestin only" oral contraceptives[14] and postcoital estrogens for introception.[15] Their mechanism of action is believed to be an altering of tubal motility. Other factors implicated include advanced maternal age, pelvic endometriosis, and previous abortion. Whether abortion reduces the incidence of intrauterine pregnancy but not extrauterine ones, or if it predisposes to ectopic implantation, is controversial.

The frequency of presenting symptoms and signs from five recently published series were reviewed (Table 23:2).[4–6,16,17] Relatively few patients presented with the classic triad of pain, uterine bleeding, and an adnexal mass. Abdominal pain was the most common complaint, but it varied in location, being unilateral or bilateral in the lower abdomen, generalized, upper abdominal, in the back or in the vagina. In only a small percentage of patients was it present for more than a week. Shoulder pain, secondary to diaphragmatic irritation from blood, was present in a minority of women. Abnormal vaginal bleeding was noted frequently, occurring as the hormonal support of the decidua became inadequate. In most cases it was not heavy, in contrast to the profuse bleeding that may occur with an incomplete abortion.

Findings on physical examination were also nonspecific. An adnexal mass was not a universal finding and when found, it commonly consisted of a blood clot or a corpus luteum cyst rather than a tubal gestation. Systemic signs of shock were noted less frequently in recent series as advances in ancillary diagnostic modalities made early diagnosis more common. Uterine enlargement, produced by increased vascularity and development of the decidua, may mimic an early intrauterine pregnancy and was not infrequent.

Patients usually were afebrile. Orthostatic changes in blood pressure were noted infrequently in the absence of hypovolemic shock.

Laboratory studies, with the exception of HCG assays, were of minimal diagnostic value. Peripheral hematocrit measurements correlated poorly with the presence or volume of hemoperitoneum.[4] However, serial assessments can, on occasion, be useful.

Culdocentesis

Culdocentesis is used to identify patients with hemoperitoneum. In a positive study, nonclotting blood is aspirated from the cul-de-sac, with a hematocrit greater than 15 percent. Occasional false negative results occur because of obliteration of the cul-de-sac from previous inflammatory disease or endometriosis, insufficient blood in the peritoneal cavity for recovery, and from severe intraabdominal hemorrhage in which the blood clots after removal. When the tube is not ruptured or no blood passes out of the fimbria, culdocentesis will be falsely negative. Eighty-two to ninety-five percent of patients who underwent a culdocentesis in the five series reviewed had positive studies. False positive results are rare but they can occur as a result of inadvertent trauma to a blood vessel or blood refluxed from the uterine cavity. Occasional patients will have a hemoperitoneum produced by other abnormalities.

When should culdocentesis be performed? If the diagnosis is believed unlikely, aspiration may be delayed until after HCG and sonographic results have been evaluated. These studies may preclude the need for culdocentesis. The degree of clinical suspicion establishes the sequence and rapidity with which ancillary modalities are needed.

Uterine Curettage

Dilatation and curettage or menstrual extraction are not routinely used for evaluating patients suspected for a tubal pregnancy, unless vaginal bleeding is significant, because these procedures can interrupt an intrauterine gestation. However, in those women desiring termination of their pregnancies who are clinically stabile, curettage is a rapid, effective, and accurate way to establish the presence of an intrauterine gestation. Tissue obtained is floated in saline to permit observation of villi or a frozen section is examined. Neither the absence of trophoblastic tissue nor the presence of Arias Stella reaction in curettings is sufficient to confirm the diagnosis of tubal pregnancy.

Chorionic Gonadotropin Assays

The early diagnosis of ectopic pregnancy has been made possible by the development of sensitive and specific assays for the beta subunit of HCG. Previously, standard slide or tube urinary pregnancy tests were negative in a substantial minority of patients with ectopic pregnancies. The lower sensitivity of these tests (700 to 1,500 mIU/ml) was inadequate to confirm the diagnosis of pregnancy on many occasions. Radioreceptor assays (sensitivity 100 to 200 mIU/ml) confirmed the presence of a pregnancy in approximately 90 percent of patients with extrauterine conceptions. Specific radioimmunoassays (sensitivity 1.5 to 10 mIU/ml) are widely available and permit detection of pregnancies seven to nine days after conception and advanced laboratory methods have substantially shortened assay times.

By using radioimmunoassays, numerous investigators have reported 99 to 100 percent accuracy in the diagnosis of pregnancy.[18,19] Furthermore, screening patients can exclude two-thirds of patients by being negative.[7,20] Further development in HCG assay technique is occurring with the introduction of commercial immunoassays having a sensitivity comparable to radioreceptor assays. Recently, the diagnostic efficacy of a sensitive (250 mIU/ml) latex agglutination-inhibition tube test was compared to the serum radioimmunoassay.[21] Although the latter was more accurate, the ease and rapidity of the urinary assay and its low cost made it a practical screening method. The development of monoclonal antibody–based enzyme immunoassay techniques for HCG determination in urine offers still further sensitivity. More information can be obtained regarding the quality of a pregnancy by evaluating HCG titer progression and regression curves. While the doubling time for HCG in a normal intrauterine gestation during the first eight weeks of pregnancy is approximately two days,[22] the daily increment in eight patients subsequently found to have ectopic gestations was less than 13 percent.[23] Others have suggested that HCG titers should increase more than 66 percent over 48 hours in a normal pregnancy.[24] Abnormal titer progression reflects the limited ability of trophoblastic tissue located in the fallopian tube to increase HCG production with advancing gestation. Unfortunately, impaired HCG production also may be noted with abnormal intrauterine gestations.

Non-HCG Markers of Trophoblastic Activity

Although advances in methodology make beta HCG assays extremely sensitive and the results rapidly available, single measurements and even serial assessments are sometimes incapable of distinguishing ectopic from intrauterine gestations. Therefore, other markers of trophoblastic activity have been evaluated in conjunction with HCG assays.

Assays for pregnancy-specific beta-1 glycoprotein have comparable sensitivity and diagnostic efficacy to those for beta HCG but they are not superior in distinguishing ectopic gestations or advantageous when used in association with HCG evaluations.[19,21,25] Placental lactogen and cystine aminopeptidase assays cannot detect early pregnancy.[21] Pregnancy-associated plasma protein A, a glycoprotein of placental origin does not consistently appear in the maternal circulation until approximately 30 days after conception, thus limiting its usefulness in distinguishing between normal and abnormal early gestations. In a single case it was reported to be persistently undetectable in a patient with an ectopic gestation of greater than six weeks of age.[26]

Alpha-fetoprotein (AFP) may help to diagnose tubal pregnancy. There is frequently a breakdown in the fetal-maternal barrier, permitting small amounts of fetal serum to enter the maternal circulation. In a small series of patients with ectopic gestations, all had detectable amounts of AFP and two of five had grossly elevated levels.[27] This assay might be useful in evaluation of patients with a positive beta HCG assay of low titer and questionable gestational age.

Ultrasonography

In patients suspected of having an ectopic pregnancy with a positive HCG assay, ultrasonography may help in the evaluation by confirming the presence of an intrauterine gestation; the rare occurrence of an associated heterotopic pregnancy cannot be excluded. Ultrasonography can usually demonstrate an intrauterine gestational sac by five to six weeks and confirm fetal cardiac activity at seven to eight weeks.

Recent reports of pseudogestational sacs being falsely interpreted as intrauterine pregnancies have raised concerns about the accuracy of the procedure.[28] When intrauterine bleeding causes sloughing of the decidua, this artifact occurs. It is possible to distinguish it from a true intrauterine pregnancy by noting the presence of a double decidual ring prior to recognition of an intrauterine embryo. The two concentric rings are thought to be composed of the decidua parietalis and the adjacent decidua capsularis. In a large retrospective review, 59 of 60 patients with double rings had intrauterine pregnancies, whereas of 68 who lacked this finding, only four had normal intrauterine pregnancies. The remainder had either ectopic or abnormal intrauterine gesta-

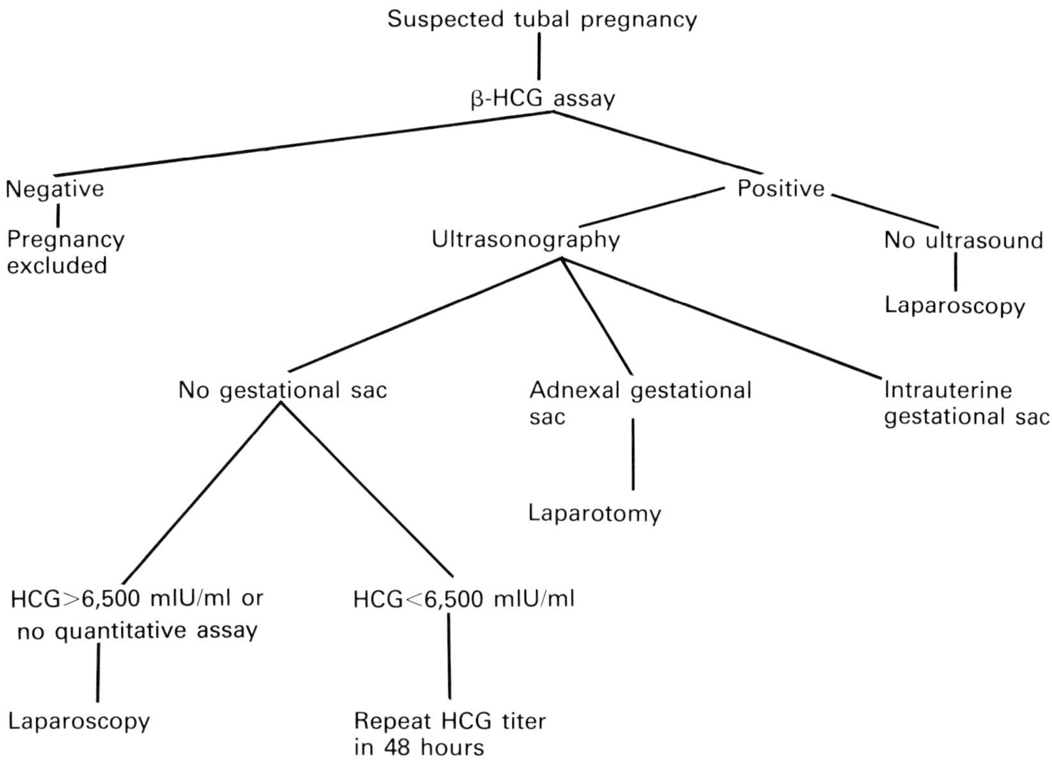

FIGURE 23:1—*Protocol for diagnosing tubal pregnancy.*

tions.[29] Clearly the equipment used and the skill of the ultrasonographer affect the accuracy of this technique.

In only 15 percent of ectopic gestations can a diagnosis be definitively made on the basis of sonographic findings.[30] Diagnostic criteria include the presence of a gestational sac or fetal cardiac activity in the adnexa, and fluid in the cul-de-sac without evidence of an intrauterine gestation. Recently, the use of more advanced equipment has enabled the diagnosis of an ectopic gestation to be correctly made in 8 of 9 patients and excluded in 22 of 23 in one series.[31] The only misdiagnosis was in a patient with a ruptured tubal pregnancy, which is not an uncommon error with ultrasound.

Diagnostic Scheme

Knowledge of the relationship of HCG titers to findings on ultrasonography permits the development of a protocol to identify and exclude more accurately those patients who are not pregnant (Fig. 23:1). Women who are clinically stabile without hemoperitoneum and whose pregnancy tests are positive should have sonography. If an intrauterine gestational sac is seen, an ectopic pregnancy is essentially excluded. Similarly, the presence of an adnexal gestational sac excludes the need for further diagnostic studies. Individuals with positive pregnancy tests, in the absence of a gestational sac, can be divided into two subgroups: (1) patients with serum concentrations of beta HCG $> 6{,}500$ mIU/ml should have laparoscopy to rule out an ectopic pregnancy; (2) patients with serum concentrations of beta HCG $<$ 6,500 mIU/ml can be followed by serial quantitative assays to assess deviation from the normal pattern established for intrauterine gestations.

The use of such a protocol can delay

the diagnosis of ectopic pregnancy in 13 percent of patients and identify incorrectly 15 percent of those with intrauterine gestations.[32] However, by following this diagnostic scheme, it was possible to increase the preoperative diagnostic accuracy to 93 percent while reducing the incidence of ruptured ectopic gestation by over 40 percent at the Cook County Hospital.[23] Obviously, patients with a clinical picture of a ruptured ectopic gestation require immediate operative intervention.

Laparoscopy

Laparoscopy is a definitive diagnostic procedure unless the view and mobility of the pelvic structures are obstructed by pelvic adhesions. In addition, a very early tubal gestation can be too small to enable its recognition. The two puncture technique is necessary for the successful observation of the pelvis; no intrauterine elevator is used because it might interrupt a normal nidation. Unless both tubes are observed from cornu to fimbria, a laparotomy should ensue. Approximately 1 percent of patients have a technically inadequate laparoscopy and 50 percent of them have ectopic gestations.[33]

References

1. Dorfman SF: Deaths from ectopic pregnancy, United States, 1979 to 1980. *Obstet Gynecol*, 62:334, 1983.
2. Rubin GL, Peterson HB, Dorfman BF, et al: Ectopic pregnancy in the United States, 1970 through 1978. *JAMA*, 249:1725, 1983.
3. Sherman D, Langer R, Sadovsky G, et al: Improved fertility following ectopic pregnancy. *Fertil Steril*, 37:497, 1982.
4. Alsuleiman SA, Grimes EM: Ectopic pregnancy; A review of 147 cases, *J Reprod Med*, 27:101, 1982.
5. Brenner PF, Roy S, Mishell DR: Ectopic pregnancy; A study of 300 consecutive surgically treated cases. *JAMA*, 243:673, 1980.
6. Weinstein L, Morris MB, Dotters D, et al: Ectopic pregnancy—A new surgical epidemic. *Obstet Gynecol* 61:698, 1983.
7. Bryson SCP: β- subunit of human chorionic gonadotropin, ultrasound, and ectopic pregnancy: A prospective study. *Am J Obstet Gynecol*, 146:163, 1983.
8. St John RK, Blout J, Jones OG: Pelvic inflammatory disease in the United States: Incidence and trends in private practice. *Sex Trans Dis*, 8:56, 1981.
9. Weström L: Incidence, prevalence, and trends of acute pelvic inflammatory disease and its consequence in industrialized countries. *Am J Obstet Gynecol*, 138:880, 1980.
10. Kumar J, Oxorn H: Ectopic pregnancy following tubal sterilization. *Can Med Assoc J*, 119:156, 1978.
11. McCausland A: High rate of ectopic pregnancy following laparoscopic tubal coagulation failures. *Am J Obstet Gynecol*, 136:97, 1980.
12. Schoen JA, Nowak RJ: Repeat ectopic pregnancy, a 16-year clinical survey. *Obstet Gynecol*, 45:542, 1975.
13. Snowden R: The Progestasert and ectopic pregnancy. *Br Med J*, 2:1600, 1977.
14. Smith M, Vessey M, Bounds M, et al: Progesterone only oral contraception and ectopic gestation. *Br Med J*, 4:104, 1974.
15. Morris JM, Van Wagenen G: Introception: The use of post-ovulatory estrogens to prevent implantation. *Am J Obstet Gynecol*, 115:101, 1973.
16. Kitchin JD III, Wein RM, Nunley WC, et al: Ectopic pregnancy: Current clinical trends. *Am J Obstet Gynecol*, 134:870, 1979.
17. DeCherney AH, Minkin MJ, Spangler S: Contemporary management of ectopic pregnancy. *J Reprod Med*, 26:519, 1981.
18. Schwartz RD, DiPetro DL: β-HCG as a diagnostic aid for suspected ectopic pregnancy. *Obstet Gynecol*, 56:197, 1980.
19. Seppälä M, Venesmaa P, Rutanen EM: Pregnancy-specific beta-1 glycoprotein in ectopic pregnancy. *Am J Obstet Gynecol*, 136:189, 1980.
20. Hussa RO: Clinical utility of human chorionic gonadotropin and α-subunit measurements. *Obstet Gynecol*, 60:1, 1982.
21. Braunstein GD, Asch RH: Predictive value analysis of measurements of hu-

man chorionic gonadotropin, pregnancy specific β_1-glycoprotein, placental lactogen, and cystine aminopeptidase for the diagnosis of ectopic pregnancy. *Fertil Steril*, 39:62, 1983.

22. Corson SL, Batzer FR, Schlaff S: A comparison of serial quantitative serum and urine tests in early pregnancy. *J Reprod Med*, 26:611, 1981.
23. Hosseinian AH, Morales WA, Kulkarni B: Evaluation of the usefulness of serum HCG and ultrasound for detection of ectopic pregnancy. Unpublished data, 1983.
24. Kadar N, Caldwell BV, Romero R: A method of screening for ectopic pregnancy and its indications. *Obstet Gynecol*, 58:162, 1981.
25. Kaupila A, Rantakylä P, Huhtaniemi I, et al: Trophoblastic markers in the differential diagnosis of ectopic pregnancy. *Obstet Gynecol*, 55:560, 1980.
26. Sinosich MJ, Smith DH, Grudzinskas JG, et al: The prediction of pregnancy failure by measurement of pregnancy-associated plasma protein A (PAPP-A) following in vitro fertilization and embryo transfer. *Fertil Steril*, 40:539, 1983.
27. Cederqvist LL, Killackey MA, Abdel-Latif N, et al: α-Fetoprotein and ectopic pregnancy. *Br Med J*, 286:1247, 1983.
28. Weiner CP: The pseudogestational sac in ectopic pregnancy. *Am J Obstet Gynecol*, 139:959, 1981.
29. Nyberg DA, Laing FC, Filly RA, et al: Ultrasonographic differentiation of the gestational sac of early pregnancy from the pseudogestational sac of ectopic pregnancy. *Radiology*, 146:755, 1983.
30. Lawson TL: Ectopic pregnancy: Criteria and accuracy of ultrasonic diagnosis. *Am J Roent*, 131:153, 1978.
31. Gleicher N, Giglia RV, Deppe G, et al: Direct diagnosis of unruptured ectopic pregnancy by real-time ultrasonography. *Obstet Gynecol*, 61:425, 1983.
32. Kadar N, DeVore G, Romero R: Discriminatory HCG zone: Its use in the sonographic evaluation for ectopic pregnancy. *Obstet Gynecol*, 58:156, 1981.
33. Esposito JM: Ectopic pregnancy: The laparoscope as a diagnostic aid. *J Reprod Med*, 25:17, 1980.

24

Laparoscopy for Infertility and Pelvic Pain

Donald E. Pittaway and
Jamil A. Fayez

Although used to investigate and treat a multitude of disorders, laparoscopy is most often performed to confirm or rule out pelvic abnormalities that may be responsible for infertility or for pelvic pain.[1] In addition, laparoscopy may be necessary on an emergency basis following abdominal trauma or surgical complications such as perforation of the uterus during hysteroscopy or during a dilatation and currettage. In this chapter, we address the preoperative evaluation and counseling of women with infertility or pelvic pain and the technical aspects of laparoscopy.

The Infertile Patient

The goals of an infertility evaluation are to ascertain the causes of infertility, and depending on the findings, to provide the couple with therapeutic options and prognosis. To accomplish these goals, several factors (male, ovulatory, cervical, uterine, tubal, peritoneal) must be systematically investigated (Table 24:1). When such an evaluation has been completed, a cause for the infertility will be found in more than 90 percent of the couples.[2]

The laparoscopic examination is an important part of any infertility evaluation since tubal and peritoneal factors account for approximately 30 to 40 percent of infertility.[3] However, the preoperative evaluation should be completed first to rule out other causes of infertility. Delaying laparoscopy will allow time and opportunity for a small percentage of couples to conceive during the evaluation. Information provided to the couple such as the fertile period of the cycle, the adverse effects of lubricants, the therapeutic effects of hysterosalpingography or the correction of ovulatory dysfunction may result in a pregnancy and avoid an unnecessary operation. Furthermore, when laparoscopy reveals tubal occlusion, peritubal adhesions, or endometriosis, the best estimate of the prognosis cannot be provided to the couple without

The Fallopian Tube: Basic Studies and Clinical Contributions, edited by Alvin M. Siegler, M.D. Mount Kisco, New York: Futura Publishing Company, Inc. © 1986.

Table 24:1

Summary of the Preoperative Infertility Evaluation

Factor	Evaluation: Initial	Evaluation: Secondary
Male	Semen analysis Postcoital test	Antisperm antibodies Mucus penetration Hamster egg penetration
Ovulatory	History Basal temperature Endometrial biopsy	
Cervical	Papanicolaou smear Postcoital test	Antisperm antibodies Mucus penetration
Uterine	Hysterosalpingogram Endometrial biopsy	Office microhysteroscopy(?)
Tubal	Hysterosalpingogram	
Peritoneal	Hysterosalpingogram	

a consideration of all aspects of the case.

Since there are several excellent descriptions of the evaluation of infertility,[3–5] it is not our intent to present a detailed summary. An evaluation of infertility must be thorough and succinct with the preoperative portion usually completed within six to eight weeks in an ovulatory patient (Table 24:1). During the initial visit, the history of the couple is particularly important and special attention should be paid to age, duration of infertility, medical or surgical conditions, and any previous infertility evaluation or therapy. A gynecologic examination should be performed, including a Papanicolaou smear and blood tests for rubella immunity. The infertility evaluation should be explained to the couple and a plan formulated for the necessary tests.

Ovulation is presumed in women with regular cycles (30 $\pm$ 4 days and a basal body temperature chart is used to assist in the scheduling and interpretation of certain tests. A semen analysis is scheduled early in the evaluation since approximately 40 to 50 percent of infertility is caused by a male factor. Depending on the time of the menstrual cycle, the next step is scheduled, i.e., hysterosalpingography (postmenstrual), postcoital test (preovulatory), and endometrial biopsy, (a few days prior to the anticipated menses). If a test is abnormal, it is repeated as needed or evaluated further with additional studies such as antisperm antibody or mucus penetration tests (Table 24:1). Treatment is recommended to correct any problems that may be discovered. Further evaluation of abnormal hysterosalpingograms by laparoscopy is necessary to confirm the abnormality and to discover its extent. Approximately 56 to 75 percent of women in whom no cause for infertility is found during the preoperative evaluation will be shown to have peritubal adhesions or endometriosis when laparoscopy is performed.[6,7] Consequently, no infertility evaluation is considered complete without a laparoscopic examination.

The Patient with Pelvic Pain

Pain is the primary complaint in approximately 25 percent of all patients (ex-

Table 24:2

Possible Causes of Pelvic Pain

Gynecologic		
Tubal	*Nontubal*	*Nongynecologic*
Ectopic pregnancy	Abdominal pregnancy	*Gastrointestinal*
Endometriosis	Adenomyosis	Appendiceal disease
Hydrosalpinx	Cervicitis	Diverticulitis
Peritubal adhesions	Endometriosis	Gastroenteritis
Salpingitis	Endometritis	Inflammatory bowel disease
Torsion of the adnexa	Malignancy	Intestinal fistula
Torsion of a hydatid cyst	Menstruation	Intestinal obstruction
Tubal carcinoma	Mittelschmerz	Irritable bowel syndrome
	Ovarian cyst	Malignancy
	Pelvic congestion	Ruptured viscus
	Pelvic inflammatory disease	Volvulus
	Postoperative adhesions	*Urologic*
	Ruptured corpus luteum	Trigonitis
	Torsion of ovarian cyst	Ureteral obstruction
	Uterine descensus	Urinary tract infection
	Uterine myomata	*Musculoskeletal*
		Neurological
		Psychogenic

cluding visits for contraception) presenting to a nonspecialized gynecologic practice,[8] and is a major indication for diagnostic endoscopy.[1] The cause of pelvic pain is frequently misdiagnosed prior to laparoscopic examination, and the discomfort may be gynecologic, nongynecologic or combined (Table 24:2). Consequently, the evaluation of pelvic pain requires a thorough history and physical examination, laboratory and radiological tests when the cause is obscure. Frequently, in cases of chronic or recurrent pain, therapeutic trials with medication before laparoscopy are indicated.

The history and physical examination of a patient with pelvic pain are the most important aspects of the evaluation. The physician should ask about the location and the quality of the pain, any associated symptoms or signs, and whether it is acute, chronic, or recurrent. Past medical and surgical histories may be relevant, as is the association of pain with menses or sexual intercourse. The physical examination may confirm the presumptive diagnosis suspected by the historic information.

When the diagnosis remains obscure after a thorough history and examination, the completed workup should include laparoscopy. The diagnostic approaches to acute and chronic pelvic pain have been described in detail.[8–10] The physician must decide whether the pain requires an immediate operation (i.e., to rule out tubal pregnancy). If no operation is warranted, then other laboratory and radiological tests may be needed. Consultation with other medical and surgical specialists may be beneficial. When the diagnosis is still not certain and medication has not alleviated the pain, then a laparoscopy should be performed. Frequently with endometriosis or adhesions, not only does the laparoscopy reveal the cause of the pain but therapeutic laparoscopic techniques relieve the symptoms. In patients with pain of suspected psychogenic origin, organic causes must first be eliminated by including a laparoscopic examination before referring the patient for psychological evaluation.

Laparoscopy

Preoperative counseling of the patient considering laparoscopy should include an explanation of the technique, the types of information that can be obtained, the benefits, risks, and potential complications, and alternative approaches to the problem. If therapeutic laparoscopy is anticipated, these techniques should be discussed, including the possibility of a laparotomy which may be a planned extension of the laparoscopy, as required, to treat the problem or an emergency procedure if a complication occurs. Contraindications to a laparoscopy include generalized peritonitis, ileus and bowel obstruction, hiatal or abdominal hernias, tuberculous peritonitis, and severe cardiopulmonary disease. Large intraabdominal masses, extensive intraabdominal adhesions, extreme obesity, and advanced pregnancy are considered relative contraindications.

Laparoscopy may be performed as either an outpatient or inpatient procedure in a patient less than 40 years of age without any significant medical illnesses (ASA Class I). However, when therapeutic laparoscopy is anticipated, admittance to the hospital is preferred. Approximately 80 to 90 percent of patients will be able to leave the hospital within four to six hours postoperatively. The availability of an efficient outpatient surgical section, the relative cost, and the patient's preference will often influence whether admittance is arranged preoperatively.

Although local anesthesia has been used for certain laparoscopic sterilization procedures[11] and regional anesthesia has been employed,[12] general anesthesia with endotracheal intubation is preferable for diagnostic and operative laparoscopy.[13] The techniques of general anesthesia for laparoscopy have been tailored for fairly rapid postoperative recovery and provide the necessary analgesia and relaxation for obtaining an adequate pneumoperitoneum and for performing laparoscopic procedures which may include manipulation of the pelvic organs, chromopertubation, fulguration or vaporization, lysis of adhesions, tubal surgery, drainage or aspiration of cysts, and irrigation (and suction) of the pelvic structures.

The instruments, operating room preparation, and techniques of laparoscopy have been previously summarized.[6,14–16] In general, the techniques must maximize safety and provide the necessary information. These include adequate observation of the pelvic and abdominal structures and, for therapeutic laparoscopy, sufficient access, exposure, and retraction of pelvic structures so that procedures can be performed effectively and safely. At least two punctures are required, the first for the laparoscope and a second midline suprapubic site for manipulation, retraction, or positioning of pelvic viscera. A third puncture is required occasionally and is placed laterally in either lower quadrant after transillumination to locate large subcutaneous vessels.

The laparoscopic examination must be systematic and thorough. The use of photography, standardized forms, or classifications for documenting the pelvic findings such as those available from the American Fertility Society (1985)[17] are recommended. If therapeutic operative techniques are performed, these procedures must be completely described.

Postoperatively the findings, type of procedures, and postoperative instructions are explained to the patient after she is lucid. The consequences of the findings, the prognosis, and follow-up therapy are outlined but an in-depth discussion of these topics is deferred to the first postoperative visit.

References

1. Chamberlain G, Brown JC: Gynaecological laparoscopy. Report of the Confi-

dential Enquiry into Gynaecological Laparoscopy, Royal College of Obstetricians and Gynaecologists, London, 1978.
2. Drake T, Tredway D, Buchanan G, et al: Unexplained infertility. *Obstet Gynecol*, 50:644, 1977.
3. Hammond MG, Talbert LM: Infertility. Chapel Hill: Health Sciences Consortium, 1981.
4. Glass RH: Infertility. In Yen SSC, Jaffe RB (Eds): *Reproductive Endocrinology*. Philadelphia: WB Saunders, 1978: p. 398.
5. Wentz AC: *Manual of Gynecologic Endocrinology and Infertility*. Baltimore: Williams and Wilkins, 1979.
6. Corson SL: Operating room preparation and basic techniques. In Phillips JM (Ed): *Laparoscopy*, Baltimore: Williams and Wilkins, 1977: p. 88.
7. Wood GP: Laparoscopic examination of the normal infertile woman. *Obstet Gynecol*, 62:642, 1983.
8. Renaer M: *Chronic Pelvic Pain in Women*. Berlin: Springer-Verlag, 1981.
9. Cope Z: *Cope's Diagnosis of the Acute Abdomen*, revised by William Silen, 16th ed. New York: Oxford University Press, 1983.
10. Beal JM, Raffensperger JC: *Diagnosis of Acute Abdominal Disease*. Philadelphia: Lea & Febiger, 1979.
11. Wheeless CR: Outpatient laparoscopy sterilization under local anesthesia. *Obstet Gynecol*, 39:767, 1972.
12. Aribarg A: Epidural analgesia for laparoscopy. *J Obstet Gynaecol Br Commonw*, 80:567, 1973.
13. Fishburne JI, Keith L: Anesthesia. In Phillips JM (Ed): *Laparoscopy*. Baltimore: Williams & Wilkins, 1979: p. 69.
14. Wheeless CR: Laparoscopy. In Mattingly RF (Ed): *Telinde's Operative Gynecology*, 5th ed. Philadelphia: JB Lippincott, 1977: p. 549.
15. Corson SL: Use of the laparoscope in the infertile patient. *Fertil Steril*, 32:359, 1979.
16. Cohen MR: Gynecologic laparoscopy. In Sciarra JJ (Ed): *Obstetrics and Gynecology*, vol. 1. Hagerstown, MD: Harper & Row, 1981.
17. American Fertility Society, Revised classification of endometriosis: 1985. *Fertil Steril*, 43:351, 1985.

III

Sterilization

Editorial Comments

Voluntary sterilization is the most prevalent method of regulating fertility but there remains a compelling need for developing new methods that are safe, effective outpatient procedures. Hosseinian, and Hamou and his coworkers have described their current use and evaluation of the hysteroscopic approach to the uterotubal ostia.

Hysteroscopy

For more than a century, physicians have searched for a way to occlude the fallopian tubes at their uterotubal junction. The width of the ostia in the intramural segment is less than 0.5 mm; the endosalpinx is lined with low-columnar cells. The three-layered surrounding muscular wall is the thickest area of the fallopian tube and this intramural segment is about 2 cm in length. Although no anatomical sphincter has ever been discovered, hysterosalpingograms can identify the intramural segment as a small triangle whose base is toward the uterus with straight or convex side walls and the apex points at the tubal isthmus. An interruption in the continuity of contrast material usually occurs at the base of the triangle and separates the intramural segment from the uterine cornua. An anatomical basis for this radiological finding seems to be a mucosal fold at the transition between the endometrium and endosalpinx that is often seen during hysteroscopy.

Sterilization at the uterotubal ostia has been by indirect transcervical techniques and through direct observation by hysteroscopy. As early as 1849, Froriep[1] infused a solution of silver nitrate into the uterine cavity to occlude the ostia. Kocks in 1878[2] reported his early attempts at transcervical sterilization by cauterizing the ostia at the cornua. Similar techniques, with specially designed probes and balloons without benefit of direct observation, have been reported. Since permanent tubal occlusion occurred in only 80 percent of these patients, the results were considered unacceptable.

The endoscopic approach to the tubal ostia for sterilization was initially suggested by von Mikulicz-Radecki and Freund in 1927.[3] They cited the need to destroy the endosalpinx and part of the myometrium to prevent recanalization following cauterization of the intramural segments of experimental animals. A few

The Fallopian Tube: Basic Studies and Clinical Contributions, edited by Alvin M. Siegler, M.D. Mount Kisco, New York: Futura Publishing Company, Inc. © 1986.

of these operations were done on women and followed soon afterwards with a hysterectomy to study the tissue effects of coagulation.

Schroeder[4] reported the results of hysteroscopic tubal sterilization by electrocoagulation and hysterosalpingograms done two weeks postoperatively in two women. Since the radiological study showed tubal patency, the sterilizaton procedure was considered inadequate; the patients were subsequently sterilized at laparotomy. Although Norment[5] described fulguration of the cornual ostia under hysteroscopic control, he never disclosed the number of patients treated or the results.

The potential advantage of hysteroscopic sterilization is the avoidance of hospitalization, general anesthesia, entering the peritoneal cavity, and an abdominal scar. In 1973 a workshop on hysteroscopic sterilization was convened in Minneapolis where 17 experts discussed this new technique[6] with the anticipation that it would prove safe, effective, and easily learned. The consensus was that patients had to be treated between days five and nine of the cycle because it seemed difficult to locate the tubal opening routinely during the secretory phase. When the uterotubal ostium is clearly seen, it is easy to insert a probe and perform electrocoagulation. Probably 75 to 100 operations were needed before ostial identification became consistent. The active end of the probe was between 5 and 8 mm long and 1 to 2 mm wide but no consensus emerged at this symposium on the electrosurgical factors involved.

Carbon dioxide, dextran, polyvinylpyrrolidone, dextrose 5 percent, and physiological saline had all been used to distend the uterine cavity during the procedures.

The number of operations performed grew slowly and cautious optimism continued to be expressed. Sugimoto[7] performed 38 procedures but no follow-up results were noted. Neuwirth[8] described hysteroscopic electrosurgical sterilization, with dextran 32 percent as the distending medium in 93 patients, and found that three patients had both tubes patent and 16 others had at least one open tube postoperatively, a patency rate of 20 percent. In 1976, Quinones and coworkers[9] reported 930 hysteroscopic electrosurgical tubal sterilizations under paracervical block. The patients had to be in the follicular phase and the silastic-tip electrode was inserted 6 mm into the intramural segment. Electrocoagulation was precise, 25 watts at the end of the probe for 8 to 10 seconds. Vaginitis, cervicitis, myomas, or uterine abnormalities that distorted the cavity were contraindications to the procedure. Patients were discharged 20 minutes postoperatively and only a few minor complications occurred. Temporary contraception, either intrauterine devices (IUDs) or oral contraceptives, were advised until a hysterosalpingogram taken 12 to 14 weeks postoperatively confirmed occlusion. Hysterosalpingograms were performed on 552 women; 115 (17.3 percent) showed unilateral or bilateral patency. These women were resterilized by the same technique and 112 (98 percent) of them subsequently had bilateral tubal occlusion. No pregnancies occurred in 513 patients who had bilateral occlusion and were followed for one year. Of the six pregnancies reported from the entire group, three occurred in the interstitial segment.

Lindemann and Mohr[10] observed at least one patent tube on hysterosalpingography in 33 of 124 women 12 weeks postoperatively. They believed that functional sterility resulted from destruction of the tubal "sphincter" preventing the fertilized ovum from remaining in the tube long enough for maturation. Since histologic studies of some cauterized segments showed significant endosalpingeal destruction, it was speculated that a postoperative pregnancy might represent a failure to detect patency by hysterosalpingography because recanalization was unlikely. In a subsequent report on 580 patients studied postoperatively with hysterosalpingography, Lindemann[11] noted that 14 percent had at least one patent tube. Rimkus and Semm[12] reported results from 50 operations, with 49 of their patients having follow-up hysterosalpingograms. At least one patent tube was seen in 61 percent, in two instances the thermal probe perforated the uterus, and five intrauterine pregnancies occurred. The hysterosalpingograms in these women do not show the intramural segment whereas after tubal sterilization by either laparoscopy or laparotomy this region is opacified.

Hysteroscopic sterilization with electrocoagulation fell into disfavor because of a high tubal patency rate and pregnancies postoperatively, and reports of serious complications.[13] In a collaborative study, investigators reported between 6 and 298 operations (a total of 773) with an overall failure rate of 33 percent. Even in 349 women whose hysterosalpingograms showed closed fallopian tubes bilaterally, 11 pregnancies were reported. Second sterilizations were done in 27 percent of the patients and a persistent patency was noted in 18 percent of these women. Sixteen patients had a third sterilization by hysteroscopy and three continued to show some patency. The major complications included seven uterine perforations, six ectopic pregnancies, seven bowel damages and peritonitis; one mortality was caused by an unrecognized bowel perforation. Only 25 percent of the patients were followed for more than six months. The report concluded that hysteroscopic electrosurgical sterilization was not simple or reliable. It required a highly skilled gynecologist and a special time in the patient's cycle. There was no objective endpoint, electrodes and generators were unpredictable, and the influence of the medium surrounding the electrode was undetermined.

Tubal plugs can be created by flowing a catalyzed liquid silicone polymer into the oviduct through a silicone rubber obturator tip positioned at the tubal ostium. The formed-in-place plug becomes bonded to the tip, resulting in a flexible structure that is larger in diameter at both ends than it is in the isthmus, thus remaining in place to effect tubal occlusion.

Corfman and Taylor[14] were the first to mention the concept of silicone plugs. Experiments with rabbits were reported by Hefnawi and associates[15] who demonstrated that this approach did not interfere with ovarian function, produced no salpingitis, and the procedure was reversible. The antifertility efficacy of the plug was 100 percent when the device was in the isthmus but declined greatly if the plug only filled the ampulla. Unfortunately many experimental animals expelled the cured plugs into the peritoneal cavity. Rakshit's technique[16] involved filling the entire uterine cavity with silastic material with flow into the oviducts, and an antifertility efficacy after 11 months to two years. Erb[17] developed special instruments, combinations of ingredients and techniques to form effective plugs, providing a practical approach.[17]

Although the successful tubal occlusion with these plugs has been noteworthy, problems and concerns remain. These include the need for a follow-up pelvic x-ray or hysterosalpingogram to evaluate the continuity of the plug and to detect any migration. Other problems at the time of hysteroscopy include uterotubal spasm, inadequate observation of the ostia because of mucus or blood and the failure to obtain parallel axis.[18]

The benefits of the new procedure include its being an office procedure done under paracervical block with minimal discomfort in most cases,[19] few patients are not acceptable candidates, the risks and complications are minimal, expenses are less than those encountered with traditional sterilization procedures, and most patients can return to normal daily activities on the day of the operation. When abnormal plugs are formed, they can be removed at hysteroscopy and normal plugs placed. Hysteroscopic sterilization remains experimental and no evidence exists at present that subsequent removal of plugs or devices will result in tubal patency and subsequent normal intrauterine pregnancy.

Temporary (Reversible) Sterilization

Methods of temporary or reversible sterilization have been described for almost a century but it was unusual to find reports of attempts made to reverse them.[20–46] Innovators expressed optimism that their operation would give the patient who changed her mind about the sterilization the opportunity to become fertile again. Initial sterilization required a laparotomy, some methods had unacceptable failure rates, and a second laparotomy was needed to reverse the procedure.

Meeker and Roth describe a tubal plug and clip method which was successfully reversed in baboons. The plugs were inserted at a minilaparotomy, clipped in place, and subsequently removed.

Several authors described sterilization by fimbrial fixation into a new location and designed the operation for temporary sterilization. However, burying of fimbria often failed as a method of sterilization, fimbria tended to adhere to the broad ligament, and the technique for reversal required a major abdominal operation (Table III:1).

If reversible sterilization is developed, it must be viewed as temporary contraception. The importance of reversibility and the acceptance of sterilization have not been definitely ascertained. The concept of reversibility might enhance the popularity and acceptability of sterilization helping to eliminate some religious and cultural objections. Nevertheless, the thrust and wisdom to develop reversible methods of sterilization are questionable for several reasons: (1) there is a large disparity between the number of sterilizations performed and the number of requests for reversal; (2) in developing countries the current demand for permanent sterilization exceeds the capacity to deliver these services; (3) the enrollment of women into an experimental program designed to test the efficacy of a reversible method is ethically unfeasible.

Current Sterilization Methods and Complications

Ansari and his colleagues, and Barwin have briefly reviewed current sterilization techniques performed at laparotomy and laparoscopy. The latter has proven safe and effective in the hands of well-trained surgeons in appropriate settings. It is done by open or closed methods, with either a single or double puncture technique, under local or general anesthesia, with electrocoagulation, tubal rings, or clips. However, outside of major urban centers, and especially in the postpartum patient, minilaparotomy with the Pomeroy technique appears to be superior in terms of failures and complications.

Riedel and coworkers continue to demonstrate by histologic, histochemical, and electromicroscopic examinations that the amount of tissue destroyed during sterilization by electrocoagulation and bipolar techniques operated at lower coagulation currents is insignificant compared to the destruction caused by the monopolar method.

A comprehensive review by Peterson and coauthors focuses on immediate and delayed complications of female sterilization. Of special interest is the analysis of results from the Collaborative Review of Sterilization (CREST) in which 12 hospitals or outpatient surgical facilities in six U.S. cities participated in a prospective cohort study since 1978.

Patients occasionally manifest gynecologic and psychological problems in the so-called post-tubal ligation syndrome. The patient's attitude toward menstruation is a difficult factor to evaluate and clearly any possible claim of menstrual dysfunction after sterilization must be assessed in this light. Thus far, the only consistent finding in women complaining of this "syndrome" is a history of heavy menses prior to sterilization often masked by the use of oral contraceptives.

The evidence concerning ovarian steroidogenesis postoperatively has been conflicting and it is difficult to understand the mechanism for interference with the ovarian blood supply by the uncomplicated application of a ring or clip. Indeed, in several studies following a hysterectomy in younger women who had ovarian conservation, normal ovulatory cycles continued in most patients. There is no

Table III:1

Sterilization Procedures Devised for Reversibility in Women

Year	*Author*	*Technique*
1897	Buettner[20]	Infundibulectomy with serosal covering.
1905	Rissmann[21]	Cornual wedge resection, tube left intact.
1911	Pana[22]	Peritoneal exclusion of ovary.
1913	Selheim[23]	Extraperitonealization of fimbria into broad ligament.
1913	DeTarnowsky[24]	Distal stumps anchored into subserosal canal on posterior wall.
1913	Holzapfel[25]	Tubal transection 22 cm from uterus and distal ends placed into broad ligament.
1915	Stoeckel[26]	¾ of tube placed into rectus fascia and abdominal muscle.
1917	Nürnberger[27]	Tube placed in inguinal canal between abdominal muscles and fascia.
1919	Turenne[28]	Fimbriated end placed into posterior leaf of broad ligament.
1921	Hellendall[29]	Subcutaneous extraperitonealization of tubes.
1921	Wessel[30]	Extraperitonealization of ovaries into inguinal canal.
1923	Freund[31]	Submucosal extraperitonealization of tubes into anterior vaginal wall.
1934	Aldridge[32]	Extraperitonealization of distal ends of tubes into broad ligament.
1967	Skouvaklis[33]	Resection of small intramural-isthmic segment.
1969	Wood and Leeton[34]	Ovariotexy with ovaries placed into silastic bags and then into broad ligament.
1971	Oberli and Rieben[35]	Resection of small intramural isthmic segment.
1976	Brueschke[36]	Hysteroscopic placement of reversible occlusive devices.
1976	Camelo et al.[37]	Ovariotexy.
1976	Koschnick and Magnus[38]	Vaginal application of plastic clips.
1976	Brun and Ducarme[39]	Ovariotexy.
1978	Mahgoub[40]	Extraperitoneal anterior transposition of ovaries below round ligaments.
1978	Sugimoto[41]	Intratubal contraceptive.
1981	Steptoe[43]	Intratubal devices placed by laparoscope.
1981	Chang[44]	Transection of tubes; cauterization of transected ends.
1982	Tierzi and Zanno[45]	Salpingodeviation; fimbriated ends placed into broad ligament.
1983	Reed and Erb[42]	Hysteroscopic occlusive blocking device.
1983	Taylor and Hamou[46]	Hysteroscopic placement of occlusive device.

increase in menstrual disorders subsequent to surgical tubal sterilization in women when compared to a similar nonsterilized group who solved their multiparity problems by vasectomy. Women who have irregular vaginal bleeding prior to sterilization might select another method of birth control to solve their combined problem.

Accidental pregnancies seem to increase during the years following sterilization so that true pregnancy rates really cannot be ascertained after only the first postoperative year. After five years, most of the pregnancies will have occurred and at least half of them will be extrauterine. Interestingly enough in most series, pregnancy is uncommon during the first year but its incidence can increase to almost 1 in 100 operations after seven years. The majority of ectopics occur in the distal tubal segment by fertilization from a sperm passing through a fistula in the proximal segment and finding its way into the fimbriated end. Tubal coagulation without division has a very low failure rate. Tuboperitoneal fistulas can result from tubal division after cautery, following fimbriectomy or even after salpingectomy. Properly placed mechanical devices, clips, or falope rings are associated with a failure rate of less than 0.5 percent.

Intestinal damage caused by bipolar cautery is generally less extensive than that from using a unipolar technique. Following the serosal injury caused from a bipolar instrument (if it is small and shallow), the patient can be observed. On the other hand, laparotomy and excision of the burned area with suturing of the defect is appropriate if the injured area appears more involved.

With a unipolar current, the extent of the damage is more difficult to assess and wider margins must be resected because tissue necrosis can occur as far as 5 cm from the visible burn. Irrigation, drainage, and antibiotic therapy are indicated in such instances.

Approximately 600,00 women are sterilized in the United States each year and although death is rarely associated with the operation, it has been reported in about 4 per 100,000 operations. Almost half of the deaths have resulted from anesthetic complications, other deaths were caused by either postoperative sepsis or hemorrhage.

References

1. Froriep R: Zur Vorbeugung der Nothwendigkeit des Kaiserchnitts und der Perforation. *Notiz Geb Naturund Heilk,* 11:9, 1849.
2. Kocks J: Eine neue Methode der Sterilisation die Frauen. *Zentralb Gynäkol,* 2:617, 1878.
3. Mikulicz-Radecki F, Freund A: Ein neues Hysteroskop und seine praktische Anwendung in der Gynäkologie. *Geburtsh Gynäkol,* 92:13, 1927.
4. Schroeder C: Über den Ausbau und die Keistungen der Hysteroskopie. *Arch Gynäkol,* 156:407, 1934.
5. Norment WB: The hysteroscope. *Am J Obstet Gynecol,* 71:426, 1956.
6. Sciarra JJ, Butler JC, Speidel JJ: *Hysteroscopic Sterlization.* New York: Intercontinental Medical Book Corp., 1974.
7. Sugimoto O: Hysteroscopic sterilization by electrocoagulation. In Sciarra JJ, Butler JC, Speidel IG (Eds): *Hysteroscopic Sterilization.* New York: Intercontinental Medical Book Corp., 1974.
8. Neuwirth RS: *Hysteroscopy.* Philadelphia: WB Saunders, 1975: p. 64.
9. Quinones R, Alvarado A, Ley E: Hysteroscopic sterilization. *Int J Gynecol Obstet,* 16:27, 1976.
10. Lindemann HJ, Mohr J: Tubensterilisation per Hysteroskop. *Sexulmedizin,* 3:122, 1974.
11. Lindemann HJ: Hysteroskopie. In Frangenheim H (Ed): *Die Laparoskopie in der Gynäkologie, Chiurgie und Pädiatrie.* Stuttgart: G. Thieme, 1977.
12. Rimkus V, Semm K: Hysteroscopic sterilization, a routine method? *Int J Fertil,* 22:121, 1977.
13. Darabi K, Richart RM: Collaborative study on hysteroscopic sterilization procedures. *Obstet Gynecol,* 49:48, 1977.
14. Corfman PA, Taylor HC: An instrument for transcervical treatment of the oviduct and uterine cornua. *Obstet Gynecol,* 27:880, 1966.
15. Hefnawi F, Fuchs A, Laurence KA: Control of fertility by temporary occlusion of the oviduct. *Am J Obstet Gynecol,* 99:421, 1967.
16. Rakshit B: Attempts at chemical blocking the fallopian tube for female sterilization. *J Obstet Gynaecol* (India), 20:618, 1970.
17. Erb RA, Davis RH, Kyriazia GA, et al: Device and technique for blocking the fallopian tubes. *Contemp Ob/Gyn,* 3:92, 1974.
18. Reed TP, Erb RA: Tubal occlusion with silicone rubber: An update. *J Reprod Med,* 25:25, 1980.
19. Cooper JM, Houck RM, Rigberg HS: Hysteroscopic tubal occlusion with formed-in-place silicone plugs: A clini-

cal review. *Obstet Gynecol*, 62:587, 1983.
20. Buettner O: Sterilisation mittles Tubendurchschneidung nach Laparotomie. *Zentralb Gynäkol*, 21:1227, 1897.
21. Rissmann P: Die Methoden zur Herbeifuhrung der weiblichen Sterilitat. *Zentralb Gynäkol*, 19:116, 1905.
22. Pana M: Contributo anatomo-patologico alla studio dell" esclusione ovarica della cavita abdominale. *Ann di Ostet*, 33:341, 1911.
23. Selheim O: Schwangershafts Unterbrechung und Sterilisation in einer Sitzung auf abdominalem Wege. *Monat Geburtsh Gynäkol*, 38:166, 1913.
24. DeTarnowsky G: Tubal reimplantation. A new conservative operation for sterilization in women. *JAMA*, 60:1221, 1913.
25. Holzapfel OP: Zur Technik der tubaren Sterilisierung. *Geburtsh Gynäkol*, 74:189, 1913.
26. Stoeckel W: Die extraperitoneale Tubenverlagerung als Methode der Sterilisierung. *Zentralb Gynäkol*, 39:161, 1915.
27. Nürnberger L: *Die sterilisierenden Operationen an den Tuben und ihre Fehlschlage*. Leipzig: JA Barth, 1917.
28. Turenne A: Temporary sterilization of the female. *Surg Gynecol Obstet*, 29:577, 1919.
29. Hellendall H: Eine neue Methode zur temporaren Sterilisierung. *Zentralb Gynäkol*, 45:822, 1921.
30. Wessel O: Eine neue Methode der zeitweiligen Sterilisation der Frau auf operativem Wege. *Zentralb Gynäkol*, 42:75, 1921.
31. Freund H: Die temporare Sterilisation. *Geburtsh Gynäkol*, 47:277, 1923.
32. Aldridge AH: Temporary sterilization with subsequent pregnancy. *Am J Obstet Gynecol*, 27:741, 1934.
33. Skouvaklis M: Sterilisation tubaire interstitielle selon Skouvaklis. *Bull Féd Gynécol Obstèt Franç*, 19:5, 1967.
34. Wood EC, Leeton J: Sterilization by ovariotexy: A reversible technique. *Lancet*, 2:1213, 1969.
35. Oberli H, Rieben G: Tubensterilisation, Versagerquote und Moglichkeit der operativen Refertilisierung. *Schweiz Med Wschr*, 101:1699, 1971.
36. Brueschke EE: Reversible occlusive devices. *J Reprod Med*, 17:103, 1976.
37. Camelo AA, Garcia J, Neto A: A practical method for reversible sterilization in women. *Excerpta Med*, 370:229, 1976.
38. Koschnick KF, Magnus J: Zur ambulaten vaginalen Tubernsterilisation mit dem Kunstoffclip unter besonderer Berucksichtigung der Reversibilitat. *Zentralb Gynäkol*, 98:1518, 1976.
39. Brun G, Ducarme AM: L'ovaire aprés ovariotexie. *J Gynecol Obstet Biol Reprod*, 5:957, 1976.
40. Mahgoub S: Mahgoub's operation: A reversible method of sterilization. *Fertil Steril*, 29:466, 1978.
41. Sugimoto O: *Diagnostic and Therapeutic Hysteroscopy*. Tokyo: Igaku-Shoin, 1978: p. 208.
42. Reed TP III, Erb R: Hysteroscopic tubal occlusion with silicone rubber. *Obstet Gynecol*, 61:388, 1983.
43. Steptoe PC: Endoscopic sterilization. In Hodgson JE (Ed): *Abortion and Sterilization*. New York: Academic Press, 1981: p. 439.
44. Chang MCE: Abdominal sterilization. In Hodgson JE (Ed): *Abortion and Sterilization*. New York: Academic Press, 1981.
45. Tierzi I, Zanno C: Un metodo originale di sterilizazione chirurica reversible feminile: la salpingodeviazione. *Minerva Ginecol*, 34:797, 1982.
46. Taylor PJ, Hamou JE: Hysteroscopy. *J Reprod Med*, 28:389, 1983.

25

History of Tubal Sterilization

Alvin M. Siegler

The history of tubal sterilization, like the history of medicine, describes some of the trials and failures of the early pioneers (Table 25:1). A recapitulation and awareness of their attempts add immeasurably to the fascination with this subject. In 1809, Haighton[1] reported a series of experiments on animal impregnation by dividing rabbit fallopian tubes. Dr. James Blundell[2] (Fig. 25:1), in his *Lectures on the Principles and Practice of Midwifery* given at Guy's Hospital in London, suggested that tubal resection could be performed during cesarean section or as an interval procedure for the purpose of sterilization:

> *[I]f you intercept the contact between the semen and the rudiments, you insure sterility. . . . To preclude the possibility therefore, of a second need for the incision, before closing the abdomen (after performing a cesarean section), the operator, I conceive, ought to remove a portion, say one line, of the Fallopian tube, right and left, so as to intercept its caliber—the larger blood vessels being avoided. Mere divisions of the tube might be sufficient to produce sterility, but further removal of a portion of the tube appears to be surer practice. I recommend this precaution, therefore, as an improvement of the operation.*

In lecture XXVII, entitled *Means of Superseding the Cesarean Operation*, Blundell[2] suggested a method for interval sterilization by laparotomy:

> *In my opinion, there is: for if a woman were in that condition, in which delivery could not take place by the natural passage, provided she distrusted the circumstances in which she was placed, I would advise an incision of an inch in length in the linea alba above the symphysis pubis; I would advise further, that the fallopian tube on either side should be drawn up to this aperture; and, lastly, I would advise, that a portion of the tube should be removed, an operation easily performed, when the woman would, forever afterward, be sterile; all this, after due consideration, circumstances not forbidding. But the abdominal incision—that is bad:—true; but the Cesarean incision, that is worse. Is not that true also?*

Blundell's vivid description of a "mini-laparotomy" is quite precise. He described this procedure as early as 1824.[3] It is difficult to imagine that he did not perform this operation, but in none of his voluminous contributions to the medical literature could any specific acknowledgment be found.

Aware of the dangers of laparotomy, Froriep[4] described a different method of

The Fallopian Tube: Basic Studies and Clinical Contributions, edited by Alvin M. Siegler, M.D. Mount Kisco, New York: Futura Publishing Company, Inc. © 1986.

Table 25:1

Significant Historical Developments in Tubal Sterilization

Haighton[1]	1809	Tubal section in rabbits.
Blundell[2,3]	1828	Suggested partial salpingectomy during cesarean section and as interval procedure.
Froriep[4]	1849	Transuterine application of silver nitrate to uterine horns.
Lungren[6]	1880	Tubal ligation performed with silk during repeat cesarean section.
Kehrer[9]	1897	Tubal ligation with catgut and partial resection performed vaginally.
Mikulicz-Radecki and Freund[11]	1927	Hysteroscopic sterilization by cauterization of tubal ostia.
Power and Barnes[12]	1941	Peritoneoscopic tubal fulguration.

tubal sterilization in 1849. Using the transcervical approach, he introduced silver nitrate into the uterine cavity to stricture the upper uterine angles (tubal ostia) by chemical cauterization.

As surgical techniques improved and more women survived cesarean sections, physicians became concerned about the rising incidence of repeat cesarean section and the added maternal risks of reoperation. One of the accepted methods was to induce premature labor. Another approach was to remove the ovaries during the cesarean section or to remove the uterus after delivery.

In 1875 Dr. Samuel Smith Lungren,[5] of Toledo, Ohio (Fig. 25:2) reported a technique of cesarean section in the *Ohio Medical and Surgical Reporter.* He performed this operation on a Mrs. K, a native of Bavaria, who had a contracted pelvis. He used silver wire sutures to close the uterine incision. On May 22, 1880, Lungren performed a repeat cesarean section on the same patient. He presented this case report one month later in Milwaukee, Wisconsin, at the Thirty-Third Session of the American Institute of Homeopathy, of which he was a member. The case was published in the *Transactions* the same year.[6] Lungren intended to remove both ovaries during the surgery to prevent further pregnancies. He wrote:

[U]pon exposing the uterus, search was made for the silver sutures placed there five years previously, they were seen under the peritoneum, but without any signs of irritation from their presence. It was considered best not to remove them, as hemorrhage might be troublesome from the uterus at that point after closing the abdominal wound. The right ovary resembled in color varicose veins; the left was normal. It was the intention first to remove both ovaries during the operation, but decided, after mature consideration, that the risk would be lessened and the same result would be accomplished by tying both Fallopian tubes with strong silk ligatures about one inch from the uterus.

The following year, this report was published in the *American Journal of Obstetrics* under the title, "A Case of Cesarean Section Twice Successfully Performed on the Same Patient."[7] The tubal ligation was carried out shortly after entering the abdominal cavity and before the uterine incision was made. Of added significance was the fact that the patient had survived a second cesarean section, an accomplishment that had been recorded only six times previously in American medicine.[8]

Tubal ligations became more frequent after 1897. Kehrer,[9] of Heidelberg, Germany, described his method of sterilization by tubal resection through an anterior colpotomy. In the ensuing years innumer-

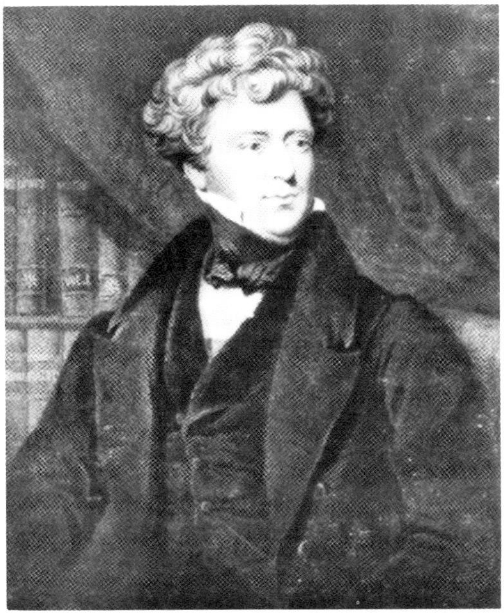

FIGURE 25:1—*Dr. James Blundell (1790–1877) suggested tubal ligation for sterilization.*

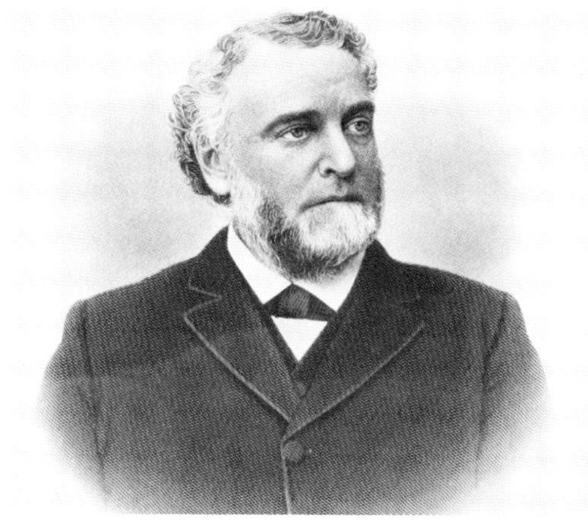

FIGURE 25:2—*Dr. Samuel Smith Lungren (1827–1892) is credited with performance of the first tubal ligation for sterilization.*

able reports were published about different forms of tubal sterilization, and in 1911 Stolz[10] had collected 199 references on this subject.

In 1927 Mikulicz-Radecki and Freund[11] were the first to use a hysteroscope for tubal sterilization. They used a "curettoscope," constructed by Freund in 1924, which enabled lavage of the uterine cavity and the introduction of a probe for excision and cauterization. These authors named the procedure "non-bloody sterilization." Working on uteri that were already extirpated or were subsequently to be removed, they cauterized the intramural parts of the fallopian tubes. The tissues were examined histologically, and these authors concluded that it was not sufficient merely to destroy the tubal mucosa. To prevent further recanalization, the muscularis layer needed to be coagulated as well.

Although laparoscopic tubal sterilization has been an increasingly common method of interval sterilization in the last decade, at least a quarter of a century seems to have elapsed between its earliest application and subsequent popularity. In 1941, Power and Barnes[12] used a laparoscope for tubal sterilization. They described a 1 cm incision made through the skin under local anesthesia, just below and left of the umbilicus and carried through the rectus sheath. After induction of a pneumoperitoneum with a small rubber hand pump, the peritoneoscope was inserted into the abdominal cavity. A fallopian tube was grasped with a biopsy forceps near the cornu and fulgurating current applied until a 1 cm segment of the tube was blanched. Neither the number of patients operated on nor the follow-up course was noted.

These physicians were torch bearers who handed down a rich legacy. Their concepts and ideas regarding techniques for tubal sterilization were innovative and daring for their time.

References

1. Haighton J: An experimental inquiry concerning animal impregnation. *Philos Trans R Soc Lond* 18:112, 1809.
2. Blundell J: *Lectures on the Principles and Practice of Midwifery*. London: Charles Severn, 1842.

3. Blundell J: Lectures on the gravid uterus, and on the disease of women and children. Lecture VI. *Lancet* 1:257, 1828.
4. Froriep R: Zur Vorbeugung der Nothwendigkeit des Kaiserschnitts und der Perforation. *Notiz Geburtshilfe Natur- und Heilkd* 11:9, 1849.
5. Lungren SS: Cesarean section-case. *Ohio Med Surg Reporter* 9:207, 1875.
6. Lungren SS: Cesarean section. In *Transactions of the Thirty-Third Session of the American Institute of Homoeopathy*, Milwaukee, June 15–18, 1880: p. 432.
7. Lungren SS: A case of cesarean section twice successfully performed on the same patient. *Am J Obstet* 14:78, 1881.
8. Harris RP: The operation of gastro-hysterotomy. *Am J Med Sci* 75:313, 1878.
9. Kehrer FA: Sterilisation mittels Tubendurchschneidung nach vorderem Scheidenschnitt. *Centralblatt Gynäkol* 21:961, 1897.
10. Stolz M: Die Sterilisation des Weibes. *Samml Klin Vortraege Gynaekol* 222–224:699, 1911.
11. Mikulicz-Radecki Fv, and Freund A: Ein neues Hysteroskop und seine praktische Anwendung in der Gynäkologie. *Z Geburtsh Gynäkol* 92:13, 1927.
12. Power FH, and Barnes AC: Sterilization by means of peritoneoscopic tubal fulguration. A preliminary report. *Am J Obstet Gynecol* 41:1038, 1941.

26

Hysteroscopic Sterilization

Abdol H. Hosseinian

Technical advances in endoscopic methods and an ever increasing demand for a safer sterilization technique encouraged investigators to use hysteroscopy to obstruct the interstitial tubal segment. The advantages of hysteroscopic techniques, such as elimination of the need for general anesthesia, avoiding a laparotomy or laparoscopy and an abdominal scar, are the promising aspects of this method of sterilization. The initial euphoria with hysteroscopic electrocoagula of the tubal ostia was dampened by failure rates and occurrence of complications, including one

In this chapter various techniques of hysteroscopic sterilization are reviewed based on two major categories: (1) the nondestructive techniques in which the uterotubal ostia are occluded mechanically with plugs or devices placed through the hysteroscope, and (2) the destructive techniques in which the interstitial tubal segment is destroyed either by electrocoagulation or by injection of sclerosing substances.

Nondestructive Techniques

Since 1975, the author has been exploring the safety and effectiveness of mechanically blocking the tubal ostia through hysteroscopy with a uterotubal junction blocking device (UTJD), which can be implanted in or removed from the tubal ostia by a device carrier. The reversibility potential of the procedure has been one of the prime objectives of this technique. The original UTJD was made of a polyethylene plug, which measures 10 mm in length with a diameter of 1 mm at the tip and 2 mm at the base. Since the polyethylene plug is quite rigid and the possibility of tissue injury and tubal perforation was feared, the composition of the plug was subsequently changed to silicone rubber (Fig. 26:1). Both of these plugs have been investigated in animal experimentation using baboons as the test animal and in selected women.[2–4]

Two metallic components are attached to the plugs: (1) four anchoring

The Fallopian Tube: Basic Studies and Clinical Contributions, edited by Alvin M. Siegler, M.D. Mount Kisco, New York: Futura Publishing Company, Inc. © 1986.

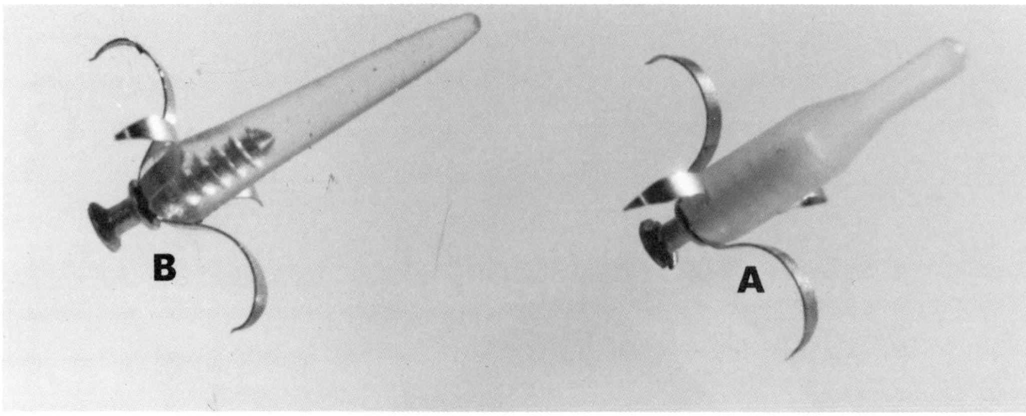

FIGURE 26:1—*Uterotubal junction blocking devices. (A) polyethylene device; (B) silicone device.*

spines, delicately made of elgiloy, serve to fix and keep the device in place by penetrating the adjacent myometrium; (2) the assembly screw, made of stainless steel, attaches the anchoring spines to the plug and provides a grasping base for the device carrier. The UTJD is carried through a straight operating channel of a hysteroscope by a device carrier which can implant in or remove the plug from the uterotubal junction. In primate studies, the efficacy of the device for contraception was found to be 100 percent using 21 baboons for a minimum of eight breedings (Table 26:1). The reversibility potential of the technique was investigated by hysteroscopic removal of the device in 15 baboons. Of these animals, eight became pregnant, achieving a total of 12 pregnancies (Table 26:2). It should be noted that the incidence of infertility in baboons in captivity is approximately 30 percent.

Clinical trials with UTJD have been conducted in two phases. During phase I, the capability of the plug to occlude the uterotubal junction and the extent of tissue reaction were investigated in 33 women. Since all of the subjects had been prescheduled for hysterectomy for unrelated gynecologic conditions, we could only assess the efficacy of the procedure for a short time (two to six months). No adverse side effects such as bleeding or uterine cramps were reported during the period of study. Effective closure (Fig. 26:2) was achieved in 91 percent of the tubes, only one pregnancy occurred in this phase of the study (Table 26:3). The reversibility potential of this technique was also examined in 20 women (Table 26:4). Ninety percent of the tubes regained their patency (Fig. 26:2) after hysteroscopic removal of the device. All women in this study underwent hysterectomy. Histologic studies of the uterotubal junction showed expansion of the tubal lumen and flattening of the cells of the endosalpinx, in addition to minimal to moderate tissue reaction around the anchoring spines (Fig. 26:3).

In phase II, the author studied long-term efficacy of the method as a permanent sterilization procedure with reversibility potential. Eleven volunteers underwent implantation of the hysteroscopic device under paracervical block. Proper device implantation in some of the subjects in this phase, as well as in phase I of the clinical trials, was difficult mainly because of the rigid hysteroscope. It appears that proper implantation can be achieved only by bringing the device and the tip of the carrier in parallel axis with the tubal lumen at the uterine cornu (Fig. 26:4). Assumption of such a position in some women could be difficult, or even impossible, when the tubal ostia are too laterally positioned. Five patients became pregnant. Two of them did not follow the research

Table 26:1

*Results of Hysteroscopic Implantation of Devices in Baboons**

Factor	*Results*
Failures	1 (one-sided)
Duration of implantation	8–27 months
Pregnancies	None
Expulsions	
polyethylene	None
silicone	2 animals

*Polyethylene devices were implanted in 7 animals, and silicone devices were implanted in 14 animals.[4]

Table 26:2

*Reversal of Fertility after Hysteroscopic Removal of Devices from 15 Baboons**

Type of device	*No. pregnancies*†
Polyethylene	3
Silicone	5

*Polyethylene devices were implanted in six animals and silicone devices were implanted in nine animals. One to eighteen breeding cycles were required.[4]
†There were twelve pregnancies in eight animals.

Table 26:3

*Hysteroscopic Implantation of Uterotubal Junction Blocking Devices in Human Volunteers**

Event	*No.*
Tubal closures	58 (91%)
Expulsions	0
Pregnancies	1
Duration of implantation	2–6 months
Complications	2†
Tissue reaction	minimal to moderate

*64 devices implanted in 33 subjects.[3]
†One vaginal cuff infection; one wound infection.

Table 26:4

Hysteroscopic Removal of Uterotubal Junction Blocking Devices in Human Volunteers[3]

Event	*No.*
Number of devices removed (from 20 subjects)	40
polyethylene	20
silicone	20
Tubal patencies (after removal of devices)	36 (90%)
Tubal closures (after removal of devices)	4
polyethylene	2
silicone	2

protocol while the other three procedures should be considered as technical failures.

Although the technique proved 100 percent effective in baboons in terms of tubal occlusion, as well as contraception (in some animals after more than two years of follow-up), the long-term efficacy in women was disappointing. The disparity of results can be explained by the differences in the shape and the size of the uterine cavity and the accessibility of the uterotubal junctions in women and baboons. The uterine cavities in the baboons are much smaller, making the uterotubal junctions easily accessible for proper alignment and device implantation through the rigid hysteroscope (Fig. 26:5). In women, however, when ostia are too laterally situated, alignment between the device and the tubal lumen through the rigid hysteroscope becomes technically difficult or even impossible. Improper device implantation not only results in a higher rate of tubal patency, but also can lead to uneven device fixation, resulting in future dislocation. This may explain the

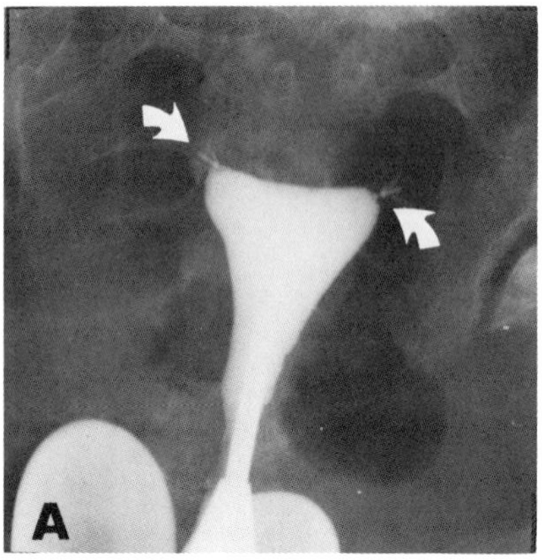

FIGURE 26:2A—*Hysterosalpingography with devices in place shows bilateral proximal tubal obstruction (arrows).*

three technical failures observed in phase II of the clinical trials. Because of the shape of the UTJD, the size of the tubal ostia should not influence the results between baboons and women. A suitable steerable hysteroscope can eliminate the alignment difficulties encountered with the rigid hysteroscope and help to reduce the chances of technical failures. Further investigations with this device await the development of such a hysteroscope.

Formed-in-place silicone rubber plugs

In this technique, liquid silicone polymer and a catalyst are instilled hysteroscopically into the fallopian tube through a specially designed dispenser. The material solidifies in situ and conforms to the oviductal lumen without distorting, adhering, or causing inflammatory reaction in the surrounding tissue. Following the ini- tial animal studies in rabbits[5] and monkeys,[6] clinical trials have been undertaken.[7,8] At the time of reporting,[8] a total of 965 subjects from different centers had undergone this method of sterilization. Successful bilateral occlusion was achieved in 791 cases (82 percent), while 13 pregnancies were reported. There has been only one ectopic preg-

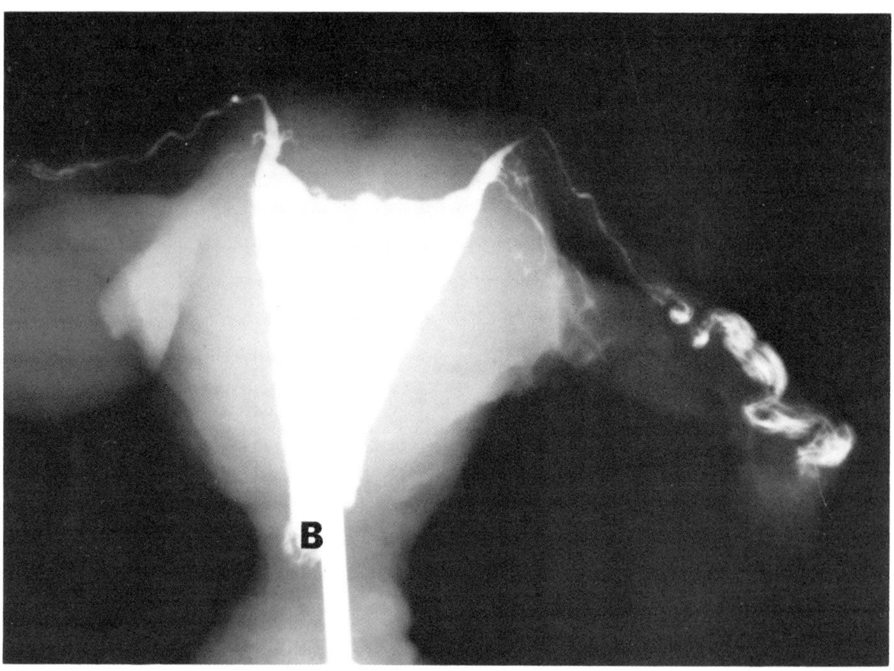

FIGURE 26:2B—*Hysterosalpingography after removal of devices shows patent tube in extirpated specimen.*

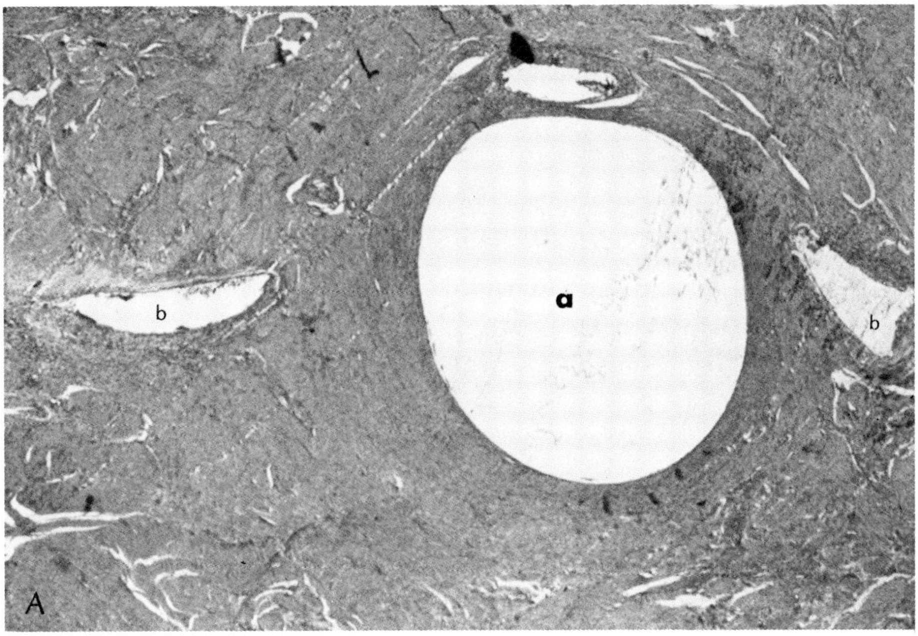

FIGURE 26:3A—*Site of the plug (a) and site of the spine (b).*

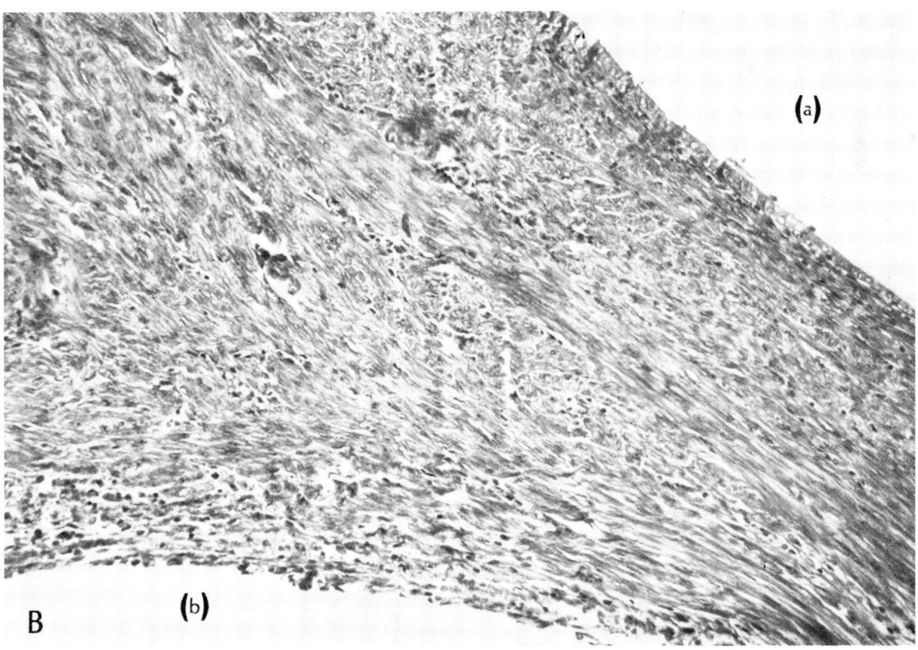

FIGURE 26:3B—*Higher magnification showing site of the plug (a) and site of the spine (b).*

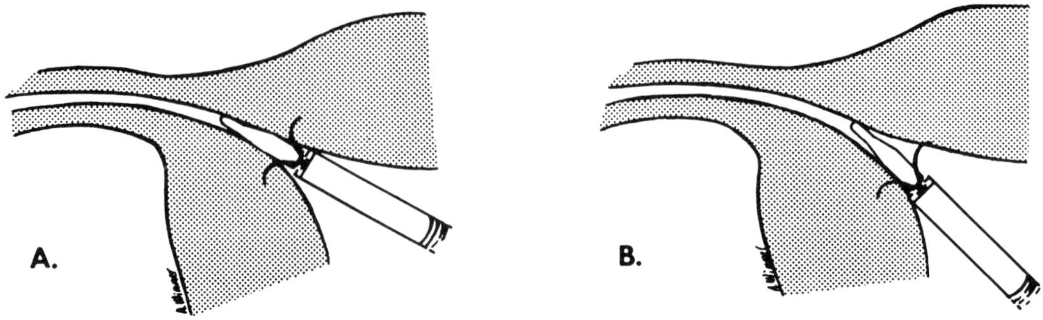

FIGURE 26:4—*Proper (A) and improper (B) alignment of the device and the tip of the carrier are seen at the time of device implantation.*

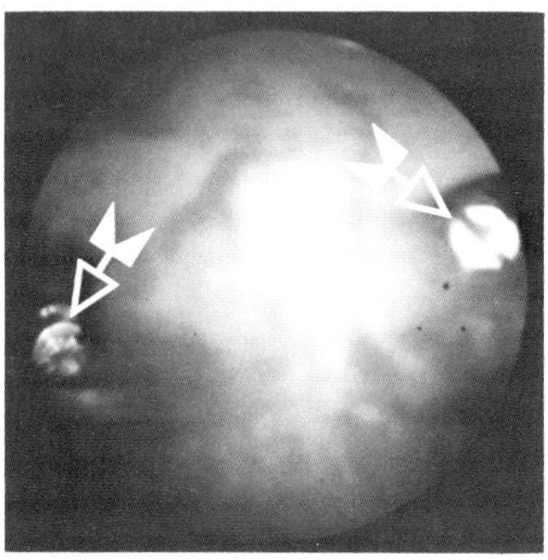

FIGURE 26:5—*Implanted UTJD (arrows) is noted at baboon's uterotubal junctions.*

nancy in a fallopian tube on the side of an improper plug. Another 63 major or minor complications have been reported in the series.

The investigators believe that the results could be improved further by exclusion of patients with possible tubal abnormalities from this form of sterilization and by the postoperative radiological evaluation of the shape of the plugs. The attractive features of this method are the same as other nondestructive hysteroscopic sterilization techniques. However, its reversibility potential has never been demonstrated in women. The animal experimentation in rabbits[5] for reversibility potential was extremely limited and under different technical application. In that experiment, seven rabbits were mated 31 days following the removal of the plugs that had been in place for 200 days, and two animals became pregnant after a single mating.

The P-block

This device of Brundin consists of a prefabricated skeleton of nylon 6 on which a hydrogelic body has been anchored (Fig. 26:6A). The device is placed hysteroscopically through a catheter that also contains a flexible plunger. It is hydrated by the body fluids after insertion and retains a good memory of the shape during swelling. The P-block is retained in situ by polymeric protrusions, hydratings, and swelling of the plug after insertion.[9]

Brundin's smaller P-blocks, called Mark 1 to 6, were inserted during the first phase of the investigation. Because of the high incidence of expulsion, perforation, and pregnancy, the investigator subsequently modified the device which is called Mark 7. Hysteroscopic insertion of Mark 7 in 35 women achieved bilateral tubal occlusion in 15, while insertion was impossible in another 15. Subsequent pregnancies occurred in four women and in one case, devices were removed because of bleeding. While the paucity of the side effects and tissue reaction with this technique is encouraging, the inability to insert the device in over 42 percent of the women and the incidence of pregnancy despite apparent bilateral tubal occlusion are major sources of concern. One of the problems appears to be related to the difficulties in the proper placement of the P-block in the intramural part of the oviduct. The author believes that with the improvement of the insertion device now in progress and new plugs (Fig. 26:6), the results of this technique should improve.

Craft's uterotubal ceramic plug

In 1976, Craft[10] reported on the feasibility of hysteroscopic implantation of ceramic plugs at the uterotubal junctions. The composition of this ceramic plug was pure alpha alumina: the central solid core having a porosity of 3.5 percent which extended for approximately 5 mm beyond the head to facilitate application, and the outer head having a porosity of 30 percent and measuring approximately 7 mm in length and 2 mm in width at its widest point (Fig. 26:6B).

Craft selected porous ceramic because animal experiments in orthodontic and orthopedic research had shown that this material provides a stable support system which allows tissue ingrowth within the porous matrix without inflammation or foreign body reactions. Results of inserting porous ceramic plugs into the uterotubal junction of eight rabbits for six weeks showed histologic evidence of tissue ingrowth in three but the ceramic plug was securely in place in only one animal.

Satisfactory hysteroscopic insertion of the plug was accomplished in 10 of 15 patients undergoing immediate hysterectomy. No subsequent studies have been reported.

Sugimoto's silicone rubber intratubal contraceptive device (ITCD)

Sugimoto's device is made of silicone rubber and measures 10 mm long and 1.2 mm in diameter. To prevent spontaneous expulsion from the tubes, the device has notches every 1.5 mm. To prevent slipping into the tube and to provide grasping base for its removal, there are two flanges near the base of the device (Fig. 26:6C). For device implantation, two or three devices are inserted into the introducer, which is a teflon tube with an extruding wire plunger. After the introducer is positioned hysteroscopically with the tubal opening, the device is pushed into the tube by the plunger. The device can also be removed through the hysteroscope.

Sugimoto's device has been tested in 32 women scheduled for hysterectomy.[11] Unilateral spontaneous expulsion occurred in three cases. Long-term follow-up studies are needed to evaluate its efficacy as a contraceptive method.

Brueschke's plugs

Two types of uterotubal junction blocking devices have been studied by Brueschke and his associates. The type 1 device, consisting entirely of silicone rubber, was only partially successful because it buckled occasionally at the time of implantation. The type 2 device consisted of the same silicone rubber, but had, in addition, a flexible metallic stiffening core (Fig. 26:6D). Metallic retention anchors provided the means for device fixation.

Brueschke's plug was implanted through their specially designed steerable hysteroscope in baboons and in extirpated human uteri, in addition to the acute implantation of devices in 21 patients scheduled for hysterectomy.[12,13] Despite Brueschke's plans for short- and long-term implantation of the device, testing has not continued.

Other devices

There are at least five other devices that have been proposed for hysteroscopic tubal insertion, but none of those has been studied in women. The Popp Claw de-

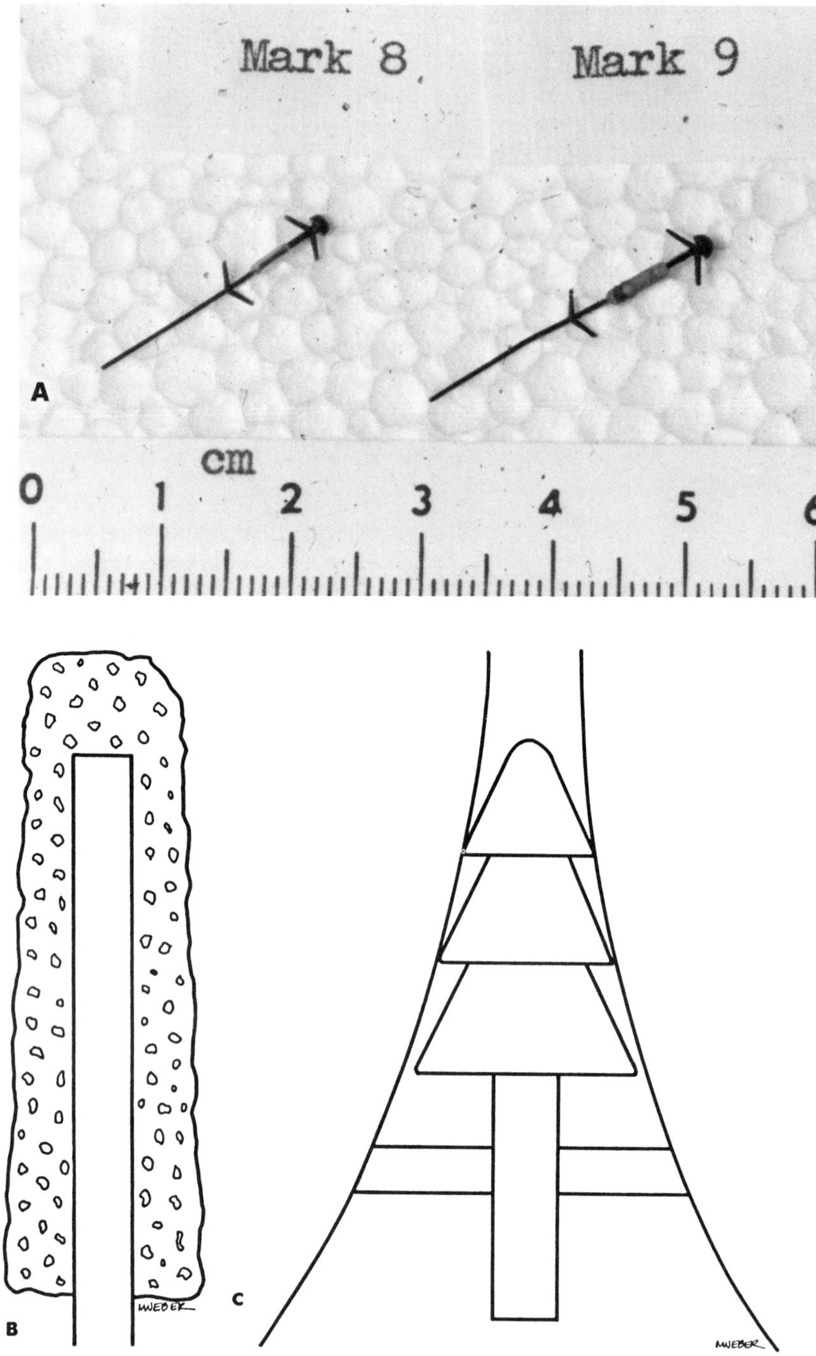

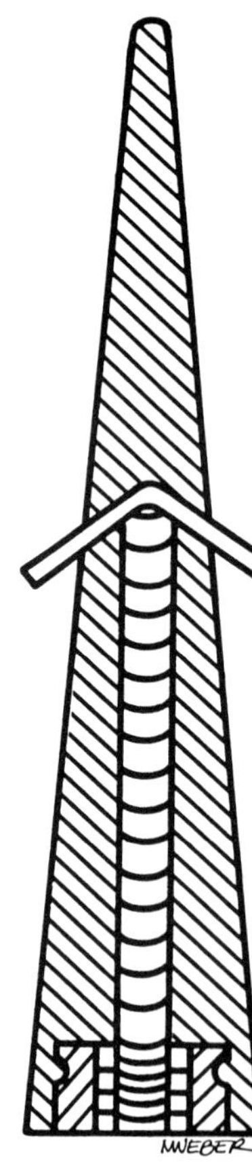

FIGURE 26:6—*Other types of tubal plugs.* (A) *Brundin's newer P-block plugs.* (B) *Diagrammatic representation of Craft's uterotubal ceramic plug.* (C) *Sugimoto's silicone rubber ITCD.* (D) *Brueschke's plug with metallic stiffening core.*

vice[14] and the Popp intratubal devices[15] were used in rats with poor results. Polymer block and metal alloy intratubal devices, which were inserted through the fimbrial ends in pigtail monkeys,[16] and Porto's plug, which has never been tested in either animals or women,[17] are some of the other devices.

Destructive Techniques

Electrocoagulation

Electrocoagulation of the tubal cornua under hysteroscopic control was first reported five decades ago. However, it was not until the early 1970s that this nonincisional method of tubal occlusion gained worldwide popularity. Techniques used by different investigators varied from one another by the choice of distending mediums,[18–20] the size and shape of the electrodes, as well as the coagulating power and the duration of cautery. The initial enthusiasm abated rather rapidly after isolated reports of major complications[1] and later publication of the results of the collaborative study.[21] Ten investigators from five countries participated in the survey with series ranging from 6 to 298 cases. Of the total 773 operations in the survey, 524 were tested for tubal patency. A discouraging 175 (33 percent) failures (patency of one or both tubes) were reported. Even in 349 patients in whom the tubes had appeared closed bilaterally by hysterosalpingography, 11 pregnancies occurred. This might imply recanalization of the tubes after closure, inadequacy of patency tests used, or the reopening of the blocked tube by patency test.[18] In the series, 25 major complications were reported (3.2 percent), including 7 uterine perforations, 3 intestinal injuries with peritonitis, acute peritonitis in 4, ectopic pregnancies in 8, and 3 miscellaneous complications; there was one death from bowel perforation and peritonitis. The minor complications, a total of 40 (5.2 percent), included in the order of frequency: bleeding or menstrual irregularities, cramps, pain, dizziness, and endometritis. There was considerable variation in the rate of failures (from 12.5 to 82.8 percent), as well as complication rates (from 0 to 37.5 percent) among the investigators.

The investigators concluded that this procedure should be performed under highly controlled conditions by physicians with extensive experience. Of the major investigators, only Quinones and his collaborators continued with tubal electrocoagulation under hysteroscopic control. In 1976, they reported their results in a series of 800 patients.[22] Only 513 cases were studied with hysterosalpingography. Bilateral tubal occlusion was achieved in 84.5 percent at the first attempt. A second electrocoagulation increased the overall tubal occlusion rate to 98.8 percent in 487 patients. These investigators reported data with respect to 1,284 hysteroscopic tubal electorocoagulation procedures with an overall bilateral tubal occlusion rate of 80 percent.[14] In their opinion, the following factors had a negative influence on the results: (1) performance of the procedure beyond the eighth day of the menstrual cycle; (2) teaching more than one person and hence lengthening the time of the procedure; and (3) uterine abnormalities.[22] They believed that the size of the electrode did not influence success in their series, but a ball tip seemed to have a negative influence. Cylindrical tip electrodes, which were not introduced further than 5 mm, were preferable. Transistorized coagulating units delivering 25 watts for 8 seconds improved the results and avoided excessive cauterization which could lead to thermal intestinal injuries, perforation, and peritonitis.

Sclerosing agents

Transcervical application or instillation of various chemicals such as gelatin-resorcinol-formaldehyde (GRF),[23] silver nitrate,[24] quinacrine,[25,26] methyl cyanoacrylate (MCA),[27] phenol-atabrine paste (PAP),[28] and phenolmucilage[29] and a number of other less promising agents have been used for nonsurgical tubal occlusion. It was contended that a direct injection of a sclerosing agent into the intramural tubal segment under hysteroscopic observation should increase the rate of success. However, hysteroscopically injected 50 mg of quinacrine in each tubal cornu through a catheter resulted in only 6 bilateral tubal occlusions in 16 patients who were subsequently tested for tubal patency by hysterosalpingography.[30] Surprisingly, it was a lower efficacy rate than 50 percent bilateral tubal occlusion which occurred after a single transcervical application of quinacrine.[25] Instead of hysteroscopic injection of chemicals, efforts have been directed toward designing simple and practical methods for transcervical application of sclerosing agents for large-scale, nonsurgical sterilization programs.[27,31,32]

Conclusion

Despite the attractive features of hysteroscopic sterilization and the painstaking efforts by a number of investigators over a decade, the ideal method is yet to be developed. The following three methods appear more promising, assuming the shortcomings associated with each of them could be resolved:

1. The future of the formed-in-place silicone rubber plugs depends on establishing their long-term efficacy and further modifications resulting in reduction in the number of failures and complications. However, the reversibility potential of this technique still remains speculative.
2. The only nondestructive tubal plug with proven high reversibility rate is the uterotubal junction blocking device, whose future depends on the development of a suitable steerable hysteroscope for proper device implantation.
3. Electrocoagulation of the tubal cornua was associated with an unacceptably high failure rate and both major and minor complications. The problems of recanalization and ectopic pregnancies are also disturbing features. Only the skill and experience of the gynecologist can minimize the rate of failures and complications associated with this technique.

Acknowledgments: The author expresses sincere appreciation to Dr. Jan Brundin for providing advance information and photographs of his latest plugs, and Mrs. Diane Krier-Morrow, M.B.A., Director, Administration, PARFR, for supplying some of the photographs related to the uterotubal junction blocking devices.

References

1. Israngkun C, and Phaosavasdi S: Hysteroscopic sterilization in 296 cases. In Sciarra JJ, Droegemueller W, Speidel JJ (Eds): *Advances in Female Sterilization Techniques.* Hagerstown, MD: Harper & Row, 1976: p. 148.
2. Hosseinian AH, Lucero S, and Kim MH: Hysteroscopic implantation of UTJ blocking devices. In Sciarra JJ, Droegemueller W, Speidel JJ (Eds): *Advances in Female Sterilization Techniques.* Hagerstown, MD: Harper & Row, 1976: p. 169.
3. Hosseinian AH, Lucero S, and Zaneveld LJD: Hysteroscopically delivered tubal plugs. In Sciarra JJ, Zatuchni GI, Speidel JJ (Eds): *Reversal of Sterilization.* Hagerstown, MD: Harper & Row, 1978: p. 241.
4. Hosseinian AH, and Morales WA: Clinical application of hysteroscopic sterilization using uterotubal junction blocking devices. In Zatuchni GI, Shelton JD, Goldsmith A, et al (Eds): *Female Transcervical Sterilization.* Hagerstown, MD: Harper & Row, 1983: p. 234.
5. Davis RH, Erb R, Kyriazis GA, et al: Fallopian tube occlusion in rabbits with silicone rubber. *J. Reprod Med* 14:56, 1975.
6. Davis, RH, Platt, HA, Moonka DK, et al: Chronic occlusion of the monkey fallopian tube with silicone polymer. *Obstet Gynecol* 53:527, 1979.
7. Reed TP, and Erb RA: Hysteroscopic oviductal blocking with formed-in-place silicone rubber plugs. II. Clinical studies. *J Reprod Med* 23:69, 1979.

8. Reed TP: Formed-in-place silicone plugs: Improvements and limitations. In Zatuchni GI, Shelton JD, Goldsmith A, et al (Eds): *Female Transcervical Sterilization*, Hagerstown, MD: Harper & Row, 1983: p. 270.
9. Brundin J: Hydrogel tubal blocking P-block. In Zatuchni GI, Shelton JD, Goldsmith A, et al (Eds): *Female Transcervical Sterilzation*, Hagerstown, MD: Harper & Row, 1983: p. 240.
10. Craft I: Uterotubal ceramic plugs. In Sciarra JJ, Droegemueller W, Speidel JJ (Eds): *Advances in Female Sterilization Techniques*. Hagerstown, MD: Harper & Row, 1976: p. 176.
11. Sugimoto O: *Diagnostic and Therapeutic Hysteroscopy*. Tokyo: Igaku-Shoin, 1978: p. 208.
12. Brueschke EE, Zaneveld LJD, Wilbanks GD, et al: A steerable hysteroscope and mechanical tubal occlusive devices. In Sciarra JJ, Droegemueller W, Speidel JJ (Eds): *Advances in Female Sterilization Techniques*. Hagerstown, MD: Harper & Row, 1976: p. 182.
13. Brueschke EE, Fadel HE, Mayerhofer K, et al: Transcervical tubal occlusion with a steerable hysteroscope: Implantation of devices into extirpated human uteri. *Am J Obstet Gynecol* 127:118, 1977.
14. Sciarra JJ: Hysteroscopic approaches for tubal closure. In Zatuchni GI, Labbok MH, Sciarra JJ (Eds): *Research Frontiers in Fertility Regulation*. Hagerstown, MD: Harper & Row, 1980: p. 270.
15. Popp LW, Schultz S, and Lindemann HJ: Intratubal devices in rats: An experimental model. In Siegler AM, Lindemann HJ (Eds): *Hysteroscopy, Principles and Practice*. Philadelphia: JB Lippincott, 1983: p. 247.
16. Richart RM, Neuwirth RS, Nuwayser ES, et al: Evaluation of polymer block and metal alloy intratubal device in pigtail monkeys. *Contraception* 18:459, 1978.
17. Porto R: Pneumohysteroscopy: Instrumentation and technique. In Sciarra JJ, Butler JC Jr, Speidel JJ (Eds): *Hysteroscopic Sterilization*. New York: Intercontinental Medical Book Corporation, 1974: p. 51.
18. Quinones R, Alvarado A, and Aznar R: Tubal electrocoagulation under hysteroscopic control. In Sciarra JJ, Butler JC Jr, Speidel JJ (Eds): *Hysteroscopic Sterilization*. New York: International Medical Book Corporation, 1974: p. 95.
19. Lindemann HJ: Transuterine tubal sterilization by CO_2 hysteroscopy. In Sciarra JJ, Butler JC Jr, Speidel JJ (Eds): *Hysteroscopic Sterilization*. New York: International Medical Book Corporation, 1974: p. 61.
20. Neuwirth RS, Richart RM, Israngkun C, et al: Hysteroscopic sterilization. In Sciarra JJ, Butler JC Jr, Speidel JJ (Eds): *Hysteroscopic Sterilization*, New York: International Medical Book Corporation, 1974: p. 121.
21. Darabi KF, and Richart RM: Collaborative study on hysteroscopic sterilization procedures. *Obstet Gynecol* 49:48, 1977.
22. Quinones R, Alvarado A, and Ley E: Hysteroscopic sterilization: Follow-up of 800 cases. In Sciarra JJ, Droegemueller W, Speidel JJ (Eds): *Advances in Female Sterilization Techniques*. Hagerstown, MD: Harper & Row, 1976: p. 162.
23. Grode GA, Pavkov KL, and Falb RD: Feasibility study on the use of a tissue adhesive for the non-surgical blocking of fallopian tubes. Phase I: Evaluation of a tissue adhesive. *Fertil Steril* 22:552, 1971.
24. Richart RM, Taylor HC, and Neuwirth RS: Experimental studies of fallopian tube occlusion. In Richart RM, Prager D (Eds): *Human Sterilization*. Springfield, IL: Charles C Thomas, 1972: p. 260.
25. Zipper J, Stachetti E, and Mendel M: Human fertility control by transvaginal application of quinacrine on the fallopian tube. *Fertil Steril* 21:581, 1970.
26. Zipper J, Edelman D, Cole LP, et al: Overview of clinical trials with quinacrine. In Zatuchni GI, Shelton JD, Goldsmith A, et al (Eds): *Female Transcervical Sterilization*. Hagerstown, MD: Harper & Row, 1983: p. 94.
27. Richart RM, Neuwirth RS, Nilsen PA, et al: The effectiveness of the FEMCEPT method and preliminary experience with radio-opaque MCA to enhance clinical acceptability. In Zatuchni GI, Shelton JD, Goldsmith A, et al (Eds): *Female Transcervical Sterilization*. Hagerstown, MD: Harper & Row, 1983: p. 212.
28. Wu YH, Qian PL, and Tien SP: Nonsurgical procedures for manual instillation of a phenolatabrine paste (PAP) for

female tubal occlusion. In Zatuchni GI, Shelton JD, Goldsmith A, et al (Eds): *Female Transcervical Sterilization*. Hagerstown, MD: Harper & Row, 1983: p. 151.

29. Zheng HG, and Chen XH: A study of phenol-mucilage-induced tubal occlusion for sterilization (analysis of the results in 4,784 cases). In Zatuchni GI, Shelton JD, Goldsmith A, et al (Eds): *Female Transcervical Sterilization*. Hagerstown, MD: Harper & Row, 1983: p. 162.
30. Alvarado A, Quinones R, Aznar R: Tubal instillation of quinacrine under hysteroscopic control. In Sciarra JJ, Butler JC Jr, and Speidel JJ (Eds): *Hysteroscopic Sterilization*. New York: International Medical Book Corporation, 1974: p. 85.
31. Laufe LE, and Wheeler RG: Quinacrine IUD's. In Zatuchni GI, Shelton JD, Goldsmith A, et al (Eds): *Female Transcervical Sterilization*. Hagerstown, MD: Harper & Row, 1983: p. 115.
32. Wheeler RG: Delivery systems for applying quinacrine as a tubal closing agent. In Zatuchni GI, Shelton JD, Goldsmith A, et al (Eds): *Female Transcervical Sterilization*. Hagerstown, MD: Harper & Row, 1983: p. 105.

27

Hysteroscopic Placement of Nylon Intratubal Devices for Potentially Reversible Sterilization

Jacques Hamou, Franco Gasparri, Ettore Cittadini, Gianfranco Scarselli, Antonio Perino, and Luca Mencaglia

As an alternative to surgical methods of female sterilization by laparoscopy or minilaparotomy, work has progressed on the development of nonsurgical methods. Research has focused on transcervical methods in which tubal occlusion is obtained by chemical agents (phenol-based compounds, quinacrine, or methyl cyanoacrylate—MCA)[1–3] cryotherapy,[4] electrocautery[5,6] or tubal blocking devices.[7–12] Of the chemical agents, MCA has been widely tested and appears to have the potential of becoming a simple and effective method of nonsurgical sterilization. The drawback of this procedure is that multiple applications of MCA are needed to obtain tubal closure in about 30 percent of women. The use of phenol-based compounds and quinacrine may cause untoward effects. The use of electrocautery has been associated with serious complications and cryotherapy has not proved to be a practical, transcervical method.

The use of improved hysteroscopes has facilitated the development of procedures in which the tubes can be occluded by intratubal placement of various types of plugs. All of the tubal plugs that have been tested were designed to provide a reversible method of sterilization. Clinical trials with the P-block plug[8] (a hydrogelic co-polymerized device) were designed to block the isthmic portion of the uterotubal junction device, and a silicone device with metallic protusions to prevent expulsion[7] gave unsatisfactory results. The most widely tested tubal plug has been the catalyzed silicone polymer plug which is placed in the tubes through a specially designed dispenser.[9,10] The silicone solid-

The Fallopian Tube: Basic Studies and Clinical Contributions, edited by Alvin M. Siegler, M.D. Mount Kisco, New York: Futura Publishing Company, Inc. © 1986.

ifies in the tubes, forming a plug. The only other plug that has been largely evaluated in women is the nylon intratubal device of Hamou.[11,12] This chapter describes the preliminary results with this device.

Material and Methods

Since March 1982, studies have been carried out with the Hamou intratubal device (ITD) to evaluate techniques of insertion and placement, complications, frequency of device displacement and expulsion, and its effectiveness in preventing pregnancy. The present prospective study was conducted to evaluate the most recent ITD modifications designed to overcome problems experienced with other prototypes of the same device.

The ITD is inserted into the fallopian tube under direct vision with a specially designed hysteroscope. It consists of a soft strand of surgical nylon with a 1 mm diameter. At each end of the nylon strand (about 28–30 mm long) there is a loop with an "elastic memory." The loops prevent expulsion of the ITD into the uterine cavity and its migration along the fallopian tube. The ITDs are inserted with hysteroscopic control. The endoscope is 4 mm in diameter with panoramic as well as contact capabilities and with different magnifications (from $\times$ 1 to $\times$ 150). Thehysteroscope is inserted into an operative sheath which has a 6.5 mm outside diameter. Light is provided by a 150 watt cold light source through a fiberoptic cable. The uterine cavity is distended by continuous CO_2 flow delivered at a rate of 30 ml/min and with a maximal pressure of 90 mmHg.[11,12] Procedures were usually scheduled for the early proliferative phase of the menstrual cycle and were performed by three experienced hysteroscopists. Because of the small diameter of the operative sheath, the procedure generally can be performed without the need for premedication and general anesthesia although in the present study, we elected to use anesthesia for 80 of the procedures (general 12; local 68). General anesthesia was more frequently used during the initial procedures until the operators became familiar with the technique of ITD insertion.

The hysteroscopic technique is the same as the one used for routine diagnostic examination.[11,12] The cervix is grasped with a single-toothed tenaculum, and the hysteroscope, with two ITDs contained in the insertion catheter, is inserted into the cervical canal under direct visual control. A careful examination is made of the uterine cavity to rule out abnormalities that might preclude correct placement of the ITD. The end of the insertion catheter is brought within about 3 mm of the tubal ostia (Fig. 27:1) and the ITD is inserted into the interstitial portion. The second ITD is placed in the other tube in the same manner without removing the microhysteroscope from the uterus (Figs. 27:2 and 27:3). The ITDs may be removed at any time by grasping and gently pulling, under hysteroscopic control, the proximal loop of the ITD.

Women were informed about the experimental aspects of the study and they were requested to use a barrier contraceptive method until correct placement of the ITDs was confirmed by hysteroscopic examination during the proliferative phase of their next menstrual cycle. Patients who had correct bilateral placement were continued in the study and followed every three months for one year. A repeat hysteroscopic examination was scheduled at the final visit (Fig. 27:4).

Data pertaining to the hysteroscopic procedures and follow-up of the subjects were recorded on standard forms and analyzed by one of the authors. The data were analyzed using standard statistical procedures.

Results

All women were generally healthy and without known contraindications to hysteroscopy. Most of them were 35 years or older, parity 1 or 2, and had terminated their last pregnancy at least three years before the procedure. The majority of

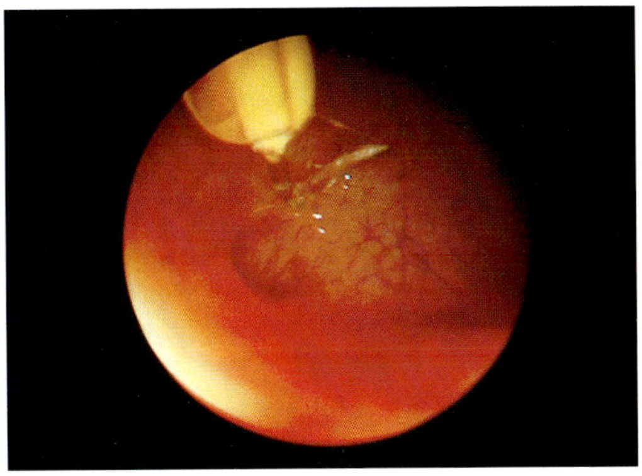

FIGURE 27:1—*Closeup view of the uterotubal orifice and of the distal end of the device.*

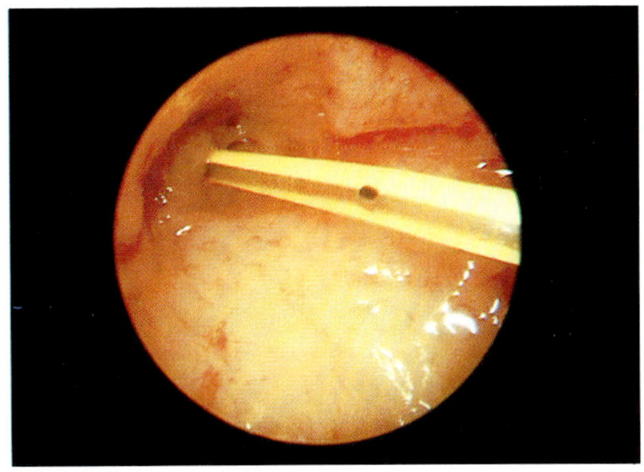

FIGURE 27:2—*Hysteroscopic observation during the release of the ITD.*

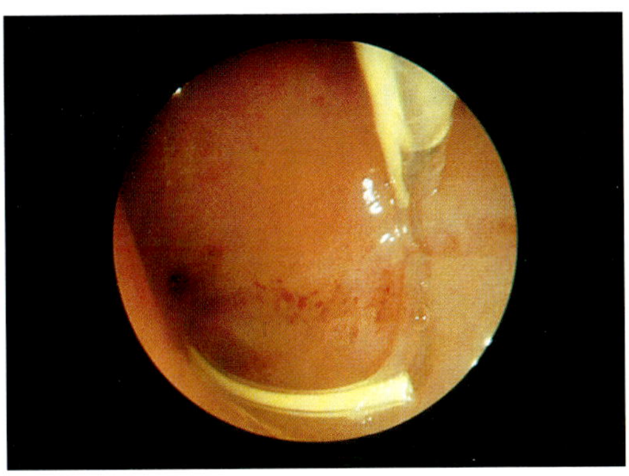

FIGURE 27:3—*The ITD has been completely released.*

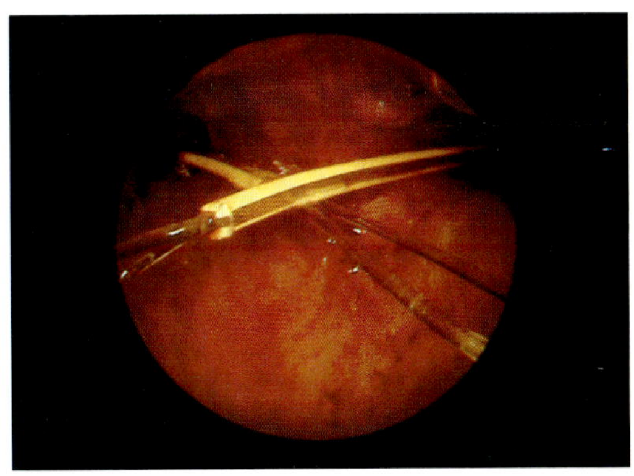

FIGURE 27:4—*Hysteroscopic control one month after the insertion. Both devices are in place.*

women had used IUDs or oral contraceptives in the three months prior to hysteroscopy.

Difficulties in performing the hysteroscopic sterilization procedures occurred in eight (4.8 percent) patients. For two of these cases bilateral placement of the ITDs was not achieved. There were five others in addition to these two cases for whom bilateral ITD placement was not obtained. Nearly 9 percent of the tubal ostia were atretic but not occluded, but in only one woman, atretic tubal ostia prevented insertion of the ITDs.

There were no serious complications that required hospitalization of patients. The most frequently reported complaint was pelvic pain. Two women had their ITDs removed; one woman with a submucous myoma had used an IUD before insertion of ITDs, and she had complained of severe dysmenorrhea. Following ITD insertion, her dysmenorrhea did not improve. Her ITDs were removed without difficulty and she later had a myomectomy. Two patients complained of adnexal tenderness. Diagnostic laparoscopies were performed on both of them and no evidence of any inflammatory reaction was found. The ITDs of one were removed without difficulty; the other patient continued to use her ITDs.

Sixteen (9.6 percent) women expelled or displaced one or both ITDs. Fourteen of these explusions or displacements occurred within two months following insertion. For each of the other two women, one ITD had been expelled at the hysteroscopic examinations performed eight and nine months after the initial procedures. For most patients the distance between the tubal ostia and the end of the ITD after it was placed was estimated by the operator; this distance was 8 to 10 mm for about 70 percent of the uteri. No relationship was found between this distance and the expulsion and displacement rate of the ITDs.

More than 1,471 cycles have been observed without any other form of contraception. Only one intrauterine pregnancy occurred six months after insertion, even though hysteroscopic control had shown that the devices were apparently in place.

Comment

The results of this preliminary study with the ITD are encouraging. Complications from the procedure were infrequent. Placement of the ITDs could not be achieved in only 5 percent of the women and 9.6 percent had at least one ITD displaced or expelled. Two patients became pregnant after removal of ITDs. In the first instance, the ITDs were removed three months after their insertion because of intermenstrual pelvic pain, and the patient became pregnant two months later. The second patient, after two years of contraception with ITDs, wanted the devices removed so that she could become pregnant. Pregnancy occurred the month after removal of the tubal devices.

These results compare very favorably with those from studies that have been evaluated with the formed-in-place silicone plugs.[9,10] In a series of 1,058 women who requested this procedure, bilateral placement of the plugs could not be achieved in nearly 9 percent of the women for various anatomical reasons. Of the remaining women, bilateral tubal occlusion was obtained in 82 percent. No cases of reversibility were reported in these studies.[9,10]

The advantages of the hysteroscopic technique of sterilization are that the procedure can be performed as an outpatient procedure in an office setting; it is atraumatic and avoids the inconvenience of an abdominal incision, general anesthesia, and hospitalization. The procedure appears to be reversible by removal of the ITDs. Whether prolonged use of the ITDs adversely affects the endosalpinx or alters the likelihood of pregnancy has not been completely established. The first task has been to develop an effective method of hysteroscopic sterilization that has the potential for reversal.

The principal disadvantages of the procedure are that a skilled hysteroscopist is required; the equipment is expensive but can also be used for routine other hysteroscopic procedures. About 10 percent of women had ITDs expelled or displaced. Modifications of the insertion procedure, to assure a better anchorage of the devices, with an insertion of more than 10 mm beyond the tubal ostia may result in a reduced expulsion or displacement rate. Further follow-up of the women enrolled in the study will provide additional information to ascertain whether expanded trials of the ITD should be undertaken.

References

1. Richart RM, Taylor HC, and Neuwirth RS: Experimental studies of fallopian tube occlusion. In Richart RM, Prager D (Eds): *Human Sterilization*. Springfield, IL: Charles C Thomas, 1972: p. 360.
2. Goldsmith A, and Edelman DA: Nonsurgical methods of female sterilization. In Sciarra JJ (Ed): *Obstetrics and Gynecology*, vol. 6. Philadelphia: Harper & Row, 1985.
3. Zipper J, Stachetti E, and Mendel M: Human fertility control by transvaginal application of quinacrine on the fallopian tube. *Fertil Steril* 21:251, 1970.
4. Sciarra JJ: Hysteroscopic approaches for tubal closure. In Zatuchni GI, Labbok MH, Sciarra JJ (Eds): *Research Frontiers in Fertility Regulation*. Hagerstown, MD: Harper & Row, 1980: p. 270.
5. Quinones R, Alvarado A, and Anzar R: Tubal electrocoagulation under hysteroscopic control. In Sciarra JJ, Butler JC, Speidel JJ (Eds): *Hysteroscopic Sterilization*. New York: International Medical Book Corp., 1979: p. 95.
6. Quinones R, Alvarado A, and Ley E: Hysteroscopic sterilization: Followup of 800 cases. In Sciarra JJ, Droegemueller W, Speidel JJ (Eds): *Advances in Female Sterilization Techniques*. Hagerstown, MD: Harper & Row, 1976: p. 162.
7. Hosseinian AH, and Morales WA: Clinical application of hysteroscopic sterilization using uterotubal junction blocking device. In Zatuchni GI, Shelton JD, Goldsmith A, et al (Eds): *Female Transcervical Sterilization*. Hagerstown, MD: Harper & Row, 1983: p. 234.
8. Brundin J: Hydrogel tubal blocking device: P-block. In Zatuchni GI, Shelton JD, Goldsmith A, et al (Eds): *Female Transcervical Sterilization*. Hagerstown, MD: Harper & Row, 1983: p. 240.
9. Erb RA: Hysteroscopic tubal occlusion procedure with formed-in-place silicone plugs. In Zatuchni GI, Shelton JD, Goldsmith A, et al (Eds): *Female Transcervical Sterilization*. Hagerstown, MD: Harper & Row, 1983: p. 245.
10. Reed TP: Formed-in-place silicone plugs: Improvements and limitations. In Zatuchni GI, Shelton JD, Goldsmith A, et al (Eds): *Female Sterilization*. Hagerstown, MD: Harper & Row, 1983: p. 270.
11. Scarselli G, Mecaglia L, and Hamou JE: *Atlante di Microcolpoisteroscopia*. Palermo: Cofese, 1981.
12. Hamou JE: Autres applicationes de la microhystéroscopie. In Hamou JE (Ed): *Hystéroscopie et Microcolpohystéroscopie*. Palermo: Cofese, 1984: p. 241.

28

Reversible Tubal Sterilization

C. Irving Meeker and
Wilfrid Roth

Sterilization is the most widely used method of fertility control. It is being employed by young couples with small families as well as by single individuals. This has led to an increasing demand for reversal as the desire for pregnancy recurs. In a global sense, the lack of ready reversibility is a constant deterrent to many couples who would choose sterilization except for their concern about the permanent nature of the procedure.

An attempt has been made to quantify the importance of reversibility as a specific aspect of sterilization.[1] While the study was based on a hypothetical question, which limited the value to some extent, the magnitude of the response must be taken seriously. It was reported that if current methods of sterilization were predictably reversible, even though abdominal surgical procedures were required, then the number of patients who would seriously consider sterilization would almost double (an increase of 95 percent). Further, the proportion of patients who expressed an intention to undergo sterilization eventually increased from 22 to 62 percent (an increase of 178 percent). The study involved more than 1,000 patients in the southwestern United States. In countries such as India, where many believe it is essential to replace the eldest son should the child die, or China, where families are allowed to have only one child, any permanent method of sterilization will always be resisted by a large portion of the population.

The importance of reversibility has long been recognized and historically there have been several techniques devised with reversibility as a major goal. Although some of these sterilizations were reversed, none was sufficiently simple, safe, effective, or predictably reversible to receive widespread favor. To date there is no method of sterilization in clinical use that is reversible, even in animals, except by a major operative procedure. There are several techniques under study that have the potential for reversal in women but their evaluation has only been reported in other animals.

Methods of Historical Interest

Aldridge procedure

One of the earliest methods of "temporary sterilization" was described in 1934.[2]

The Fallopian Tube: Basic Studies and Clinical Contributions, edited by Alvin M. Siegler, M.D. Mount Kisco, New York: Futura Publishing Company, Inc. © 1986.

The fimbria were buried between the leaves of the broad ligament and sutured in place. This sterilizing procedure had an unacceptably high failure rate and the fimbria often became adherent to the broad ligament. Consequently, it was difficult to release them without damage and another abdominal operation was needed for reversal.

Fimbriotexy

Laufe[3] modified the Aldridge procedure by placing a silicone rubber cap over the fimbria in a small group of rabbits. Pregnancies were achieved after removal of the caps in these animals. In a further modification of this approach, Droegemueller et al.[4] used a stocking of polytetrafluoroethylene (PTFE) to protect the fimbria and then buried both the stocking and the enclosed fimbria in the broad ligament. With baboons as a model, there were no failures during six months and more than 50 percent of the animals conceived after removal of the fimbria from the stockings for reversal. Human studies have not been undertaken.

Ovariotexy

The ovaries were placed in silastic pouches which were then buried in the broad ligament in six women.[5] There were no early problems with the technique but reversibility has not been reported.

Tubal clips

A wide variety of clips have been designed for temporary and permanent tubal occlusion.[6,7] The first reported use of clips involved a one-inch tantalum clip on each tube for sterilization.[8] The technique was described as rapid, simple, and safe. However, the problems associated with the use of clips became evident in studies with rhesus monkeys.[9] If clips were applied too tightly, the tissue would undergo necrosis and the tube would be transected. If less pressure was applied, the tube would reopen since tissue tends to shrink under pressure, thus restoring tubal patency. These problems have been largely corrected with the newest clip devices, such as Hulka-Clemmons, Bleier, and Filshie types.

Maghoub's operation

A less complicated approach was described in which the ovaries were passed forward through a window in the broad ligament to lie under the round ligament.[10] There were no failures among 30 women followed for four years and one successful reversal. It would seem likely that failures will occur since the ovum is released into the peritoneal cavity, although it is anterior to the broad ligament.

Intratubal splints

Intratubal splints were designed and placed in 26 women for sterilization.[11] These silastic rods were placed laparoscopically using a triple puncture technique and were secured in place by Weck hemoclips. The splints migrated into the peritoneal cavity in 3 of 26 patients; two pregnancies followed, one being intrauterine and the other in the tube. Other clips were to be tested and while removal of the splints for planned pregnancy is theoretically possible, there are no reported data on reversibility.

Methods in Current Clinical Use

Essentially all current methods for female sterilization cause some tubal destruction or significant tubal damage. These vary from hysterectomy and salpingectomy to injection of sclerosing material through the cervix into the uterotubal junction. In many instances there is no possibility of reversal.

A variety of sterilization procedures enable reversal through the use of advanced operative techniques designed to restore the luminal continuity. The possibility of successful reversal appears greatest when the smallest tubal segment is damaged, at least 4 to 5 cm of tube remains after the repair, and the sterilization is done in the tubal isthmus about 1 cm from the uterine serosal surface. Properly placed clips in the tubal isthmus will damage only 2 to 3 mm of tube, allowing an excellent opportunity for anastomosis. Success or failure also may be inversely related to the time interval between the sterilization and its attempted reversal.

Fimbriectomy and extensive unipolar or bipolar electrocoagulation leave the least chance for a successful reversal.

Several hysteroscopic sterilization techniques are available. Only the uterotubal junction blocking device (UTJD) and the formed-in-place silicone rubber plugs offer a potential for reversal. Both methods are office procedures and do not require a major operation for either implantation or removal. The major disadvantage is that they require considerable skill and experience and highly specialized equipment, thus limiting their use in less developed countries. The reversibility of the UTJD has been demonstrated in animal studies but not in women. The results of clinical trials in women were so disappointing (50 percent failure rate) that they have been suspended until a steerable hysteroscope is developed.[12]

The formed-in-place silicone rubber plugs were successfully placed in 82 percent of patients accepted for this procedure. An additional 9 percent, of more than 1,000 patients requesting the plugs, were refused the operation because of tubal disease or a fixed retrodisplaced uterus.[13] There have been no pregnancies reported in the most recent series of patients who had proper bilateral placement of plugs for as long as 38 months of use.[14] Although designed with a loop for their removal, there are few published data on reversibility in women.

New Methods

Tubal plug and clip

This method was designed specifically to be simple, safe, effective, and to offer a high probability of reversal. It consists of a small teflon plug introduced through the fimbria and secured in place with a teflon clip. In the initial studies, nonabsorbable suture was used to secure the clip. The plugs were designed to overcome the basic problem of all clips or ties intended to occlude the tube by pressure. When a clip or suture is placed on the tube, the compressed tissue eventually shrinks, thus allowing the tube to reopen (Fig. 28:1). If too much pressure is used, the tube is cut, leaving one or both ends open. The notched plugs make it possible to occlude the tube and compress the wall against the plug, thus maintaining the obstruction even with the normal shrinkage of tissue.

The teflon clip was designed to secure the plug in place (Fig. 28:2). This clip was quickly covered with a fibrinous exudate, as is seen with any foreign body. For removal, the clip can be dissected free from the fibrin covering, opened, and lifted away from the tube. Then the plug is either squeezed out or removed through a small tubal incision.

In studies on baboons, plugs were inserted and left in place for 12 months. Ten of 18 animals became pregnant and delivered normally within 12 months of removal of the plug. Six of these 18 animals conceived and delivered a second time. There were no unplanned pregnancies in over 480 breeding cycles in 86 animals with plugs in place.[15,16] The expected pregnancy rate for baboons in that facility was approximately 60 percent per year with regular breeding so that the 55.6 percent pregnancy rate in the reversal series approached the expected rate.

A successful reversal of this technique was demonstrated in baboons. The devices did not migrate or move while in situ. The method clearly was effective in

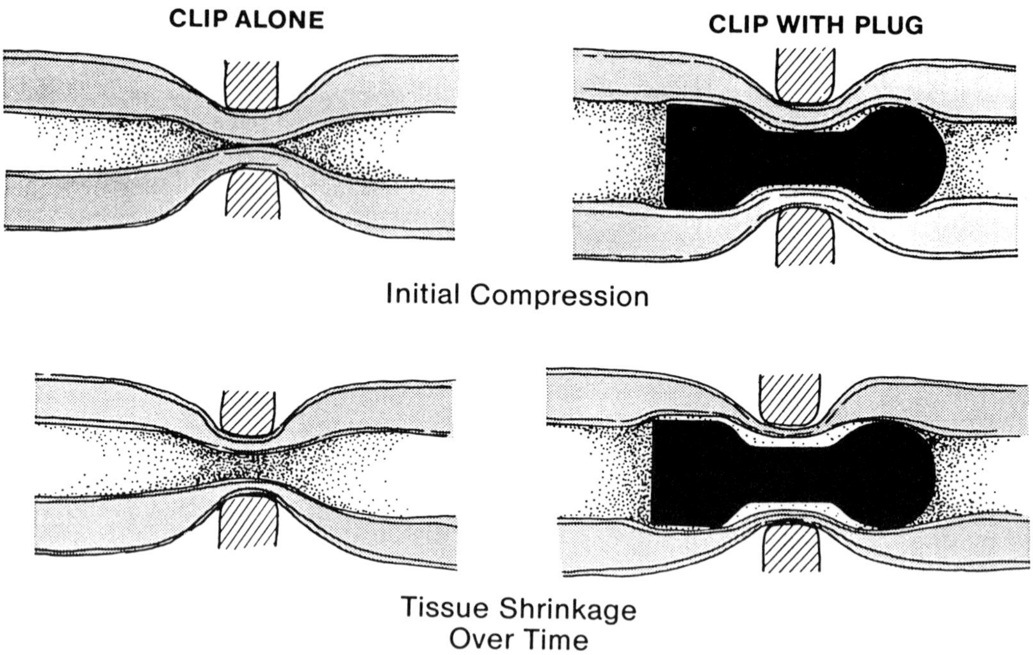

FIGURE 28:1—*Principle upon which the notched tubal plug and teflon clip was designed. As tissue shrinks, lumen reopens if only the clip is used. The notched plug overcomes this problem.*

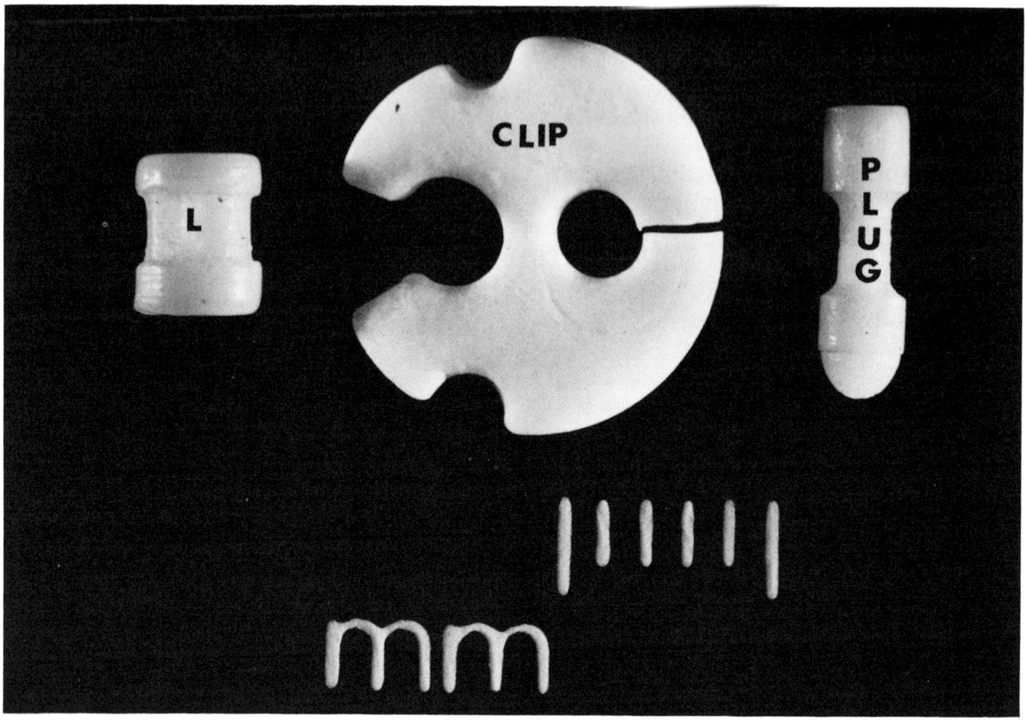

FIGURE 28:2—*Lock (L), clip, and plug are seen with a millimeter scale.*

the primate model. The advantages of this method are its simplicity and efficacy. The plugs can be inserted through a minilaparotomy as an outpatient (one-day) procedure. No special instruments or skills are required other than those necessary to enter the peritoneal cavity.

Comment

There are many simple, safe, and effective sterilization methods and most of them can be reversed in selected instances. Except for the hysteroscopic methods described above, the others require a laparotomy and tuboplasty for reversal. These procedures are costly and their availability is limited, even in developed countries. They are not even a possibility for most of the sterilized women in the world. The potential advantage of the "plug and clip" is the simplicity of reversal. Neither special instruments nor special skills are needed and only a 4 cm abdominal incision is required.

The major disadvantage of the "plug and clip" technique is the need to perform a minilaparotomy for sterilization and another for its reversal because it can not be done laparoscopically. However, such an operation requires a short hospitalization, and is available in almost any institution. A second problem is possible inadvertent tubal damage or transection while removing the clip. This "worst case" situation still allows an optimal alternative of conventional anastomosis since only 2 to 3 mm of tube are compromised by the clip. The technique fulfilled all the original objectives, in the primate model, and it is now ready for the initial human trials.

Although it is not necessary to guarantee reversibility, a reasonably high probability of success is required to make sterilization acceptable to a large group of women who would not otherwise accept it.

The central problem of reversibility, without the need for tubal reanastomosis, is not so much with the occlusive device as with the method of securing the device in place. The clip presented in the present study, made of a biologically inert material, allows removal without further tubal damage. It is this ease of application, as well as the possibility of simple reversal, that represent the greatest potential benefit of this method for women.

It is difficult to test reversibility in women. It is possible to examine this question in an animal model using the study design described here. Although one cannot extrapolate from any animal model to human subjects, the high rate of reversibility in this primate model would seem to justify clinical trials at this time. These will be designed initially to determine safety and efficacy. Potential reversibility will make sterilization an acceptable alternative to many women who do not plan to have more children. However, the possibility that this or any other technique of surgical sterilization will be offered to women who wish to maintain their long-term fertility is remote at best. To do so would require that both the sterilization and reversal procedures be safe and reasonably simple to perform, that the cost be competitive with current methods of contraception, and finally, that the expected success with reversal be greater than 75 to 80 percent.

References

1. Shain RN: The potential impact of reversibility on selection of sterilization. *Contraception* 22:227, 1980.
2. Aldridge AH: Temporary surgical sterilization with subsequent pregnancy. *Am J Obstet Gynecol* 27:741, 1934.
3. Laufe LE: The fimbrial prosthesis: Part I: Evaluation of micro-surgical technique. In Sciarra JJ, Zatuchni GI, Speidel JJ (Eds): *Reversal of Sterilization.* Hagerstown, MD: Harper & Row, 1978: p. 220.
4. Droegemueller W, Chvapil M, and Christian CD: Modern modified Aldridge procedure. In Sciarra JJ, Zatuchni GI, Speidel JJ (Eds): *Reversal of Sterilization.* Hagerstown, MD: Harper & Row, 1978: p. 224.
5. Wood EC, and Leeton J: Sterilization by ovariotexy: A reversible technique. *Lancet* 2:1213, 1969.

6. Wortman J, Hulka J, and Piotrow T: Laparoscopic sterilization with clips. *Population Reports*, Series C #4, 45–52, 1974.
7. Wortman J: Tubal sterilization, review of methods. *Population Reports*, Series C #7, 73–96, 1976.
8. Evans TN: Simplified method for sterilization of the female. *Am J Obstet Gynecol* 66:393, 1953.
9. Neuman HH, and Frick HC: Occlusion of the fallopian tubes with tantalum clips. *Am J Obstet Gynecol* 81:803, 1961.
10. Mahgoub S: Mahgoub's operation: A reversible method of sterilization. *Fertil Steril* 29:466, 1978.
11. Steptoe PC: The potential use of intratubal stents for reversible sterilization. In Sciarra JJ, Droegemueller W, Speidel JJ (Eds): *Advances in Female Sterilization Techniques*. Hagerstown, MD: Harper & Row, 1976: p. 91.
12. Hosseinian AH, and Wilson AM: Clinical application of hysteroscopic sterilization using uterotubal junction blocking devices. In Zatuchni GI, Shelton JD, Goldsmith A, et al (Eds): *Female Transcervical Sterilization*. Hagerstown, MD: Harper & Row, 1983: p. 234.
13. Reed TP III: Hysteroscopic sterilization: Silicone elastic plugs. *Clin Obstet Gynecol* 26:313, 1983.
14. Reed TP III, and Erb R: Hysteroscopic tubal occlusion with silicone rubber. *Obstet Gynecol* 61:388, 1983.
15. Meeker CI: A tubal occlusive device in monkeys. In Sciarra JJ, Zatuchni GI, Speidel JJ (Eds): *Reversal of Sterilization*. Hagerstown, MD: Harper & Row, 1978: p. 226.
16. Meeker CI, and Roth W: A tubal plug and clip method for female sterilization. *Obstet Gynecol* 65:430, 1985.

29

Laparoscopic Tubal Sterilization

Amir H. Ansari, Jaroslav J. Marik, and John G. Moore

Laparoscopic sterilization in the United States is the most common method of interval tubal sterilization. Complications are infrequent when an experienced surgeon performs the procedure. The disadvantages include the need for special training in diagnostic laparoscopy, the frequent need for general anesthesia, and the expensive equipment which must be properly maintained.

Although Anderson in 1937,[1] and Power and Barnes in 1941[2] published the first reports describing sterilization by laparoscopic tubal fulguration, most of the pioneer work with laparoscopy was done by Palmer[3] and Steptoe.[4]

Laparoscopic sterilization presently is accomplished using thermal or mechanical techniques.

Initially with unipolar methods, multiple points of coagulation are done in the isthmic portion of the tube so as to destroy approximately 3 cm of tubal length. This may be accomplished by using an appropriate coagulation forceps introduced either through the operating laparoscope or through secondary trocar sleeves. Under direct observation, the physician can observe blanching, swelling, and finally collapse and dehydration of the coagulated area. The electrical current is concentrated at the tip of the grasping forceps. The current also has a tendency to seek other leads to complete the connection with the ground plate and therefore may "jump" to adjacent areas during the operative procedure. In the early 1970s, it was believed that transection of the coagulated area increased the efficacy of the procedure. Some surgeons advise multiple transections but there is no evidence that this approach is an improvement over coagulation techniques alone.

Soderstorm and Smith[5] introduced the method of partial tubal resection which guaranteed pathological confirmation of the extirpated tissue. This technique required an insulated rectal polyp snare placed through a secondary trocar. When the snare was drawn tightly around the knuckle of the tube, the electrocoagulation current was applied until adequate hemostasis occurred. Complete closure of the snare transected the base of the specimen. Marik and coworkers[6] described the use of Semms' biopsy for-

The Fallopian Tube: Basic Studies and Clinical Contributions, edited by Alvin M. Siegler, M.D. Mount Kisco, New York: Futura Publishing Company, Inc. © 1986.

ceps to excise the tubal specimen with a cutting current. Since surgical specimens are no longer essential to prove the adequacy of the laparoscopic tubal sterilization, these techniques are not used.

With the bipolar method introduced by Rioux and Cloutier,[7] the unipolar ground plate was eliminated. The current runs only between the grasping jaws of the forceps and thus, with an isolated ground circuitry unit, there is no possibility of alternate paths of ground seeking. One jaw of the forceps is the active electrode and the other jaw is the ground electrode. The current density is quite confined and the spread of electrocoagulation is less than with unipolar forceps. Since only low-voltage, high-frequency units can be used with the forceps, the safety of the procedure is increased. This method of tubal electrocoagulation has become the preferred technique for sterilization with the use of electrosurgical energy. It is essential that at least three contiguous areas of the tube are coagulated. Bipolar coagulation has proved to be a safe and efficient method of tubal sterilization. Its other advantages are that the coagulated area can be strictly confined to the tube without impairment of the mesosalpinx and its vessels. The rate of complications and failures is low. There is no pain postoperatively and no foreign body is introduced into the abdomen. The reversibility of this technique is probably less than that of mechanical sterilization methods. Therefore, in young women, it is preferable to use clips or bands.

Tubal sterilization with endocoagulation destroys only 5 mm of tube by means of a heating temperature of 100–110°C. The fallopian tube is grasped with a crocodile forceps and heated to 100°C for 20 seconds. The procedure is done twice and then the tube is transected.[8]

Two mechanical occlusive devices have been used with excellent results.

A Silastic ring ceveloped by Yoon and King[9] in 1975 is made of nonreactive, medical grade silastic silicone rubber (polydimethylsiloxanes with 5 percent barium sulfate). It has an inner diameter of 1 mm, an outer diameter of 4 mm, a thickness of 2.5 mm, and specific elastic power. The ring applicator consists of two cylinders that contain grasping forceps.

With a special loading device, the ring is stretched over the outer applicator cylinder. Two tongs within the cylinder are maneuvered so as to grasp the tube 4 cm from its uterine origin. The tube is pulled into the cylinder of the applicator, the ring is released, and approximately 2 cm of tube are above the ring. The banded segments are inspected to ensure proper application and adequate hemostasis. Should inadvertent bleeding occur, either additional silastic rings can be placed or bipolar cautery can be used to provide hemostasis.

The Hulka clip consists of two plastic jaws made of Lexan, hinged by a small metal pin 2 mm from one end. Each jaw has teeth on the opposite surface, and a gold-plated stainless steel spring holds the clip jaws in the open position. The first human studies of a spring-loaded clip and a single incision laparoscope clip applicator for female sterilization was published in 1975.[10] The clip is approximately 12.5 mm in length and 4 mm in width. Only 5 mm of tube are destroyed in contrast to the 2 cm using the ring. When the clip is closed, there is a 1 mm gap between the upper and lower jaws so as to prevent tearing of the tube or blood vessels. This space becomes obliterated by the action of the spring 48 to 72 hours after application. The Filshie clip has smooth jaws that are lined with rubber.[11]

Open laparoscopy[12] is the endoscopic method of observing the peritoneal cavity through a minilaparotomy incision. The technique is viewed as a minilaparotomy with endoscopic instruments. With the open method, the abdomen is entered initially under vision with a small incision and then it is insufflated. With the closed method, the abdomen is insufflated with a Veress needle and then entered blindly with careful penetration with a sharp trocar. The aspects of both methods are similar except the fascia is sutured closed in the open technique after removal of the subumbilical trocar.

Laparoscopy for an average patient in

a large city in the United States done by a skilled gynecologist with the assistance of trained personnel is an effective, rapid, and safe method of tubal sterilization. Laparoscopy also plays a crucial role in the introduction of sterilization services into less developed countries. There is a time and place for each technique and it is incumbent on the physician and the patient to discuss the alternative methods, choosing the method that best suits the patient's situation.

References

1. Anderson ET: Peritoneoscopy. *Am J Surg* 35:136, 1937.
2. Power FH, and Barnes AC: Sterilization by means of peritoneoscopy tubal fulguration: A preliminary report. *Am J Obstet Gynecol* 41:1038, 1941.
3. Palmer MR: Essais de stérilisation tubaire coelioscopique par électrocoagulation isthmique. *Bull Fed Soc Gynécol Obstét* 14:298, 1962.
4. Steptoe PC: *Laparoscopy in Gynecology.* London: ES Livingstone Ltd., 1967.
5. Soderstrom RM, and Smith MR: Tubal sterilization: A new laparoscopic method. *Obstet Gynecol* 38:152, 1971.
6. Marik JJ, Friedman S, and Tyler ET: A simple technique of laparoscopic tubal sterilization. *J Reprod Med* 15:109, 1975.
7. Rioux JE, and Cloutier D: A new bipolar instrument for laparoscopic tubal sterilization. *Am J Obstet Gynecol* 119:737, 1974.
8. Semm K: Endocoagulation: A new field of endoscopic surgery. *J Reprod Med* 16:195, 1976.
9. Yoon IB, and King TM: A preliminary and intermediate report on a new laparoscopic tubal ring procedure. *J Reprod Med* 15:54, 1975.
10. Hulka JF, Omran KF, Phillip JM, et al: Sterilization by spring clip: A report of 1,000 cases with a 6 month follow-up. *Fertil Steril* 26:1122, 1975.
11. Filshie FM, Casey D, Pogmore JR, et al: The titanium/silicone rubber clip for female sterilization. *Br J Obstet Gynaecol* 88:655, 1981.
12. Hasson HM: Open laparoscopy: A report of 150 cases. *J Reprod Med* 12:234, 1974.

30

Tubal Coagulation Techniques in Animal Models with Follow-up Morphological and Endocrinological Studies

Hans-Harald Riedel,
Kurt Semm, and
Günter Corts-Kleinwort

Sterilization Techniques and Ovarian Metabolism

For over 100 years tubal sterilization procedures have been described in the medical literature. When all the variations are considered, over 1,000 different techniques have been developed. The use of different coagulation techniques for tubal sterilization include monopolar and bipolar high-frequency endocoagulation and CO_2 laser vaporization. These result in varying degrees of mesosalpingeal destruction and subsequent disruption of the nervous and vascular supplies to the ovaries, depending largely on the method.[1–17] In 1981 we proved that a significant relationship existed between the extent of the destroyed area during tubal coagulation and the occurrence of menstrual disorders or premature menstrual complaints.[7–9]

Differing results have been reported in the literature regarding the frequency of these late complications, especially when dealing with detectable hormonal changes following tubal sterilization. Radwanska and coauthors[18] and Donnez and colleagues[19] reported a significant drop in the average progesterone concentrations in patients sterilized with the Pomeroy technique or by electrocoagulation.[16] In similar studies this reduction

The Fallopian Tube: Basic Studies and Clinical Contributions, edited by Alvin M. Siegler, M.D. Mount Kisco, New York: Futura Publishing Company, Inc. © 1986.

Table 30:1

Distribution of Rabbits according to the Coagulation Method, Tissue Temperature, and Current Output

Method of coagulation	*°C/sec or Watt/sec.*	*# animals/group*
Endocoagulation	(1) 120°C/20 sec.	7
	(2) 140°C/40 sec.	7
Monopolar, HF coagulation	(3) 32 W/20 sec.	7
	(4) 68 W/20 sec.	7
Bipolar, HF coagulation	(5) 12 W/20 sec.	7
	(6) 23 W/20 sec.	7
Control		7

HF = high frequency.

in progesterone levels was not evident.[20–21]

The endocoagulation of Riedel and Semm did not cause measurable differ ences in the pre- and postoperative progesterone or estradiol (E_2) levels.[11,22–24] McComb et al.,[25] and also Koninckx and his group[26] reported that a disruption of the vascular anastomoses between the ovaries and the uterine horns could destroy normal ovulation following microsurgical fimbriectomy of white New Zealand rabbits. The changes resulted from the disruption of neuroendocrine connections between the tube and ovary. Therefore the role of the autonomic system for the regulation of ovarian functions was shown to be of particular importance.[3,11,14,25] Halme and coauthors[27] performed bilateral salpingectomies on nine rabbits. Compared to a normal control, no changes in the number of corpora lutea, ovarian weight or average progesterone concentrations were evident.

Different Coagulation Techniques in the Rabbit Model

Pelviscopy or a laparotomy was performed on 370 New Zealand white rabbits followed by coagulation of the distal uterine horns with unipolar, bipolar, or endocoagulation methods or CO_2 laser. The laser was performed at 20 or 40 watts and approximately 2 seconds were required for a complete severing of each uterine horn. The endocoagulation of the uterine horns was achieved at temperatures between 120°C and 140°C with coagulation times of 20 to 40 seconds, using the Semm endocoagulator and the crocodile clamp. For monopolar and bipolar coagulation, the Eschmann TD 311 and the Martin MC electrosurgical instruments, respectively, were used. Monopolar coagulation was performed at a current of 32 to 68 watts and at coagulation times ranging from 10 to 50 seconds while bipolar technique was carried out at 10 to 50 seconds.

At the time of the operations the rabbits weighed 2.5 to 4.5 kg. A general anesthesia was carried out by using nembutal (30–40 mg/kg body wt.) which was injected intravenously into a marginal vein of the ear (Table 30:1).

Approximately 1.2 liters of CO_2 were insufflated intraperitoneally into each animal; the intraabdominal pressure was 6–8 mmHg. The pelviscopies were performed with the same instruments used for women and were carried out using the security measures specified by Semm. Chloramphenicol (50 mg/day for 5 days) was prophylactically administered for nearly all the animals postoperatively.

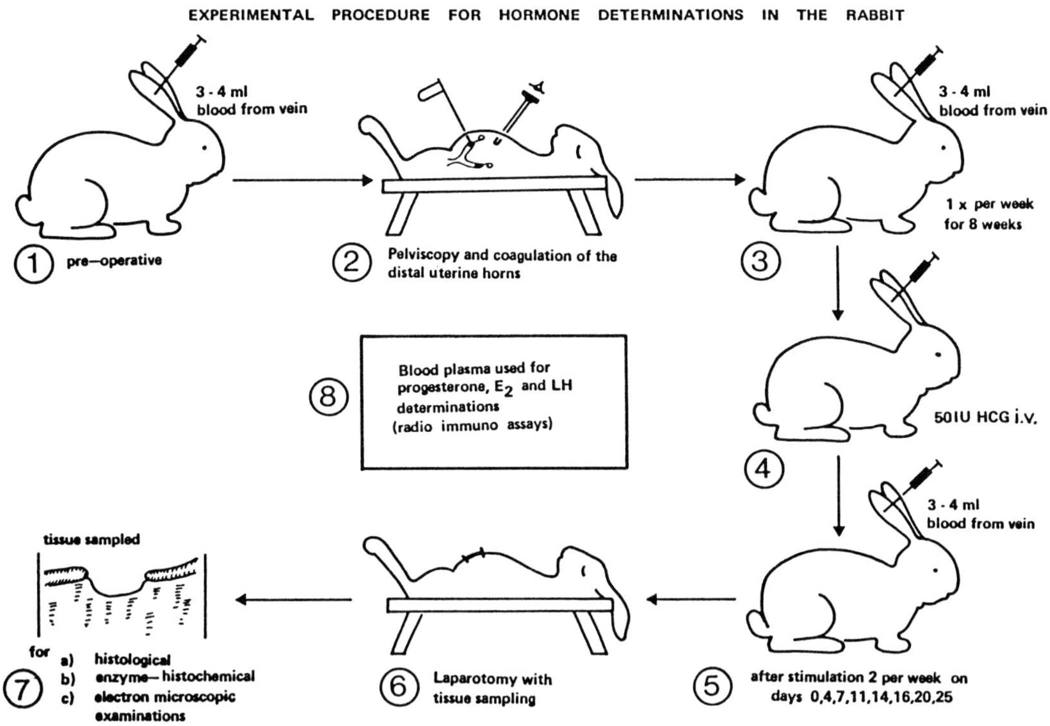

FIGURE 30:1—*Experimental procedure for hormone measurements in the rabbit.*

Laparotomy was performed after 1, 2, 4, 8, or 12 weeks. Following a macroscopic description, photodocumentation and measurement of the amount of destroyed tissue, the uterine horns were excised. In addition to the normal histologic and electron microscopic evaluation, 5 μ thick cyrostat sections were examined for the presence of nine different enzymes, of which ATPase, 5-nucleotidase, basic and acid phosphatase, acid and unspecific esterase and diaminopeptidase were measured.

Hormone Examinations in the Rabbit Model

Progesterone, E_2 and luteinizing hormone (LH) levels were measured in 49 New Zealand rabbits before and after stimulation with 50 I.U. HCG intravenously. All the rabbits used for the endocrine studies were individually caged. Blood samples were taken from a marginal vein in the ear before operation and eight weeks postoperatively following different coagulation techniques. At the end of this period, the rabbits were stimulated by injecting 50 I.U. HCG intravenously to provoke a pseudopregnancy. During this poststimulation phase, blood samples were taken twice each week on days 4, 7, 11, 14, 16, 20, and 25 (Fig. 30:1).

Tissue Damage in Relation to the Coagulation Technique

Measurable endocrinological changes would not be expected following the precise execution of tubal sterilizaton by endocoagulation, since none of the mesosalpingeal vessels or nerves is destroyed. Endocoagulation is strictly lim-

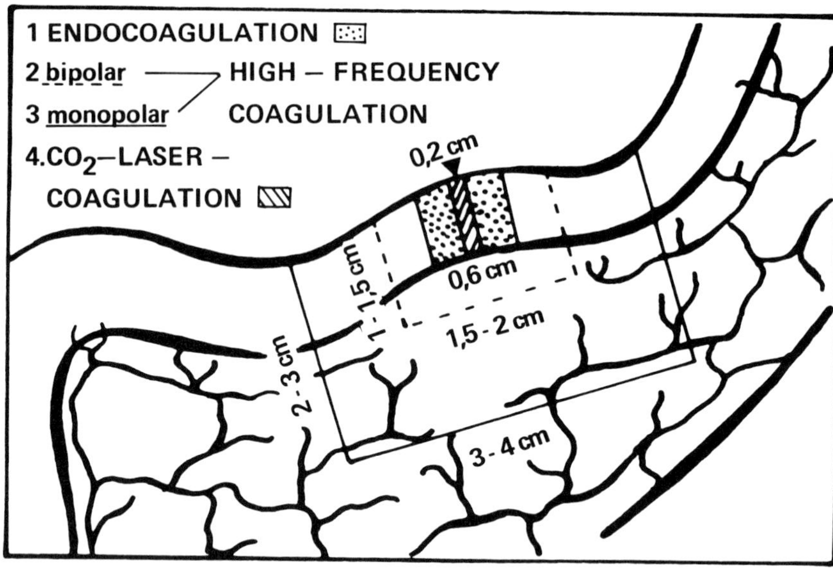

FIGURE 30:2—*Areas of tissue damage after the use of different coagulation techniques.*

ited to tubal tissue, whereas monopolar high frequency current technique destroys 3–4 cm of tubal tissue but also 2–4 cm of mesosalpinx.[7–11]

Limited destruction is impossible when sterilization is performed with the high frequency current technique even when it is carried out at lower coagulating temperatures and for shorter periods of time. Some portion of the mesosalpinx is always damaged (Fig. 30:2). By using the bipolar technique at a current output of only 10 watts for tubal sterilization, it is possible to avoid extensive damage of the mesosalpinx, if the coagulation time is less than 20 seconds. In this case the complete severing of the fallopian tubes is necessary, as with endocoagulation to prevent recanalization.

Through the use of unipolar high-frequency coagulation, extensive destruction of the uterine horns and the surrounding mesosalpingeal tissue occurred after a coagulation time of only 10 seconds. Thus, coagulation for only a few seconds leads not only to a white coloring of the tissue 2 to 3 cm around the coagulated uterine horn but also to its disruption. The smoke caused by laparoscopic coagulation with monopolar high-frequency current limited the visibility of the operative site significantly so that in several cases superficial burning of the intestine took place. The damage resulted in adhesions between the intestine and the genital organs, however, and there was no intestinal perforation (Fig. 30:3).

During laparotomy one to four weeks after unipolar coagulation, most of the tissue was necrotic; after eight to twelve weeks the uterine horns consisted mainly of a thin fibrous tissue. Moreover, considerable destruction of the mesosalpingeal tissue was noted (Fig. 30:4).

With the bipolar technique, in which we used the coagulation forceps developed by Hirsch, the smoke was less and destruction of tissue localized. However, a negative aspect was the adherence of the coagulated tissue to the forceps. Examinations following bilateral coagulation after four to twelve weeks showed a destroyed mesosalpingeal area (approximately 1–2 cm in size) and a swelling of the distal uterine horns that was comparable to a hydrosalpinx.

With the Sharplan 733 CO_2 laser, we separated the uterine horns using a power output of 20 or 40 watts. The adjoining mesosalpingeal tissue was not in-

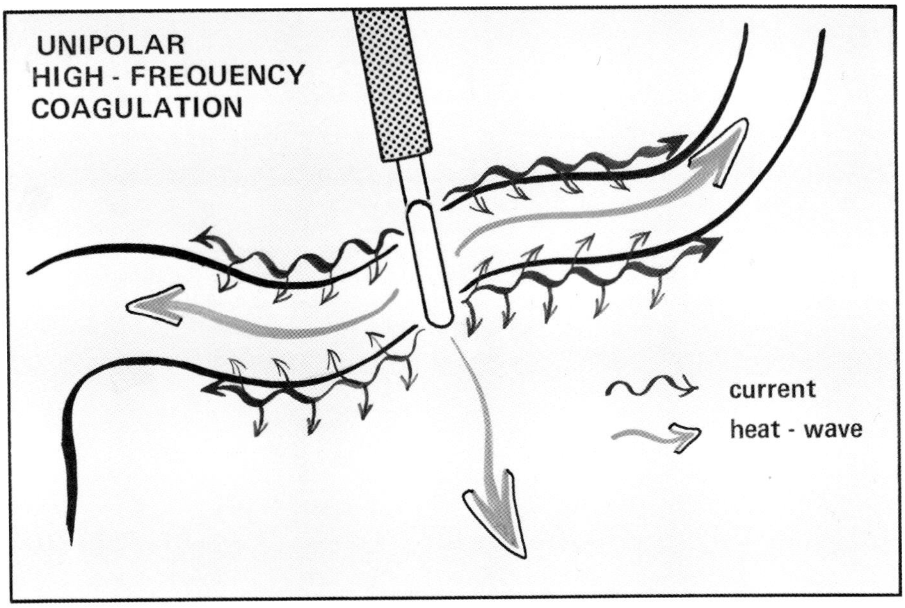

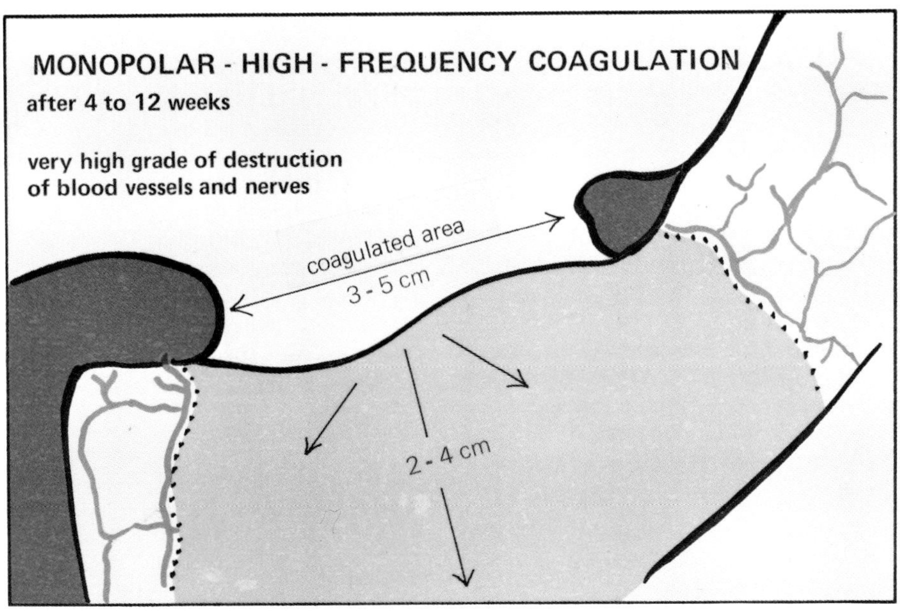

FIGURE 30:3—*Technique of unipolar current coagulation of rabbit uterine horns* (top) *and area of tissue destruction* (bottom).

jured. In two instances (especially in the case of thick uterine horns) the CO_2 laser did not provide sufficient hemostasis.

On the basis of the results reported by Tadir et al.[29] in 8 out of 23 cases (34.8 percent) laser sterilization is not efficient because a high rate of recanalization occurs.[11,30]

Using endocoagulation with a forceps temperature of 120°C and coagulation for 20 seconds, coagulation of the uterine horns occurred without complications. During the "second-look" operations, a

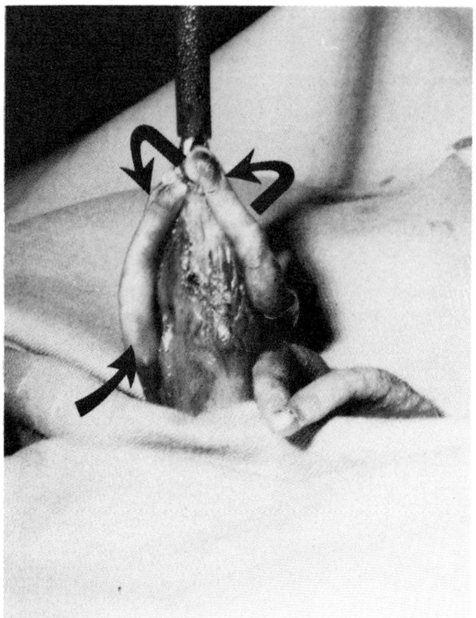

FIGURE 30:4*a*—*Unipolar coagulation of rabbit uterine horns. Extensive destruction of both uterine horns* (curved arrows) *and mesosalpinx.*

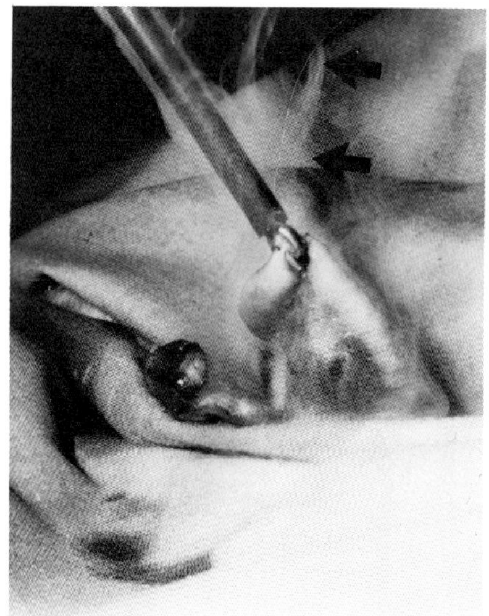

FIGURE 30:4*b*—*Formation of smoke during unipolar coagulation.*

complete division (of approximately 0.5 cm) of the uterine horns was evident and the technique had no effect on the mesosalpingeal tissue. Although we deliberately did not use the hooked scissors in the coagulated area to divide the uterine horns, spontaneous recanalization did not occur.

Hormonal Results after Different Coagulation Techniques

The primary vascular supply of the uterine horns in New Zealand rabbits is located much deeper within the mesosalpinx than is the case in human fallopian tubes. During coagulation with the monopolar technique, however, the uterine artery is nearly always destroyed. This was clearly demonstrated not only macroscopically but also by our histologic and enzyme histochemical analyses.

Results of hormonal studies,[25–27] in ovarian blood supply, and the weights of ovaries[30–33] on 49 New Zealand rabbits showed large variations. After stimulation of the animals with 50 I.U. HCG intravenously the control group showed a clear rise in average progesterone levels of 12.69 ± 6.02 ng/ml up to the 11th day of pseudopregnancy followed by a gradual decrease in concentrations returning to basal levels from days 14 to 25. Although the average basal progesterone concentrations were nearly identical in all groups, the progesterone concentrations after stimulation were lower in the two groups of animals whose horns were coagulated with monopolar current than in the other groups (Fig. 30:5).

At monopolar coagulation currents of 32 and 68 watts, the average progesterone concentrations on day 11 of 7.84 ± 1.68 and 7.66 ± 2.6 ng/ml, respectively, were significantly lower than control levels. Similar differences were evident on days 4, 7, 14, and 16.

Conclusions

Examination of the tissue destroyed during laparotomy by histologic, histochemical, and electron microscopic exam-

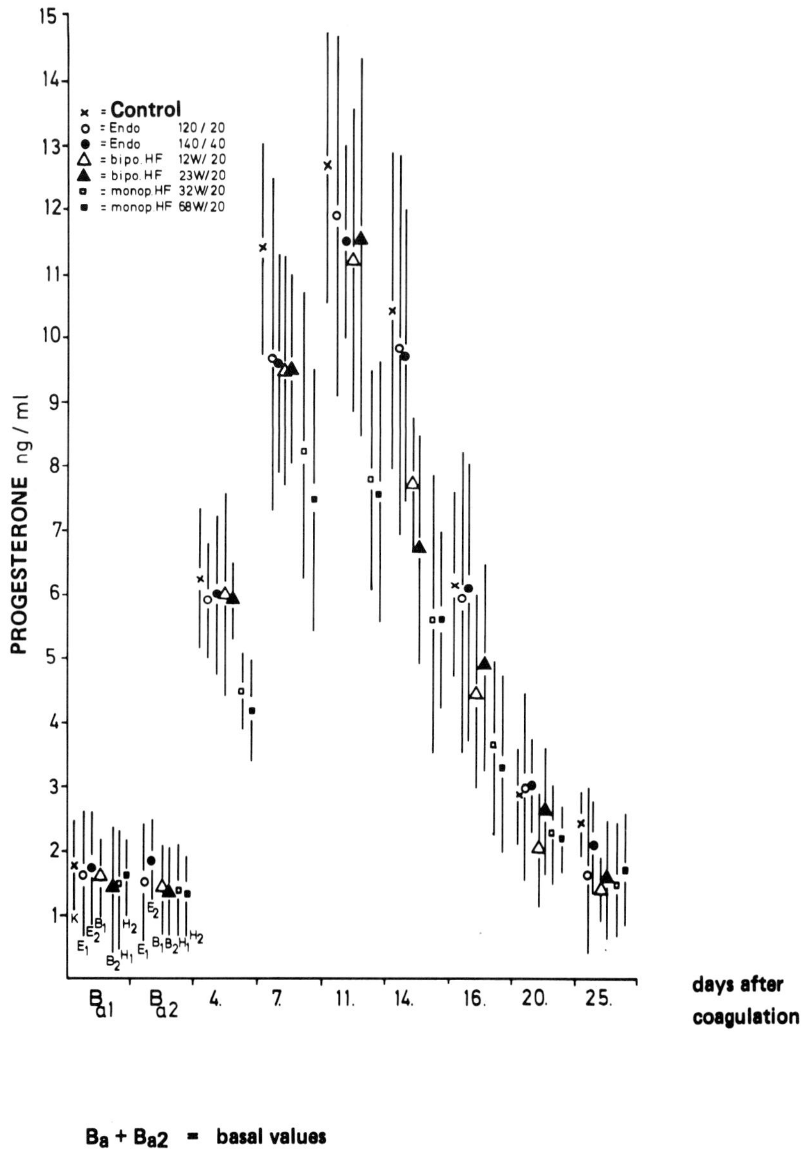

FIGURE 30:5—*Progesterone levels after different coagulation techniques.*

inations revealed that the extent of tissue destruction during sterilization by endocoagulation or bipolar techniques operated at lower coagulation currents was insignificant compared to the destruction caused by the monopolar technique.[4,7–11,28,34]

Differences in the extent of the coagulated zone could not be correlated with the experience of the surgeons, but was dependent on the coagulation temperature reached by the tissue and the duration of coagulation. Large variations in the course of blood vessels and nerves occur in individual species. Therefore, experiments performed on small groups of animals may not be significant and particularly since they are carried out only for a few months.[11,26,31,33,35] No definite conclusion regarding the effect of different sterilization techniques on ovarian metabolism can be drawn from these experiments. The occurrence of measurable hormonal changes immediately following sterilization of a patient has little significance. For example, women who had preoperative progesterone levels in the upper normal range experienced no drop in progesterone or E_2 concentrations below normal even after reduction of the ovarian blood supply.[2,9,11,12,19,20,24,36] However, women whose preoperative hormone levels were in the lower range, postoperatively, on the average of two and a half to three years later, experienced menstrual disorders and measurable hormonal changes. As observed by several investigators,[18–20] disturbances in ovarian metabolism following tubal sterilization by electrocoagulation or the Pomeroy techniques can be explained by the disruption of tubal and uterine blood flow.[4,11,12,19–22,36]

References

1. Battig CG: Electrosurgical burn injuries and their prevention. *JAMA* 204:1025, 1968.
2. Corson SL, Hamilton HPT, and Bolognese RJ: Electrical considerations of laparoscopic sterilization. *J Reprod Med* 11:1, 1973.
3. Esposito JM: Electrical burn of the abdominal wall as a complication of fallopian tube cautery. *Fertil Steril* 24:158, 1973.
4. Frangenheim H: Wie sicher sind die einzelnen Methoden der laparoskopischen Tubensterilisation? *Geburtsh Frauenheilkd* 40:398, 1980.
5. Garite TJ, and Gunning JE: Enter the thermal cautery. *Contemp Obstet Gynecol* 11:99, 1978.
6. Hirsch HA: Verbrennungen bei der laparoskopischen Tubensterilisation und Möglichkeiten ihrer Vermeidung. *Geburtsh Frauenheilkd* 34:345, 1974.
7. Riedel H-H, and Semm K: There is no place in gynecological endoscopy for unipolar or bipolar high-frequency current. *Endoscopy* 14:51, 1982.
8. Riedel H-H, Ahrens H, and Semm K: Late complications according to method. *J Reprod Med* 26:353, 1981.
9. Riedel H-H, Ahrens H, and Semm K: Spätkomplikationen nach Anwendung unterschiedlicher Sterilisationstechniken: Ein Vergleich zwischen der unipolaren Hochfrequenzsterilisation und der Endokoagulationstechnik nach Semm. *Geburtsh Frauenheikd* 42:273, 1982.
10. Riedel H-H, Müller L, Mosler H, et al: Devitalisierung und Hämostase durch destruktive Wärme: Ergebnisse enzymhistochemischer und histologischer Untersuchungen an Eileiter präparaten nach Gewebskoagulation mit Endokoagulation oder Hochfrequenz. *Zentralb Gynäkol* 104:489, 1982.
11. Riedel HH, and Semm K: An initial comparison of coagulation techniques of sterilization. *J Reprod Med* 27:261, 1982.
12. Rioux JE: Late complications of female sterilization: A review of the literature and a proposal for further research. *J Reprod Med* 19:329, 1977.
13. Semm K: Endocoagulation: A new and completely safe medical current for sterilization. *Int J Fertil* 22:238, 1977.
14. Semm K: Statistical survey of gynecological laparoscopy/pelviscopy in Germany till 1977. *Endoscopy* 2:101, 1979.
15. Semm K, and Philipp E: Eileiterre generation post sterilisationem. *Geburtsh Frauenheilkd* 39:14, 1979.
16. Schwimmer AB: Electrosurgical burn injuries during laparoscopy sterilization. *Obstet Gynecol* 44:526, 1974.
17. Te Breutl W, and Boeminghaus F: Harnleiterläsion bei laparoskopischr Tubensterilisation. *Geburtsh Frauenheilkd* 37:572, 1977.
18. Radwanska E, Berger G, and Hammond J: Luteal deficiency among women with normal menstrual cycles, requesting reversal of tubal sterilization. *Obstet Gynecol* 54:189, 1979.
19. Donnez J, Wauters M, and Thomas K: Luteal function after tubal sterilization. *Obstet Gynecol* 57:65, 1981.
20. Alvarez Sanchez F, Segal SJ, Brache V, et al: Pituitary-ovarian function after tubal ligation. *Fertil Steril* 36:606, 1981.
21. Corson SL, Levinson CJ, Batzer FR, et

al: Hormonal levels following sterilization and hysterectomy. *J Reprod Med* 26: 363, 1981.

22. Sorensen T, Ladehoff P, Lindholm P, et al: Follicular stimulating hormone, luteinizing hormone and estrogen levels before and after female sterilization. *Acta Obstet Gynecol Scand* 60:559, 1981.
23. Helm G, and Sjöberg NO: Progesterone levels before and after laparoscopic tubal sterilization using endothermal coagulation. *Acta Obstet Gynecol Scand* 62:63, 1983.
24. Ladehoff P, Lindholm P, Qvist K, et al: Gonadotropin and estrogen levels before and after laparoscopy sterilization. *Acta Obstet Gynecol Scand* (in press).
25. McComb PF, Bourdage RJ, and Halbert SH: Suppressed ovulatory function and oviductal microsurgery in the rabbit. *Fertil Steril* 35:481, 1981.
26. Koninckx PR, Heyns WJ, Corvelyn PA, et al: Delayed onset of luteinization as a cause of infertility. *Fertil Steril* 29:266, 1978.
27. Halme J, Rong ZJ, Wing R, et al: The removal of fallopian tubes has no adverse effect on subsequent ovarian functions in rabbits. Presented at the 10th Annual Meeting of the American Association of Gynecologic Laparoscopists, Phoenix, Arizona, 1981.
28. Kastendieck E, and Mestwerdt W: Tierexperimentelle und klinische Aspekte zur Technik der laparoskopischen Tubensterilisation. *Geburtsh Frauenheilkd* 33:971, 1973.
29. Tadir Y, Kaplan I, Zuckermann Z, et al: Laparoscopic CO_2 laser sterilization. *Proceedings III*. World Congress on Human Reproduction, Berlin, 1981, p. 429.
30. Okano K, Matsumoto K, Kotoh K, et al: Progestins in the ovarian vein blood of nonpregnant and pregnant rabbits before and after gonadotropic stimulation. *Endocrinol Japan* 13:438, 1966.
31. Shaikh AA, and Harper MJK: Ovarian steroid secretion in estrous, mated and hCG-treated rabbits, determined by concurrent cannulation of both ovarian veins. *Biol Reprod* 7:387, 1972.
32. Eaton LW, and Hilliard J: Estradiol-17 β, progesterone and 20 -hydroxypregn-4-en-3-one in rabbit ovarian venous plasma. I. Steroid secretion from paired ovaries with and without corpora lutea; Effect of LH. *Endocrinology* 89:105, 1971.
33. Beyth Y, and Winston RML: Ovum capture and fertility following microscopical fimbriectomy in the rabbit. *Fertil Steril* 35:464, 1981.
34. Larbig J, and Goeldner E: Measurement of temperature in laparoscopic tubal sterilisation. *Endoscopy* 6:233, 1974.
35. Weiner S, Wright KG, and Wallach EE: The influence of ovarian denervation and nerve stimulation on ovarian contractions. *Am J Obstet Gynecol* 128:154, 1977.

31

Tubal Sterilization at Laparotomy

B. Norman Barwin

Despite the development of newer techniques of contraception, sterilization provides a safe method for permanent contraception.[1,2] For some women, the birth control pill and the intrauterine contraceptive device are unsuitable or contraindicated.[3] There may be medical, psychiatric, or social indications that tubal sterilization is the method of choice for the prevention of pregnancy. In view of the growing world population, elective sterilization is becoming increasingly popular as a method of limiting family size.[4]

Female sterilization dates back to Hippocrates who proposed sterilization to avoid "perpetration of insanity through heredity" in the 4th century B.C.[5] Tubal sterilization was first carried out by Lungren in 1880[6] in Toledo, Ohio, although initially suggested by Blundell in 1842.[7] Since then, over 100 surgical techniques have been reported for the sterilization of women,[8] including partial or total tubal resection, simple ligation, implantation, and occlusion by electrocauterization or the injection of sclerosing agents. Clips and rings have also been applied. Such a variety of methods reflects current practices indicating that no single method is applicable to all women who request sterilization. Each case must be individually assessed and the suitable technique applied.[9]

Counseling

A woman should not be sterilized without her informed consent, including an adequate discussion and counseling describing the advantages and disadvantages of sterilization compared with temporary methods of contraception.[10] Despite increasing success with microsurgery for reversal of some sterilizing operations, successful reversal cannot be guaranteed. The patient must understand and accept that sterilization is irreversible unless a major operation is done.[11,12] Sterilization should never be undertaken as a temporary method of contraception. In general, the patient should not be sterilized in a stressful situation since she may later regret such a decision. The younger the patient, the greater the need for caution prior to sterilization.[11]

Selection of Procedure

The ideal method of sterilization does not exist and the choice of method de-

The Fallopian Tube: Basic Studies and Clinical Contributions, edited by Alvin M. Siegler, M.D. Mount Kisco, New York: Futura Publishing Company, Inc. © 1986.

pends on many factors.[13] A significant systemic disease may increase the risks of operation and general anesthesia. The age of the patient may indicate a technique that allows the best opportunity of reversal should circumstances change. Sterilizing methods need not necessarily be destructive. Different techniques are indicated for postpartum and interval sterilizations. Previous pelvic surgery and the experience of the surgeon also influence the selection of procedure. Indeed, vasectomy may prove a safer alternative in certain instances.

Not all patients are suitable for laparoscopic tubal sterilization and some surgeons are not experienced in the various laparoscopic techniques. Laparoscopy has an increased risk in the patient with respiratory problems or previous abdominal surgery. There is difficulty in retrieving tubal tissue for diagnostic and legal purposes. Perforation of internal viscera, hemorrhage, and electrosurgical injuries from cauterization techniques have been reported.[9] However, the newer clip and ring techniques and open laparoscopy avoid many of these problems.[14–16] When gynecologic symptoms or pelvic abnormalities exist, hysterectomy may be the method of choice for sterilization.[17]

Sterilization by Laparotomy

Most laparotomy techniques for female sterilization involve ligation or excision of a portion of the fallopian tube which may be its proximal, middle, or fimbrial segments.[18] Crushing techniques predispose to tubal fistula.[19,20]

Tubal ligation can be undertaken in conjunction with pregnancy[21] (postabortal or postpartum) or as an interval procedure unrelated to pregnancy.[15] Tubal ligation performed at the conclusion of a cesarean section does not add any risk beyond the primary procedure.[22] The methods include partial resection, electrocoagulation, or occlusion by clips and rings.[14] Postpartum sterilization is advantageous because the delivery and the sterilization can be done during the same hospitalization.[23] However, patients who have sterilization performed in conjunction with a delivery, especially after cesarean section, are more likely to regret the decision in the future compared to those who have it done as an interval procedure.[11,12]

The subumbilical incision gives best access to the fallopian tubes and is often easier because the fundus is at the umbilicus.[15] The risk of periumbilical minilaparotomy and morbidity ranges from 2 to 4 percent.[24] The most common complications directly attributable to the procedure are wound infection and hemorrhage.[1]

The Pomeroy technique

This method is simple and can be done by the abdominal or vaginal route.[25] The fallopian tube is grasped in its midportion with a Babcock clamp and the elevated loop tied off at its base with a plain catgut #0 suture (Fig. 31:1). A 1–2 cm segment is removed ensuring that the loop is not resected too close to the ligature. The transected ends retract and the edges eventually become 1 to 2 cm apart.

The Irving method

This procedure involves transection of the tube near the ampullary-isthmic junction and subsequent burying of either or both stumps.[28] The fallopian tube is divided at the ampullary-isthmic junction; the tubal stumps are tied, leaving the ends of the sutures long. By blunt dissection, a tunnel is made in the anterior or posterior wall of the myometrium and the proximal tubal segment is pulled into this opening and sutured in place. The distal tubal stump may or may not be buried into the leaves of the broad ligament. This procedure is very effective but cannot be used as an interval operation (Fig. 31:2). A modification of the Irving technique is to divide

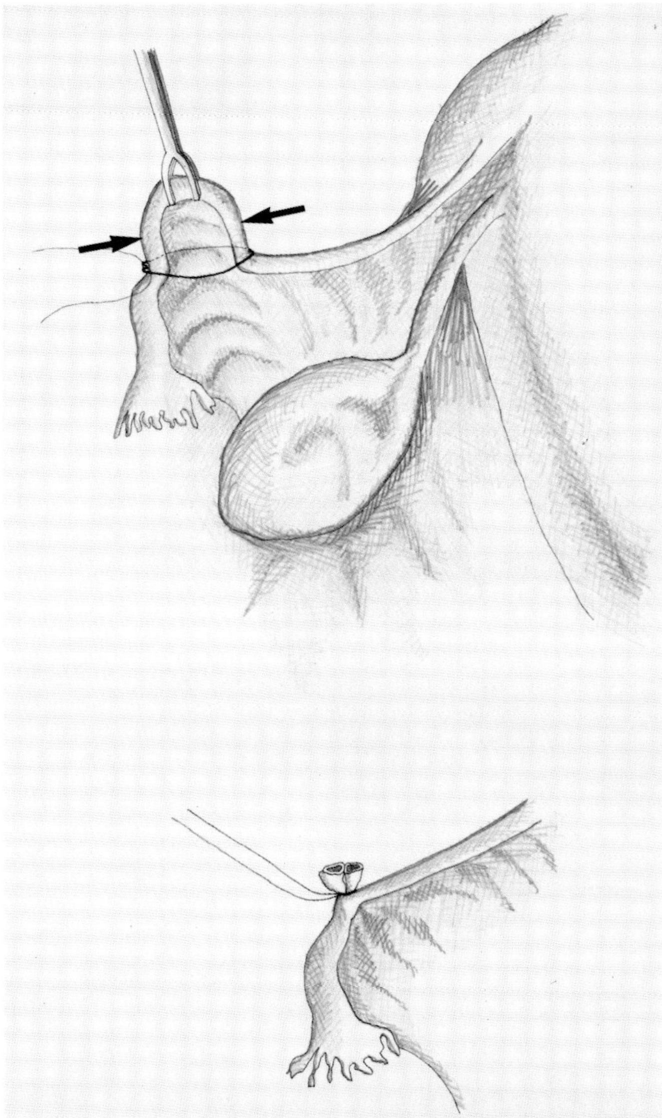

FIGURE 31:1—Top: *Midsegment of tube is grasped with a Babcock clamp and elevated. The knuckle of tube is tied with a plain catgut suture. Arrows indicate area for tubal transection.* Bottom: *The ligated tubal segment has been resected.*

the tubes in their isthmic portion and bury both ends in the pockets of the mesosalpinx (Fig. 31:3).

The Kroener technique

The technique of fimbriectomy involves placing two nonabsorbable sutures near the fimbriated end followed by resection of the fimbria (Fig. 31:4).[29] The procedure can be performed either abdominally or vaginally and ligation and hemostasis are accomplished simultaneously.

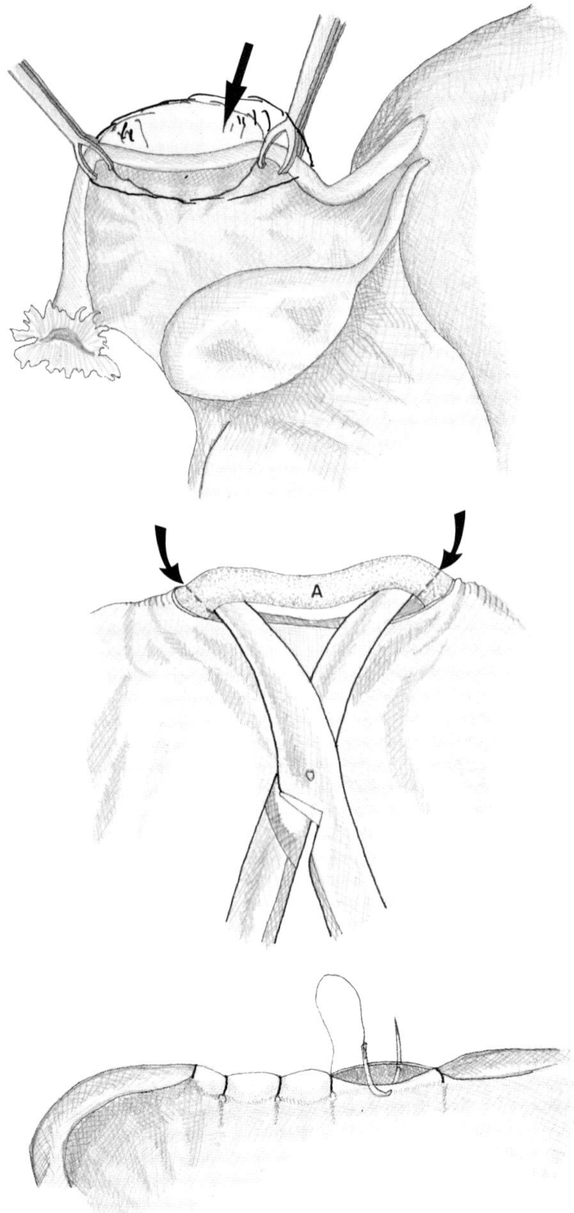

FIGURE 31:2—Top: *Elevation of tubal midsegment following submucosal injection in the region of the tubal ampulla causing swelling (arrow).* Middle: *The serosa has been incised with scissors exposing the myosalpinx. Both portions* (arrows) *are ligated and the segment* (A) *excised.* Bottom: *Continuous suture following resection of tubal segment. The defect in the mesosalpinx is closed.*

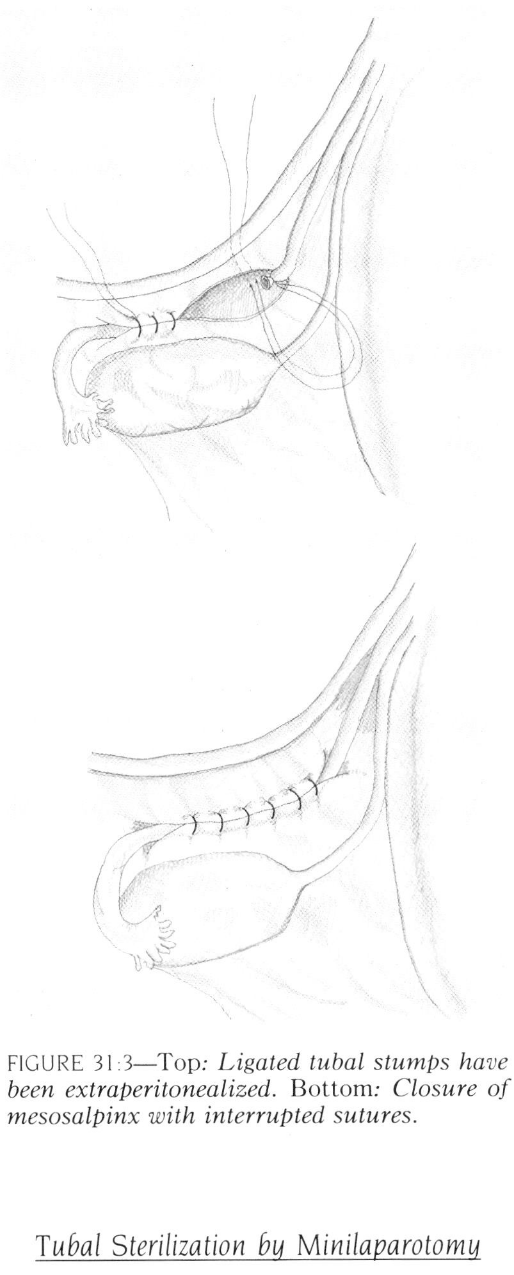

FIGURE 31:3—Top: *Ligated tubal stumps have been extraperitonealized.* Bottom: *Closure of mesosalpinx with interrupted sutures.*

Tubal Sterilization by Minilaparotomy

The minilaparotomy has been used for a long time for puerperal sterilization and is also an alternative to the laparoscopic approach for postabortal or interval sterilization because the technique requires less training and equipment compared to the laparoscopic procedure.[9] The procedure requires 10 to 30 minutes and it can be performed either under local or general anesthesia, on an outpatient basis.

A suprapubic transverse or longitudinal incision of 2 to 3 cm is made, although in a thin patient a 1 cm longitudinal incision may be used.[26] Retraction of the incision is achieved by a small abdominal rake or small vaginal speculum. The uterus is elevated with an intrauterine elevator or probe (placed prior to the abdominal incision) so that the uterus is closer to the abdominal wall. Uterine manipulation brings the tube into view so that it can be grasped with a Babcock clamp or blunt hook. Sterilization is possible by partial tubal resection, occlusive devices such as bands or clips, or electrocoagulation. The procedure can be difficult if the patient is obese or has had previous abdominal operations resulting in adhesions or uterine fixation.[30]

Complications

A failed sterilization resulting in a pregnancy could be considered a complication and an undesirable result. Cheng and coworkers[22] reported that the failure rate (expressed as the ratio of the number of failures to the number of sterilizations, expressed as a percentage), was 0.48 percent. The length of follow-up after sterilization was not noted. The cumulative failure rate was defined in terms of observation time at which pregnancy could possibly be identified. They noted that the failure rate at 12 months was 0.47, 0.81 percent at 24 months, and 0.85 percent at 36 months. Penfield[9] found that the incidence of ectopic pregnancies relative to intrauterine pregnancies following all methods of tubal ligation was approximately 25 percent. Most pregnancies occur during the first year following sterilization and are detected in the first trimester.[8]

In a review of 29,000 sterilizations, Garb reported an overall failure rate of 0.71 percent. Fistula formation with the Madlener method and cornual resection resulted in the highest failure rates, while postpartum sterilization and sterilization

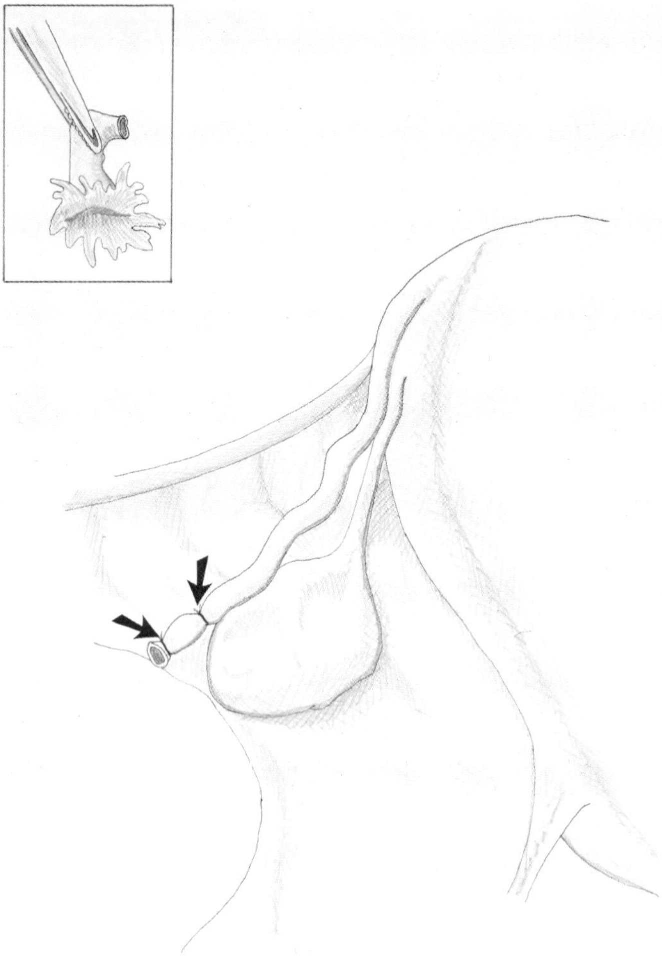

FIGURE 31:4—*Two nonabsorbable sutures at infundibulum* (arrows) *and distal segment has been resected.* Inset: *Resected infundibular portion of tube.*

with cesarean section also resulted in increased failure rates.[3] Most failures are caused by an operator's error.

With minilaparotomy, hematoma, injury to adjacent organs, and uterine perforation occur in 1 to 3 percent.[30] The risk of complications is greatly increased when laparotomy sterilization is carried out because of some systemic disease contraindicating pregnancy.[13] Major complications from sterilization vary from one to six per one hundred procedures. The collaborative review of sterilization (1977) reported that 0.6 percent of patients sterilized by laparoscopic methods were rehospitalized, as compared to 1.4 percent from laparotomy techniques. In this same report, the overall complication rate was 2 percent in the laparoscopy group as compared to 5.8 percent in the laparotomy group.

The long-term morbidity from minilaparotomy was 0.5 per 100 as compared to 1.5 per 100 with laparoscopy, while the mortality was 1 in 4,000 as compared with 1 in 12,000 with minilaparotomy.[30]

The most serious complications were infection and hemorrhage[31] and the risk of venous thrombosis. Incisional bleeding is usually easily controlled with pressure or a few additional sutures. The rare instance of abdominal bleeding may necessitate a repeat laparotomy. Superficial or deep infections may require antibiotics but prophylactic antibiotics are rarely indicated. Subsequent incisional hernia or intestinal obstruction were rare complications.[32,33]

The allegation that menstrual dysfunction is caused by tubal ligation has been investigated by many authors but little evidence of a cause and effect relationship has been established.[34,35] Carefully controlled prospective studies will be necessary to ascertain whether sterilization increases the risk of gynecologic abnormalities in such women.

Peel and Potts[23] reported that less than 5 percent of patients who were sterilized later expressed regret. Many women reported improved health and better relationships because of the reduced fear of unwanted pregnancy. Stock[33] noted that 5 percent of women who had been sterilized considered reversal and that 1 percent actually had the reversal procedure. Some women had divorced and remarried. Other reasons included the death of a child and an inability to accept the permanent character of sterilization. Essentially, reversals are sought because of major changes in life situations.[10,12] In general, the potential for reversal is directly proportional to the amount of tube remaining. This information can only be ascertained by careful review of the operation and pathology reports, and from a laparoscopy. All the procedures described in this chapter are designed to be irreversible and should be offered only to patients who seek permanent sterilization.

References

1. Chamberlain G, and Brown JC: *Gynaecological Laparoscopy: The Report of The Working Party of the Confidential Enquiry into Gynaecological Laparoscopy.* London: The Royal College of Obstetricians and Gynaecologists, 1978: p. 114.
2. Aubert JM, Lubell I, and Schima M: Mortality risk associated with female sterilization. *Int J Gynaecol Obstet* 18:406, 1980.
3. Seiler JS: The evolution of tubal sterilization. *Obstet Gynecol Surv*, 39:177, 1983.
4. Bordahl PE: Tubal sterilization: A historical review. *J Reprd Med* 30:1, 1985.
5. Finch BE, and Green H: *Contraception through the Ages.* Springfield, IL: Charles C Thomas, 1964.
6. Lungren SS: A case of caesarean section twice successfully performed on the same patient, with remarks on the time, indications and details of the operation. *Am J Obstet Gynecol* 14:78, 1881.
7. Blundell J: *Lectures on the Principles and Practice of Midwifery.* Philadelphia: Ed Barrintton & Geo D Hawell, 1842.
8. Garb AE: A review of tubal sterilization failures. *Obstet Gynecol Surv* 12:291, 1957.
9. Penfield AJ: *Female Sterilization by Minilaparotomy or Open Laparoscopy.* Baltimore: Urban and Schwarzenberg. 1980.
10. Stepan J, Kellog EH, and Piotrow PT: Legal trends and issues in voluntary sterilization. *Population Reports,* Series E, #6, 1981.
11. Gomel V: Profile of women requesting reversal of sterilization. *Fertil Steril* 30:39, 1978.
12. Winston RML: Why 103 women asked for reversal of sterilization. *Br Med J* 2:305, 1977.
13. Evans TN: Sterilization of women. In Hafez ESE, Evans TN (Eds): *Human Reproduction: Conception and Contraception.* Hagerstown, MD: Harper & Row, 1973: p. 383.
14. Hulka JF, Omran K, and Lieberman BA: Laparoscopic sterilization with the spring clip: Instrumentation development and current clinical experience, *Am J Obstet Gynecol* 135:1016, 1979.
15. Soderstrom RM, and Yuzpe AA: Female sterilization. *Clin Obstet Gynecol* 6:1, 1979.
16. Yoon I, and Poliakoff SR: Laparoscopic tubal ligation: A followup report on the Yoon Falope ring methodology. *J Reprod Med* 23:76, 1979.
17. Williams EL, Jones HE, and Merrill

RE: Subsequent course of patients sterilized by tubal ligation: Consideration of hysterectomy for sterilization. *Am J Obstet Gynecol* 61:423, 1951.

18. Overstreet E: Techniques of sterilization. *Clin Obstet Gynecol* 7:109, 1964.
19. Madlener M: Über sterilisierende Operationen an den Tuben. *Zentralb Gynäkol* 13:380, 1919.
20. Gomel V: Microsurgical reversal of female sterilization: A reappraisal. *Fertil Steril* 33:587, 1980.
21. Tietze C: Induced abortion and sterilization as methods of fertility control. *J Chron Dis* 18:1161, 1965.
22. Cheng MCE, Wong YM, Rochat RW, et al: Sterilization failures in Singapore: An examination of ligation techniques and failure rates. *Stud Fam Plann* 8:109, 1977.
23. Peel J and Potts M: *Textbook of Contraceptive Practice.* London: Cambridge University Press, 1969.
24. Shepard MK: Female contraceptive sterilization. *Obstet Gynecol Surv* 29:739, 1977.
25. Lull CB, and Mitchell RM: The Pomeroy method of sterilization. *Am J Obstet Gynecol* 59:1118, 1950.
26. Uchida H: Uchida's abdominal sterilization technique. *Proc 3rd World Congr Int Fed Obstet Gynecol* (Vienna) 1:26, 1961.
27. Uchida H: Uchida tubal sterilization. *Am J Obstet Gynecol* 121:153, 1975.
28. Irving FC: Tubal sterilization. *Am J Obstet Gynecol* 60:1101, 1950.
29. Kroener WF Jr.: Surgical sterilization by fimbriectomy. *Am J Obstet Gynecol* 104:247, 1969.
30. Soonawala RP: Minilaparotomy sterilization. In van Lith D, Keith LG, van Hall EV (Eds): *New Trends in Female Sterilization.* Chicago: Year Book Medical Publishers, 1983: p. 125.
31. Penfield AJ: Needle and trocar injuries. In Phillips JM (Ed): Laparotomy. Baltimore: Williams & Wilkins, 1977: p. 7.
32. Noble AD: Female sterilization: Long term effects. In Sciarra JJ, Zatuchni GI, Speidel JJ (Eds): *Controversy in Fertility Control,* Hagerstown, MD: Harper & Row, 1978: p. 102.
33. Stock RJ: Evaluation of sequelae of tubal ligation. *Fertil Steril* 29:169, 1978.
34. Fortney JA: A new approach to measuring menstrual pattern change after sterilization. *Am J Obstet Gynecol* 147:830, 1983.
35. Alderman B: Menstrual loss after tubal ligation. *Lancet* 2:103, 1975.

32

Complications of Tubal Sterilization

Herbert B. Peterson, Gary S. Grubb, Frank DeStefano, and George L. Rubin

Worldwide, over 60 million women have undergone tubal sterilization. In the United States alone, over 5 million women had tubal sterilizations in the 1970s.[1] With so many women involved, any important complications of sterilization must be clearly understood. This is particularly true since most tubal sterilizations are performed electively on young, healthy women.

In 1978, to ascertain better the risks of tubal sterilization, the Centers for Disease Control (CDC) began the Collaborative Review of Sterilization (CREST), a prospective multicenter, observational study. At approximately the same time, it developed a national surveillance program to identify and investigate deaths attributable to sterilization. These two research efforts are ongoing but both have already yielded useful information concerning sequelae of tubal sterilization. Initially we will provide background information necessary to interpret results of these efforts and will then review what CREST and the mortality surveillance program have suggested about early complications of tubal sterilization. Later we will detail available data from CREST concerning late complications, including changes in menstrual function, the risk of hysterectomy, the risk of regret, and failure of sterilization. Complications reported by others will also be reviewed.

Background

The history of sterilization—Safety studies

Most studies of the complications of tubal sterilization have been reported by individual surgeons or medical centers using differing definitions of complications. Further, most of these reports are of single procedures and do not allow for comparison of safety by timing with respect to pregnancy, surgical approach, method of tubal occlusion, or anesthetic technique.

The Fallopian Tube: Basic Studies and Clinical Contributions, edited by Alvin M. Siegler, M.D. Mount Kisco, New York: Futura Publishing Company, Inc. © 1986.

A few national or multicenter studies have been performed that discuss complications of tubal sterilization in a way allowing for some comparison. These include previously noted studies from CDC and two prospective studies performed in the United Kingdom, one by the Royal College of Obstetricians and Gynaecologists[2] which was limited to laparoscopic sterilization, and the other in two large family planning clinics where a variety of procedures were analyzed.[3] In addition, Family Health International (formerly International Fertility Research Program) has performed a large multinational study in 23 countries most of which are classified as developing countries.[4]

The Collaborative Review of Sterilization (CREST)

Since 1978, 12 hospitals or outpatient surgical facilities in six U.S. cities have participated in this prospective cohort study. All the hospitals are affiliated with university medical centers. When the study is completed, it will include over 12,000 women who have undergone tubal sterilization. In addition, there are plans to enroll an appropriate number of nonsterilized women as controls. An attempt will be made to follow all participants for a minimum of five years.

At each hospital where women are enrolled, trained nurse interviewers identify all women 15 to 44 years of age who are scheduled for tubal sterilization and attempt to contact them to request their participation in the study. Those who agree to participate must sign a consent form.

The same standard questionnaire is used at each hospital. Women are interviewed preoperatively to obtain demographic, pregnancy, contraceptive, and medical data. Details of the operation are recorded and information on the patient's postoperative course is obtained from hospital charts. The nurse interviewers attempt to contact all participants by telephone four to eight weeks later to obtain details on their recovery. Thereafter they are contacted at yearly intervals for five years.

For comparability, six categories of intraoperative and postoperative complications have been defined so as to enable a comparison of anesthetic and surgical techniques by using objective, clearly defined outcomes that are not subject to variability in interpretation and are not related to a particular sterilization method.

Sterilization mortality surveillance

In 1979, CDC began surveillance of death associated with tubal sterilization to ascertain why deaths occur and their possible prevention. Deaths have been identified through two sources. The first has been a nationwide epidemiological surveillance effort which includes reporting to CDC by individual clinicians, state health departments, medical examiners' offices, and professional societies.[5] The second source was from the Commission on Professional and Hospital Activities (CPHA).

The CPHA annually collects information on approximately 40 percent of the patients discharged from hospitals in the United States. It has performed computer file searches to locate deaths that are temporally associated with tubal sterilizations performed in member hospitals. When death was so identified, the CPHA has contacted the administrator of the hospital involved to request permission for CDC to obtain details about the patient's death.[6] Once a death was reported, CDC obtained detailed information to ascertain the clinical circumstances. When possible, details were obtained from physicians caring for the patient. Complete, pertinent medical records were always requested.

For each death, a detailed clinical summary was prepared with all identifying information removed. The summary was presented to a panel of physicians who decided whether the patient's death

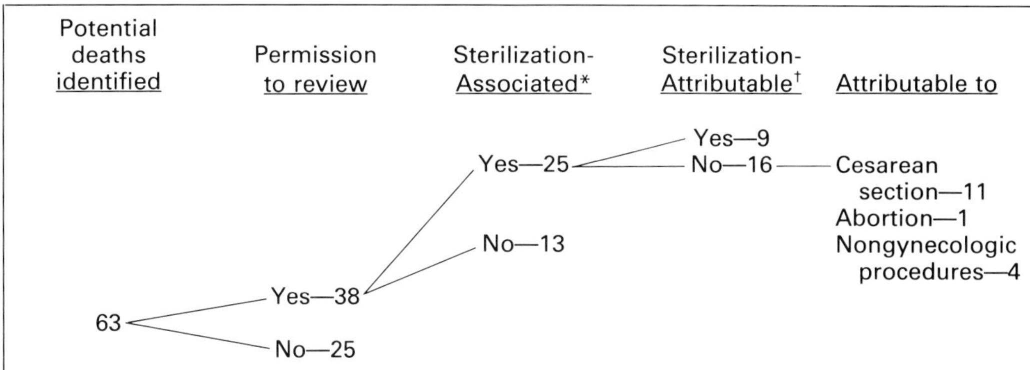

*Death occurring within 42 days of tubal sterilization or complications leading to death first occurred within 42 days of tubal sterilization.
†Tubal sterilization was a major factor contributing to death.

FIGURE 32:1—*Flow chart illustrating the progression from identification of potential deaths to determination by review of whether deaths were sterilization-attributable.*

was caused by sterilization and if so, the most likely cause of death.

Early Complications

General considerations

Tubal sterilization is a safe surgical procedure but safe relative to what? The answer depends on the comparison of tubal sterilization to (1) other surgical procedures, (2) other methods of fertility control, (3) the risks of pregnancy, and (4) individual circumstances. For example, in certain settings some women may be at greater risk from complications of pregnancy than from sterilization. In some parts of Bangladesh, the maternal mortality rate is 570 deaths per 100,000 live births, whereas the case-fatality rate for tubal sterilization is 16 per 100,000 procedures.[7] Even in developed countries, some women may be at greater medical risk from pregnancy than they are from surgical procedures to prevent pregnancy. Clearly, the safety of tubal sterilization must be considered in relative terms, but in the aggregate tubal sterilization can be considered a relatively safe operation.

Mortality

Risk of death

To obtain an accurate estimate of the risk of dying from tubal sterilization, CDC investigators combined an analysis of national data on the number and characteristics of sterilizations performed with a review of medical records of women whose deaths were identified as being associated with sterilization. We then refined this estimate, by detailed clinical reviews, to include just those deaths attributable to sterilization.[6]

Data for calculating case fatality rates in the CDC study were based on information for the years 1977 and 1978. Sixty-three potential deaths were identified and permission was obtained to review 38 of them (Fig. 32:1). Of these 38, 25 were associated with sterilization (a complication leading to death occurred within 42 days of the tubal sterilization). In only 9 of these 25 was sterilization a major factor contributing to death. Using these nine deaths as a numerator and estimating a denominator based on data from the National Center for Health Statistics, we calculated a case-fatality rate of approximately 4 per 100,000 procedures. The four deaths did not allow for a calculation of case-fatality rates by various surgical approaches, methods of occlusion, or anesthetic techniques. The overall case-fatality rate of 4 per 100,000 is similar to that obtained by the American Association of Gynecologic Laparoscopists in its 1975 membership survey of laparoscopic sterilizations, which reported a rate of 2.5 per 100,000 procedures.[8] However, this rate is less than the 10 per 100,000 reported from a prospective study of laparoscopic procedures conducted by the Royal College of Obstetricians and Gynaecologists in the United Kingdom.[2]

Causes of deaths

The voluntary reporting of deaths to CDC has enabled us to find out why they occur and methods of prevention. Twenty-nine deaths reported to CDC were attributable to tubal sterilization from 1977 to 1981 (Table 32:1) and about 3 million tubal sterilizations were performed during this time. Applying case-fatality rates for tubal sterilization of approximately 4 per 100,000, as many as 108 deaths may have occurred. If this projection is correct, then our surveillance identified 27 percent of the projected deaths attributed to sterilization. General comparisons of risks between laparoscopy and laparotomy or between interval and postpartum sterilization cannot be made. Complications from general anesthesia accounted for 11 of the 29 deaths. Sepsis and hemorrhage caused death in seven and four women, respectively. Ten of the women who died had underlying medical conditions.[5]

Hypoventilation was an important factor contributing to 6 of the 11 anesthetic deaths and none of these women had been intubated prior to sterilization. Seven women died from complications of general anesthesia while undergoing laparoscopic sterilization and 4 had not been intubated. Hypoventilation has been reported as a leading cause of anesthetic deaths for a variety of surgical procedures.[9] Endotracheal intubation, particularly for laparoscopic sterilization, has been suggested to prevent hypoventilation.[10]

From this study it is not possible to make generalizations about the comparative safety of local and general anesthesia but other information is available on this issue. In 1981, the CDC reported that complications of anesthesia were the leading cause of abortion related deaths and that the risk of death associated with induced abortion was greatest with use of general anesthesia.[11] Tubal sterilization, like abortion, is generally an elective procedure performed on healthy young women. Although any surgical procedure carries certain risks, it appears that for tubal sterilization, as for abortion, the greatest risk of death is that associated with the anesthesia used for the procedure.

Of the seven deaths caused by sepsis, three were attributed to thermal intestinal injury associated with use of unipolar coagulating devices. More than 100 nonfatal thermal intestinal injuries have been previously reported with the use of unipolar instruments. Unipolar electrocoagulation includes the patient as part of the electrical circuit (Fig. 32:2), whereas bipolar coagulation, developed as an alternative by Rioux and Cloutier,[12] only includes the structure between the grasping forceps as part of the electrical circuit. Because unipolar coagulation is apparently associated with a greater risk of electrical accidents than bipolar coagulation without any demonstrated greater efficacy, CDC has questioned the need for continuing its use in tubal sterilization.[13]

Major vessel lacerations are a catastrophic consequence of laparoscopic sterilization. Three deaths related to such lacerations were reported in this study, one each attributable to insertion of the Veress needle, trocar, and scalpel. Numerous suggestions have been made for minimizing risks in needle and trocar insertion. Most of these include careful attention to anatomical landmarks and insertion of the needle and trocar in the midline at an angle toward the pelvis while the anterior abdominal wall is elevated.[14] Details of the three deaths sug-

Table 32:1

*Deaths Attributable to Tubal Sterilization by Cause of Death, United States, 1977–1981**

Cause of Death	*Surgical Approach*	*Age*	*Concurrent pregnancy termination*	*Preexisting conditions*
Anesthesia	Laparoscopy	24	No	Obesity
Anesthesia	Laparoscopy	28	No	None
Anesthesia	Laparoscopy	27	No	None
Anesthesia	Laparoscopy	32	No	None
Anesthesia	Laparoscopy	41	No	Obesity, hypertension, asthma
Anesthesia	Laparotomy	19	Vaginal delivery (twins)	Obesity
Anesthesia	Laparotomy	27	Vaginal delivery	None
Anesthesia	Laparotomy	27	Vaginal delivery	Obesity, hypertension
Anesthesia	Laparotomy	22	Vaginal delivery	Astrocytoma
Anesthesia	Laparotomy	36	Hysterotomy abortion	Obesity, hypertension
Anesthesia	Laparoscopy	33	No	None
Sepsis	Laparoscopy	27	No	None
Sepsis	Laparoscopy	41	No	None
Sepsis	Laparoscopy	22	No	None
Sepsis	Laparoscopy	26	No	None
Sepsis	Laparotomy	27	Vaginal delivery	None
Sepsis	Colpotomy	39	No	None
Sepsis	Open laparoscopy	35	No	None
Hemorrhage	Laparoscopy	39	No	None
Hemorrhage	Laparoscopy	38	No	None
Hemorrhage	Laparoscopy	31	No	None
Hemorrhage	Laparotomy	35	Vaginal delivery	None
Myocardial infarction	Laparoscopy	35	No	Oral contraceptive use
Myocardial infarction	Laparotomy	33	No	Obesity, history of chest pain
Myocardial infarction	Laparotomy	37	Vaginal delivery	None
Mesenteric vein thrombosis	Laparotomy	24	No	Oral contraceptive use
Complication of Eisenmenger's syndrome	Laparotomy	19	No	Eisenmenger's syndrome
Pulmonary embolus	Laparoscopy	43	No	None
Complete heart block	Laparoscopy	28	No	None

*Adapted from Peterson et al.[5]

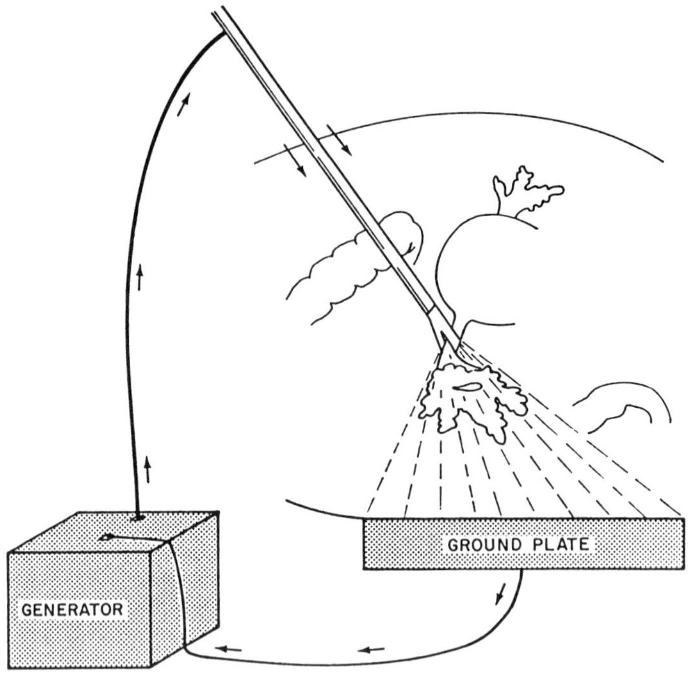

FIGURE 32:2—*The unipolar laparoscopy system. Electric current* (arrows) *passes through the operating instruments to the jaws of the forceps, which together constitute the active electrode. The current coagulates the grasped tube and spreads radially through the patient's body toward the ground plant (return electrode). The patient's body is therefore part of the electrical circuit.*

gest that when major vessel injury occurs, prompt recognition and treatment are necessary to prevent death.

The use of oral contraceptives at the time of sterilization may have contributed to two of the deaths. Oral contraceptives have been shown to cause at least a threefold increase in the risk of postoperative thromboembolism.[15] Because of this increased risk, package inserts for oral contraceptives sold in the United States suggest discontinuation of use at least one month before major elective surgery. Obviously, a decision to discontinue oral contraceptives before sterilization must be based not only on the potential risk of thromboembolic disease but also on the risk of pregnancy. Some of the contraceptive effect of oral contraceptives persists for a few months after use has stopped.[15] Thus for a motivated user of barrier methods, stopping oral contraceptives and using a barrier method for the month before sterilization may be the safest option. Obviously, given the possible risks of pregnancy, any decision to stop oral contraceptives should be individualized.

A review of the 29 deaths suggests that the use of endotracheal intubation when general anesthesia was used, particularly for laparoscopic sterilization, might have prevented some deaths. Others might have been avoided by safer use of unipolar coagulation or by using alternative techniques. Careful insertion of the needle and trocar during laparoscopy or use of alternative techniques, such as minilaparotomy or open laparoscopy, might have averted three of the hemorrhagic deaths. Finally, when it is otherwise clinically appropriate, discontinuation of oral contraceptives before sterilization might have prevented other deaths.

Morbidity

Standard categories of complications—CREST

Tubal sterilizations can be performed using a variety of surgical approaches, methods of tubal occlusion, and anesthetic techniques. In order to allow for comparison, six standard categories of intraoperative and postoperative complications were defined for use in CREST:

a. Unanticipated major surgery: any laparotomy, repair of a perforated viscus, or repair of major blood vessel that was performed intraoperatively or postoperatively during the same hospitalization, that was not planned and was necessary because of a problem related to the tubal sterilization.

b. Transfusion: any intraoperative or postoperative blood transfusion.

c. Febrile morbidity: oral temperature 38 .0°C or higher on at least 2 postoperative days, excluding the first 24 hours after surgery.

d. Life-threatening event: any intraoperative or postoperative cardiac or respiratory arrest, myocardial infarction, pulmonary embolus, anaphylactic shock, or disseminated intravascular coagulation.

e. Rehospitalization: readmission to a hospital between the time of discharge and the follow-up interview because of a complaint or problem that the women perceived to be related to the tubal sterilization.

f. Death: death or complication leading to death occurring within 42 days of surgery.

These categories of complications were chosen because they represent life-threatening events or can reasonably be expected to result in increased morbidity. They also are clearly defined outcomes that are not subject to much variability in interpretation and are not related to a particular sterilization technique. These six standard categories of complications will be used in the following discussion of early complications.

General observations

One of the difficulties in studying the relative safety of tubal sterilization by surgical approach, method of occlusion, and anesthetic technique is that most of the serious complications of sterilization are relatively rare. Unfortunately, some of these rare conditions, for example thermal intestinal injury and major vessel laceration, are potentially fatal. It is thus important to understand any differences in these risks between techniques. Doing so is difficult, however. Assuming a maximal estimated rate of major vessel laceration of one per 1,000 procedures with conventional laparoscopy and 90 percent study power to detect a twofold increase in the risk of major vessel laceration between an alternative technique and the conventional approach, one would have to study at least 30,000 women undergoing each approach to show that there was no statistically significant twofold increase in the risk of major vessel laceration with use of the alternative technique. Since such large-scale studies are uncommon, decisions regarding risks of rare events must be based heavily on theoretical concerns and case reports of complications in addition to the results of comparative studies discussed below.

Surgical approach

Although postpartum sterilizations are generally performed by a subumbilical laparotomy incision, interval sterilizations are often performed by conventional laparoscopy, open laparoscopy, or minilaparotomy.

The CREST participants include women who had each of these surgical approaches, but most women enrolled have had interval conventional laparoscopic sterilization. Since few data are available for women undergoing open laparoscopy, the discussion will be limited to those women who have undergone

Table 32:2
Interval Laparoscopic Sterilization Complications, CREST, 1978–1981*

Complication	*Number*	*Rate*†
Unintended major surgery‡	37	1.1
Rehospitalization	16	0.5
Febrile morbidity	7	0.2
Transfusion	0	0
Life-threatening event	0	0
Death	0	0
One or more complications	58	1.7

*Includes 3,500 procedures done by electrocoagulation or silastic bands, identified by the Collaborative Review of Sterilization.
†Per 100 procedures.
‡In all cases this was an unintended laparotomy.
Adapted from De Stefano et al.[16]

interval conventional laparoscopy and interval laparotomy.

Conventional laparoscopy: In an analysis of 3,500 women who underwent interval laparoscopic tubal sterilization by electrocoagulation or silastic banding, 1.7 percent had at least one complication in one of the six standard categories (Table 32:2).[16] The most frequent complication was major surgery; in all cases this was a laparotomy. Of 37 unplanned laparotomies, 4 were performed to control bleeding, 3 because of some other complication, 1 because of equipment malfunctioning, and 29 because of technical difficulties. Of the women who underwent laparotomy because of technical difficulties, 66 percent had pelvic or abdominal adhesions as compared with 18 percent of the women who did not undergo laparotomy. Sixteen women were rehospitalized for the following reasons: pelvic infections (3), heavy vaginal bleeding (3), pregnancy (3), abdominal/pelvic pain (2), completion of the tubal sterilization (2), peritonitis secondary to a bowel burn (1), bronchitis (1), and depression (1). Febrile morbidity occurred in seven women: one had septicemia, two had urinary tract infections, and four had no specific source of infection identified. No woman required intraoperative or postoperative blood transfusion and no life-threatening events or deaths occurred.

Certain women appeared to be at increased risk for interval laparoscopic sterilization. Of 18 potential surgical risk factors for laparoscopic sterilization examined, only 6 appeared to be statistically significant predictors of having one of the six standard complications (Table 32:3). Five of these are patient characteristics that can be identified preoperatively: diabetes, history of abdominal or pelvic surgery, pulmonary disease, history of pelvic inflammatory disease (PID), and obesity. For previous abdominal or pelvic surgery and history of PID, the complications noted were usually attributable to the presence of abdominal or pelvic adhesions.

The rates of major complications for interval laparoscopic sterilizations in CREST are similar to those in other national studies. The only other large prospective study of laparoscopic sterilization in a developed country was conducted by The Royal College of Obstetricians and Gynaecologists in the United Kingdom during 1976–1977.[2] The only category of complications comparable to the categories in CREST was that of procedures requiring laparotomy. In the Royal College study, the laparotomy rate was 1.2/100 laparoscopic sterilizations, almost identical to the rate of 1.1/100 procedures found in CREST. The only national information available in the United States on complications of laparoscopic sterilization comes from membership surveys conducted by the American Association of Gynecologic Laparoscopists (AAGL).[17] The rates of laparotomy done to treat complications in the 1976 and 1979 AAGL surveys were 2.7/1,000 procedures and 1.8/1,000 procedures, respectively. In CREST, the comparable rate of laparotomy done because of a complication was 2.0/1,000 procedures.

Table 32:3

*Complication Rates for Interval Laparoscopic Sterilization by Presence or Absence of Selected Preoperatively Identifiable Factors, CREST, 1977–1981**

Complication rate (per 100)

Factor	*Unintended major surgery*	*Rehospital-ization*	*Febrile morbidity*	*One or more com-plications*	*Relative risk† of one or more complications (95% conf. int.)*
Diabetes mellitus					
No	1.0	0.4	0.2	1.6	1 (referent)
Yes	4.3	4.3	0	8.5	5.4 (2.2, 13.3)
Anesthesia					
Local	0	0.4	0	0.4	1 (referent)
General	1.3	0.5	0.2	1.9	5.2 (1.5, 18.3)
Previous abdominal or pelvic surgery					
No	0.6	0.4	0.2	1.1	1 (referent)
Yes	2.3	0.8	0.3	3.1	2.7 (1.7, 4.5)
Pulmonary disease‡					
No	1.0	0.3	0.2	1.4	1 (referent)
Yes	1.9	1.6	0.5	3.8	2.7 (1.5, 4.8)
History of PID					
No	1.0	0.5	0.1	1.5	1 (referent)
Yes	1.7	0.4	1.7	3.4	2.2 (1.1, 4.6)
Percent ideal body weight§					
$<$120%	0.7	0.4	0.1	1.2	1 (referent)
$\geqslant$120%	1.7	0.7	0.3	2.5	2.1 (1.3, 3.4)

*Includes 3,500 procedures done by electrocoagulation or silastic bands, identified by the Collaborative Review of Sterilization.
†Unadjusted, calculated by dividing the rate when the factor is present by the rate when the factor is not present (referent category).
‡History of asthma, bronchitis, or emphysema.
§Hamwi's formula (7).
Adapted from De Stefano et al.[16]

Laparotomy: Minilaparotomy is a term generally used to describe a suprapubic transverse incision variously characterized as from 1.5 to 5.5 cm. It has been presumed by some that minilaparotomy is safer than conventional laparotomy primarily for two reasons: (1) the technique can be used with local anesthesia; and (2) the incision is smaller than one generally used for conventional laparotomy.

CREST is the only study in the English-language literature to have compared the relative morbidity of laparotomy by incisional length.[18] Of 340 women undergoing interval sterilization by laparotomy, 282 were included in the analysis reported here. The study excluded three women whose incisions were extended intraoperatively because of complications. It also excluded 55 women who had surgery other than dilatation and curettage of the uterus concurrent with tubal sterilization. Women who had a laparotomy with an incisional length of from

Table 32:4

*Length of Abdominal Incision and the Risk of Complications of Tubal Sterilization by Laparotomy**

Length of incision (cm)	*No. of patients*	*Complication rates per 100 procedures*	*Relative risk*
1–4	85	3.5	1.0
5–6	109	3.7	1.0
≥7	54	11.1	3.1
Unknown	34	8.8	0

*Adapted from Layde et al.[18]

1 to 4 cm had a complication rate of 3.5/100 procedures, whereas women with an incisional length greater than 7 cm had a complication rate of 11/100 procedures (Table 32:4). The complication rates noted were adjusted for all other important risk factors studied.

The CREST study cannot at this point be used to evaluate definitively the relative safety of the alternative surgical approaches. Although the CREST complication rate from minilaparotomy is almost twice that noted for conventional laparoscopy, the comparison may not be completely valid because the laparotomies were performed in institutions that generally performed laparoscopic sterilizations. It is thus possible that the patients who underwent minilaparotomies were at higher risk than those who underwent laparoscopic sterilization. Further, as will be discussed, use of general anesthesia for laparoscopic sterilizations in CREST is associated with greater morbidity than is the use of local anesthesia. In CREST, too few minilaparotomies were performed with local anesthesia to allow for adjusting morbidity risk by anesthetic techniques, so some or all of the observed difference in risk may be attributable to anesthetic technique.

Finally, as noted earlier, it is difficult, even in a large prospective study, to detect differences in rare events. Thus, we would not expect to detect important differences in risks of events such as major vessel laceration or visceral injury between minilaparotomy and conventional laparotomy or conventional laparoscopy.

Method of Tubal Occlusion: Because of the relatively small number of salpingectomies in CREST to date, it is difficult to compare the safety of salpingectomy with that of the laparoscopic methods of occlusion. In CREST to date, the interval laparoscopic methods, unipolar and bipolar coagulation, silastic bands, and clips have not been strongly associated with important differences in complications. Both types of electrocoagulation carry some higher risk for at least one of the six standard complications than does silastic banding, which carries a slightly higher risk than application of spring clips, but to date none of these differences is statistically significant. Among the electrocoagulative procedures in CREST, those done with unipolar instruments carry a similar risk of complications to those done with bipolar instruments.

It seems contradictory that the mortality surveillance noted previously suggests a higher risk of serious morbidity for unipolar coagulating devices than for other methods. The apparent contradiction is possibly related to the relative frequency of the events being studied. For example, it is estimated that thermal bowel injuries with unipolar coagulating devices may occur in 1/1,000 procedures.[13] Given the relative rarity of thermal bowel injury, as well as the concerns already noted, it is easy to see why a study with only 3,000 to 4,000 patients analyzed to date would not reveal any important difference in risk by method of occlusion.

Anesthesia: As noted previously, complications of general anesthesia appear to be the single leading cause of sterilization-attributable deaths in the United States. In CREST participants undergoing laparoscopy, those having general anesthesia had a fourfold greater risk of one of the standard complications than did those having local anesthesia, even after adjustment was made for other known risk factors. The use of local anesthesia may act in part as a surrogate for other risk factors that we could not identify. For example, most of the difference in risk by type of anesthesia was related to unplanned laparotomies. Perhaps women who were less likely to have complications were selected for use of local anesthesia. Operator skill could not be controlled for in the reported CREST analysis. The lower complication risk for procedures performed under local anesthesia may have been attributable to these procedures being done by surgeons with greater skill. Still, in combination with other sterilization studies, including the mortality studies noted previously, the type of anesthesia used appears to be a major determinant of both morbidity and mortality from laparoscopic sterilization.

Late Complications

General considerations

Appreciably more is known about the early complications of tubal sterilization than about potential late sequelae. Both theoretical concerns and actual studies, however, suggest the possiblity of potential late health consequences of sterilization. The four greatest concerns are (1) changes in menstrual function, (2) risk of hysterectomy, (3) risk of regret, and (4) failure of sterilization.

These concerns have been addressed incompletely in the literature to date. Further, many available studies have methodological limitations that make it difficult to interpret results. Most have been hampered to varying degrees by small study size, limited follow-up, and lack of adequate control groups. In addition, in most studies of late sequelae, only poststerilization information has been collected so that comparison with presterilization status is not possible. Only a few of the studies of late complaints have taken into account possible confounding factors such as previous contraceptive use.

The CREST study is not without methodological concerns, but it has been able to overcome many of the limitations that have affected previous studies. The study is large and has good follow-up (over 80 percent at three years). The fact that women are interviewed preoperatively to ascertain factors such as menstrual status avoids any influence that sterilization may have had on recall of events occurring before sterilization. Other biases have been minimized by use of a standard methodology with a standard questionnaire and standard definitions of complications. Further standardization for differences in numerous clinical and demographic characteristics enables us to ascertain the association between study groups and study outcomes of interest without the influence of other factors.

Menstrual changes after tubal sterilization

Since a report in 1951 of an increased incidence of menstrual disturbances among women who had undergone tubal sterilization, the existence of a "posttubal syndrome" has been postulated.[19] Abnormalities reported after tubal sterilization included a spectrum of menstrual disorders: (1) irregular menstrual cycles, (2) more and less frequent menstrual periods, prolonged menstrual bleeding, increased menstrual flow, (3) intermenstrual bleeding or spotting, and (4) dysmenorrhea. Although various studies have shown that

Table 32:5

Menstrual Pain Preoperatively and Two Years Postoperatively, by Method of Tubal Sterilization; Collaborative Review of Sterilization (CREST)*

Methods of tubal sterilization	Not severe preoperatively: Not severe postoperatively	Not severe preoperatively: Severe postoperatively	Severe preoperatively: Not severe postoperatively	Severe preoperatively: Severe postoperatively	Percentage of women with severe pain: Preoperatively	Percentage of women with severe pain: Postoperatively
Unipolar coagulation	542	166†	110†	136	25.8	31.7
Bipolar coagulation	324	90†	142†	69	33.8	25.4
Silastic bands	344	81†	110†	81	31.0	26.3
Other	119	38	36	44	33.8	34.6
Total	1329	375	398	330	29.9	29.0

*The Collaborative Review of Sterilization, September 1978 to January 1982; 24 women with unknown responses were excluded

†The number of women who changed from not severe preoperatively to severe postoperatively is significantly different from the number who changed from severe preoperatively to not severe postoperatively, as determined by McNemar test ×2 (p = .0009 for unipolar coagulation; p = .0008 for bipolar coagulation; p = .04 for silastic bands).

From De Stefano et al.[20]

tubal sterilization may increase the likelihood of any or all of these disorders, all such studies have had methodological limitations. Further, their results have been variable and often conflicting.

We studied 2,456 women in a preliminary analysis of menstrual function in CREST particpants two years after sterilization.[20] Each woman served as her own control, and her menstrual function at the two-year follow-up interview was compared with menstrual function at the preoperative interview. Duration of menstrual bleeding, menstrual cycle length, cyclic regularity, amount of menstrual bleeding, menstrual pain, and intermenstrual bleeding were examined. At two-year follow-up, for all menstrual variables, most women had no changes from their preoperative assessment. In general, for those women who had changes in any of the six menstrual characteristics, the percentages of favorable and adverse changes were approximately equal. The sole exception was found among women who had unipolar electrocoagulation procedures. In that group the percentage of women with severe pain postoperatively was significantly greater than the percentage with severe pain preoperatively following other procedures (Table 32:5). It should be stressed that these findings are preliminary and for two-year follow-up only. One other recent study performed by Family Health International (FHI) had one-year follow-up findings similar to those in CREST. The only published prospective study with longer-term follow-up is one conducted in the United Kingdom.[3] In that large study of more than 2,000 women undergoing tubal sterilization, a control group of women whose husbands had undergone vasectomy was used for comparison. The two groups were not substantially different in the likelihood of hospitalization for menstrual problems up to five years after tubal sterilization.

To date, a major strength of CREST has been the ability to compare the methods of tubal occlusion with respect to likelihood of subsequent menstrual change. Some laboratory evidence suggests that the various methods of tubal occlusion may have different effects on luteal function.[21,22] CREST should be able to compare sterilization methods epidemiologically, allowing for correlation with laboratory findings. To date, however, CREST has not been able to answer the more general question, "Does tubal sterilization cause an increase in the likelihood of menstrual changes?" To address that question carefully, nonsterilized controls are required. Thus, plans for expansion of CREST include an appropriate group of nonsterilized controls. At the completion of the expanded CREST study, substantial evidence should be available to address whether or not tubal sterilization in general causes menstrual changes and, if so, whether there are important differences related to method of tubal occlusion.

Risk of hysterectomy after sterilization

In part, because of the menstrual problems addressed previously, there is concern that tubal sterilization may increase the likelihood of subsequent hysterectomy. In several small studies that followed women for from one to ten years, crude hysterectomy rates varied from 5/1,000 procedures at one year[23] to 187/1,000 procedures at ten years.[24] Since tubal sterilization and hysterectomy are both very common procedures (over 5 million tubal sterilizations and 5 million hysterectomies were performed in the United States in the last decade alone), many women who undergo tubal sterilization will subsequently undergo hysterectomy. It is obvious that a certain number of women have these as independent events. Whether or not tubal sterilization actually increases a woman's risk of having a hysterectomy is at issue. Further, whether certain women are at particular risk is an important concern.

Two recent studies,[25,26] both using data from hospital discharges, the former from Scotland and the latter from England, suggested that an increased risk of hysterectomy does occur after tubal sterilization. A third study, a prospective one by Vessey[3] in the United Kingdom, involved 2,243 women undergoing tubal sterilization. Women whose husbands had undergone vasectomy were used as controls. No increased likelihood of hysterectomy was found for up to five years after sterilization.

Few studies have examined the relationship between tubal sterilization and subsequent hysterectomy in detail. Whether there are patient characteristics or tubal occlusive methods that are selectively associated with an increased risk is unknown. Only one other study, a multinational one conducted by Family Health International,[27] has examined patient risk factors. In that study, certain factors, for example heavy menstrual flow occurring preoperatively, increased the likelihood of subsequent hysterectomy. No studies have been done to ascertain whether methods of tubal occlusion may be related to the risk of subsequent hysterectomy.

When completed, CREST should be able to help us to find out whether or not tubal sterilization increases the risk of subsequent hysterectomy and, if so, whether differences in risk are related to the method of tubal occlusion. At present, we have been able only to examine risk factors for subsequent hysterectomy. In a preliminary analysis of 4,000 CREST participants, followed for 15 months after sterilization, 1.6 percent underwent hysterectomy.[28] Women with histories of menstrual complaints, leiomyomata, ovarian cysts, or endometriosis before tubal sterilization had 2.4-, 4.7-, 11.5-, and 12.8- fold increased risks of hysterectomy within 15 months after sterilization, respectively. Women with two or more of these risk factors had a 13.7-fold increased risk. However, most women with these risk factors did not undergo hysterectomy. Thus, a longer term of follow-up and comparison with nonsterilized controls will be necessary to decide whether relationships observed to date represent actual late risks. This information will be important in adequately counseling women with gynecologic complaints at the time sterilization is requested.

Regret after sterilization

A number of studies[29–31] have suggested that regret after tubal sterilization is not rare, occurring in as many as 2 to 4 percent of women. Regret in these instances is varyingly defined or not defined. Further, few studies have followed women at more than one time in order to assess changes in the rate of regret over time.[29]

It is important not only to ascertain the likelihood and degree of regret following sterilization, but also to find out whether or not there are preoperatively identifiable patient characteristics which might predict the likelihood of regret. Several studies have documented determinants of regret. Divorce and remarriage are the reasons most commonly given by women for regret in descriptive analyses of women who request reversal of sterilization.[32] To evaluate determinants of regret adequately, studies must compare women who regret sterilization with those who do not regret sterilization, that is, they must have a suitable referent group. Most studies in which such comparisons are made, however, have not evaluated risk factors for regret. Of those that have, most have examined young age and low parity as determinants. Approximately equal numbers of studies supported[30,31,33] and refuted[30,34] these characteristics as significant determinants.

In CREST, we have been able to use standard methods to compare women who did and did not regret sterilization at one- and two-year follow-up interviews.[35] Of 5,024 women enrolled in the study, 2.0 percent regretted having been sterilized at one year after the procedure compared with 2.7 percent at two years. Using a multivariate analysis to identify risk factors for regret, we found that almost all risk factors were more closely associated with regret at one year than at two years postoperatively. A desire for more children and menstrual complaints after sterilization were the reasons most frequently given for regret within the two-year follow-up. In the two-year follow-up, appreciably fewer women who expressed regret did so for reasons related to menstruation.

We examined preoperatively determinable characteristics of women who regretted sterilization. The only risks for regret that were statistically significant at two years after sterilization were age less than 30 and the performance of sterilization concurrent with cesarean section in white women. These risk factors were more closely associated with fertility-related regret than with menstruation-related regret. In contrast to several other studies that did not control for the effects of age, low parity did not appear to be an important risk factor. Women undergoing sterilization after vaginal delivery had 1.5- and 1.7-fold higher risks of regret at one and two years, respectively, than women having an interval sterilization. This difference, however, may be related to chance alone and further study will be necessary to find out whether an important difference exists. Interestingly, all women who regretted having a sterilization after vaginal delivery had their sterilizations within 36 hours of delivery, as compared with 65 percent of those without regret.

It should be stressed that the previous discussion is applicable only to the likelihood of regret within two years after sterilization. In the study, to date, preoperatively determinable risk factors for regret became less closely associated with regret from the first to the second year. This suggests that postoperative life changes (for example, divorce and remarriage) may be stronger influences on regret with increasing time after sterilization. We will be able to test this hypothesis when five-year follow-up data are available.

Sterilization Failure

Sterilizations are intended to prevent pregnancy permanently, and the extent to which they do that and whether or not efficacy varies according to tubal occlusive methods used is important. Sterilization failure can result in intrauterine pregnancy which is unintended and usually unwanted; even more important, such failure can result in ectopic pregnancy which is life-threatening. There is some limited evidence that variation in the risk of intrauterine and ectopic pregnancy may be related to the tubal occlusive method used.

Few good data are available that carefully address the likelihood of sterilization failure. The few existing comparative studies have methodological concerns, but two studies have provided particularly useful information. One was a multinational study by Family Health International (FHI)[4] and the other was a study in Singapore.[31] These investigations demonstrated that studies of sterilization failure must have long follow-up and, in analysis, must account for patients lost to follow-up and variation in length of follow-up. A high follow-up rate is particularly important in evaluating the efficacy of various tubal occlusive methods. With low follow-up rates, one cannot be certain that the failures identified were representative of those occurring among all methods, thus making a comparison of tubal occlusive methods difficult. In these two studies, follow-up rates were less than 35 percent in one and not reported in the other. Even so, both the FHI multinational study and Cheng's study suggest that the likelihood of failure may differ depending on the tubal occlusive technique used. In the FHI study, life table pregnancy rates were calculated for 12,000 women. Cumulative failure rates per 100 women at 12 months were 0.23 for interval coagulation, 0.44 for interval tubal ring, and 0.19 for interval Rocket clip procedures. In Cheng's report, cumulative failure rates at 12 months were 0.23 and 3.61 per 100 women for abdominal and laparoscopic procedures, respectively. However, only 221 laparoscopic procedures were examined. Several reports have suggested that tubal sterilization may increase a woman's risk of subsequent ectopic pregnancy.[36,37] Another report[38] provides strong evidence that this is not the case. Rather, tubal sterilization appears actually to decrease the *absolute* risk of ectopic pregnancy because it significantly decreases the risk for pregnancy overall. Should a woman become pregnant after sterilization, however, the *relative* likelihood of ectopic pregnancy is increased. Additionally, a membership survey of the American Association of Gynecologic Laparoscopists[17] suggested that there may be a difference in risk of ectopic pregnancy after sterilization by method of tubal occlusion, with the coagulation techniques (which involve more extensive destruction) resulting in a greater likelihood of ectopic pregnancy than the mechanical occlusive techniques (silastic bands and clips).

At the time of this writing, 7,040 CREST participants have been followed for at least 24 months after sterilization and a total of 58 pregnancies have been identified. These pregnancies will be discussed as luteal phase pregnancies and true sterilization failures, including both intrauterine and ectopic gestations.

Luteal phase pregnancy has been defined in CREST as a pregnancy that occurred in a woman with a history of poststerilization amenorrhea whose estimated date of ovulation was before or on the date of sterilization. A total of 20 such luteal phase pregnancies have been reported to date.[39] Of these 20, 14 (70 percent) occurred among the 16.5 percent of CREST participants who were sterilized after their estimated date of ovulation and who had used barrier methods, rhythm, or withdrawal in the month before sterilization. Comparison of the characteristics of women having luteal phase pregnancies with those of other study participants suggests that the performance of sterilization before the estimated time of ovulation will prevent nearly all luteal phase pregnancies. The estimated date of ovulation in CREST participants was, by definition, easy to calculate in patients with regular cycles. However, even for women with irregular cycles, there were no participants who had luteal phase pregnancies in which sterilizations were performed prior to their date of ovulation as estimated by adding 14 days to the first day of the last menstrual period.

Thus, optimal timing of sterilization is the most effective strategy in preventing luteal phase pregnancy. Even if sterilization is not optimally timed, women who use the more effective methods of contraception (oral contraceptives and IUDs) are at relatively low risk of luteal phase pregnancy. Only 3 of 20 women with luteal phase pregnancies used oral contraceptives or IUDs before sterilization. For the group at highest risk of luteal phase pregnancy, that is, women whose sterilizations are performed after their estimated date of ovulation and who use barrier methods, rhythm, or withdrawal in the previous month, additional preventive measures for luteal phase pregnancy would include pregnancy testing and dilatation and curettage (D&C). However, it should be noted that D&C will not terminate all early conceptions.[39] In fact, of the 17 women who had luteal phase pregnancies and who were not using oral contraceptives or an IUD, 3 had D&Cs performed concurrently with their sterilizations. In summary, luteal phase pregnancies can, in all likelihood, be prevented by optimal timing of sterilization. Backup measures such as D&Cs for sterilizations that are not so timed cannot be expected to prevent luteal phase pregnancy with certainty.

Of 7,040 CREST patients studied for at least 24 months, 38 have had sterilization failures, for a crude failure rate of 5.4 per 1,000 procedures at 24 months. Although the different methods appear possibly to vary in efficacy, with coagulation techniques being somewhat more effective in preventing intrauterine pregnancy than the mechanical techniques, these differences are not statistically significant at present. Study power is too limited to date to expect to detect statistically significant differences between methods of tubal occlusion.

Summary

While millions of tubal sterilizations have been performed, most have occurred over the past decade. Thus, there has been relatively little time to study late complications of sterilization. A substantial number of studies have been reported, however, which suggest that sterilization is in general a safe operation. The CDC's sterilization mortality surveillance program suggests that death attributable to tubal sterilization is rare but that deaths do occur and in some instances may be preventable. CREST, along with other comparative studies, has shown that major morbidity attributable to tubal sterilization is likewise uncommon. There is some evidence that early complications may vary by surgical approach, method of tubal occlusion, and anesthetic technique. Some of the more serious complications, however, are fortunately rare, which makes it difficult, even in large comparative studies, to document differences in risk. Thus, it is important in evaluating relative safety to complement knowledge from comparative studies with clinical impressions, theoretical concerns, and individual reports of complications.

Comparatively few data are available that carefully address risks of late complications. Of those studies with the fewest methodological concerns, most suggest that tubal sterilization does not cause an increase in adverse menstrual changes up to two years after sterilization. Continued comparative studies will be necessary to ascertain whether such increased risks occur at a later time. Evidence concerning whether tubal sterilization increases the risk of subsequent hysterectomy is contradictory, but further follow-up of women in CREST should provide additional useful information. Regret after tubal sterilization is fortunately infrequent but does occur. Determinants of regret in CREST participants at two years after sterilization have been identified and further follow-up will help us to discern whether risk factors for regret can be ascertained preoperatively so that counseling may be of optimal benefit.

Finally, in part because sterilization failure is relatively rare, no definitive data exist to allow accurate comparison of the risk of pregnancy by method of tubal occlusion. Available data from CREST and other studies suggest that luteal phase pregnancy is generally preventable if sterilization is optimally timed but that backup measures such as D&C are not always effective. A determination of whether use of different methods of tubal occlusion results in a difference in absolute risk of one type of gestation or another (intrauterine or ectopic pregnancy) will require longer-term follow-up in CREST and a more accurate determination of failure rate by method of occlusion.

References

1. Centers for Disease Control: *Surgical Sterilization Surveillance; Tubal Sterilization and Hysterectomy in Women Ages 15–44, 1979–1980.* Atlanta: CDC, September 1983.
2. Chamberlain G, and Brown JC (Eds): *Gynaecological Laparoscopy: The report of the working party of the confidential enquiry into gynaecological laparoscopy.* London: The Royal College of Obstetricians and Gynaecologists, 1978.
3. Vessey M, Huggins G, Lawless M, et al: Tubal sterilization: Findings in a large prospective study. *Br J Obstet Gynaecol* 90:203, 1983.
4. Bhiwandiwala PP, Mumford SD, and Feldblum PJ: A comparison of different laparoscopic sterilization occlusion techniques in 24,939 procedures. *Am J Obstet Gynecol* 144:319, 1982.
5. Peterson HB, DeStefano F, Rubin GL, et al: Deaths attributable to tubal sterilization in the United States, 1977 to 1981. *Am J Obstet Gynecol* 146:131, 1983.
6. Peterson HB, DeStefano F, Greenspan JR, et al: Mortality risk associated with tubal sterilization in United States hospitals. *Am J Obstet Gynecol* 143:125, 1982.
7. Grimes DA, Peterson HB, Rosenberg MD, et al: Sterilization-attributable deaths in Bangladesh. *Int J Gynaecol Obstet* 20:149, 1982.
8. Phillips J, Hulka J, Keith D, et al: Laparoscopic precedures: A national survey for 1975. *J Reprod Med* 18:219, 1977.
9. Taylor G, Larson CP Jr, and Prestwich R: Unexpected cardiac arrest during anesthesia and surgery. An environmental study. *JAMA* 236:275, 1976.
10. Fishburne JI, and Keith L: Anesthesia. In Philips JM (Ed): *Laparoscopy*, Baltimore: Williams & Wilkins, 1977: p. 69.
11. Peterson HB, Grimes DA, Cates W Jr, et al: Comparative risk of death from induced abortion at 12 weeks' gestation performed with local versus general anesthesia. *Am J Obstet Gynecol* 141:763, 1980.
12. Rioux JE, and Cloutier D: A new bipolar instrument for laparoscopic tubal sterilization. *Am J Obstet Gynecol* 119:737, 1974.
13. Peterson HB, Ory HW, Greenspan JR, et al: Deaths associated with laparoscopic sterilization by unipolar electrocoagulating devices, 1978 and 1979. *Am J Obstet Gynecol* 139:141, 1981.
14. Peterson HB, Greenspan JR, and Ory HW: Death following puncture of the aorta during laparoscopic sterilization. *Obstet Gynecol* 59:133, 1982.
15. DeStefano F, Peterson HB, Ory HW, et al: Oral contraceptives and postoperative venous thrombosis. *Am J Obstet Gynecol* 143:227, 1982.
16. DeStefano F, Greenspan JR, Dicker RC, et al: Complications of interval laparoscopic tubal sterilization. *Obstet Gynecol* 61:153, 1983.
17. Phillips J, Hulka JF, Hulka B, et al: 1979 AAGL Membership Survey. *J Reprod Med* 26:529, 1981.
18. Layde PM, Peterson HB, Dicker RC, et al: Risk factors for complications of interval tubal sterilization by laparotomy. *Obstet Gynecol* 62:180, 1983.
19. Williams EL, Jones HE, and Merrill RE: The subsequent course of patients sterilized by tubal ligation. *Am J Obstet Gynecol* 61:423, 1951.
20. DeStefano F, Huezo CM, Peterson HB, et al: Menstrual changes after tubal sterilization. *Obstet Gynecol* 62:673, 1983.
21. Radwanska E, Berger GS, and Hammond J: Luteal deficiency among women with normal menstrual cycles requesting reversal of tubal sterilization. *Obstet Gynecol* 54:189, 1979.
22. Donnez J, Wauters M, and Thomas K: Luteal function after tubal sterilization. *Obstet Gynecol* 57:65, 1981.
23. McCann MF, and Kessel E: International experience with laparoscopic sterilization follow-up of 8500 women. *Adv Plann Parenth* 12:199, 1978.

24. Muldoon MJ: Gynecological illness after sterilization. *Br Med J* 1:84, 1972.
25. Templeton AA, and Cole S: Hysterectomy following sterilization. *Br J Obstet Gynaecol* 89:845, 1982.
26. Cooper PJ: Risk of hysterectomy after sterilization. *Lancet* 1:59, 1983.
27. Chi IC, and Feldblum PJ: Hysterectomy after interval laparoscopic sterilization. *Lancet* 1:848, 1982.
28. Kendrick JS, Rubin GL, Lee NC, et al: Hysterectomy performed within one year after tubal sterilization. *Fertil Steril* (in press).
29. Cooper P, Gath D, Rose N, et al: Psychological sequelae to elective sterilization: A prospective study. *Br Med J* 284:461, 1982.
30. Alderman B: Women who regret sterilization. *Br Med J* 2:766, 1977.
31. Cheng MCE, Cheong J, Khew KS, et al: Psychological sequelae of sterilization in women, in Singapore. *Int J Gynaecol Obstet* 15:44, 1977.
32. Gomel V: Profile of women requesting reversal of sterilization. *Fertil Steril* 30:39, 1978.
33. Leader A, Galan N, George R, et al: A comparison of definable traits in women requesting reversal of sterilization and women satisfied with sterilization. *Am J Obstet Gynecol* 145:198, 1983.
34. Alder E, Cook A, Gray J, et al: The effects of sterilization: A comparison of sterilized women with the wives of vasectomized men. *Contraception* 23:45, 1981.
35. Grubb GS, Peterson HB, Rubin GL, et al: Regret after decision to have a tubal sterilization. *Fertil Steril* (in press).
36. Wolf GC, and Thompson JN: Female sterilization and subsequent ectopic pregnancy. *Obstet Gynecol* 55:17, 1980.
37. Lubell I, Neuwirth RS, and Frischer R: A hidden risk: Extrauterine pregnancy after tubal sterilization. *Adv Plann Parenth* 13:24, 1978.
38. DeStefano F, Peterson HB, Layde PM, et al: Risk of ectopic pregnancy following tubal sterilization. *Obstet Gynecol* 60:326, 1982.
39. Grubb GS, and Peterson HB: Luteal phase pregnancy and tubal sterilization. *Obstet Gynecol* (in press).
40. Grimes DA, and Peterson HB: Routine performance of dilation and curettage at the time of laparoscopy. *J Reprod Med* 27:213, 1982.

IV

Tuboplasty

Editorial Comments

Many infertile women with diseased fallopian tubes are poor candidates for tuboplasty because of a history of pelvic tuberculosis, a recent adnexal infection with residual pelvic tenderness, advanced age (over 40 years), obesity (over 200 lbs), seminal inadequacy, poor sperm migration, or ovular dysfunction. Some women refuse the operation because the chances for a successful outcome are not good enough.

The results of preoperative tubal testing influence the selection of patients. The prognosis is affected by the cause of the tubal abnormality, the location and type of obstruction, the severity of associated periadnexal adhesions, and the operative technique.

As a consequence of changing social mores and contraceptive technology, more women have developed tubal obstruction. The rising incidence and prevalence of sexually transmitted diseases and iatrogenic sterility resulting from sterilization account for a large proportion of occluded and damaged tubes.

Results from conventional nonoperative tests for tubal patency, such as uterotubal insufflation and hysterosalpingography, sometimes are misleading or disagree. The accuracy of these diagnostic procedures depends on the physician's technique, a careful interpretation, and an awareness of their limitations. Repeated failure of carbon dioxide to pass through tubes at 200 mmHg and to produce subsequent shoulder pain suggests obstruction. However, a positive test indicated by passage of carbon dioxide at normal pressures followed by shoulder pain can occur in the presence of dilated occluded ampullae or with extensive peritubal adhesions, thus leading to an erroneous diagnosis.

Salpingography can reveal the size of a distally obstructed tube but not the condition of its fimbriae or the degree of tubal or ovarian fixation. Persistent, localized pelvic collections observed on the follow-up x-ray film suggest a hydrosalpinx. Such tubes are found to be normal at laparoscopy in fewer than 10 percent of the patients. The largest discrepancies between the findings of these two tests relate to the inability of the salpingogram to detect periadnexal adhesions accurately. For the diagnosis of proximal obstruction, it is important to be aware of the amount of contrast medium used, the presence of leakage at the junction of the cannula and the external os, the resis-

The Fallopian Tube: Basic Studies and Clinical Contributions, edited by Alvin M. Siegler, M.D. Mount Kisco, New York: Futura Publishing Company, Inc. © 1986.

tance to instillation of the liquid, and the patient's complaint of pain. The demonstration of intramural or isthmic shadows can influence the selection of the type of tubal repair.

Laparoscopy is used to search for tubal patency or to locate the site of obstruction by chromopertubation, to evaluate tubes for possible tuboplasty, and to lyse peritubal adhesions. Tubes showing filling and peritoneal spilling of the contrast medium on the delayed film, following a recent hysterosalpingogram, rarely are found occluded at laparoscopy.

A concise update of the merits and limitations of various diagnostic procedures has been provided by Ansari. Ascending and descending tests are described as well as operative procedures.

Salpingoscopy is the most recent endoscopic method used to evaluate the endosalpinx. Mencaglia and coworkers, and Cornier have described their technique and findings. It is possible to see intratubal adhesions, an atrophied or scarred tubal lining, and web-like patterns. In selected instances adhesions can be cut and removed.

To gynecologists, microsurgery implies optical magnification with either a magnifying loupe or operative microscope, gentle handling of tissue and constant irrigation of the operative site with appropriate solutions, hemostasis with bipolar cautery, lysis of adhesions and tubal incisions with a unipolar microelectrode or laser, the use of fine sutures, and microsurgical instruments. Magnification permits the performance of intricate maneuvers with precision and minimal trauma.

Special considerations apply to the use of microsurgery in gynecology. The surgeon should be familiar with the range of infertility disorders and have good knowledge of the principles of microsurgical tuboplasty. The first tuboplasty is the one most likely to succeed and it may be the patient's only chance for pregnancy. Prolonged procedures lasting over four hours predispose tissues to drying and trauma, leading to a greater incidence of postoperative adhesions.

This operative technique, involving the use of optical magnification, miniaturized instruments, and fine sutures, requires special skills that can be acquired with patience, practice, perseverance, proper preparation, and sufficient clinical opportunity. The ideal training is a preceptorship in a clinical setting that gives the gynecologist the opportunity for continued, weekly exposure to patients who have need for tubal repair. The literature on the subject has a good deal of current fundamental information. Workshops can augment the didactic and practical experience. Familiarity with the instruments and sutures can be gained by practice in the laboratory using the loupe and the microscope. Learning to tie knots with these fine sutures is a most important skill and the number of hours of practice will vary with the individual surgeon. Perseverance and the conviction that microsurgical principles make a difference in the outcome of fertility surgery are important ingredients. In addition to experimental animals, surgical gloves, placental blood vessels, and extirpated fallopian tubes are good structures on which techniques for anastomosis may be practiced.

Extensive studies have been performed on various sizes and types of sutures to evaluate their holding strength, resistance to breakage on direct pull, provocation of granulomatous reactions, and reaction to methods of sterilization. Polyglycolic acid sutures have a more clearly defined time for absorbability (two weeks) than protein collagen sutures (15 days to 2 months). Nylon, a polyamine, is depolymerized in tissue and slowly absorbed. When knots are tied correctly, it is always possible to remove excess thread to the level of the knot without its becoming untied. Although biodegradation eventually takes place, it does not occur until long after healing.

Fine needles require careful handling and the surgeon must be aware of the position at which they can best be grasped by the needle holder or forceps. This can be done by observing their penetration and exiting from tissue under magnification. Needles are held at about their center or point of balance and not at the tip. The directional stability is lost if the needle is held too close to the shank. Tissue damage results from a needle that does not penetrate well or pass easily. Needles for microsurgery should be tapered with a 3–6 mm cord length, a curvature of about 135°, and a wire diameter of 50–150 μm. Larger needles and sutures of 7-0 are easily manipulated and tied; they are certainly acceptable in performance of most microsurgical procedures. Generally, the swaged needles are three to four times the diameter of their respective threads. The size of suture material is important because it influences the time necessary for completing the operation, and it may influence the success of the anastomoses. Very fine sutures (above 8-0) do not improve the patency rate significantly, require more meticulous care in handling, and increase the duration of the operation. The thread should be colored for contrast and not too long to prevent easy handling.

Leader and Taylor did not find any significant difference between the absorbable sutures if tensile strength, wound strength, and tissue reaction are compared, despite the fact that Dexon® remains in tissue longer than Vicryl® or PDS®. Other methods for tissue approximation such as CO_2 or fibrin glue have not proved superior to microsutures.

The microsurgical approach to overcoming tubal occlusion is reviewed by Owen who reports on the largest series of anastomosis operations done for reversal of a previous sterilization. Cohen and Angle have described the step-by-step procedure for anastomosis for tubal obstruction caused by inflammatory disease.

Evans and Ansari have presented an alternative approach to blockage at the uterotubal junction in their chapter on tubal implantation. Both techniques of cornual and posterior fundal uterine openings are described for situations in which the entire intramural segment is blocked so that the tubocornual anastomosis is not fea- sible. For distal tubal obstruction, fimbrioplasty, Roland has continued to maintain that his splint enables more women to achieve pregnancy subsequently and, more importantly, few tubal gestations were noted in his series.

Therapeutic laparoscopic procedures from myomectomy to oophorectomy have been reported by Semm. His skills and fine equipment have enabled him to reduce the number of laparotomies for removal of tubal gestations, lysis of pelvic adhesions and fimbrioplasty. Semm has detailed a review of these techniques with accompanying illustrations so that one can follow the methods described without difficulty.

Assessing results from tuboplasty remains difficult and some of the problems in evaluation are described by Chamberlain.

Since the turn of the 20th century, procedures used to restore patency to occluded tubes and the criteria for expressing and analyzing results have varied. Operations for tuboperitoneal causes of infertility must be carefully analyzed, and the extent of tubal damage assessed to enable physicians to evaluate their own work and the studies of others. In this way, the most suitable patients will be selected, the distribution of procedures in a series ascertained, the operative techniques individualized, and standards for success evolved. The polemics about the duration of follow-up required for inclusions of a given patient in a series are yet to be resolved. Patients not evaluated postoperatively by tubal patency tests are considered closed tube failures if no conception occurs. For obvious reasons, all patients operated on must be included in a series, even those who have had tuboplasty only a short time before the published report, since some women do conceive within the first few months postoperatively.

In tubal reconstructive surgery, it is well known that a wide discrepancy exists between anatomical postoperative patency and pregnancy and most physicians would agree that the only measure of success is a subsequent delivery.

It is very difficult to evaluate or compare results without a method of classification; the following classification was developed and agreed on by many reproductive surgeons at the 10th World Congress of Fertility and Sterility held in Madrid in 1980. It is based primarily on the type of tubal repair without consideration of the cause of the obstruction or exact surgical technique.

1. *Lysis of periadnexal adhesions (salpingolysis ovariolysis)*, classified according to adnexa with the least abnormality
   a. minimal: 1 cm of tube or ovary involved (<⅓)
   b. moderate: partially surrounding tube or ovary
   c. severe: encapsulating peritubal or periovarian adhesions (or both) (>⅔)
2. *Lysis of extraadnexal adhesions*
   a. minimal
   b. moderate
   c. severe
3. *Tubouterine implantation*
   a. isthmic: implantation of isthmic segment
   b. ampullary: implantation of ampullary segment
   c. combination: different type of implantation on right and left sides
4. *Tubotubal anastomosis*
   a. interstitial (intramural)-isthmic
   b. interstitial (intramural)-ampullary
   c. isthmic-isthmic
   d. isthmic-ampullary
   e. ampullary-ampullary
   f. ampullary-infundibular (fimbrial)
   x. combination: different type of anastomosis on right and left tubes
5. *Salpingostomy (Salpingoneostomy):* surgical creation of a new tubal ostium
   a. terminal
   b. ampullary
   c. isthmic
   x. combination: different type of salpingostomy on right and left tubes
6. *Fimbrioplasty* (reconstruction of existent fimbria)
   a. by deagglutination and dilatation
   b. with serosal incision (for completely occluded tube)
   x. combination: different type of fimbrioplasty on right and left tubes
7. *Other reconstructive tubal operations* (the type should be specified)
8. *Combination of different types of operations*
   a. *bipolar*: for occlusion at both proximal and distal end of tube (specific procedures should be stated)
   b. *bilateral*: different operations on the right and left sides (specific procedures should be stated)

An important modification of Group 1. Lysis of periadnexal adhesions was developed by Hulka and colleagues who staged pelvic adhesions by their extent, density and vascularity (Hulka et al.: *Fertil Steril* 30:661, 1978). Most significant was the extent (more or less than one-half of the ovarian surface covered) rather than the nature of the adhesions. When removal of stage II adhesions (over one-half of the ovary covered) was required, in addition to repair of a distally occluded tube, an intrauterine pregnancy rarely followed.

Most of us would agree that in classifying procedures involving a tubal anastomosis, two separate systems are relevant: one in which the cause of occlusion has resulted from a previous sterilization and the other from occluded tubes caused by salpingitis isthmica nodosa, luminal fibrosis, endometriosis, chronic salpingitis, tubal polyps, or tuberculosis.

To be acceptable to the gynecologist, the classification must be relatively simple to follow and editors of medical journals should not accept manuscripts for publication unless they conform to the agreed-on guidelines.

All of the relevant information can be incorporated onto one sheet with appropriate illustrations and information for coding (Fig. IV:1a). It should include, obviously, the patient's name and her age. The influence of the age of the patient is difficult to evaluate. Increasing age is associated with longer intervals since sterilization, ovulatory disturbances, and older partners. In the absence of such cofactors, counseling as to medical and social implications of parenthood at or beyond age 40 is appropriate. The type of sterilization can influence the technique of repair but, thus far, it has not been possible to state with any degree of certainty that one particular method of sterilization is more "reversible" than another. Although bipolar coagulation has replaced the unipolar method for the most part, many women now seeking re-

REVERSAL OF STERILIZATION CLASSIFICATION

Patient's Name:____________________ Age:________

Type of Sterilization:____________________ Date:________

Screening Laparoscopy: Yes ________ No ________ Date: ________

Tuboplasty:____________________ Date:________

Segment Length (cm)

	Before Repair		After Repair
	Proximal	Distal	
R			
L			

Anastomosis:

	IM-IS	IM-AM	IS-IS	IS-AM	AM-AM	OTHER
R						
L						

Implantation:

Segment Length (cm)

	After Repair		Location in Uterus	
	Isthmic	Ampulla	Posterior	Cornua
R				
R				

Salpingoneostomy:

Segment Length (cm) After Repair

R

L

FIGURE IV:1*a*—*Code sheet for reversal of sterilization (*front*).*

versal had undergone sterilization when the unipolar approach was the more common technique. It is important to perform laparoscopy as a screening procedure if any coagulation method was used or whenever the operative report is not available and inconsistent with the pathology report. Based on this form, we still cannot obtain an accurate reversibility rate because that requires a knowledge of the number of women who sought consultation for reversal and who were ultimately operated on with a successful outcome.[1] Few authors have included in their results of reversal of sterilizations the original procedure used to sterilize the patient or the interval until tubal operation for reversal of sterilization. Electron microscopic studies have shown relative atrophy of the tubal epithelium in the proximal stumps of women sterilized more than five years prior to reversal. Vasquez et al.[2] did scanning electron microscopy on 26 specimens and generally noted increased abnormalities with increasing intervals between sterilization and sterilization reversal. These included flattening of longitudinal folds, deciliation, and polyposis. Disorders in the tubal isthmus occurred with chronic occlusion. The operating microscope helps to define the extent of polyposis.

The next section in this classification proposal concerns anastomosis with the description of the right and left fallopian tubes, the lengths in centimeters of the proximal and distal segments before repair and after completion of the operation-(Fig. IV:1a).

McComb and Gomel[3] designed studies to measure the effect of tubal length on fertility in the rabbit. The animals were subjected to microsurgical resection of different lengths of fallopian tube involving the isthmus in each case. Fertility rates were significantly lower following anastomosis of remaining segments only after 40 percent of the tubes had been removed. In a follow-up study,[4] these investigators attempted to ascertain the influence of ampullary length on infertility. Based on the results of the new studies, these authors suggested that the length of the distal tubal remnant (ampulla) may influence fertility more than the length of the proximal tubal segment.

This section on lengths of segments is a check on the type of anastomosis. A proximal segment measuring less than 5 cm obviously includes only isthmus and a distal segment measuring 3 or 4 cm includes ampulla. Several studies[5] have been published on the significance of the length of the extrauterine portion of tube on completion of the operation but more data are needed. The classification of the type of anastomosis follows and it is fairly straightforward. These include intramural-isthmic, intramural-ampullary, isthmic-isthmic, isthmic-ampullary and ampullary-ampullary. Other possibilities are double anastomoses and anastomosis of opposite tubal segments.

Since operations for reversal of sterilization other than anastomosis are also possible, including implantation and salpingoneostomy, they are included in the proposal.

There are several studies[6,7] on the reversal of sterilization in which tubal implantations were done. Several types are possible involving either the isthmus or ampullary portion of the tube and either a cornual or posterior fundal incision. Once again, the length of the extrauterine tubal segment should be measured and its new location in the uterine wall indicated.

Salpingoneostomy is done for reversal of a previous fimbriectomy.[8] The length of the extrauterine tubal segment following repair should be noted. Novy[9] suggested that salpingoneostomy in such women should have at least 8 cm or more of tube, a positive rugal pattern on hysterosalpingogram, minimal peritubal adhesions, and an ampullary width of greater than one centimeter. Laparoscopy is essential in these patients prior to attempting sterilization reversal.

Equal-sized lumens occur in isthmic-isthmic or ampullary-ampullary anastomoses. The other three categories involve unequal-sized lumens. The schematic representations of these procedures are included on the form so that the physician can quite readily mark the type of procedure performed.

Although it is uncommon to encounter significant periadnexal adhesions in reversing previous sterilization procedures, their presence should be noted. However, it is not necessary to use the point system. The performance of additional pelvic procedures or associated pathology should be listed (Fig. IV:1b). The arrangement used in the endometriosis classification is quite acceptable.

The impact of microsurgery on gynecology has involved repair of previously sterilized tubes and under ideal circumstances about 60 percent of patients operated on subsequently achieve a term pregnancy. However, one of the dangers of such success can leave the impression with patients or physicians that sterilization is not to be considered permanent. Success cannot be guaranteed and extrauterine pregnancies occur with increased frequency in repaired tubes. Associated

Ovarian Adhesions		**<⅓ Enclosure**	**⅓–⅔ Enclosure**	**>⅔ Enclosure**
R	Filmy			
	Dense			
L	Filmy			
	Dense			

Tubal Adhesions

R	Filmy
	Dense
L	Filmy
	Dense

Additional Pelvic Procedure:____________________________________

Associated Pathology:____________________________________

Guidelines

Tubal segments should be measured in centimeters (cm) before and after repair. Over 95% of all reversal procedures will fit into one of these categories. Points are not given for tubal or ovarian adhesions as they rarely influence the outcome of these procedures. Sometimes it is difficult to categorize the site of anastomosis but a thought about equal and unequal segments might be helpful.

Diagram of Procedure

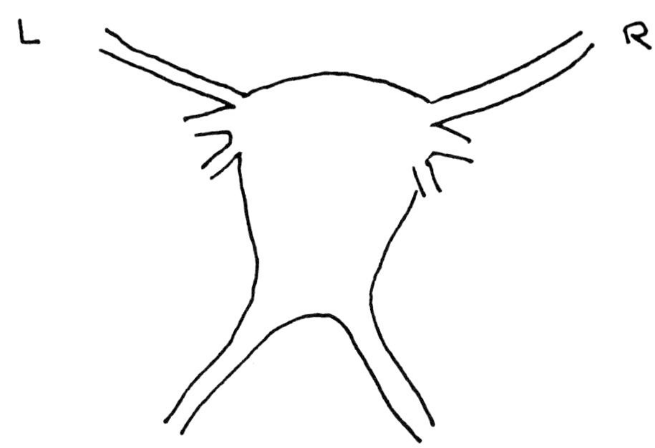

FIGURE IV:1*b*—*Code sheet for reversal of sterilization* (back).

abnormalities in the occluded segments have been reported by Rock and colleagues,[10] that included salpingitis isthmica nodosa, fibrosis, chronic salpingitis, and even hydrosalpinx. In a recent paper, Hulka, Peretz, and myself collected contributions on the subject of reversal of sterilization as they appeared in the literature. This search uncovered few series of more than 50 cases with the percentage of live births varying from 48 percent to 78 percent, the occurrence of tubal pregnancy ranging from 1.7 percent to 6.5 percent. Since about 5,000 reversal proce-

A CLASSIFICATION OF TUBO-TUBAL ANASTOMOSIS
(Except for Reversal of Sterilization)

Patient's Name:________________ Age:________________

Screening Laparoscopy: Yes______ No______ Date:________________

Tuboplasty:________________ Date:________________

Segment Length (cm)

	Before Repair		After Repair	
	Proximal	Distal	Proximal	Distal
R				
L				

Anastomosis:

	IM-IS	IM-AM	IS-IS	IS-AM	AM-AM	Other
R						
L						

Ovarian Adhesions		**$<1/3$ Enclosure**	**$1/3$–$2/3$ Enclosure**	**$>2/3$ Enclosure**
R	Filmy			
	Dense			
L	Filmy			
	Dense			

Tubal Adhesions	
R	Filmy
	Dense
L	Filmy
	Dense

FIGURE IV:2a—*Code sheet for tubo-tubal anastomosis* (front).

dures are estimated to be performed annually and fewer than 1,000 have been reported in the literature, it is obvious that most sterilization reversals are being done by the "silent majority" of gynecologists.

Another system of classification is needed for anastomosis operations performed because of pathological rather than iatrogenic occlusion (Fig. IV:2a). These procedures have a different prognosis from those done on women having a reversal of a sterilization. These patients must have a screening laparoscopy to ascertain the condition of the tube beyond the point of its proximal obstruction.

It is possible that associated tubal operations may be required in instances of bipolar obstruction; different procedures may be performed on opposite tubes. The classification for adhesions is the same as seen in the form for reversal of sterilization. We would suggest including a category entitled "Pathology Report." The list-

PATHOLOGY REPORT

	Normal	Luminal Fibrosis	Isthmica Nodosa	Chronic Salpingitis	Endometriosis	Other
R						
L						

Associated Pathology:______________________________

Additional Pelvic Procedure:______________________________

Guidelines

Fimbrioplasty means identifiable fimbriae were present. Salpingoneostomy means a new opening was created into a totally occluded, smooth distal segment. Tubal segments should be measured in centimeters (cm) before and after repair. Points are not given for tubal or ovarian adhesions as they probably do not influence the outcome of anastomosis procedures. Sometimes it is difficult to categorize the site of anastomosis but a thought about equal and unequal segments might be helpful.

Diagram of Procedure

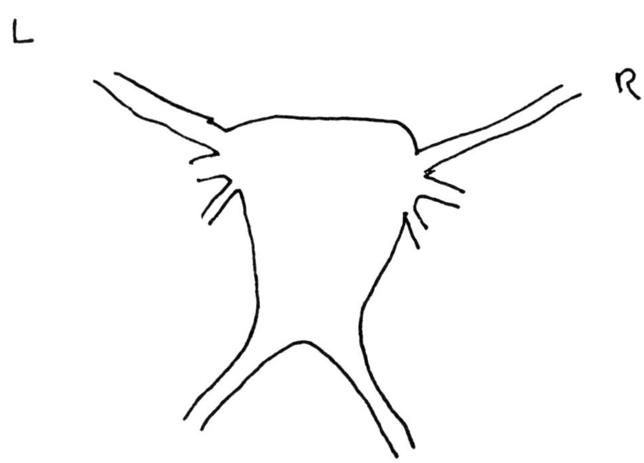

FIGURE IV:2*b*—*Code sheet for tubo-tubal anastomosis* (back).

ings are luminal fibrosis, chronic salpingitis, salpingitis isthmica nodosa, endometriosis, normal fallopian tube, and other. In at least 10 percent to 15 percent of specimens submitted for histologic examination in patients with proximal tubal obstruction, no histologic cause for the obstruction is found (Fig. IV:2b).

Various methods used to reduce or minimize formation or reformation of adhesions have been described by Larsson. The value of many agents described seems theoretically valid but the published results of studies with the agents are often inconclusive or contradictory.

Factors producing postoperative intraperitoneal adhesions include trauma, infection, ischemia, and reaction to foreign bodies. It is presumed that peritoneal trauma leads to inflammation with increased capillary permeability, serosanguineous exudate, and deposition of fibrin. Ischemia results in the suppression of fibrinolysis, the consequences of which lead to proliferation of fibroblasts and development of permanent fibrous adhesions. Therefore, vigorous attempts at reperitonealization of large defects create tension and further ischemia leading to adhesions. With a good blood supply, adequate plasminogen activator and plasmin help to lyse the fibrin; mesothelial cells are recruited, stromal cells are transformed, and healing occurs. The formation of postoperative adnexal adhesions following conservative adnexal surgery can cause infertility and the presence of these adhesions represents a major factor in failed tuboplasty.

One therapeutic regimen designed to increase the chances of pregnancy following tuboplasty is postoperative hydropertubation, the purposes of which are to flush exudate or blood out of the recently manipulated oviduct, to maintain patency of the repaired tube, and to deliver medication directly to the operative site. In most instances hydropertubation is used following repair of the distally occluded tube, although some physicians advocate its use even following tubal anastomosis.

Hydropertubations described in the literature vary in the frequency and intervals of the injection and in the quantity and quality of the fluid instilled. Their efficacy remains unclear because of the wide variety of "cocktails" and other concomitant medications. Commonly used combinations of fluid contain antibiotics, enzymes, corticosteroids, and Dextran®, although there is little evidence that local therapy is more effective than systemically administered drugs.

Hydropertubation may cause a patient discomfort if the fluid is excessive or injected too quickly. Even with strict sterile precautions it is not possible to prevent some bacterial contamination. In a collaborative study, a series of patients who were operated on for distal tubal occlusion received either no hydrotubation, or 50 ml of lactated Ringer's, or cortisone plus lactated Ringer's for the first three postoperative days and then on the day of discharge from the hospital. Subsequent follow-up ascertained that there was no difference in pregnancy rates among the three groups.

Antibiotics

Surgeons who perform tuboplasty use various amounts and types of antibiotics prophylactically. Such therapy has been used perioperatively in special gynecologic and obstetric procedures in patients who have no clinical evidence of infection.

The precise mechanism by which the antibiotic is presumed to reduce postoperative infectious morbidity in these women remains unclear since tuboplasty is hardly ever associated with significant bacterial contamination. Until recently, ampicillin was the most commonly used antibiotic.

To study the role of prophylactic antibiotics, 85 patients who were admitted for tuboplasty to the Downstate Medical Center in Brooklyn, New York, were divided into two groups: 40 patients in one group received two grams of cephalosporin I.M. two hours preoperatively and then every six hours after the operation for a total dose of 18 grams. This regimen of antibiotics would be considered long-term prophylaxis. The other 45 patients were not given antibiotics. The profiles of the two groups were similar and the postoperative results were not significantly different. Postoperative wound infections occurred in one patient from each group and three women developed urinary tract infections. Based on these findings, the merits of antibiotic prophylaxis in women having tuboplasty should be reevaluated because of recent operative innovations and the relative infrequency of postoperative febrile morbidity.

In the final section both Martin and Tadir, who are experienced endoscopists and well trained with the laser, emphasize the importance of learning to control the effects of laser by manipulating lenses, power, duration of exposure, and backstops. Maximal power density (greatest tissue impact) is at the beam's focal point. Laser power for gynecologic surgery averages approximately 30 watts or more, although each type of laser interacts differently with tissues.

Carbon dioxide laser penetrates tissue only 0.1 mm, in contrast to Argon laser (0.8 mm) and Nd:YAG laser (4.2 mm). The CO_2 beam can make precise, knife-like incisions with reasonable hemostasis and permits careful depth control. The beam can be directed to the tissue site either by an articulated arm and handpiece or by a micromanipulator (joystick) connected to an operating microscope. The latter produces 0.5 mm spots at focal distances of 250 to 300 mm. The typical focal length for the handpiece delivery system is between 50 and 100 mm.

It is probably best to apply laser techniques after learning with a preceptor and then proceed from its use in the lower genital tract into laparotomy. Laparoscopic use should be delayed until the physician develops a skill in the other two areas.

Removing smoke and carbon is not simple and causes some problems during their evacuation from the abdomen during laparoscopy. A special system is needed or else the abdomen is constantly deflated and one's vision becomes obscured.

The still unanswered questions are: the long-term possible untoward effects from carbon; improved fertility rates because of the use of laser in selected instances; the advantages of laser over the microelectrode needle and electrosurgery; the specific procedures that the tubal surgeon can do more effectively.

The Committee on Gynecologic Practice of the American College of Obstetricians and Gynecologists issued a state-of-the-art opinion in April 1984 concerning carbon dioxide laser which reads as follows:

> Laser is an acronym for light amplification by stimulated emission of radiation. It consists of an instrument, varying in power, that is often coupled with a colposcope and is used to destroy abnormal tissue.
>
> The laser beam, when used for tissue incision or destruction, is an alternative to hot or cryo cautery or electrodesiccation of lesions of the cervix, vulva, or vagina. It is useful in limited situations that require precise destruction of abnormal tissue. Current data suggest it is useful in treating cervical, vulvar, and vaginal intraepithelial neoplasia and condyloma accuminatum, but long-term follow-up is not yet available.
>
> Special training, as well as competence in colposcopy, is needed to learn laser therapy. The limitations and advantages of laser therapy are still being determined and clinical application should be restricted at this time to those appropriately trained physicians who have developed and adhere to a strict protocol and system of long-term follow-up. It is recommended at present that this technology not generally replace other widely used procedures with comparable clinical efficacy.
>
> The carbon dioxide laser is classified as clinically applicable* for limited use as described above, based on the following implications:
>
> A. Risk/benefit: Safe use of the instrument is dependent on the physician's knowledge of the indications, precautions, and limitations of the technology.
>
> B. Cost implications: The laser is an expensive instrument, and cost effectiveness relative to other treatment modalities is unknown.
>
> The laser has been used through the laparoscope for vaporization of adhesions and endometriotic lesions. It has also been employed for tissue incision and vaporization of adhesions in reconstructive operations of the fallopian tube and in surgery for endometriosis. The use of this modality for infertility surgery requires competence in microsurgery and special training in the proper use of the laser.
>
> There are no firm data at present that suggest a decrease in postoperative adhesions or improved pregnancy rates associated with the use of this modality. There is a risk of inadvertent damage to adjacent structures. The use of laser for

infertility surgery should be considered as investigative* in that it is not yet proven as an effective clinical procedure.

Classifications

- Experimental: Techniques that have been largely confined to laboratory and/or animal research.
- Investigative: Techniques that have progressed to limited human application but lack wide recognition as proven and effective procedures in clinical medicine.
- Clinically applicable: Techniques that have been accepted as clinically effective procedures for general or limited use based on risk/benefit and cost implications.

References

Carter R, Krantz KE, Hara GS, et al: Treatment of cervical intraepithelial neoplasia with the carbon dioxide laser beam: A preliminary report. *Am J Obstet Gynecol* 131:831, 1978.

Dorsey JH, Diggs ES: Microsurgical conization of the cervix by carbon dioxide laser. *Obstet Gynecol* 54:565, 1979.

Dorsey JH: Cervical conization by the carbon dioxide laser. *Pelvic Surg* 1:1, 1980.

Stafl A., Wilikinson EJ, Mattingly RF: Laser treatment of cervical and vaginal neoplasia. *Am J Obstet Gynecol* 128:128, 1977.

Summary

Selecting the patient for tubal surgery and choosing the trained physician are the two main factors affecting results. Proper infertility studies should not be omitted in shortcuts to the operating room. Hysterosalpingography affords a luminal study and it can delineate the longitudinal folds in the ampulla. The presence of these dark lines with water-soluble media augur for a significantly better prognosis than those distally obstructed tubes that show a homogeneous opacification. Laparoscopy is an important procedure before tubal repair in most, but not all, instances.

A plethora of manuscripts have been appearing on the surgical management of obstructed or distorted fallopian tubes. A diversity of approaches suggests that the choice of the best operation for a given abnormality still is not certain.

Progress is slow in this field because so many tubes become irreversibly damaged. It might seem hackneyed to reiterate the need for constant care in conservative adnexal surgery so as to prevent iatrogenic damage and to educate and counsel patients concerning the prevention of pelvic inflammatory disease.

The improved results following tuboplasty attributed to the use of gynecologic microsurgery have been limited principally to the operation of anastomosis. As yet the evidence to indicate the superiority of laser over cautery using bipolar forceps and microelectrode needles has not been published.

33

A Review of Early Contributions to the Development of Tuboplasty

Alvin M. Siegler

An important cause of sterility is the abnormal fallopian tube, but the existence of disease in it cannot be ascertained accurately by history and pelvic examination. Occlusive tubal adhesions and strictures, and isthmic nodular salpingitis are significant nonpalpable entities. Even endoscopic observation of a grossly normal oviduct does not always detect its role as a factor in some instances of unexplained infertility. Disturbances in ciliary action, in secretion, and in contractility can prevent a successful meeting of gametes in a patent tube.

Although still incomplete, our information concerning this special organ has come a long way since one of its earliest schematic representations appeared in the anatomical writings of Giacomo Berengario (1470–1530), surgeon and anatomist. He wrote a textbook on anatomy in 1514 with illustrations in which the dissected subjects were depicted as alive. The uterus appeared as globular (Fig. 33:1) and not bicornuate, this observation casting out Galen's concept that the septate human uterus was its normal configuration.[1] Berengario did not mention the oviducts. Vesalius in his famous textbook on anatomy, *De Humani Corporis Fabrica*, published in 1543 mentioned but did not describe angulated tubal entrances into the uterus. Fame came early to Vesalius and after his appointment as Court Physician, his anatomical researches ceased. One of his most famous pupils was Gabriele Fallopio (Fig. 33:2) who succeeded Vesalius as Professor of Anatomy at Padua. His most important work, published in 1561 entitled *Observations Anatomicae*, contains the first exact description of the ovaries and tubes, the end of which reads: "wherefore since the seminal duct from its beginning to its end has a likeness of the bent-parts of this classic instrument, separate or attached, therefore it has been called by me the Uteri Tuba. These are present not only in the human body, but also in the sheep, cows and all other animals which I have dissected."[2]

The originator of the first tuboplastic operation performed primarily for the purpose of correcting organic tubal ob-

The Fallopian Tube: Basic Studies and Clinical Contributions, edited by Alvin M. Siegler, M.D. Mount Kisco, New York: Futura Publishing Company, Inc.

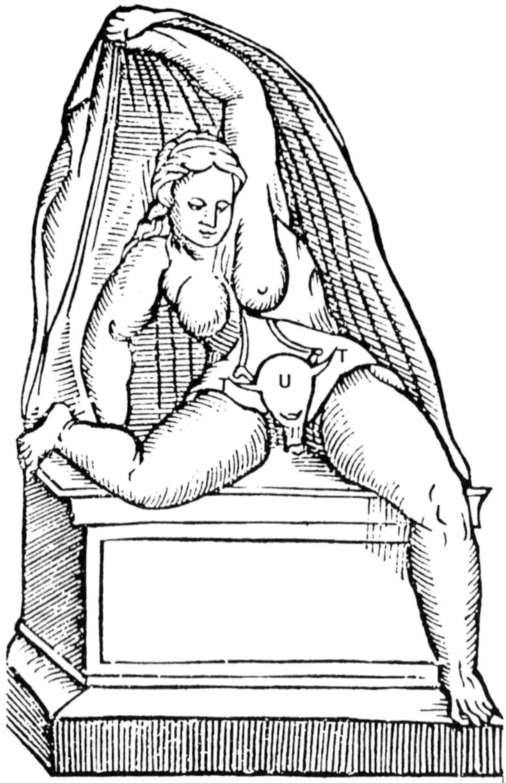

FIGURE 33:1—*A schematic representation of the uterus (U) and tubes (T) in 1530 by Berengario.*[1]

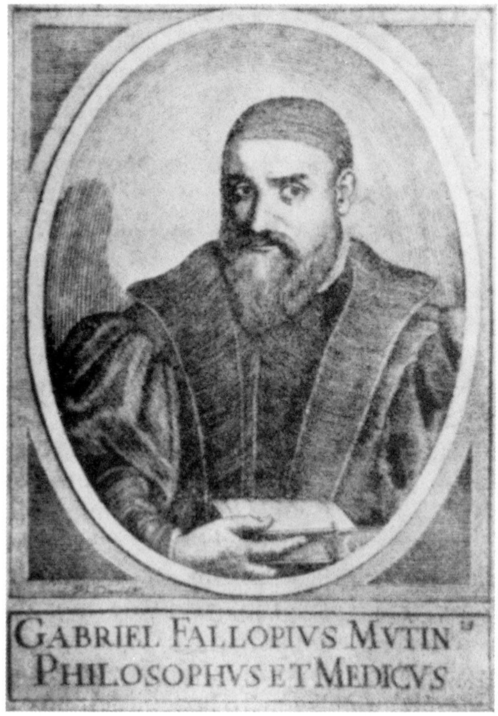

FIGURE 33:2—*Gabriele Fallopio (1523–1562).*

struction has been difficult to discover. Many gynecologists in the later part of the 19th century performed conservative adnexal operations on patients who had benign tubo-ovarian disease. In 1884 Schroeder[3] reported five tubal operations and in one of them, a tube was resected. In 1889 Skutsch[4] used the term salpingostomy to describe his procedure. Martin[5] in 1891 reported 21 ovarian and 24 tubal resections. The resected borders of the residual tubes were "hemstitched" for hemostasis. Most of the patients who were in the younger age groups retained their ability to menstruate. In his series, the first operation was done in 1883 and a spontaneous abortion resulted from the only pregnancy that followed.

The concept of conservative surgery for inflammatory disease of the pelvic organs was given further impetus by Polk[6] who in 1894 reported 78 cases. He used the term "salpingolysis" which he defined "to free tubes which had adhesions from their imprisonment." In 12 instances, he opened the tubes at the peritoneal ostia, cleaned them and stitched them back to the fimbriated rim. Four women on whom he performed combinations of salpingolysis and salpingostomy subsequently delivered at term.

In Kelly's *Operative Gynecology,*[7] published in 1898, seven conservative operations on the uterine tubes are listed:

1. The release of adherent tubes
2. The opening or resection of closed tubes
3. The emptying, cleansing, and sterilization of inflamed tubes
4. The amputation of diseased tubes

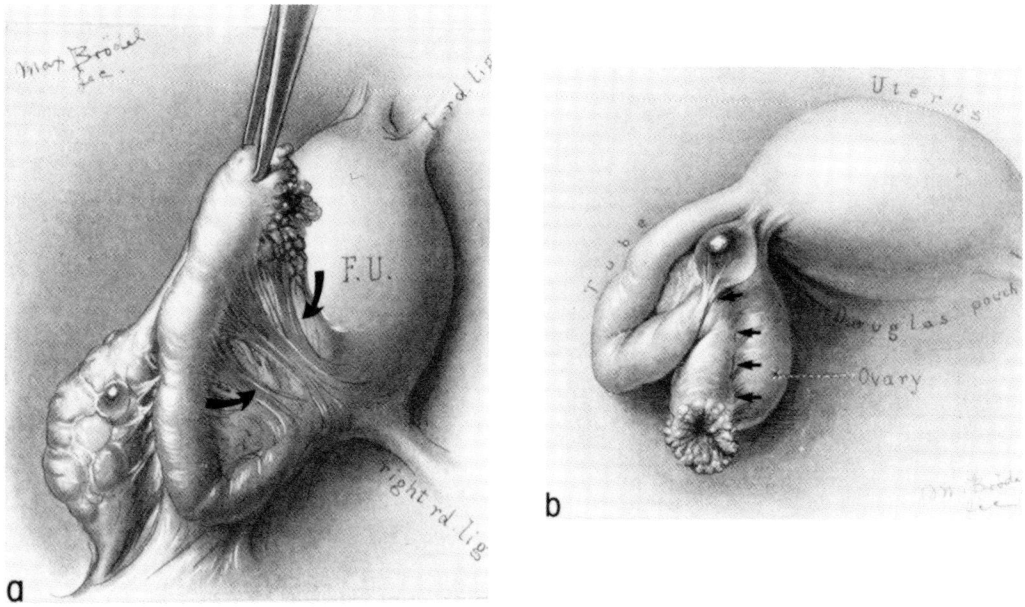

FIGURE 33:3—*Tubal distortion caused by peritubal adhesions (1898).*[7] (a) *tubouterine adhesions* (arrows); (b) *tubo-ovarian adhesions* (arrows).

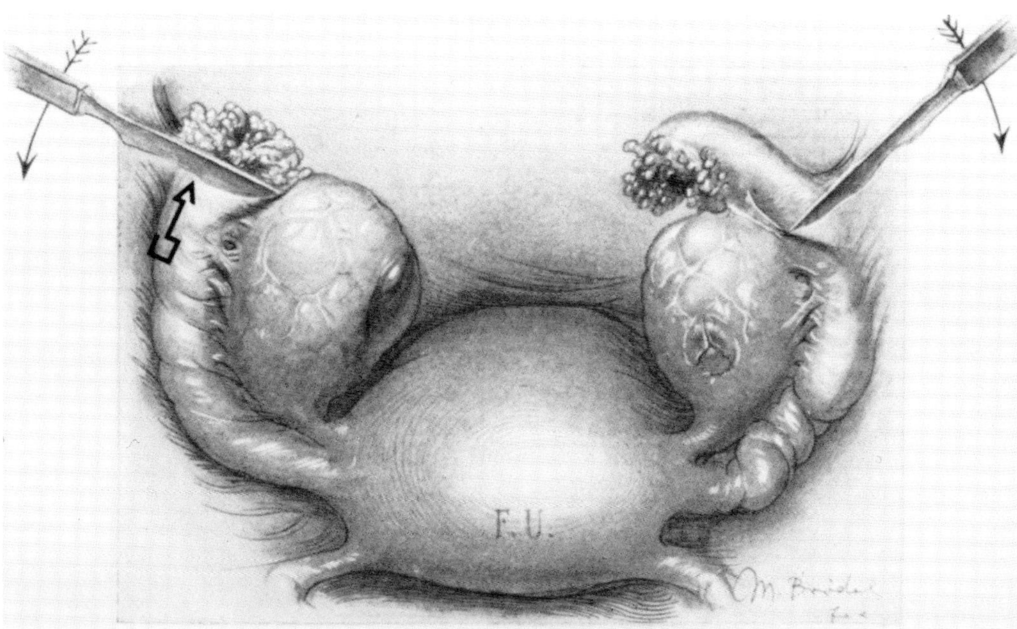

FIGURE 33:4—*Fimbrioplasty showing incision into prefimbrial scar to cure tubal stenosis (1898).*[7]

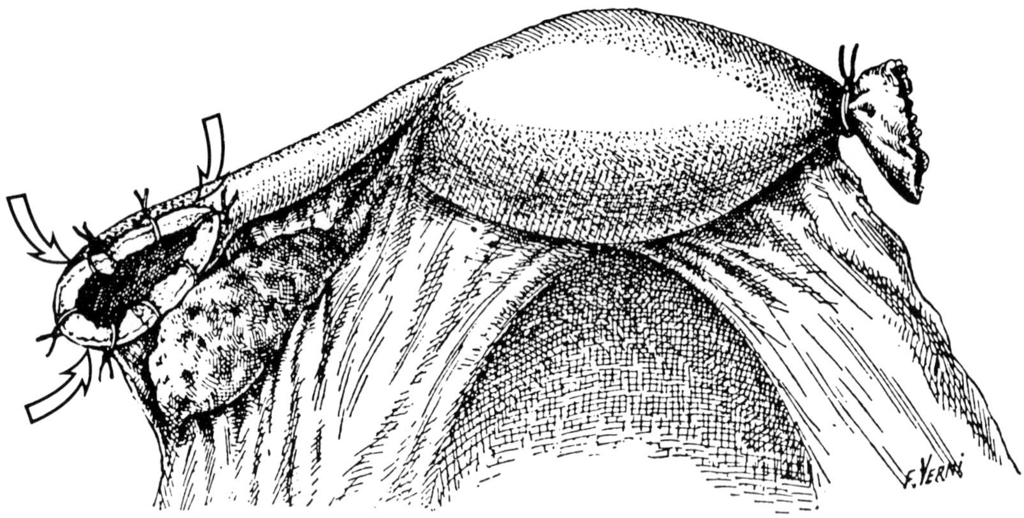

FIGURE 33:5—*Drawing of salpingostomy (*arrows*) associated with contralateral salpingo-oophorectomy. Attempted eversion of mucosal edge (1899).*[8]

5. The exsection of diseased or strictured tubes
6. The drainage of tubal abscesses
7. Preservation of the tube in the extrauterine pregnancy

For adherent tubes (Figs. 33:3 and 33:4) he advised dissection with scalpel, scissors, or sometimes with digital manipulation. In his book, Kelly probably described for the first time, a fimbrioplasty. Adhesions formed a collar behind the fimbria with a white fibrous band and this collar was divided in several places to release the fimbria.

Goullioud[8] in 1899 reviewed the salpingostomy operation and his articles contained the first drawing of the procedure as it was practiced in his era (Fig. 33:5). The next year Burrage[9] described his remote results from conservative operations on tubes and ovaries: 85 patients were followed for one year or more but no pregnancies occurred in 17 women who had had tubal resections. He described a cuff operation and a dorsal slit technique with and without amputation of the diseased part of the tube.

Gellhorn[10] noted that operations on the tubes were followed infrequently by successful conception because of poor selection of patients and recurrence of occlusion. The tubes often had microscopic evidence of destruction of the ciliated epithelium, a scarred myosalpinx, and numerous intraluminal adhesions. These tubes were damaged irreparably and conservative surgery was of little value.

In 1932 Holden and Sovak[11] described the circumcision cuff operation as it was performed in seven women (Fig. 33:6). Vaginal diathermy was given from three to four weeks preoperatively and no special devices were used to maintain the newly formed ostium. No live births were reported postoperatively. Halban[12] described the terminal salpingostomy without formation of a cuff (Fig. 33:7). Beecham and Sigman[13] poured sulfanilamide crystals into the created tubal ostia of eight patients and in seven of them the tubes remained patent postoperatively as ascertained by tubal insufflation. One woman had a term delivery.

In 1943 Gepfert[14] described a method of terminal salpingostomy without tubal resection followed by the insertion of a 4 × 6-inch sheet of allantoic membrane over the newly formed stoma (Fig. 33:8). Allantoic membrane had gained considerable favor as a cover for the brain to pre-

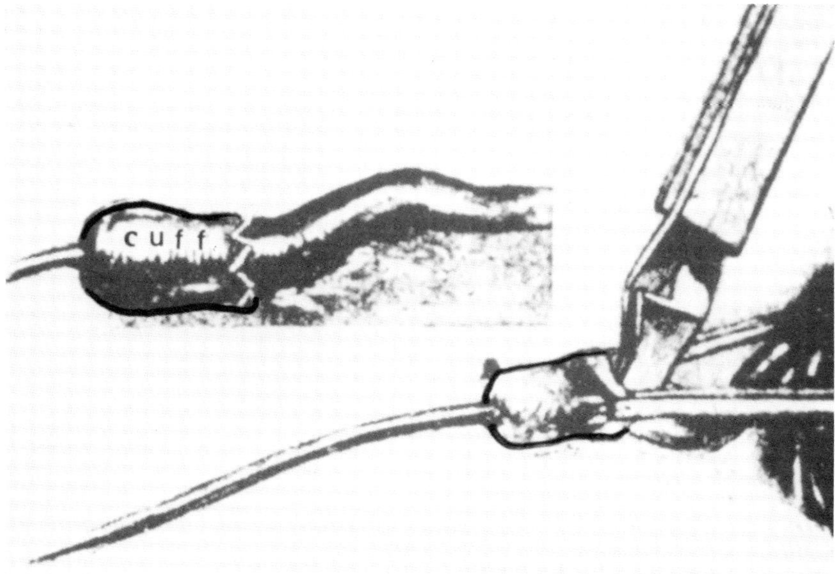

FIGURE 33:6—*Special clamp used to help form a large distal cuff (1932).*[11] *Inset shows catheter in cuffed neostomy.*

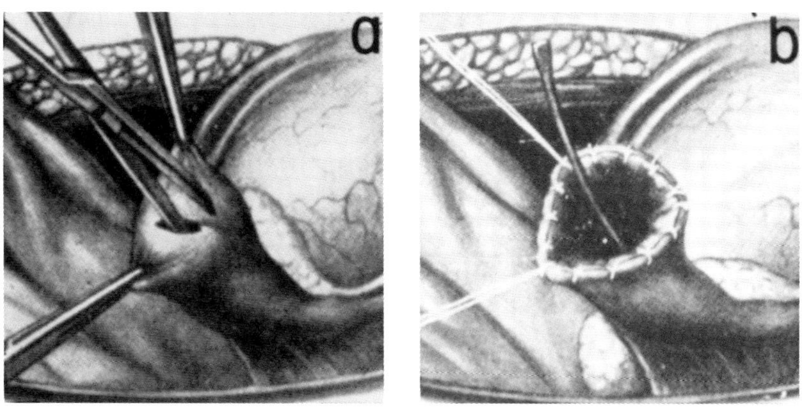

FIGURE 33:7—(a) *Opening tube with scissors for hydrosalpinx.* (b) *Repair without creation of cuff (1932).*[12]

vent the formation of adhesions in neurosurgery. Of Gepfert's 28 tuboplasties performed in the above manner, 24 were followed for six months and 18 maintained patency. Hofmann[15] had occasion to reoperate on a patient on whom a bilateral cuff operation included application of the allantoic membrane on one side. This tube was reoccluded and extensive adhesions were present. The extrauterine pregnancy was in the opposite tube. Westman[16] inserted plugs of cholesteroloxalate in the newly formed ostium and two weeks postoperatively the plugs were melted by inducing a fever of 104°F with a vaccine.

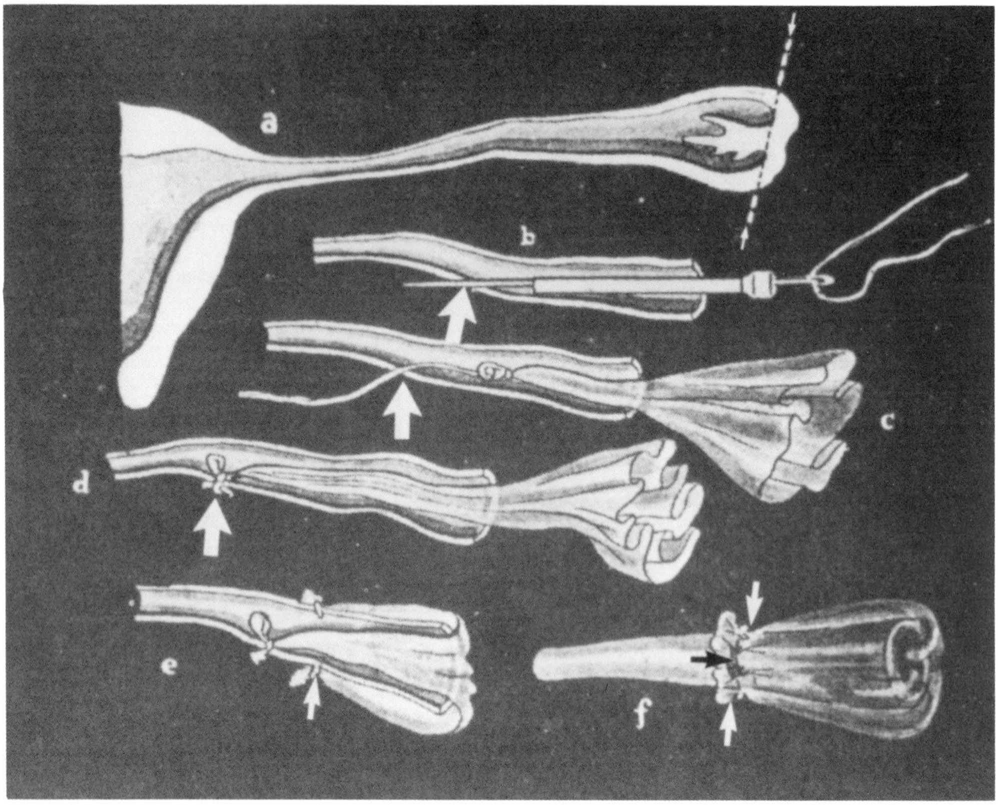

FIGURE 33:8—(a) *Occluded segment* (arrows) *removed.* (b) *Needle is passed through cannula and through tubal lumen* (arrow) *with suture tied to allantoic membrane.* (c) *Suture passed through tube* (arrow) *as membrane is pulled into lumen.* (d) *Suture is tied to tube* (arrow). (e and f) *Allantoic membrane covering resected ampullary end and fastened to tubal serosa* (arrows).[14]

Johnston[17] modified the salpingostomy by creating a tubal flap from the reopened sactosalpinx and attached it to the ovarian hilum. The location of the initial tubal incision was selected by the point of maximal crepitation when tubal insufflation was combined with the operation.

Bunster[18] summarized multiple variations of salpingostomy. These included the terminal salpingostomy of Martin, the lateral salpingostomy of Skutsch, the total linear salpingostomy of Chalier, and the transverse type of Halban and Holden and Sovak (Fig. 33:9).

Gardner[19] in 1856 described an instrument like a catheter that had an opening in its extremity for the passage of a small probe (Fig. 33:10). It was used to overcome proximal tubal obstruction. He acknowledged the risk of lacerating the mucous membrane and of forming a false passage.

The treatment of proximal tubal obstruction traditionally had been tubouterine implantation until the advent of tubocornual anastomosis. In a very comprehensive and detailed article in 1897, Ries[20] described the pathology of nodular salpingitis. In one of these patients the tubal isthmus was submitted for microscopic study and the residual portion was implanted into the uterus. The operation was performed by Dr. T.J. Watkins and named "metrosalpingoanastomosis." In 1903 Ferguson[21] described hysterosal-

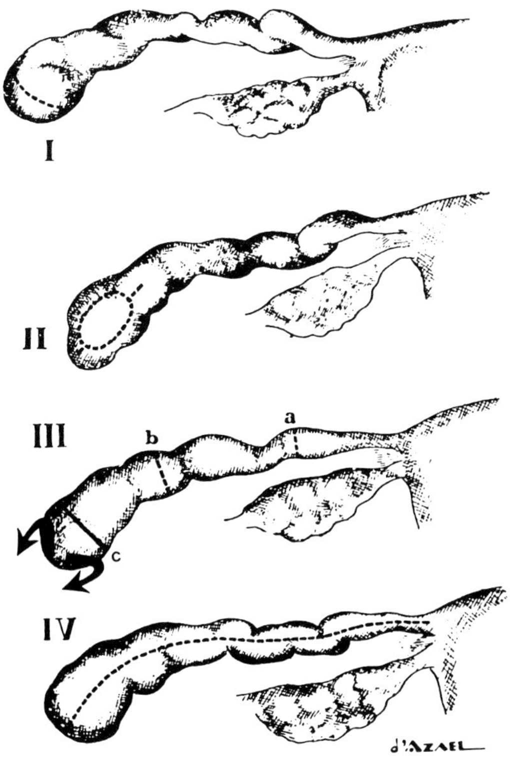

FIGURE 33:9—*Types of salpingostomy.*[18] (I) *terminal-transverse;* (II) *terminal-lateral;* (III) *isthmic* (a), *midampullary* (b), *terminal with resected segment* (c) (arrows); (IV) *linear.*

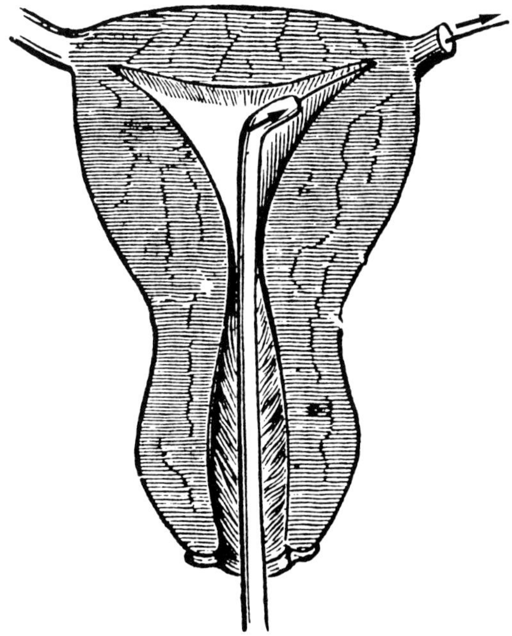

FIGURE 33:10—*Attempted passage of probes* (arrows) *through uterotubal orifice.*[19]

pingostomy and salpingostomy in six patients, one of whom subsequently conceived but aborted. In each instance there were multiple operations on the tubes and the paper had a drawing of his technique (Fig. 33:11). At operation, the tube was tested to locate the site of obstruction and the occluded segment was removed. The large sactosalpinx was amputated and the resected borders of the tube everted. The isthmic or interstitial occlusion of the cornu was excised, the tube fishmouthed, and sutures were used to draw it into the uterine cavity. Turck[22] in 1909 reported eight cases of implantation and he stated that term pregnancies occurred in two women.

During the first quarter of the 20th century the technique most commonly used was division of the tube at the point of obstruction; the occluded cornual portion was reamed out; the patent residual tube was pulled into the uterus and held there by stitches. Patency was proved by air or water insufflation from the fimbriated end. Polow[23] reported two operations in which he made a vertical incision into the anterior uterine wall and reamed out the diseased cornua. Since no sutures were used in the uterine end of the resected salpinx, the tube was pulled into the uterine cavity through the cornu with a hemostat directed through the anterior fundal incision. A few small sutures of catgut or silk were used to anchor the tubal and uterine serosa near the uterine serosal surface. The implant was tested for patency before closure of the uterine incision. Then, to maintain patency, sutures of plain catgut were passed through the lumen into the uterine cavity.

In 1948 Vltavsky[24] published results on 18 women who had tubal implantation, nine had hysterosalpingograms postoperatively. Of these, six women had at least one patent tube and two became pregnant

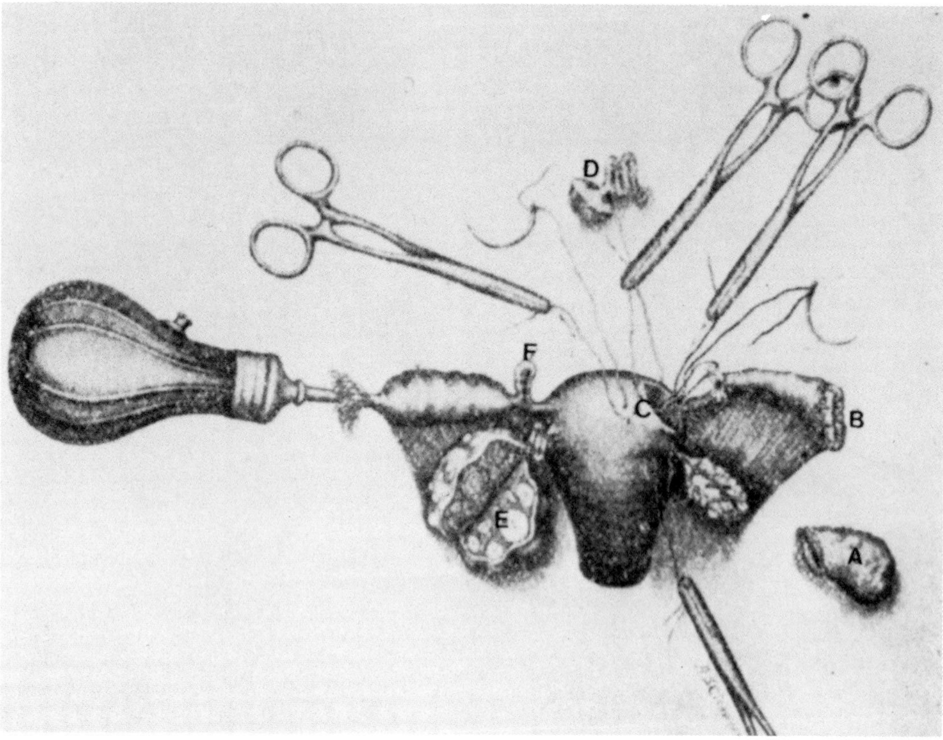

FIGURE 33:11—*Combined tubal operation, tubal testing in vivo and ovarian resection.*[21] (A) *resected part of ampulla;* (B) *cuff midampullary salpingostomy;* (C) *uterine incision prepared for implantation;* (D) *resected cornu and isthmic segment;* (E) *resection of ovary;* (F) *site of presumed proximal tubal obstruction.*

(the outcomes not stated). In the same year, Rommer[25] reported that six pregnancies (outcomes unknown) occurred in 16 women. He created a new uterine cornual opening by an incision into the serosa and then forceful insertion of a straight Kocher clamp until the uterine cavity was entered. No inert distenders were used. The next year Ingersoll[26] wrote about five women who had bilateral uterotubal implantations for cornual obstruction after which three had normal term pregnancies. No devices were used to maintain the lumen of the implant and in the two instances that failed, combinations of implantation with fimbrioplasty were done.

White[27] recorded four cases in which her technique included the lateral division of the resected residual patent tube on each side and its attachment to the uterine cavity by silk sutures. A metal probe helped to manipulate the tube into the uterus. Insufflation was performed on the tenth postoperative day and repeated after the first menstruation. Patency resulted in six of the implanted tubes and one term infant was delivered.

Concern about the potential reversibility of operations for female sterilization began soon after Kocks[28] attempted a transcervical cornual cauterization in 1878.

Lungren[29] in 1880 tied the fallopian tubes of a patient having her second cesarean section and in 1897 Kehrer[30] described tubal ligation through a colpotomy. An end-to-end anastomosis in a fowl was reported by Pearl and Surface[31] in 1908; they removed 10 cm of a hen's oviduct and repaired the cut ends with silk sutures inserted through all tubal layers. Subsequently, the bird layed eggs. Four years later Christian and Sanderson[32] reported successful isthmic-to-isthmic anastomosis in three women in whom 20-day catgut was employed as a temporary splint.

Kelly's *Operative Gynecology*[7] describes a salpingo-salpingostomy (end-to-end anastomosis) following excision of strictured or nodular areas in the tubes: "After cutting out the disease, the ends of the tube may be united by fine catgut sutures penetrating the peritoneal and muscular coats and introduced at intervals of about 2 mm." Kelly further noted that "in order to graft the isthmus onto the ampulla, it must be slit open on its dorsum to make a lumen corresponding in size to that of the ampulla to which it is to be attached."

Another type of tuboplasty or conservative procedure on the fallopian tube concerns the management of an extrauterine pregnancy. As far back as 1898, Kelly[7] indicated that salpingectomy for this entity could only be justified "when the identity of the tube is so distorted or when the tube is so far destroyed that its regeneration is impossible. There is no reason why the tube should not be freed from its adhesions, cleaned as far as possible of all clots, the rent sutured, and the tube, together with its ovary preserved."

Summary

Significant reports concerning the development of techniques for overcoming infertility caused by tubal disease have been described. It has not been possible in this resume to cite all of the contributions on this subject. The paper has been limited to the achievements before 1951.

References

1. Ricci JV: *The Genealogy of Gynecology*. Philadelphia: The Blakiston Co., 1943; p. 291.
2. Graham H: *Eternal Eve*. New York: Doubleday and Co., 1951; p. 160.
3. Schroeder C: Die Excision von Ovarian tumoren mit Erhaltung des Ovarium. *Zentralb Gynäkol* 8:716, 1884.
4. Skutsch F: Beitrag zur operativen Therapie der Tubenerkrankungen. *Zentralb Gynäkol* 13:565, 1889.
5. Martin A: Über Tuben- und Ovarialresektion. *Zentralb Gynäkol* 15:515, 1891.
6. Polk WM: The conservative surgery of the female pelvic organs. *NY State J Med* 3:182, 1894.
7. Kelly HA: *Operative Gynecology*. New York: D. Appleton & Co., 1898: p. 183.
8. Goullioud P: De la salpingostomie. *Lyon Med* 53:13, 1899.
9. Burrage WL: The remote results of conservative operations on the ovaries and tubes. An analysis of eighty five cases. *Am J Obstet* 42:195, 1900.
10. Gellhorn G: Salpingostomy and pregnancy. *Surg Gynecol Obstet* 13:10, 1911.
11. Holden FC, and Sovak FW: Reconstruction of the oviducts: An improved technic with report of cases. *Am J Obstet Gynecol* 24:684, 1932.
12. Halban J:, Gynäkologische Operationslehre. Berlin: Urban and Schwarzenberg, 1932.
13. Beecham CT, and Sigman MD: Technic for re-establishing tubal patency. *Am J Obstet Gynecol* 56:935, 1948.
14. Gepfert JR: Reconstruction of the oviducts in the human. Results obtained with the use of a new technique. *Am J Obstet Gynecol* 45:1031, 1943.
15. Hofmann TR: Salpingostomy using allantoic membrane. Case report of reoperative findings. *Fertil Steril* 1:463, 1950.
16. Westman A: A new method of preventing tubal occlusion following operations for sterility. *Gynaecologia* 122:133, 1946.
17. Johnston HW; Improved operative technic for salpingostomy. *Am J Obstet Gynecol* 55:426, 1948.
18. Bunster EM: *Trompa de Falōpio Esterilidad de Causa Tubaria*. Buenos Aires: Guillermo Kraft Ltda, 1951.
19. Gardner AK: *The Causes and Curative Treatment of Sterility with a Preliminary Statement on the Physiology of Generations*. New York: De Witt & Davenport, 1856.

20. Ries E: Nodular forms of tubal disease. *J Exp Med* 2:347, 1897.
21. Ferguson AH: Presidential address. *Med Fortnightly* 24:528, 1903.
22. Turck RC: Hysterosalpingotomy. *NY State J Med* 99:1193, 1909.
23. Polowe D: New technic for reconstruction of oviducts. *Am J Surg* 68:208, 1945.
24. Vltavsky J: Implantation of tubes; Indication, operative technic and results. *Gynaecologia* 125:347, 1948.
25. Rommer J: Surgery in treatment of sterility. *Urol Cutan Rev* 82:586, 1948.
26. Ingersoll FM: Plastic operation on fallopian tube. *N Eng J Med* 241:686, 1949.
27. White MM: Four cases of re-implantation of the fallopian tube. *J Obstet Gynaecol Brit Emp* 58:381, 1951.
28. Kocks J: Eine neue Methode der Sterilization der Frauen. *Zentralb Gynäkol* 26:617, 1878.
29. Lungren SS: A case of cesarean section twice successfully performed in the same patient with remarks on the time, indications and details of the operations. *Am J Obstet* 14:78, 1897.
30. Kehrer RA: Sterilization Mittels Tuben durchschneidung vorderem Schneidenschnitt. *Zentralb Gynäkol* 31:961, 1897.
31. Pearl R, Surface FM: Resection and end-to-end anastomosis of the oviduct in the hen without loss of function. *Am J Physiol* 22:357, 1908.
32. Christian SL, Sanderson EL: New method of anastomosing the ovarian tube or vas deferens. *JAMA* 61:2157, 1912.

34

A Review of Diagnostic Procedures for Assessment of Tubal Patency

Amir H. Ansari

Disorders of the fallopian tubes account for up to 50 percent of all causes of female infertility.[1–3] Therefore, evaluation of tubal patency and its anatomical relationships should be considered an essential examination in an infertility investigation (Table 34:1).

Rubin[4] and Carey[5] in 1914 independently described a test for tubal patency by injecting collargol into the uterine cavity and observing radiographic evidence of its passage into the fallopian tubes. This method did not prove safe and it was abandoned. A few years later, Rubin introduced the tubal insufflation test.[6] A variety of procedures have been described for evaluating tubal patency since that time. The basic concept for these tests involves vaginal or abdominal detection of substances transferred or transported through the tubes after their abdominal or uterine installation.

Nonoperative Techniques

Tubal insufflation of carbon dioxide into the uterine cavity and measurement of tubal resistance is one method (Fig. 34:1).

Positive auscultation of the lower abdomen for the so-called "jet sound" during insufflation, radiological detection of subdiaphragmatic gas, and shoulder pain are also indicative of tubal patency. However, the test is not precise and for the most part has been replaced by radiographic and endoscopic studies.

Hysterosalpingography enables observation of the uterine cavity and tubal lumen.[7–11] A No. 8 pediatric Foley catheter is inserted into the uterine cavity with the assistance of a uterine dressing forceps after preparation of the vagina and the cervix with an antiseptic solution. Inflation of the catheter balloon with 2 ml of water assures its intrauterine retention and effectively seals the internal os.[12,13] Under fluoroscopic observation, a watersoluble contrast medium is injected. The lower uterine segment, which is obliterated by the balloon of the catheter, is delineated by gradually deflating the balloon while continually injecting the contrast medium

The Fallopian Tube: Basic Studies and Clinical Contributions, edited by Alvin M. Siegler, M.D. Mount Kisco, New York: Futura Publishing Company, Inc.

Table 34:1

Summary of Procedures for Assessment of Tubal Patency

Nonoperative Tests		*Operative Tests*	
Ascending	*Descending*	*Partial Evaluation*	*Total Evaluation*
Hysterosalpingography	China ink	Culdotomy	Laparoscopy
Tubal insufflation	Starch test	Culposcopy	Laparotomy
Pneumohysterosalpingography	Radioactive transportation tests	Hysteroscopy	
Phenolsulfonphthalein	Surrogate ova	Salpingoscopy	
Methylene blue (MB) test			
Tubal scan			

into the uterine cavity (Figs. 34:2 and 34:3).

Despite enthusiastic reports by some authors of a higher pregnancy rate following a hysterosalpingogram with an oily medium, it has caused granulomatous salpingitis,[14] endometritis,[15] and oil embolism.[16,17] Occasionally, the configurations of the medium in the cul-de-sac or in a hydrosalpinx may cause confusion (Fig. 34:4).

Tubal spasm may occur during the injection of contrast medium, resulting in the misleading diagnosis of tubal obstruction.[18–20] Sublingual nitroglycerine, tranquilizers, narcotics, systemic or local isoxupurine, intramuscular and intravenous glucagon, and even general anesthesia have been used with inconclusive results.[21–24] Since 1980 the author has used intrauterine administration of 5 to 10 ml of 1 to 2 percent lidocaine prior to salpingography to avoid tubal spasms and to reduce or eliminate abdominal pain, with excellent results.[25]

The hysterosalpingogram is an important diagnostic study and should not be replaced by laparoscopy.

Pneumohysterosalpingography combines tubal insufflation (providing pneumoperitoneum) and hysterosalpingography.[26–28]

With the combined procedures the insufflated gas enables observation of the ovaries and provides information about the tubo-ovarian anatomical relationship. (Fig. 34:5).

The phenosulfonphthalein (PSP) was described in 1948 by Speck.[29] Dye could be detected in urine 30 minutes after its injection into the uterine cavity and the fallopian tubes. Since the dye was absorbed intraperitoneally and excreted by the kidneys, its detection in the urine indicated tubal patency. However, misleading results were reported as the dye also was absorbed by the endosalpinx especially in a hydrosalpinx.[30–31] Methylene blue is another dye in which the agent is injected into the uterine cavity with its recovery from the posterior cul-de-sac by culdocentesis.[32–35] A positive test indicates tubal patency.

Pertynski and associates[36] administered radioactive ^{133}Xe into the uterine cavity and measured its presence in the fallopian tubes and the abdominal cavity using a gamma camera. According to these authors, the test compared favorably with hysterosalpingography with reduction in the amount of radiation exposure.

Various other substances have been used,[37–39] such as india ink, red dye, milk, coal particles, and ascaris ova to test tubal transport. Decker and Decker placed starch particles into the peritoneal cavity either by culdocentesis, culdoscopy, or laparotomy.[40,41] Transported starch granules in the vagina, identified by a bluish discoloration when vagina and cervix were stained with iodine solution 24 hours later, indicated tubal patency.

Intraperitoneal insertion of radioactive gold and radioactive surrogate

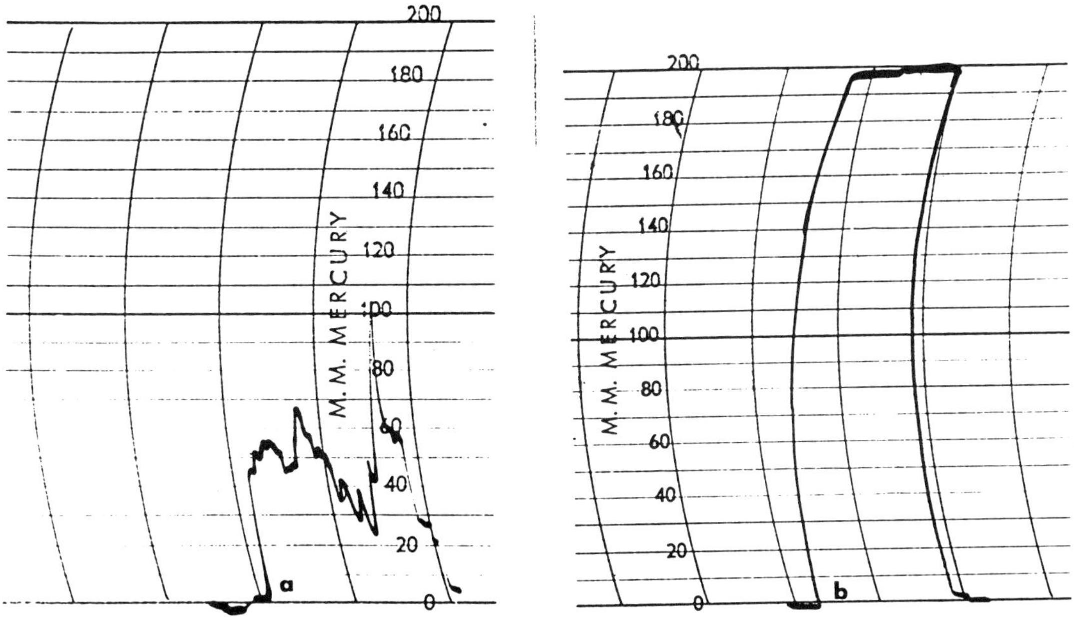

FIGURE 34:1—*Tubal insufflation recordings of* (a) *patency and* (b) *obstruction are seen.*

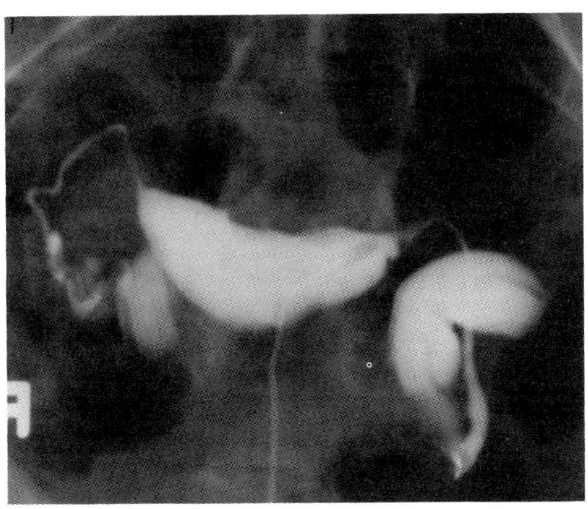

FIGURE 34:2—*The Foley catheter technique was used in this HSG and bilateral hydrosalpinges were found.*

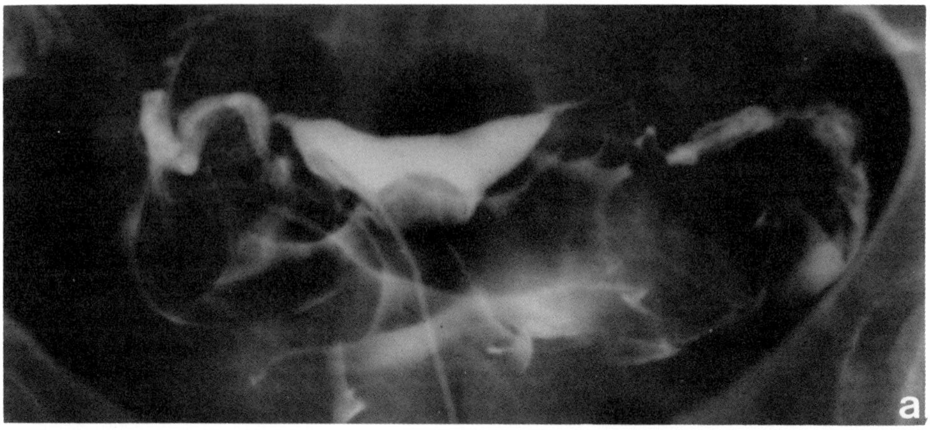

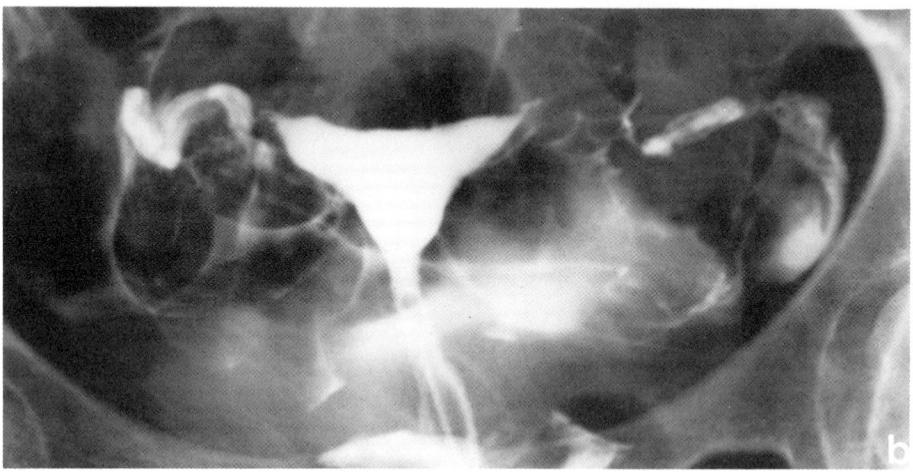

FIGURE 34:3—(a) *HSG suggests bilateral tubal patency but lower uterine segment is obscured by the balloon.* (b) *Observation of the lower uterine segment after balloon was deflated.*

ova[42,43] with detection of radioactivity in the vagina by a specially designed Geiger counter is the basis for these tests. They proved unreliable[44] as the radioactive substance was also transferred by lymphatic and blood vessels.

Operative Techniques

Observation of the fallopian tubes and assessment of their patency had been accomplished by a posterior culdotomy.[45–48] Associated complications are infection, bleeding, and potential trauma to the tubes. In 1944 Decker and Cherry[49] introduced culdoscopy and it rapidly gained popularity.[50–55] For many years it was an essential, simple method for direct observation of the fallopian tubes.

The uterotubal ostia can be seen during hysteroscopy and on occasion abnormalities in these areas are detected. Furthermore, attempts have been made to probe the tubal lumen in selected instances but as yet hysteroscopy is not used to assess tubal patency.

Laparoscopy can disclose the anatomical relationship between the fallopian tubes and ovaries and chromo-

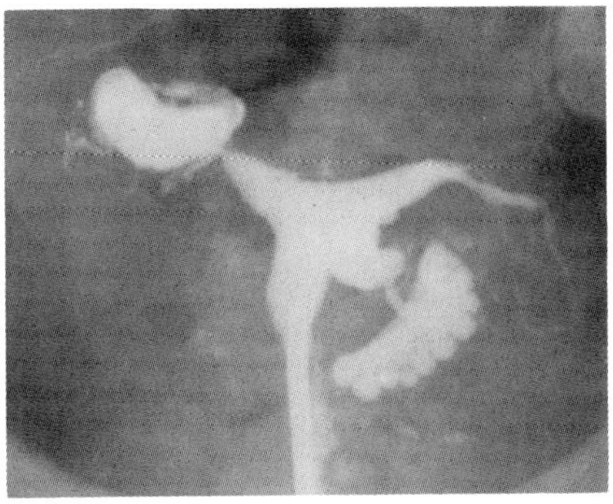

FIGURE 34:4—*HSG with oily medium shows "pearly clusters," possibly the result of interaction with peritoneal fluid in the cul-de-sac. A follow-up film in 24 hours is essential to make a definite diagnosis.*

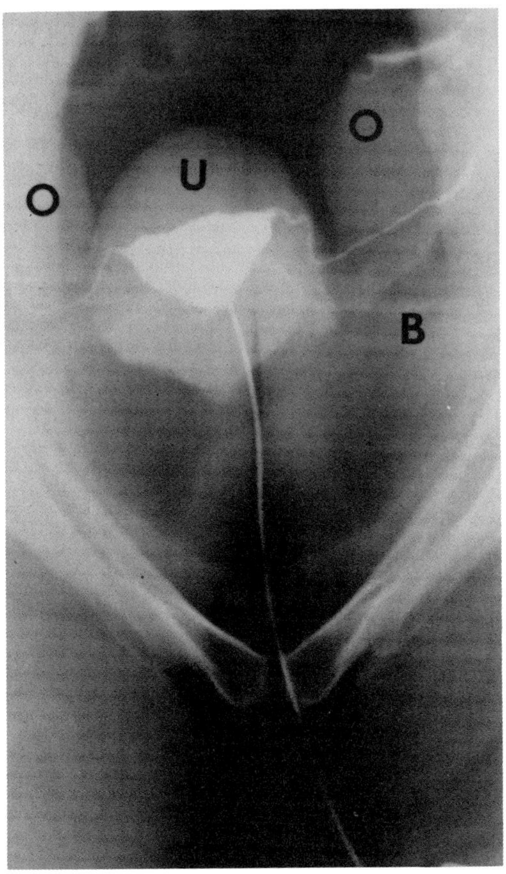

FIGURE 34:5—*Pneumohysterosalpingogram shows contrast material in the uterus and tubes. The external surfaces of the uterus (u), ovaries (o), and broad ligament are outlined with CO_2.*

pertubation provides a test for tubal patency.[56–59]

The ultimate test is done at laparotomy by injection of dilute methylene blue into the uterine cavity through a small pediatric Foley catheter which is placed into the uterine cavity prior to laparotomy. Transfundal injection using a 20 ml syringe and a 21 gauge, 2½-inch needle after occlusion of the lower uterine segment by a specially designed clamp is the alternative approach.[60,61] Difficulties from the transfundal procedure include the lack of satisfactory entrance into the uterine cavity and bleeding from the needle site. The latter is effectively controlled by cauterization of the needle during its withdrawal from the uterine fundus.[62]

Conclusion

The evaluation of tubal patency is accomplished best by hysterosalpingography and a laparoscopy.[63–67] It is imperative for the physician to be thoroughly familiar with the selected procedure, its equipment, and its interpretation. An incorrect interpretation and malfunctioning equipment may result in inaccurate diagnosis, improper treatment, and unnecessary cost.

References

1. Brown WE: Fallopian tubes in sterility. *Fertil Steril* 7:178, 1956.
2. Ansari AH: Diagnosis and management of tubal disorders. Scientific Exhibit, 13th Annual Meeting of The American Fertility Society, Hollywood, Florida, April 3–6, 1974.
3. Boyd IE: Tubal sterility; Patency test and results of operation. *J Obstet Gynaecol Br Emp* 80:142, 1973.
4. Rubin IC: Roentgendiagnostik der uterus Tumorens mit Hilfe von intrauterine collargol Injecktionen. Vorlaeufige Mitteilung. *Zentralb Gynäkol* 38:658, 1914.
5. Carey WH: Note on determination of patency of fallopian tubes by the use of

collargol and x-ray shadow. *Am J Obstet* 69:362, 1914.

6. Rubin IC: Non-operative determination of patency of fallopian tubes in sterility: Intrauterine inflation with oxygen and production of a subphrenic pneumoperitoneum: Preliminary report. *JAMA* 75:661, 1920.
7. Siegler AM: Self-retaining cannula set for hysterosalpingography. *Obstet Gynecol* 10:329, 1957.
8. Malmstrom T: A vacuum uterine cannula. *Obstet Gynecol* 18:773, 1961.
9. Hasson HM: A modified ballooned uterine elevator cannula. *J Reprod Med* 25:72, 1980.
10. Roland M, Carpenter F, and Rich J: A new water-soluble opaque medium in the study of hysterograms and hysterosalpingograms. *Am J Obstet Gynecol* 65:81, 1953.
11. Whitelaw MJ, and Miller EB: New water-soluble medium (sinografin) for hysterosalpingography. *Fertil Steril* 10:227, 1959.
12. Ansari AH, and Nagamani M: Foley catheter for salpingography, pneumography, tubal insufflation and hydrotubation. *Obstet Gynecol* 50:108, 1977.
13. Ansari AH, and Arronet GH: Pneumohysterosalpingography in infertility and related gynecologic condition: The Foley catheter technique. *Fertil Steril* 17:442, 1966.
14. Elliot GB, Brody H, and Elliot KA: Implications of "lipoid salpingitis." *Fertil Steril* 16:541, 1965.
15. Aaron JB, and Levine W: Endometrial oil granuloma following hysterosalpingography. *Am J Obstet Gynecol* 68:1594, 1954.
16. Levinson JM: Pulmonary oil embolism following hysterosalpingography. *Fertil Steril* 14:21, 1963.
17. Siegler AM: *Hysterosalpingography*. New York: Harper and Row, 1967: p. 69.
18. Buxton L, and Southam A: A critical survey of present methods of diagnosis and therapy in human infertility. *Am J Obstet Gynecol* 70:741, 1955.
19. Grant A, and Mackey R: The tubal factor in 1,122 successful sterility cases. *N Zealand Med J* 54:307, 1955.
20. Ostry EI: An investigation of tubal implantation for cornual block. *Am J Obstet Gynecol* 73:409, 1957.
21. Page EP: Use of isoxsuprine in uterosalpingography and uterotubal insufflation. *Am J Obstet Gynecol* 101:358, 1968.
22. Sher G, and Barnard PG: The alleviation of uterocornual spasm of the fallopian tubes during hysterosalpingography by intravenous administration of orciprenaline. *S Afr Med J* 50:1164, 1976.
23. Stallworthy J: Facts and fantasy in the study of female infertility. *J Obstet Gynaecol Br Emp* 55:171, 1948
24. Ansari AH, and Shimoura H: Hypotonic hysterosalpingography with glucagon. *Fertil Steril* 30:476, 1978.
25. Ansari AH: Painless hysterosalpingography with administration of local anesthetic. (Unpublished data).
26. Stein IF: Roentgenographic diagnosis in gynecology: Pneumoperitoneum. *Surg Gynecol Obstet* 42:83, 1926.
27. Stein IF: Pelvic diagnosis by roentgen visualization. *Surg Gynecol Obstet* 55:207, 1932.
28. Ansari AH: The cul-de-sac approach to induction of pneumoperitoneum for pelvic laparoscopy and pneumography. *Fertil Steril* 21:599, 1970.
29. Speck G: Phenosulfonphthalein as a test for the determination of tubal patency. *Am J Obstet Gynecol* 55:1048, 1948.
30. Rosset EM: Experience with PSP tubal patency (Speck) test. *Am J Obstet Gynecol* 60:892, 1950.
31. Williams DW, and Gering HS: Revised PSP test for tubal patency. *Fertil Steril* 19:821, 1968.
32. Ansari AH: Methylene blue test for assessment of tubal patency a new and simple technique. *Can Med Assoc J* 99:182, 1968.
33. Ansari AH: Tubal patency evaluation by the methylene blue test. *Am J Obstet Gynecol* 103:1170, 1969.
34. Ansari AH: Methylene blue (Ansari) test for evaluation of tubal patency. Proceedings of the 17th annual meeting of the Canadian Society for the Study of Fertility. Quebec City, Canada, June 1970.
35. Ansari AH: Evaluation of tubal patency by methylene blue test—A practical office procedure. *Ob Gyn Digest* 16:23, 1974.
36. Pertynski T, Radecki W, and Bialobrzeski J: Oviduct patency control by means of ^{133}Xe solution. *Nucl Med* 15:46, 1976.

37. Gyarmati E: Transtubal elimination of substances injected in the peritoneal cavity. *Riv Ital Ginecol* 16:721, 1934.
38. Conill-Serra V, Salamero F, and Trias D: Casuistica y resultados de las preubas descendentes en el estudio del factor tubarico. *Proc Second World Congr Fertil Steril* 1:927, 1956.
39. Tompkins P: Discussion of paper by I.C. Rubin "The value of uterotubal insufflation in the treatment of tubal obstruction to ovular migration." In *Proc First World Congr Fertil Steril* 2:134, 1953.
40. Decker A, and Decker WH: A tubal function test. *Obstet Gynecol* 4:35, 1954.
41. Westman AA: A contribution to the question of the transit of the ovum from the ovary to the uterus in rabbits. *Acta Obstet Gynecol Scand* 5:7, (Suppl 3) 1926.
42. Stabile A, and Leborgne FE: Radioactive gold in the study of isoperistaltic patency. *Int J Fertil* 3:139, 1958.
43. Pauerstein CJ, and Hodgson BJ: Rate of transport of radioactive ovum models through the oviducts of individual rabbits. *Am J Obstet Gynecol* 124:840, 1976.
44. Caballero A, Hurtado E, Perez-Modrego S, et al: Studies of the patency and function of apprehension and transportion of the fallopion tube with ^{198}AU. *Am J Obstet Gynecol* 90:437, 1964.
45. Beaton JH: Posterior colpotomy in diagnosis and treatment of tubal abnormalities. *Clin Obstet Gynecol* 5:816, 1962.
46. Doyle JB: Exploratory culdotomy for observation of tubo-ovarian physiology at ovulation time. *Fertil Steril* 2:475, 1951.
47. Culton YG, and Van Ostrand JR: Colpotomy as a definitive operation in ectopic pregnancy. *Obstet Gynecol* 29:279, 1967.
48. McMaster RH, and Ansari AH: Vaginal tubal ligation. *Obstet Gynecol* 38:44, 1971.
49. Decker A, and Cherry TH: Culdoscopy; New methods in diagnosis of pelvic disease—Preliminary report. *Am J Surg* 64:40, 1944.
50. Decker A: Culdoscopy in the diagnosis of pelvic disease. *Clin Obstet Gynecol* 1:610, 1958.
51. Stuermer VM: Culdoscopy and the tubal factor. *Obstet Gynecol* 25:470, 1965.
52. Cohen MR: The role of culdoscopy in infertility. *Am J Obstet Gynecol* 78:266, 1959.
53. Green TH: The role of culdoscopy in the diagnosis of tubal disorders. *Clin Obstet Gynecol* 5:799, 1962.
54. Kelly JV, and Rock J: Culdoscopy for diagnosis in infertility. *Am J Obstet Gynecol* 72:523, 1956.
55. Clyman MJ: Importance of culdoscopy in infertility. *NY State J Med* 66:1867, 1966.
56. Steptoe PC: *Laparoscopy in Gynaecology*. Edinburgh: E.S. Livingstone, 1967.
57. Neuwirth RS: Laparoscopy. *Clin Obstet Gynecol* 12:514, 1969.
58. Ansari AH: Abdominal laparoscopy and pelvic pneumography. *Ob/Gyn Digest* 13:29, 1971.
59. El-Minawi MF, Abdel-Hadi M, Ibrahim AA, et al: Comparative evaluation of laparoscopy and hysterosalpingography in infertile patients. *Obstet Gynecol* 51:29, 1978.
60. Groot-Wassink K: Abdominale Prüfung der Tubendurchgangigkeit intra Operationem (Bericht über eine praktische Uterusklemme). *Zentralb Gynäkol* 94:1559, 1972.
61. Shirodkar VN: *Contributions to Obstetrics and Gynaecology*. Edinburgh: E.S. Livingstone, 1960: p. 112.
62. Ansari AH: Tubal patency evaluation during laparotomy. (Unpublished data).
63. Holst N, Abyholm T, and Borgersen A: Hysterosalpingography in the evaluation of infertility. *Acta Radiol (Diagn, Stockh)* 24:253, 1983.
64. Duff DE, Fried AM, Wilson EA, et al: Hysterosalpingography and laparoscopy: A comparative study. *Am J Roentgenl* 141:761, 1983.
65. Portuondo JA, Echanojauregui AD, Irala JP, et al: Triple evaluation of tubal patency. *Int J Fertil* 25:307, 1980.
66. Montanari L, Bulgarelli C, and Marra A: A comparison of hysterosalpingography and laparoscopy in the investigation of infertility. *Clin Exp Obstet Gynecol* 9:66, 1982.
67. Ansari AH: Diagnostic procedures for assessment of tubal patency. *Fertil Steril* 31:469, 1979.

35

Transcervical and Retrograde Salpingoscopy: Evaluation of the Fallopian Tube in Infertile Patients

Luca Mencaglia, Jacques Hamou, Antonio Perino, and Ernelando Cosmi

Salpingoscopy is an endoscopic examination of the tubal lumen. In 1970, Mohri and coworkers[1] used a fibroscope of approximately 1 mm in diameter to examine the tubal lumen. This tubaloscope was introduced transcervically but the resolution of the optical fibers was poor because of their thin diameter. Other technical problems included difficulty in reaching the tubal lumen and insertion of very fine endoscopic fibers into the irregular channel of the intramural segment. The fragile endosalpinx could be traumatized inadvertently. Currently, retrograde salpingoscopy is preferable but a laparotomy is required for insertion of the instrument into the distal tubal opening.[2–4] The procedure is done with a 5 mm endoscope that also has the capability of magnification.

Information concerning the uterotubal ostia and proximal portion of the intramural segment can be obtained during hysteroscopy.[5] The uterotubal junction can be observed readily (Fig. 35:1). Contractions cause the tubal ostium to open and close intermittently. Cornual and intramural polyps and periostial adhesions have been noted, and the vascularity of the proximal interstitial segment has been discerned (Fig. 35:2).

The uterotubal junction sometimes is marked by a pretubal "diaphragm" appearing like a fine membrane (Fig. 35:1). It is possible to identify this area precisely after staining it with methylene blue and using $\times 20$ magnification.

The endosalpinx in its initial few millimeters is smooth with minimal vascularization, quite unlike that seen in the nearby endometrium. Increasing the flow of CO_2 during hysteroscopy can provoke uterine contractions, about once every 10 to 13 seconds.[6] This event may be caused

The Fallopian Tube: Basic Studies and Clinical Contributions, edited by Alvin M. Siegler, M.D. Mount Kisco, New York: Futura Publishing Company, Inc. © 1986.

Table 35:1

Transcervical Salpingoscopy: Endoscopic Results in 228 Infertile Patients

Abnormality	*Left ostium*	*Right ostium*
Normal uterotubal ostium	187	191
Atretic ostium	23	22
Cornual adhesions	4	3
Cornual polyps	3	3
Intramural polyps	0	2
Ostial abnormalities (other)	11	7
TOTAL	***228***	***228***

Table 35:2

Retrograde Salpingoscopy: Endoscopic Results in 30 Infertile Patients Prior to Microsurgery

Endoscopic findings	*Number*
Normal primary and secondary folds	12
Endosalpingeal sclerosis	12
Ampullary adhesions (luminal)	6
TOTAL	***30***

by irritation of the muscular fibers surrounding the uterotubal junction. If an electronic insufflator is used, the exact pressure of CO_2 necessary to provoke a tubal contraction can be measured.[6]

Periostial adhesions are thin, usually avascular, and can partially or completely cover the ostium. These adhesions can alter tubal function and occasionally cause proximal tubal obstruction. Cornual and intramural polyps can be identified hysteroscopically but their role as cause of infertility remains to be proven.[2]

Hysteroscopic examinations of the uterotubal ostia were done in 228 infertile patients and 10 percent of these women had either cornual polyps or adhesions (Table 35:1). In 14 instances these polyps were removed under hysteroscopic control. Eighteen patients who had suspected abnormalities of the uterotubal ostium had CO_2 pressure tests and 16 of them showed normal permeability. No contractions were seen in two others despite an increase in CO_2 insufflation during hysteroscopy.

Direct observation of the tubal lumen has been made possible at laparotomy by the insertion of a hysteroscope into the distal end of the tube. This examination is made before microsurgical repair of occluded tubes by the gentle introduction of the scope and distending the tube with CO_2 at a maximal flow rate of 30 ml/min (Fig. 35:3). After panoramic observation, the endosalpinx can be stained with methylene blue and $\times$ 150 magnification is used for this phase of the study (Fig. 35:4).

Using the methods described above, Hamou[6] reported that three patients had normal primary and secondary folds and in four others, sclerosis with luminal adhesions were noted. During our study of 27 women, we noted 12 instances of normal folds and vascularity, 6 of these patients becoming pregnant following tubal repair. In six other instances, ampullary adhesions (Fig. 35:5) were noted; 12 oth-

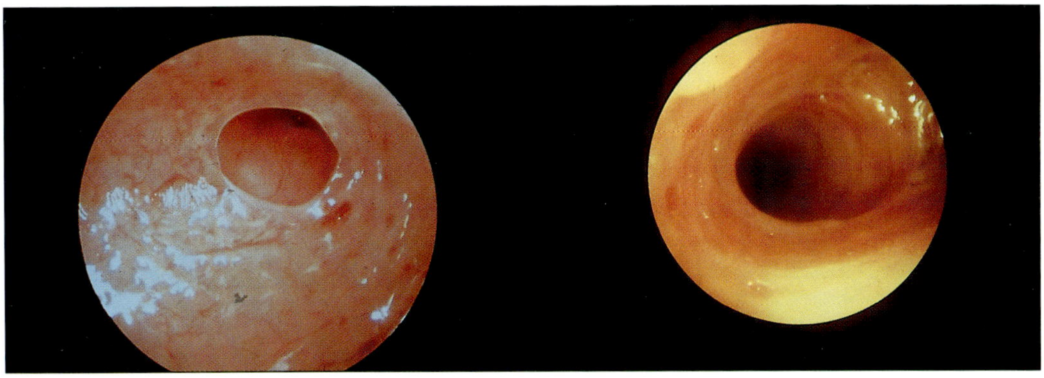

FIGURE 35:1—*Hysteroscopic views of the proximal portions of the intramural segment.*

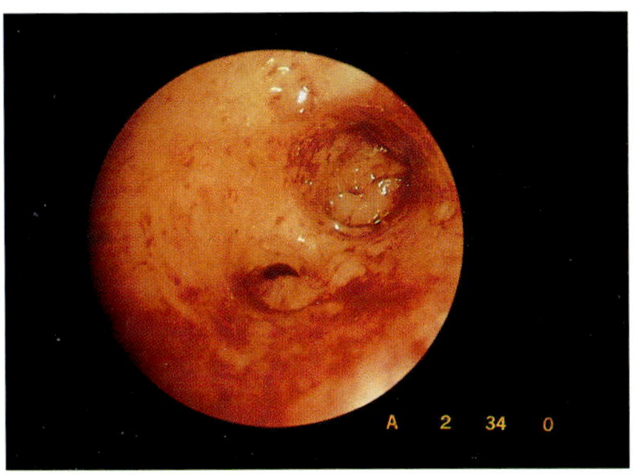

FIGURE 35:2a—*Polyp is seen in uterine cornua above uterotubal ostium.*

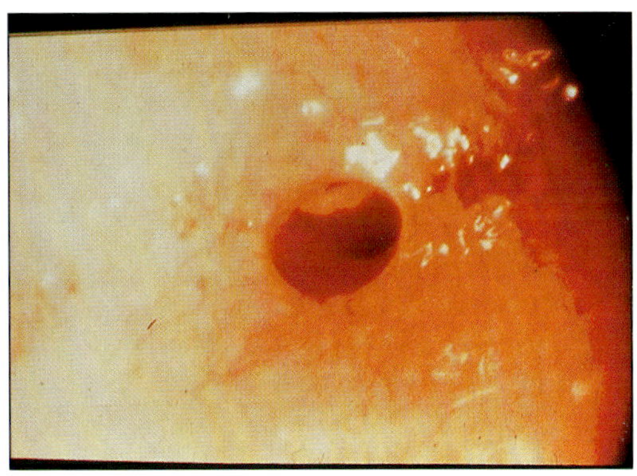

FIGURE 35:2b—*Intraluminal polyp is seen in proximal intramural segment.*

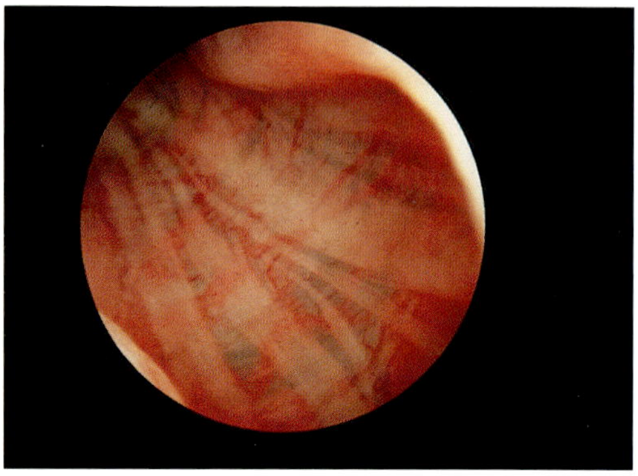

FIGURE 35:3—*Primary and secondary luminal folds are noted.*

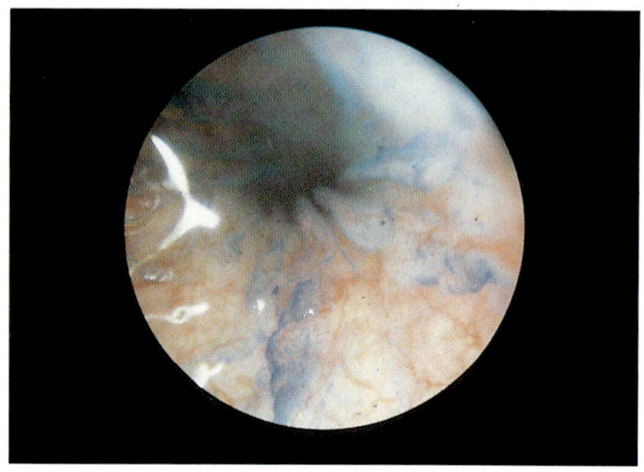

FIGURE 35:4—*Endosalpinx is stained with methylene blue.*

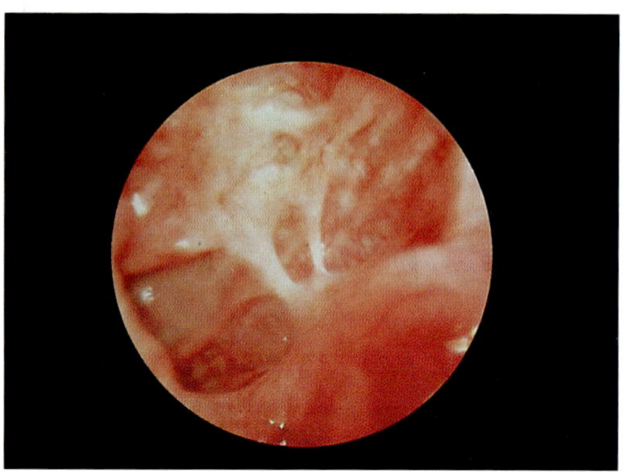

FIGURE 35:5—*Intratubal adhesions are noted.*

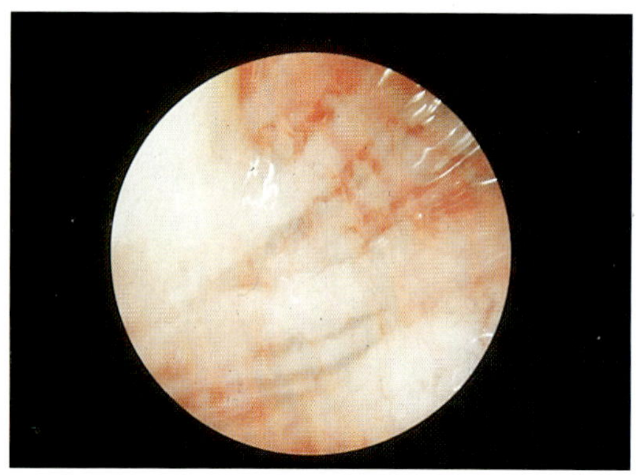

FIGURE 35:6—*Endosalpingeal sclerosis is quite evident.*

ers had areas of endosalpingeal sclerosis (Fig. 35:6) (Table 35:2).

Cornier and colleagues described the technique of fibrotuboscopy.[7] They reported a good correlation between hysterosalpingographic and endoscopic findings. No patient with an abnormal salpingogram subsequently had a normal endoscopic examination. These authors further observed a good correlation between the endoscopic result and postoperative patency and pregnancy rates following tubal repairs. In 17 women, postoperative patency was noted either by hysterosalpingography or laparoscopy and 12 of them had at least one normal tube by ampullofibroscopy. In 14 other patients, reocclusion had occurred and 12 of these women had significant luminal abnormalities endoscopically. In five women who developed tubal pregnancies, endosalpingeal sclerosis or adhesions had been seen.

Summary

It is possible to examine the tubal lumen endoscopically by either hysteroscopy or retrograde ampullary fibroscopy. Abnormalities have been described in all tubal segments, some of which can be removed under endoscopic control. In addition, it might be feasible to improve our ability, render a more accurate postoperative (postmicrosurgical tubal repair) prognosis by searching for markers such as normal folds, endosalpingeal sclerosis and adhesions.

References

1. Mohri T, Mohri C, and Yamadori F: Tubaloscope: Flexible glass fiber endoscope for intratubal observation. *Endoscopy* 2:226, 1970.
2. Henry-Suchet J: Endoscopie tubaire: Premiers résultats. *Gynécologie* 23:293, 1981.
3. Scarselli G, Mencaglia L, Tantini C, et al: Intraoperative microsalpingoscopy of the ampullar fallopian tube. *Acta Eur Fertil* 13:35, 1982.
4. Hamou JE: Microcolpohysteroscopy. A new procedure and its original applications in gynecology. *J Reprod Med* 26:375, 1981.
5. Hamou JE, and Taylor PJ: Panoramic, contact and microcolpohysteroscopy in gynecologic practice. *Curr Prob Obstet Gynecol* 4:2, 1982.
6. Scarselli G, Tantini C, Mencaglia L, et al: Microhysteroscopy and infertility. In Van der Pas H, Van Herendael B, Van Lith D, et al (Eds): Boston, MTP Press Ltd, 1983.
7. Cornier E, Feintuch MJ, and Couccara L: Fibrotuboscopie ampullaire. *J Gynécol Obstét Biol Reprod* 1:49, 1984.

36

Ampullosalpingoscopy

Edgard Cornier

Direct endoscopic exploration of the ampulla, ampullosalpingoscopy (ASC), can reveal important characteristics of the endosalpinx. I have performed this procedure in 84 patients (153 tubes) who had a microsurgical salpingoplasty and postoperative intrauterine pregnancies were obtained almost exclusively in those women who showed good mucosal folds.[1] Patients whose tubes had been altered by intraampullary scars, sclerosis, or "beehive"-shaped adhesions almost always had a poor prognosis. Either their tubes became obstructed again or they had a tubal gestation.

The technique of flexible fibroscopy permits the endoscopic exploration of the tubal ampulla.[2] This addition to traditional laparoscopy may have special merit in unexplained infertility. Interfimbrial abnormalities can be discovered using this technique.

Method

Endoscopic examination of the ampullary segment is possible with the use of a rigid hysteroscope.[3,4] The lens and its outer sheath are passed through either the fimbrial ostium or into a 5 mm opening made at the top of a hydrosalpinx. The tube is distended with saline under low pressure. Carbon dioxide is inconvenient because it seems to flatten the ampullary folds, preventing a proper exploration. In addition, the drying effect is potentially harmful. The use of a rigid hysteroscope enables the gynecologist to observe the topography and to establish prognostic correlation with a future tuboplasty. Since the endoscope is short and rigid, it can pose problems with sterilization during the examination. The end can traumatize the endosalpinx and provoke edema, preventing the continuation of the study. Distorted tubes prevent adequate observation. Therefore, a long, flexible endoscope was developed to enable the entire lumen of the ampulla to be explored without trauma.[5]

Two different fiberscopes were used: the bronchofiberscope (BF3C4 Olympus), which has a usable length of 77 cm, an external diameter of 3.5 mm, and a depth of field of 3 to 50 mm in air with an angle of vision of 55°. Its extremity can be curved with the manipulation handle and permits 160° observation on one side and 60° observation on the other. The interior of the

The Fallopian Tube: Basic Studies and Clinical Contributions, edited by Alvin M. Siegler, M.D. Mount Kisco, New York: Futura Publishing Company, Inc. © 1986.

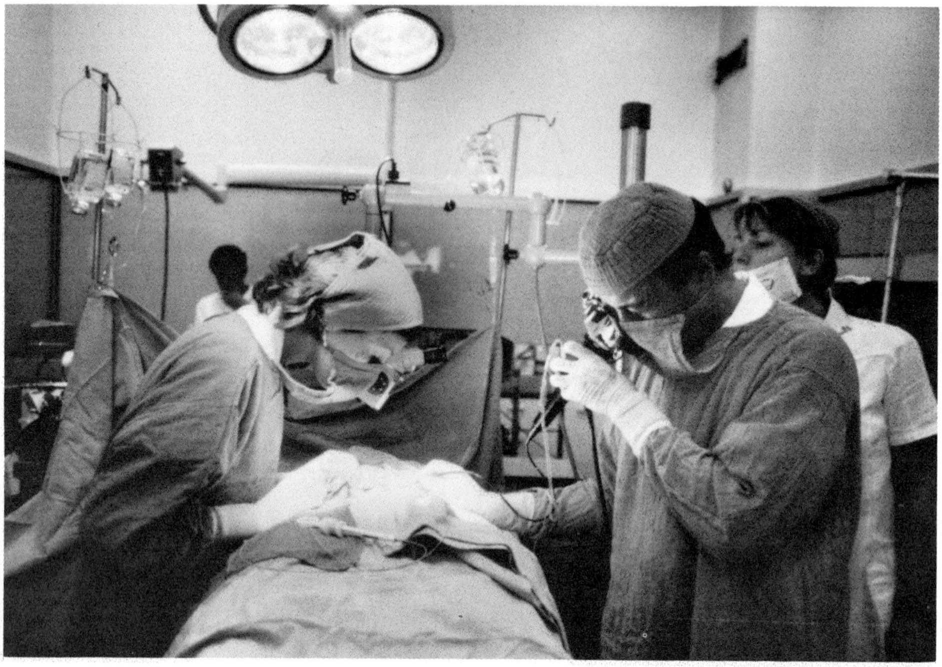

FIGURE 36:1—*Saline is being perfused and a camera is attached to the endoscope. Instruments for operative ampulloscopy can be placed through the same canal as the perfusion fluid.*

fiberscope contains a 1.2 mm wide canal which enables the passage of fluids and special instruments such as catheters and hooks.

The duodenal fiberscope (CHF4B Olympus) has a usable length of 33 cm and an external diameter of 5 mm. The depth of field in water is 3 to 50 mm with an angle of vision of 85°. The lens can be curved 160° upward. Its operational channel allows the passage of fluids and articulated instruments such as biopsy forceps and microscissors. The end of the instrument can be oriented through the full 360° by remotely turning it. Two simultaneous movements are carried out: the rotation of the holding handle, and flexing and extending the mobile extremity controlled by a lever on the handle near the lens.

The endoscopic exploration can be performed either at laparotomy during microsurgery or during a laparoscopy. After mobilizing the distal end of an occluded tube and removing periadnexal adhesions, a 5 mm opening is made at the top of the obstructed ampulla. This orifice is made in the serosa and enlarged with a special forceps to a width of 1.2 mm. The fiberscope is inserted and visually guided through the ampulla during perfusion with saline solution under low pressure (Figure 36:1). The average quantity of solution necessary for good ampullary distention and exploration of both ampullae is less than 120 ml. With the development of a waterproofed fiberscope, total sterilization of the instrument has become possible.

If luminal adhesions prevent progress of the endoscope, they can be removed by the use of microinstruments so that the entire lumen can be evaluated.

The diameter, flexibility, and orientational capabilities of the instruments enable observation of the entire ampullary lumen as far as the ampullary-isthmic junction (AIJ). The topography of the abnormal areas also can be found by trans-

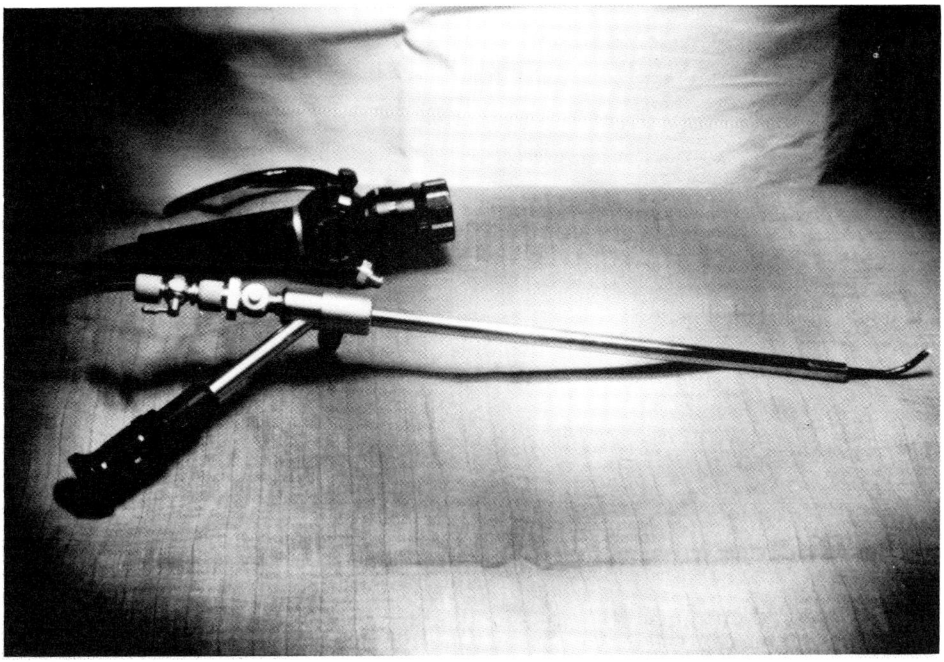

FIGURE 36:2—*The fiberscope passes through the rigid laparoscope which has a coaxial channel of 4 mm diameter.*

illumination. The location of segmental lesions is precise, permitting removal of a foreign body or a thick adhesion. The fiberscope with a diameter of 3.5 mm is inserted into the operational canal of the 4 mm laparoscope (Figs. 36:2 and 36:3). Tubal catheterization is accomplished by perfusion of saline solution which gently distends the ampulla. The end of the fiberscope is advanced under visual control to the AIJ. The examination is made by progressively withdrawing the fiberscope from this area until the tubal ostium is reached while orienting the fiberscope so as to conserve the maximal depth of field (currently 3 mm). The average duration of a laparoscopy with an ampullary salpingoscopy (ASC) is less than 30 minutes. About 120 ml of saline solution is sufficient to examine both ampullary lumina. Most of the perfusion liquid can be withdrawn at the end of the operation by direct aspiration from the cul-de-sac.

Results

Eighty-four patients had microsurgical salpingoplasty and an exploration of the ampullary lumina with a flexible fiberscope. A small abscess occurred postoperatively in one tube. The endoscope did not adversely affect tubal function since 22 postoperative intrauterine pregnancies occurred in patients who had a normal endosalpinx endoscopically. No postoperative complications were encountered in 96 patients who had fibertuboscopy under laparoscopic control.

When a laparoscopy was done following a previous ampullary endoscopic examination in seven women, the histologic evaluation of biopsy specimens from ten tubes did not reveal any evidence of trauma. The luminal exploration failed 13 times either because of tubal stenosis or severe extrinsic adhesions.

In the normal tube, the endosalpinx

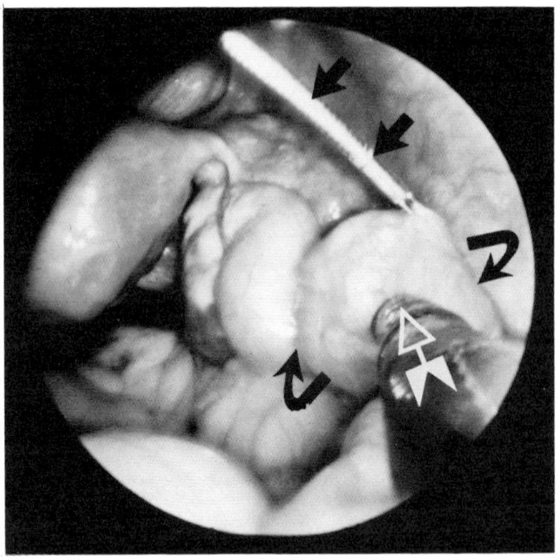

FIGURE 36:3—*The grasping forceps (*straight arrows*) and the mild distention of the ampulla (*curved arrows*) are seen. The ampulloscope (white arrows) is gently guided through the ampulla until it reaches the AIJ or encounters stenosis. Observation is performed during a slow removal of the fiberscope.*

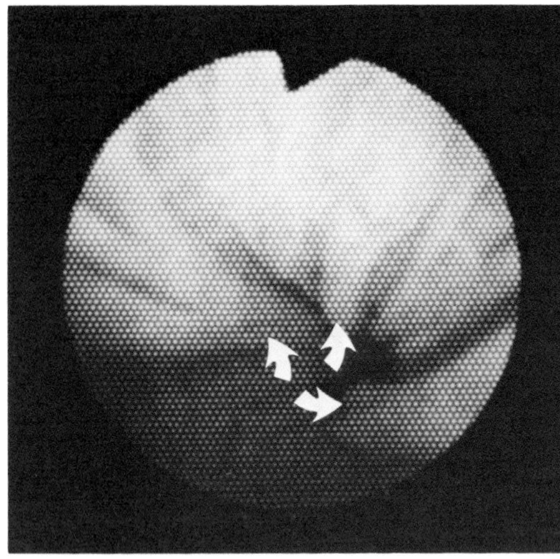

FIGURE 36:4—*Several folds (*arrows*) are seen at the AIJ.*

appeared pinkish or salmon-pink and showed parallel folds around its entire circumference that floated freely when surrounded by the perfusion medium. The size and number of folds varied according to the level at which the endoscope was placed. At the level of the AIJ, the folds were thin and short. The isthmus was visible, continuing in a gentle slope to join with the ampulla. At the midpoint of the ampulla, the folds progressively lengthened and thickened (Fig. 36:4). These folds became longer and thicker at less than 5 mm from the fimbria.

Several abnormal findings were observed. Stenoses were seen particularly at the AIJ (Fig. 36:5). Adhesions were white and fibrous and appeared in spiderweb or wheelspoke patterns, usually between atrophic folds (Fig. 36:6). Thick fringes produced a multicryptic aspect of the ampullary light (Fig. 36:7). The folds in some lumina disappeared, producing a tunnel-like aspect (Fig. 36:8). In other instances they were very small and were associated with thin adhesions. Transverse striations gave a bee's nest or cobblestone configuration to the endosalpinx. Complete atrophy around the entire circumference was occasionally encountered. Combinations of the above-mentioned abnormalities were not infrequent.

The salpingogram was analyzed before the endoscopic examination. When the salpingogram was judged either normal or equivocal, abnormalities were found in 25 percent of the women. Fifty percent of the salpingograms judged equivocal were proved to have normal rugal folds on endoscopic examination. Minor abnormalities on ampulloscopy are very difficult to detect radiographically. Of 61 tubes considered normal on salpingography, fimbrial or intraampullary abnormalities were seen in 26, a 43 percent false-negative x-ray study. In 58 instances, salpingographic findings were abnormal and ampulloscopy showed normal lumina in 23 tubes, a 40 percent error in the x-ray analysis. In 40 instances in which the salpingogram was not diagnostic, normal findings were seen at ampullosalpingoscopy in 25 instances and abnormal findings in 15 others.

A laparoscopic ASC was performed on 54 patients who had unexplained infertility. The average age of these women was

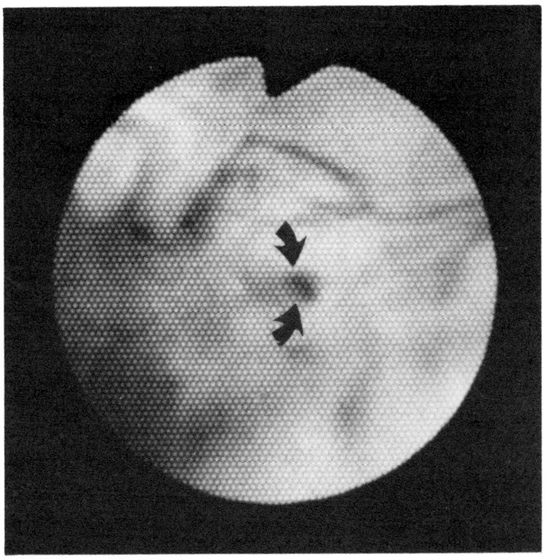

FIGURE 36:5—*Intrinsic postinflammatory stenosis* (arrows) *at the AIJ.*

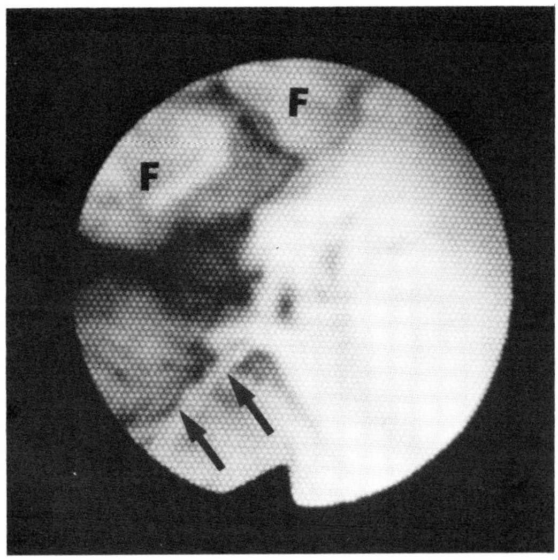

FIGURE 36:6—*Adhesions* (arrows) *and thickened fringes* (F) *are noted.*

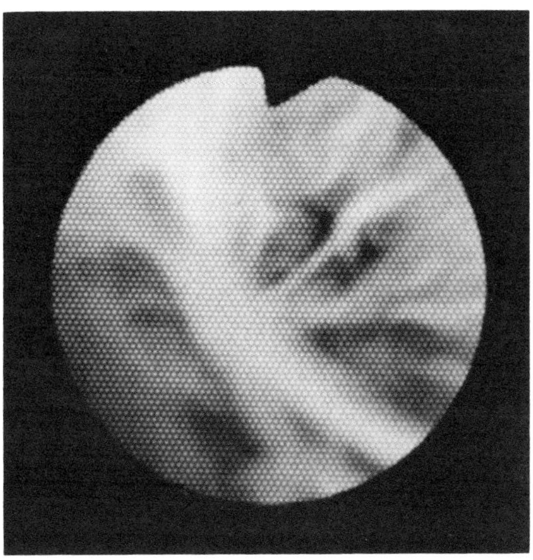

FIGURE 36:7—*Multiple ampullary adhesions are evident.*

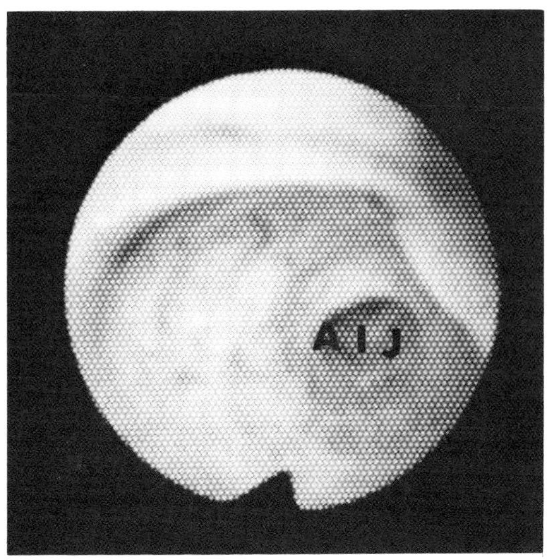

FIGURE 36:8—*Complete disappearance of the luminal folds and a hydrosalpinx is obvious.*

32 and their average length of infertility was four years. The pelvic findings on laparoscopy were normal in these patients. In 40 tubes, periostial or ampullary and fimbrial adhesions were discovered by means of an ampullosalpingoscopy. In 17 instances, these adhesions were removed by the passage of the fiberscope or by breaking them with the end of the instrument. After these operations, 11 of 17 patients became pregnant within an average of three to four months. No tubal pregnancies occurred. These findings suggest that fimbrial adhesions can cause infertility and that therapeutic ampullary salpingoscopy was a satisfactory means of

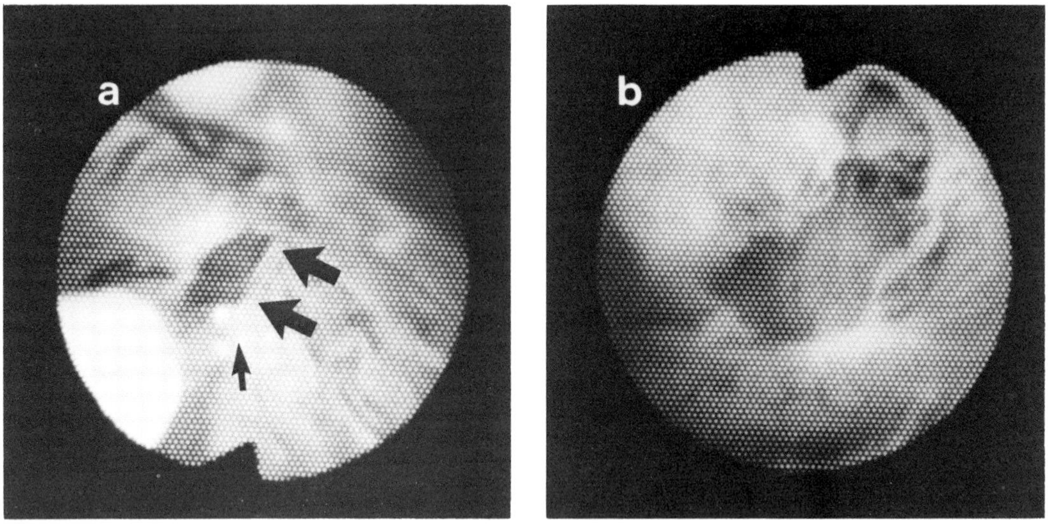

FIGURE 36:9—(a) *The forceps (*small arrow*) was introduced through the fiberscope and grasps and twists off the central white scar (*large arrows*).* (b) *The scar has been removed and the AIJ is now opened.*

therapy (Fig. 36:9). Five of the remaining 37 patients in this group became pregnant after a laparoscopy in which normal findings from an ASC were noted.

In 17 of 31 women who had a postoperative laparoscopy or hysterosalpingography, at least one tube was normal. In 12 of 14 women who had abnormal findings on ASC, the tubes became obstructed again despite microsurgical tuboplasty. Pregnancy occurred in 22 women, all of whom had normal findings on ASC in at least one tube. Eleven tubal pregnancies occurred and in each instance the ampulloscopy done before the tuboplasty had revealed luminal adhesions or endosalpingeal sclerosis. Endosalpingeal adhesions were removed during ASC carried out under laparoscopic control in 17 patients and 11 women became pregnant.[8] Similar results have been reported by others.[9]

Four patients had a history of exposure to DES in utero. They showed characteristic cervical and uterine anomalies on the hysterogram but no characteristic isthmic or ampullary images.[6,7] In two patients, the usual folds were replaced by irregular elevations giving an undulating effect to the endosalpinx. Methylene blue colored the tops of these dysmorphic fringes. In one patient, a normal intrauterine pregnancy occurred several months after the tuboscopy. Another patient exposed to DES had normal, parallel folds. This woman had postinflammatory abnormalities. These findings have not been previously described in patients who were not exposed to intrauterine DES (Fig. 36:10).

The early diagnosis of a tubal pregnancy is sometimes difficult and the laparoscopic findings are occasionally not easy to interpret because of the small size of some early ampullary pregnancies. Four patients suspected of having tubal gestations had a laparoscopy and in two women the ampulloscopy enabled the discovery of the implantation precisely and the study of ampullary changes (Fig. 36:11). In two other instances, a small amount of fluid blood was discovered but the endoscopic examination did not enable the physician to locate the ampullary gestation.

In six patients, a six-month postoperative evaluation of a fimbrioplasty was done by ASC. Ampullary adhesions had been found initially in four of them and were unchanged. In another woman who

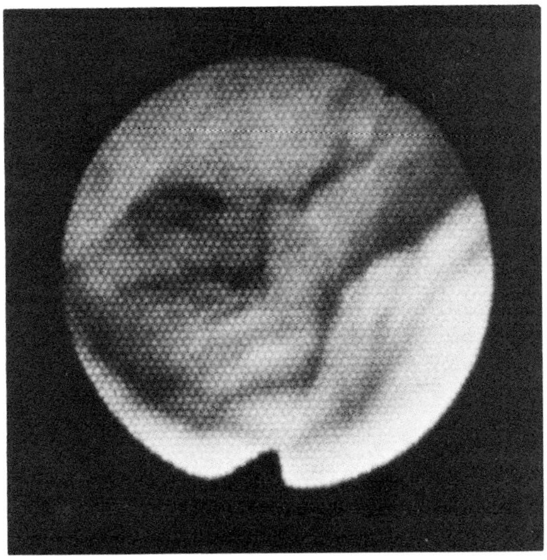

FIGURE 36:10—*The tubal lumen shows "valleys and hills" rather than normal parallel folds in a woman who was exposed to DES in utero.*

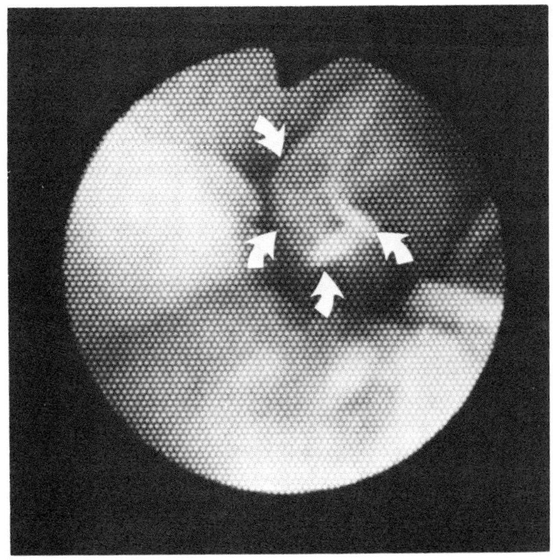

FIGURE 36:11—*An early tubal gestation* (arrows) *is seen in the ampullary lumen.*

had flattened folds because of hydrosalpinx and localized luminal adhesions, the follow-up ampulloscopy revealed normal folds with persistent adhesions. In the sixth instance, previously observed flattened folds returned to a normal configuration following ampullary salpingoneostomy. Reduction of intraluminal pressure seems to permit redevelopment of the normal surface pattern.

Conclusions

There appears to be a good correlation between the findings of ampulloscopy and success rates following tuboplasty. Whenever ampulloscopy reveals extensive adhesions at the time of tuboplasty, the prognosis for normal pregnancy is very poor and these women should be referred for consultation for in vitro fertilization. Indeed, a tubal ligation should be performed to avoid the possibility of an ectopic pregnancy. Flattened rugae caused by pressure within a hydrosalpinx eventually assume their normal configuration following ampullary salpingoneostomy.

References

1. Cornier E, Feintuch MJ, and Bouccara L: La fibrotuboscopie ampullaire. *Gynécol Obstét Reprod* 13:49, 1984.
2. Cornier E: L'ampullosalpingoscopie percoelioscopique. *Gynécol Obstét Biol Reprod* 14:459, 1985.
3. Cornier E: Intérêt pronostique de la tuboscopie per-operatoire. *Contracept Fertil Sex* 10:853, 1982.
4. Henry-Suchet J, Tesquier L, Pex JP, et al: Endoscopie tubaire ou tuboscopie: Une exploration complementaire utile dans la chirurgie repartrice des trompes. XXXIe Assises de la Ste Française de Gynécologie, Paris, Masson, 1983.
5. Cornier E: La fibroscopie en gynécologie: La fibro-hysteroscopie et la fibrotuboscopie. *Presse Méd* 11:2841, 1982.
6. DeCherney A, Cholst I, and Naftolin F: Structure and function of the fallopian tubes following exposure to diethylstibestrol during gestation. *Fertil Steril* 36:741, 1981.
7. Haney AF, Hammond CB, Joubes MR, et al: Diethylstilbestrol-induced upper genital tract abnormalities. *Fertil Steril* 31:142, 1979.
8. Cornier E: Ampullosalpingoscopy: Technique and results of permicrosurgical and percoelioscopic procedures. Abstracts XIIth AAGL Meeting, World

Congress Gynecol Endosc, 1983, p. 104.

9. Nordenskjold F, and Ahlgren M: Interfimbrial adhesions: Detection and treatment of an easily overlooked cause of infertility. Abstracts XIIth AAGL Meeting and World Congress of Gynecol Endosc, 1983, p. 21.

37

Tubal Microsurgery

Earl Owen and Amir H. Ansari

The microsurgical approach is the only rational technique for tuboplasty because, under high magnification, the surgeon can differentiate normal from abnormal tissue. Dissection, excision, and anastomosis with precision becomes possible. The results from such tubal surgery are better than from previous methods.[1]

To perform successful tubal microsurgery requires a knowledge of tubal microanatomy and physiology, an excellent operating microscope, specialized instruments and techniques, and devoted practice after training with this equipment.

Tuboplasty

The operations are planned after cessation of menses. An upper age limit must be kept in mind in view of the known complications of late-in-life pregnancies.[2] The duration of blockage does not preclude an operation. Severe pelvic fibrosis should preclude an attempt at tuboplasty. The normal health of the patient must be ascertained before recommending any pregnancy.

Indications for Microsurgery

Conservative operations on the fallopian tube should be performed under the operating microscope. These operations include: microdissection of adhesions (adhesiolysis), fimbrioplasty, neosalpingostomy, end-to-end anastomosis, correction of cornual blockage, and conservative management of tubal gestations. The operating microscope is also very useful for conservative operations for endometriosis and in removal of periovarial adhesions.

The operating microscope

This instrument has been available for over 40 years and it is now refined and reliable. Several manufacturers (Zeiss, Wild, Weck) make precision microscopes with excellent optics, allowing prolonged observation without eye strain. The motorized models have reliable motors with foot controls and they are built robustly for long usage. These manufacturers also provide backup service for their products. Twenty other manufacturers currently market less expensive operating microscopes, some with excellent features.

The Fallopian Tube: Basic Studies and Clinical Contributions, edited by Alvin M. Siegler, M.D. Mount Kisco, New York: Futura Publishing Company, Inc. © 1986.

These microscopes are designed to be used with the operator in a seated position looking forwards but having outstretched hands in a writing position in front with the feet controlling most of the microscope's functions. Considerable practice is necessary to master such a machine, enough to concentrate only on the task of tubal reconstruction. The advantages of the microscope are superb cold lighting, outstanding magnification without visual strain, foot control of almost all functions, unrivaled vision of living tissues, and excellent teaching accessories. The disadvantages include bulkiness, impractical transportation, initial expense, and the need for additional training.

Alternative to the microscope (not recommended)

The range of magnification of the headband loupe is too small for adequate observation of tubal mucosa or accurate placement of submucosal sutures. Headbands are heavy and require the operator to keep the head unnaturally still. Focusing is particularly critical. Lighting intensity cannot compare with the microscope. The light lead from the lamp runs down the back of the head and can restrict the surgeon's mobility. Loupes are only useful if the microscope is not available.

Magnifying glasses

Magnifying glasses are good and they can be useful if a microscope is not available provided the microsurgical techniques are observed. Avoid bulky, heavy long lenses which are unstable and uncomfortable. The glasses made by several firms (Keeler, Zeiss, U.S. Optical) are lightweight and wide-angled with higher magnifications. Clever designs keep the glasses securely on in difficult head positions. The maximal magnification tolerable for glasses is five times, which is really not powerful enough for microsurgery.

Selection of Instruments

A wide range of instruments is now available for tubal microsurgery. The most useful of these have long round-bodied handles that are ergonomically designed to allow control over tiny sutures deep in the pelvic cavity. Most control is provided by the concavo-convex jaws, long round bodies, and well-balanced design of the Vickers long needleholder which is part of a special set for microgynecology. This set includes a long, angulated, serrated jawed fine scissors and a similar angulated long forceps with special nontraumatic ring tips which enable anastomoses to be securely made deep in the pelvis when the uterus cannot be manipulated up into the operative wound. A flat square four-bladed retractor (the Kirschner or the Ergobionic) facilitates good exposure.

Selection of Sutures

Experienced microsurgeons use as little suture material as possible, since they know that all foreign material causes fibrosis. The actual suture can be nylon or absorbable, both of which have advantages. Knots are tied snugly and ends are cut as short as possible in an attempt to leave in as little material as possible. Nylon is nonabsorbable, retains tensile strength for many weeks and causes only a small reaction. The absorbable sutures (Dexon®, Vicryl®) tend to swell initially in the tissues but cause less reaction eventually. Catgut is not recommended for fertility operations because it swells significantly and is too reactive.

Atraumatic needles used for microsurgery are 3/8 curved. They may be fine or taper-pointed flattened central sections on their round-bodied needles, further assisting their control in placement. For most of my procedures 8-0 is used and rarely a 9-0 is preferred. In my opinion 7-0 is far too large for repair of tubes, both from the size of the needle bore and the size of the suture material, which causes five times the trauma of an 8-0 suture.

Position for Microsurgery

It is essential to be firmly placed in a comfortable position and yet have access to the pelvic cavity. Most operating tables have very little room underneath for the operator's feet and the pedals for microscope and bipolar coagulator. This can be overcome by positioning the patient halfway down the table with her legs supported by an additional table, a hand surgery table is ideal for the purpose. The microscope is positioned with its stand to one side of the operating surgeon. The operating room light (usually a ceiling mount) is directed into the pelvis and the body of the microscope positioned correctly and fully adjusted for the surgeon before hand scrubbing. I use a special operating chair, adjustable in all directions, and this is readied, as are the foot pedals, before I scrub. Leg massaging equipment is placed as soon as the general anesthetic is commenced, and then the patient is catheterized. A thin wet long gauze pack is placed high in the vagina and brought out, to lie between the patient's toes, to be used later as an indicator of the passage of dye through the tube, if necessary. If an assistant and a double microscope are available, it is essential to adjust the position, eyepieces, and seat height before preparing the patient's abdomen.

The surgeon must have had considerable experience as a microsurgeon before clinically attempting delicate operations. All the equipment and everyone's positions are checked before the surgeon leaves the room to scrub for the case. A common mistake is to fail to check the microscope's eyepieces for intrapupillary distance, since we tend to forget that other surgeons also use the microscope and change the settings to suit their own eyes and heights.

Training for Microsurgery

Delicate microsurgery requires familiarity with the equipment and confidence in technique that only comes from practice.

There are two kinds of practice: informed and haphazard. To practice correctly from the start, one should either attend a reputable "hands-on" course of instruction or learn directly from an experienced surgeon. Practicing bad habits is detrimental and will be reflected in poor clinical results. Microsurgery is not easy and the surgeon must be obsessive, meticulous, and extremely gentle because the tubal tissues are complex with a critical blood supply.

Teaching microsurgery at the Sydney Microsurgery Center for the past 17 years has not been difficult; but teaching tissue handling and wound healing has been more demanding. A change in concept must be accepted if the student surgeon is to become successful.

Microsurgical Principles in Operating

The microscope is used as an aid in observation. The cut end of the tubal mucosa is observed at the highest power available, but anastomoses are made at magnifications between 10 and 20 times. The endosalpinx is never grasped directly with metal forceps but is manipulated from the outside by gloved fingers or soft silastic coated forceps. Bleeding from cut tubal ends is controlled by bipolar coagulation under microscopic vision. Injections of weak adrenaline solution (1 to 200,000) or POR8 (ornipressin 5 IU/ml) submucosally helps reduce bleeding around the uterine cornua.

All sutures placed in tubes are neatly buried between layers. The knots at the serosal surface should be cut very short but preferably put in as deliberate buried knots. Sometimes covering with peritoneum using a delayed continuous gathering layer or a patch of peritoneum is needed.

The proximal tubal segment is tested for patency by the passage of a weak blue dye into the uterine cavity under gentle pressure. The distal segment is tested with a fine, rounded soft silastic 21 gauge catheter (angiocath) which is gently inserted and dye is injected. The passage of metal or glass rods into the tube and into the uterus to simplify anastomosis is unnecessary and can damage the endosalpinx.

All mesosalpingeal defects are repaired, bringing the peritoneal edges neatly together to avoid adhesions and prevent bowel entrapment. At the completion of these operations it is routine to irrigate the pelvic cavity with a warm normal saline solution containing 5,000 units of heparin per liter, which may reduce the occurrence of subsequent adhesions.

The Microsurgical Approach

Some important points about tubal anatomy and physiology require emphasis for those physicians contemplating the performance of tubal operations.

The tube has five anatomical segments, each with quite different functions. These are the fimbrial apparatus, the ampulla, the isthmo-ampullary junction, the isthmus, and the intramural segment. Fertilization can only take place in the ampulla within its healthy mucosal environment. To do this the ovum must get into the ampulla, which presupposes a functional opening either natural (the fimbrial apparatus), or constructed (the salpingostomy).

Even with tubal patency and a healthy mucosa, the tube cannot function successfully when external bands, kinking, fibrosis, or outside pressure cause either direct or physiological obstructions.

In distal obstruction, normal tubal secretions build up in the ampulla, the increased pressure distends it, flattens its delicate mucosa, and jeopardizes its blood supply. Even restoring patency to the fimbrial end may fail to restore function to the ampullary endosalpinx that has atrophied because of months of excessive pressure. To examine the mucosa properly requires microscopic observation with the highest power and brilliant illumination afforded only by a top-quality microscope. When diseased or fibrotic mucosa is observed, the microsurgeon can confidently excise the healthy parts of the tube, reconstruct only healthy tissue, and expect that such a tube will become functional.

Let us consider each tubal segment separately to ascertain why the results of surgery are so variable. All tubal segments must function efficiently and in harmony for them to act effectively so that a normal pregnancy becomes possible.

Fimbrioplasty

The outermost end of the tube is normally a mobile receptor capable of acting as a physiological sphincter. Its muscular pattern is thin but complex, and it works effectively in concert. Its mucosa is richly cellular and deeply channelled. The petal-like folds with their channels give a large surface area of mainly ciliated cells, arranged in tracts all beating toward the ampullary opening. It contains glandular cells secreting fluid, setting up a flow pattern for the ovum to be conveyed to its opening. A very tethered fimbriated end cannot nudge the ovary at ovulation so it is important at this site to remove even fine adhesions under careful microscope observation, for the fimbriae are supplied with an extensive and fragile blood supply. As a general rule, all pelvic adhesions should be carefully excised to avoid trauma that could lead to further formation of adhesions. Microsurgeons use either a very fine monopolar coagulation needle, a fine-pointed bipolar coagulator, or a laser beam to sever both ends of thin adhesions. After excising large adhesions, we repair the uncovered spaces wtih fine sutures, attempting to restore a smooth peritoneal serosal surface.

When infections or adhesions affect the fimbrial end, the individual fimbria may be destroyed and the opening completely or incompletely blocked. Sometimes the end is patent but nonfunctional, which can confuse the gynecologist who relies only on hysterosalpingography to assess tubal abnormalities. A stiff patent end with some destroyed fimbrial mucosa may be quite useless and would be better excised, a functional stoma microsurgically reconstructed may then allow a normal pregnancy to occur.

The fimbrial opening allows the escape of excess tubal fluid. When it is closed the fluid accumulates and damages ampullary and fimbrial mucosa. Restorative fimbrioplasty must be performed on healthy tubes covered with active mucosa on the inside and intact peritoneum on the outside. The key to an effective fimbrial operation is to observe carefully the mucosal surface with the highest power of the operating microscope. All useless mucosa is clearly seen and one should excise the unhealthy fimbria or ampulla. Any mucosa of doubtful viability should be excised by the useful technique of serrated microscissors in the right hand and a very fine pointed bipolar coagulator in the left. For a chance of pregnancy, it is essential to leave at least 3 to 4 cm of microscopically selected healthy ampulla after reconstructions in this area.

The actual reconstruction of the tubal end may be performed by any of many standard procedures and the addition of the microsurgical technique. I use the trumpet ampullostomy, so named because the completed opening resembles the open end of a trumpet rather than the appearance of multiple petals of a flower, which it replaces (Table 37:1). Short longitudinal incisions in the ampulla in the line of the tracts of ciliated cells are cut to make a series of flaps. The number of these depends on the width of the ampullary cavity which is always stretched by the previous pressure and which is usually edematous. The flaps are turned back and secured to the tubal serosa. This is done carefully with interrupted 8-0 or 9-0 sutures whose knots are buried and covered with mucosa, since only submucosa is sutured to peritoneum. This suturing requires experience; tension on the outfolded suture line will actually close off the tubal opening rather than open it. Great care must be exercised in dealing with swollen ampulla which still has cilia and is still capable of returning to normal function. If touched with metal it will bleed, and its cells are easily disrupted. The only safe ways of holding edematous diseased mucosa gently are either with gloved fingers, or with quite wide bladed forceps shielded with soft silastic tubing. These guarded forceps are useful for all delicate surgical maneuvers with fragile structures.

I have described a fimbrioplasty and its success depends on careful technique; it is performed on healthy tissue selected by microscopic observation under high power with excision of all unhealthy tissue. This aggressive approach over the last four years has produced a 34 percent pregnancy rate in bilaterally reconstructed tubes, in patients with bilateral chronic hydrosalpinx.

Salpingoneostomy and Ampullary-Ampullary Anastomosis

This is the widest part of the oviduct and it is capable of wider dilatation under pressure. It has the most complex mucosal pattern with almost equal numbers of ciliated and nonciliated cells. The mucosal lining is complexly folded and its glandular cells secrete actively following the regular menstrual cycle. Without approximately 2.5 cm of healthy ampulla, a successful pregnancy is not possible. The surgical principle is to preserve as much functional ampulla as possible. Endosalpinx and tubal serosal surface are observed under the highest power of microscope. Ampullary reconstructions are performed either as previously described for fimbrial damage, or as an anastomosis of ampulla to ampulla after excision of abnormal tissue, as a consequence of disease or following a sterilization.

We see relatively few cases of bilateral ampullary damage along with sterilization procedures. Usually ligatures have been carelessly placed and tend to include the isthmo-ampullary junction.

Table 37:1

Microsurgical Salpingoneostomy for Severe Bilateral Hydrosalpinx in 166 Women

Result	*No. of patients*	*Percentage of pregnancies*
Term pregnancy	56	34 %
Ectopic pregnancy	9	5.4%
Never pregnant	101	60.6%

Sterilization by electrocoagulation also affects this junction frequently and rarely destroys only ampullary sections. Ampullo-ampullary anastomoses are sometimes required, and although the easiest of tubal reconstructions, they still need a meticulous microsurgical technique to produce consistent success. Tubal ends are cut with serrated microscissors and bleeding from submucosal vessels is controlled with a bipolar coagulator. The anastomosis is done with interrupted 8-0 or 9-0 sutures, excluding the endosalpinx. This buries the layer of sutures. Mucosal damage and fibrosis are avoided so that the chance of a subsequent tubal pregnancy is reduced. Triple knots are made and cut very short. The ampullary mucosa often bulges out between the first few sutures and it can be excised in the usual way rather than tucked back before completing the initial layer of sutures.

Isthmo-Ampullary Anastomosis

The main principles of microsurgical repair involve a vertical incision at the isthmic end and the creation of an opening in the center of the ampulla sufficient to make the anastomosis simple and physiological. If the difference between the diameters of the segments is more than double, then the ampullary end must be partially closed and the anastomosis effected with interrupted submucosal 8-0 microsutures.

Three stay sutures are placed as triangular corner supports and the interrupted sutures between are carefully placed to avoid the endosalpinx on each side. Most of the tubal sterilization operations seen in Sydney required this type of reconstruction to restore patency, particularly after electrosurgical coagulation, where longer lengths of tube are destroyed.

Isthmic-Isthmic Anastomosis

The isthmus has a thick myosalpinx augmented at its cornual end by an additional thin, longitudinal spiral muscle. Its endosalpinx is the least complicated and its lumen relatively consistent. The isthmo-isthmic anastomosis under the microscope is relatively easy but careful observation of the freshened tubal ends is essential to ensure that all tubal layers are healthy. The reconstruction is with a few interrupted submucosal sutures, making sure the mucosa is not bunched. Since the isthmus is not critical for pregnancy, gynecologists should recommend that tubal sterilization procedures should only be performed in the isthmic segment.

A recent personal series of 252 cases of female sterilization reversal by microsurgery has been published.[3] Where the sterilization damage was confined only to the isthmus the resulting reversal operations were more rapid, easier and had an outstanding subsequent term pregnancy rate of 93.1 percent (Table 37:2). Where the sterilization was extended to other areas containing more essential anatomy, then, despite the equally metic-

Table 37:2
Microsurgical Reversal of Isthmic Sterilization Methods

Sterilization method	*No. of cases*	*Term pregnancies*	*% Term pregnancies*
Hulka clip	24	23	95.8
Falope ring	37	35	94.5
Laparoscopic cautery	7	6	85.7
Open cut & tie	5	4	80.0
TOTALS	***73***	***68***	***93.1***

Table 37:3
Microsurgical Reversal of Sterilization Performed Other Than in Isthmus Including in the Isthmo-Ampullary Junction, Cornua, and Ampulla

Site of reconstruction	*No. of cases*	*Term pregnancies*	*% Term pregnancies*
Ampulla, cornua, Isthmo-ampullary junction	179	122	68

ulous repairs, there was only a 68 percent subsequent term pregnancy rate (Table 37:3).

Intramural-Isthmic (Tubocornual) Anastomosis

The intramural segment is a highly specialized area set in uterine muscle. It is the narrowest part of the tube with an internal diameter of between 0.2 and 0.5 mm. The opening has a somewhat spiral passage, and the strong uterine muscle can contract, causing this physiological "sphincter" to close. Because of the irregular passage and delicate mucosa it is unwise to pass a probe through this area into the uterine cavity, since it will cause damage and subsequent fibrosis. Cornual occlusions are commonly the result of infection and they can be unilateral. They require exposure by serial section cutting into uterine cornual muscle at right angles to the tube. Injection of POR8 or adrenaline mixture 15 minutes prior to the sectioning will facilitate cornual surgery. The larger vessels can be seen and either tied off or coagulated. A patent tube can be detected and sutured to the patent isthmus. Patency is ascertained by occluding the cervix and filling the uterine cavity with blue dye through a thin needle inserted through the fundus. The bulging mucosa appears in the cored-out uterine muscle and allows accurate placement of interrupted 8-0 sutures from muscle to the isthmus. It is important to leave all interrupted sutures untied until each has been placed and then they are all gently snugged in and tied. This gives a satisfactory closure under full vision. When these are the only adhesions and the remaining tube is normal the results of such reconstructions are good. Fourteen bilateral cornual blocks have been reconstructed in this way, resulting in eleven term pregnancies (70 percent). Unfortunately, infection does not always affect only one area and many operations have been performed in conjunction with the repair of other occluded areas in the same tube, with poorer results.

Conclusion

Reconstructive surgery for blocked, damaged, or tethered fallopian tubes must be performed fastidiously, taking advantage of all the knowledge available concerning the tube and its reactions to trauma both natural and surgically produced. The best lighting and magnification available should be used together with a technique that does as little additional damage as possible to the remaining length of tube. For these reasons, the microsurgical technique is mandatory, and merely emphasizes, again, that excellent results in surgery will always follow an obsessive attention to detail and a meticulous technique by trained gynecologists.

References

1. Gomel V: The impact of microsurgery in gynecology. *Clin Obstet Gynecol* 23:4, 1980.
2. Owen ER, and Pickett-Heaps AA: Microsurgical basis of fallopian tube reconstruction. *Aust NZ J Surg* 47:1977.Woodruff JD, and Pauerstein C: *The Fallopian Tube.* Baltimore: Williams & Williams, 1974. Israel SL: *Menstrual Disorders and Sterility.* New York: Paul B. Hoeber Inc., 1959.
3. Owen ER: Reversal of female sterilization. Review of 252 microsurgical salpingo-salpingostomies. *Med J Aust* 141:276, 1984.

38

Tubal Anastomosis

Brian M. Cohen and
John F. Angle

The advent of gynecological microsurgery, with the introduction of the operating microscope, fine instruments, minute needles, and nonreactive sutures into modern gynecology has changed our previous concepts and understanding of tubal anastomosis.

The minute lumens of the intramural, isthmic, and isthmic-ampullary segments of the human fallopian tube were, in the past, an impediment to the possibility of restoring tubal patency at these sites. Tubal implantation was the preferred procedure in the 1940s and 1950s[1] and, indeed, the poor results following tubal anastomosis virtually contraindicated its attempt. Since Gomel[2] and Winston[3] described microsurgical techniques for tubal and tubocornual anastomosis, and their excellent results, other gynecologists have been inspired to repeat these findings.

In this chapter, we discuss the microsurgical approach to tubal anastomosis for proximal tubal obstruction. Sterilization reversal and the operation of tubal implantation are detailed elsewhere in this book. We emphasize pathological causes of proximal or midtubal obstruction and the present methods of preoperative investigation, intraoperative techniques, and postoperative care.

Preservation of the cornu and its blood supply appear to be associated with a higher incidence of postoperative pregnancy and live births. The intramural segment has major branches of the uterine artery which emerge medially from the parametrium and run into the myometrium beneath the isthmus. These blood vessels encircle the isthmus and intramural segment in vascular arcades that are found primarily in the subserosal and submucosal layers with intervening vessels (Fig. 38:1). These arteries continue to the fundus. In view of the small diameter of the tubal lumen at the cornu and isthmus (0.4–1.2 mm), magnification is required for accurate and meticulous removal of all abnormal tissue, to facilitate precise approximation of remaining normal segments, and for complete tubal reconstruction. Unquestionably, the cornu and isthmus are the prime sites for the application of gynecologic microsurgical techniques. Ischemia must be avoided by

The Fallopian Tube: Basic Studies and Clinical Contributions, edited by Alvin M. Siegler, M.D. Mount Kisco, New York: Futura Publishing Company, Inc. © 1986.

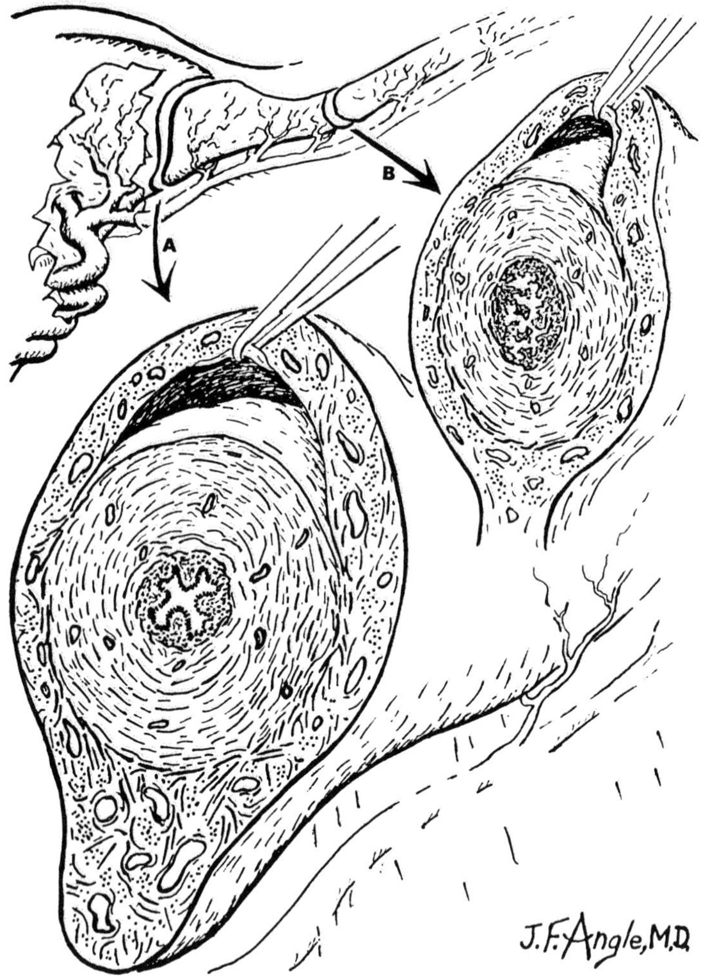

FIGURE 38:1—*The distribution of vessels is clearly seen in the intramural* (A) *and isthmic* (B) *segments.*

nondestructive methods of dissection and the judicious application of microunipolar and microbipolar electrodes.

The tuboplasty must be carried out with careful hemostasis since bleeding may be a nidus for infection and fibrin deposition, causes of subsequent adhesions and reocclusion. Precise alignment of the endosalpinx with accurate muscular apposition is essential for a successful anastomosis. The intramural segment usually has a single angulation seen during hysterosalpingography but it may appear convoluted in the extirpated uterine specimen.[4]

Causes of Proximal Tubal Occlusion

Proximal tubal occlusion may be caused by a postpartum or postabortal infection. In these cases, the distal tubal segments, the ampulla and fimbria, are usually normal. The pathologists may diagnose vascular thrombosis of the myosalpinx causing fibrosis with no histologic evidence of an infection.

Other significant causes of proximal tubal obstruction include salpingitis isthmica nodosa, endosalpingiosis, endometriosis, and rarely, tuberculosis. Congenital atresia of the proximal oviduct is unusual. Patients exposed to diethylstilbestrol (DES) in utero may have tubal anomalies resembling salpingitis isthmica nodosa or deficiencies of the myosalpinx that are associated with uterine anomalies such as a T-shaped uterus. Polyps are occasionally seen in the intramural or isthmic segments but rarely cause obstruction.

Tubal endometriosis and tuberculous salpingitis are difficult to detect preoperatively but the findings on the hysterosalpingogram and laparoscopy can be suggestive. Endometriosis is found in 5 to 63 percent of the proximal tubal segments of previously sterilized women.[5]

Additional diagnostic studies are sometimes needed so that appropriate medical therapy can be instituted. Certainly, no tuboplasty is indicated if a tuberculous cause of the tubal occlusion is detected.

Diagnosis and Preoperative Evaluation

The diagnosis of proximal tubal occlusion is usually made from a hysterosalpingogram taken during the evaluation of the infertile woman. The condition must be confirmed by a repeat radiological study, a laparoscopy with the addition of chromopertubation, and hysteroscopy. These three techniques are complementary and essential to avoid performing a laparotomy because of proximal tubal occlusion caused by spasm. With the latter condition, the cornua appear pointed on hysterosalpingography, rather than rounded since some contrast material rarely enters the intramural segment in organic occlusion.

A normal pelvis, clear ovarian surfaces, and well-defined fimbria are important positive prognostic signs, since 40 to 55 percent of these patients conceive postoperatively.[6] When the obstruction has not resulted from an infection, the live birth rate following anastomosis is even better.[7] The presence of hydrosalpinges indicating bipolar obstruction should suggest the need for further reassessment and consideration of in-vitro fertilization and embryo transfer.

During the hysteroscopic procedure, the uterotubal ostia can be observed and if they are obstructed, then tubal implantation is indicated. Microsurgical tubocornual anastomosis becomes feasible if these tubal openings are clearly discerned at hysteroscopy. A careful preoperative analysis helps the surgeon plan the strategy for each operation. The surgeon should review the hysterosalpingogram, endoscopic findings, drawings, and photographs before the operation begins.

Surgical Objectives

The objectives of microsurgical tubal anastomosis include resection of abnormal tissue and maximal preservation of healthy tube with minimal blood loss; mobilization of the distal tubal segment to facilitate anastomosis with minimal tension during the repair; and accurate alignment of the endosalopinx with precise muscular and serosal apposition of the proximal and tubal segments.

Microsurgical Dissection and Anastomosis

After adequate vaginal preparation and bladder drainage, the cervix is cleansed and grasped with a single-toothed tenaculum. A pediatric Foley catheter (no. 8) or preferably a Harris uterine injector is inserted into the uterine cavity and attached to a preloaded 50 ml syringe containing indigo carmine (diluted 1 part in 10 ml of saline). When the uterus is mobile and easily elevated against the anterior abdominal wall, a Kerlix® vaginal pack is placed in the vagina. This facilitates anterior and upward displacement of the uterus and subsequent dissection.

Laparotomy is performed through a Pfannenstiel incision using electrocoagulation. A Kirshner retractor is inserted and lint-free packs soaked in heparinized lactated Ringer's solution are applied over the retractor blades.

The uterus is elevated by the application of these packs placed in the cul-de-sac and anterior uterovesical folds. This maneuver elevates the uterine fundus close to the anterior abdominal wall and the adnexa are stabilized on these soaked pads.

The distal oviduct is examined, peritubal or periovarial adhesions are excised with the microelectrode, and hemostasis is achieved with a microbipolar coagulator. The operative sites are irrigated throughout the procedure with a solution of lactated Ringer's containing 2,000 IU of heparin, 100 mg of Solu-Cortef®, and 100 mg of ampicillin per liter. If penicillin sensitivity is suspected, the ampicillin is replaced by 100 mg of erythromycin.

Preparation of the Proximal Oviduct

Abnormal tissue is grasped with a small DeBakey-Atraugrip forceps and the initial lines of dissection are made symmetrically through the serosa on either side of the midline (Fig. 38:2). This allows specific definition of the tubal layers, avoids luminal injury, and minimizes vascular damage.

The subserosal vessels are coagulated initially with the bipolar electrode. If deep intramural resection is anticipated, the incisional lines are placed approximately 1 cm away from the entry of the tube into the uterus. This wide dissection facilitates access to the deep crater which may be necessary to identify healthy mucosa within the myometrium. Pitressin may be injected (10 IU in 20 ml saline), using a 25 to 30 gauge needle, into the myometrium approximately 1.5 to 2 cm from the tubal entry to achieve hemostasis during dissection. If the Pitressin is injected too close to the tubo-uterine junction, blanching of the entire region results and makes differentiation of ischemic tissue from fibrosis very difficult, even with the operating microscope.

Once hemostasis has been accomplished, traction is made on the myometrium and the overlying vascular serosa is displaced so that tissue planes are most evident. Vessels between the outer and inner muscular layers are identified and coagulated with the microbipolar forceps prior to tubal transection.

The dissection is carried out with an angled unipolar microelectrode needle. The obstructed tubal segment is gradually removed with a curved iris scissors or a Gomel cornual blade until the normal endosalpinx is identified. The mucosa is examined under high magnification with the operating microscope and if it appears abnormal, it is grasped again with the adjacent fibrous tissue. A 7-0 absorbable synthetic suture on a fine tapered needle is inserted twice through the proximal segment so that four symmetrical strands help to retract abnormal tissue away from the myometrium. This method enables further incisions to be made until healthy endosalpinx is seen. Adequate dissection is confirmed by the appearance of an everting endosalpinx associated with a free flow of dye injected into the uterine cavity. Partial obstruction is identified by a spiral or intermittent emission of fluid from the proximal lumen.

After a normal proximal segment has been identified and hemostasis achieved, attention is directed to the distal segment. The tubal resection avoids the adjacent mesosalpinx, thereby preserving the vessels beneath the isthmus. The fimbria are gently held with the gloved hand as the tip of a 2 ml syringe filled with indigo carmine is inserted into the tubal ostium. A moistened lint-free pad is placed beneath the tube prior to inserting the dye so that excess indigo carmine is absorbed and prevented from staining the pelvic peritoneum. As the dye is injected, the most proximal patent point is detected by a slight swelling (Fig. 38:3). When this site is identified, the overlying serosa is grasped with a fine-toothed dissecting microforceps. Only a small cap of serosa is

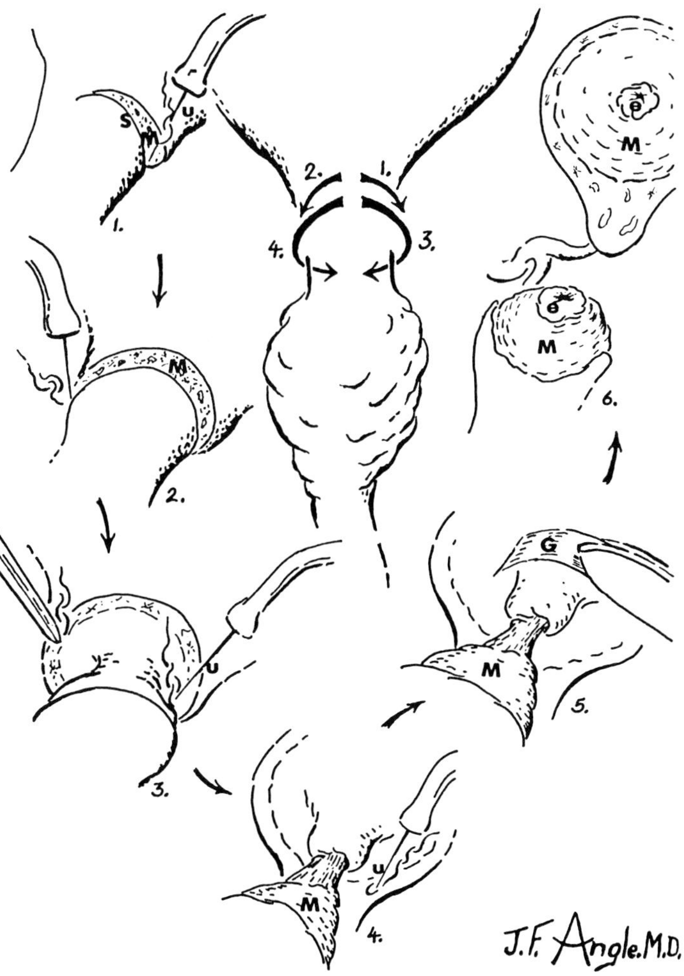

FIGURE 38:2—*Dissection of serosa (S) and muscularis (M) performed with a microunipolar electrode needle (U) carefully so as to delineate the endosalpinx (1–4) (5) A special Gomel⁺ blade (G) is used to transect the endosalpinx (E); (6) the pouting mucosa is seen.*

dissected off the distal segment using the microelectrode and a fine curved iris scissors. This technique, applied to the wide ampullary segment, preserves a small diameter identical with that of the proximal isthmic or intramural segment. Luminal disparity is avoided by perforating the distal segment bluntly with the end of a Winston "dinner fork," an intracath #18, or by a specially designed microreamer (Fig. 38:3).

If the distal portion is fibrotic, it is held with a toothed forceps and the abnormal tissue is dissected free from the healthy segment. The serosal blood vessels are identified and coagulated with microbipolar forceps. The serosa is divided symmetrically from its antimesenteric apex on either side as described previously and the tube is transected with a sharp curved iris scissors. Normal pouting endosalpinx is confirmed under the operating microscope.

In isthmo-isthmic or ampullary-ampullary anastomoses, luminal disparity does not occur and the tube is tran-

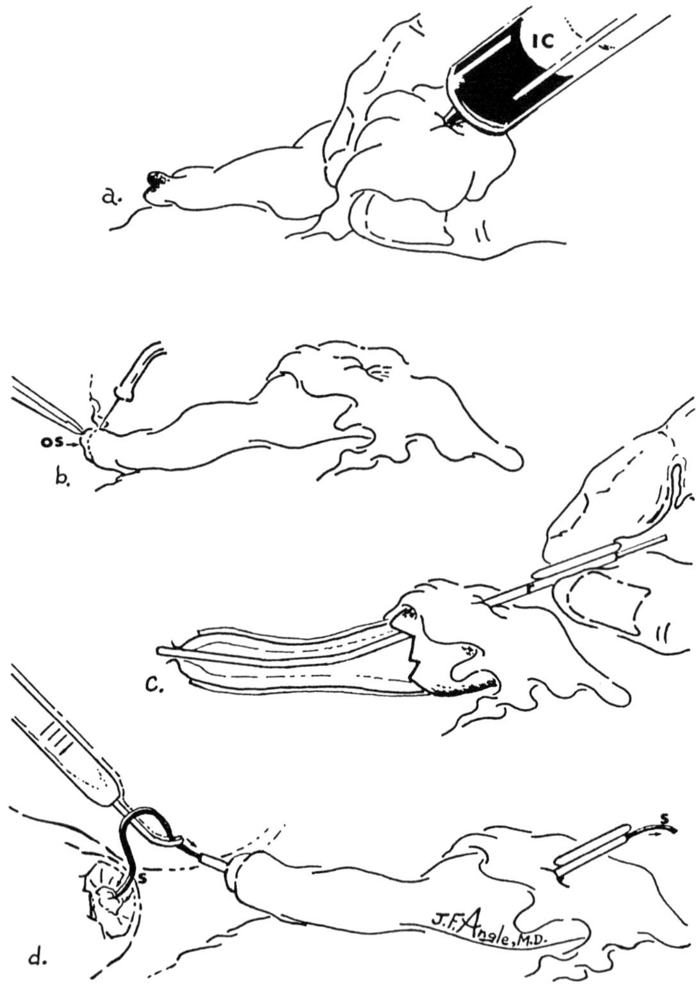

FIGURE 38:3—*Preparation of the distal segment involved:* (a) *retrograde instillation of indigo carmine (IC);* (b) *removal of a cap of occluded segment (os) with a micropolar electrode needle;* (c) *passage of a special reamer (r) through the patent tubal ends;* (d) *insertion of the splint (s) into the reamer depending on the situation.*

sected symmetrically through all layers with a curved iris scissors. A major technical problem arises whenever a large lumen must be joined to a smaller one. Luminal disparity in most cases is preventable by carefully tailoring the distal, potentially larger opening to the smaller proximal isthmic or intramural opening. Ampullary-isthmic or ampullary-intramural anastomoses imply a wide discrepancy in diameters.

Repair and Anastomosis

A 7-0 synthetic absorbable suture on a fine tapered needle is placed through the mesosalpinx to approximate the proximal and distal segments. This suture facilitates apposition of the myosalpinx and avoids tension on the anastomosis (Fig. 38:4). The first anastomotic suture is usually placed at a six o'clock position and the

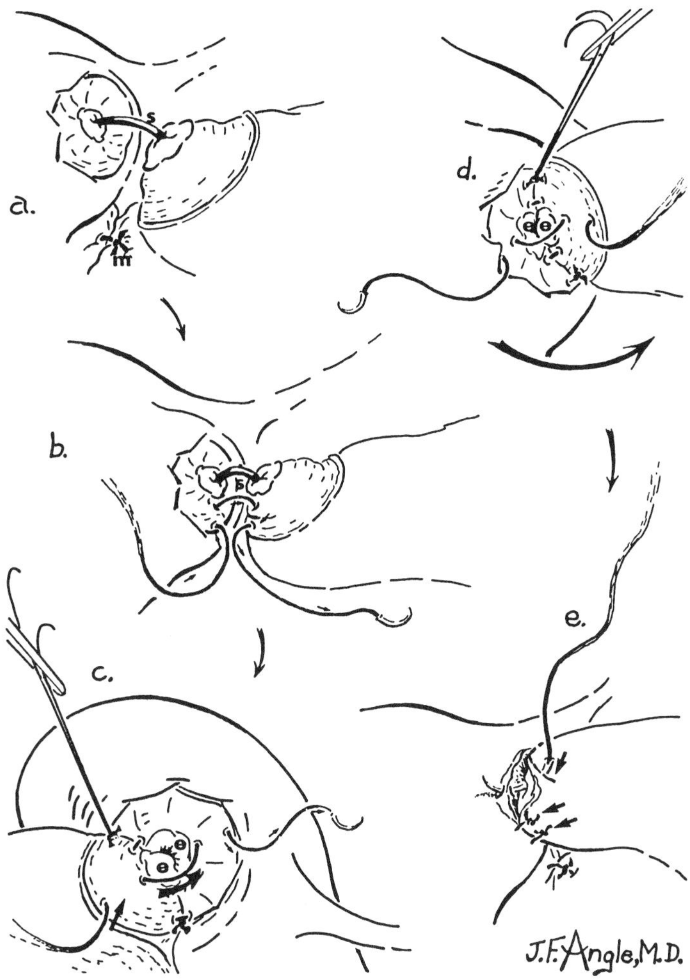

FIGURE 38:4—*Anastomosis and repair.* (a) *The suture in the mesosalpinx (m) has been tied, bringing the patent tubal ends close together. About 24 cm of splint (s) has been inserted into the uterine cavity and the other end was pulled through the fimbrial opening.* (b) *The six o'clock suture is inserted* (above) *into the myosalpinx of the isthmus and intramural segment.* (c *and* d) *Additional sutures* (arrows) *carefully approximate the endosalpinx (e) of both tubal segments.* (e) *Interrupted sutures* (arrows) *through the myosalpinx and serosa complete the operation.*

second suture is inserted at the twelve o'clock position. Once these have been tied, the twelve o'clock suture may be used to rotate the anastomosis, thereby assisting in the insertion of the remaining sutures. Upon completion of the inner layer, the overlying serosa is approximated using continuous or interrupted sutures.

If it is not possible to have direct access to the six o'clock position, sutures can be placed at the four and eight o'clock positions and subsequently, the apical and adjacent sutures are inserted. Gaps may occur despite perfect insertion of four main sutures particularly in intramural-ampullary or isthmic-ampullary anastomoses. Six or seven sutures may be necessary to achieve perfect muscular apposition in these cases. The sutures are tied gently to ensure adequate mucosal apposition associated with accurate muscular approximation. When the dissection is deep in the myometrium, identification of the lumen is sometimes difficult. A polyproplene suture (no. 0) may be placed through the proximal stump to serve as a splint. By grasping the proximal tubal segment with a fine-toothed microforceps, it is gently pulled upwards and forwards. This maneuver usually straightens the intramural segment. If there is any resistance to the passage of this splint, the procedure is abandoned to prevent iatrogenic injury. Twelve to fourteen inches are inserted into the uterine cavity. When a splint is used, the opposite end is pulled through the distal segment either directly by fastening it to the Winston "dinner fork," or through the intracath or through the microreamer which is then retracted through the fimbrial end (Fig. 38:4). This splint can be withdrawn immediately after completion of the anastomosis or removed transcervically three or four days postoperatively using a fine alligator forceps.

Whenever a tubocornual anastomosis has been completed, some of the superficial myometrium may require two or three interrupted sutures to ensure a close union and to facilitate superficial uterine and tubal apposition. Taper-cut or tapered needles are used for intramuscular sutures. Spatulated or ophthalmic cutting needles are avoided because they damage small capillaries and blood vessels close to the anastomosis.

Special Considerations

Before attempting a reversal of sterilization consequent to unipolar coagulation, a hysterosalpingogram may indicate endometriosis in the proximal stump. Adequate excision of this endometriotic tissue must be performed so that a single, patent normal lumen is present prior to completion of the anastomosis.

Whenever a multiple coagulation technique has been done for sterilization, larger segments of tube are destroyed. Occasionally, multiple anastomoses are required on a single tube. Following the use of a Hulka clip®, an isthmic-isthmic anastomosis can be completed with minimal excision of tube underneath and adjacent to the clip. Following a Pomeroy tubal ligation, there is a greater possibility of luminal disparity and not infrequently, an isthmo-ampullary anastomosis is performed. This requires dissection of a small cap of scar tissue from the ampullary segment to enable formation of a small distal lumen to correspond to that of the isthmic segment.

Salpingitis isthmica nodosa and tubal endometriosis often extend deep into the myometrium. Dissection into the cornu is often needed to identify the patent, normal proximal intramural segment. In performing this type of anastomosis, splinting facilitates the tubocornual approximation.

Whenever the occlusion is at the level of the endometrial cavity (confirmed by hysterosalpingography and hysteroscopy), dissection of the cornu should not be undertaken and tubal implantation is made in the posterior aspect of the fundus using a reamer. Preoperatively, the uterine cavity is stained with concentrated methylene blue and a large Lippes loop® attached to a sterile tape is inserted. Pitressin (2 units in 20 ml of saline) is injected into the myometrium with a 25 gauge needle at the site of the intended posterior uterine incision. This facilitates reaming out the core of uterine tissue with minimal blood loss. Since difficulty has been encountered in locating the uterine cavity from the posterior aspect of the uterus, the preoperative insertion of a Lippes loop® that divides the anterior and posterior walls of the uterus, helps to prevent trauma to the anterior endometrial surface. The loop is withdrawn prior to tubal implantation.

The fish-mouthed, previously prepared distal tubal segment is inserted into the uterine opening with the assistance of special implantation sutures. These provide a double-armed, fine taper point needle for the delicate tubal side and a large needle on the opposite end of the thread designed for penetration of the thick uterine wall with minimal trauma. (Detailed tubal implantation methods are discussed in a separate chapter.)

Postoperative Care and Follow-up

In most instances, at least 1 to 2 cm of isthmus are present so that anastomosis is possible without splinting. When minimal myometrial dissection has been carried out, conception may be attempted during the first cycle postoperatively because pregnancy can occur this early, particularly in women operated on for reversal of sterilization. When the myometrial dissection has been extensive before tubal patency is found and a tubocornual anastomosis is done, the patient is advised to avoid pregnancy for three months postoperatively to reduce the risk of possible uterine rupture. Indeed, elective cesarean delivery is advisable. Once a pregnancy has occurred, its location should be confirmed by ultrasonography at six weeks to document its intrauterine position.

Results

In analyzing the reports of results, it is important to look at the operative techniques described and the cause of the tubal obstructions. The collected series of macrosurgical and microsurgical techniques were reviewed in 1984 by Patton and Kistner (Table 38:1) who noted that the intrauterine pregnancy rate for microsurgical anastomosis was 61 percent, as opposed to 34 percent when macrosurgical techniques had been used. A significantly lower incidence of tubal pregnancy (3 percent) was observed in the microsurgical series.

Reversal of sterilization by anastomosis shows a postoperative term pregnancy rate of 60 percent. In patients who have less than 4.1 cm of tube after tubal anastomosis, Winston[8] noted a success rate of 36 percent (11 patients) whereas 62 percent of 24 patients whose residual oviducts were greater than 4 cm had intrauterine pregnancies. Silber and Cohen[9] noted that in seven patients who had postoperative tubes equal to or less than 3 cm, no pregnancies were observed. Eleven women whose residual tubes were greater than 4 cm achieved intrauterine pregnancies postoperatively. Gomel[10] showed an inverse relationship between tubal length and the interval between sterilization and the occurrence of pregnancy. When the tube was longer than 6 cm, pregnancy usually occurred within five postoperative cycles and, indeed, nine patients who conceived within the first postoperative cycles all had tubes 5.5 cm or greater. On the other hand, the interval between anastomosis and conception averaged 19.1 months in patients whose reconstructed tubes were measured at 4 cm or less. The overall average time between anastomosis and conception in his series was 10.2 months.

The incidence of pregnancy following tubal anastomosis done because of extensive abnormal proximal occlusion was 48 percent, with a 10 percent incidence of tubal pregnancy (Table 38:2). Verhoeven[11] confirmed the need for careful resection of the abnormal intramural segment. In his series, the intrauterine pregnancy rate was increased following extensive removal of the abnormal tissue with a corresponding decline in the postoperative incidence of tubal pregnancy (Table 38:3).

Microsurgical tubal anastomosis clearly has an excellent prognosis when a noninflammatory basis has been the cause of the occlusion. When the distal segment is normal, pregnancy usually occurs within 12 to 18 months of the operative procedure. The inability to conceive may be associated with reocclusion most commonly caused by inadequate excision of all of the original abnormal tissue. The incidence of pregnancy following mic-

Table 38:1

*Pregnancy following Reanastomosis for Reversal of Sterilization**

Technique	*No.*	*Pregnancy*	
		Intrauterine	*Tubal*
Macro	334	64%	23%
Micro	343	61%	3%

*From Patton and Kistner,[6] p. 275.

Table 38:2

Pregnancies following Reanastomosis for Pathological Cornual Occlusion

Author	*No.*	*Pregnancy*	
		Intrauterine	*Tubal*
Winston and Margara[8]	29	52%	3%
Gomel[10]	38	55%	5%
Verhoeven[11]	41	39%	12%
TOTAL	*108*	*48%*	*10%*

Table 38:3

Effect of Radical Resection of the Abnormal Intramural Segment on Pregnancy Rates

Technique	*No.*	*Intrauterine pregnancy*
Resect until patency	17	29%
Radical resection	24	46%

Table 38:4

Pregnancy following Anastomosis Associated with Repair of Distal Oviduct

Author	*No.*	*Pregnancy*	
		Intrauterine	*Tubal*
Winston and Margara[8]	16	25%	33%
Verhoeven[11]	17	24%	33%

rosurgical anastomosis and repair of the distal segment is poor (Table 38:4). At present it would seem that such patients should be offered in-vitro fertilization and embryo transfer.

Summary

Tubal anastomosis for proximal tubal obstruction is an operative procedure whose results have improved because of the use of microsurgical techniques. The causes of such obstructions include luminal fibrosis, chronic salpingitis, endometriosis, salpingitis isthmica nodosa, tuberculosis, and a previous sterilization. Tubal anastomosis should be followed by postoperative patency and successful pregnancies in over 60 percent of women. Tubocornual anastomosis does not weaken the uterine wall in most instances and a subsequent pregnancy does not mandate a cesarean delivery. Tubal anastomosis may be accomplished in most women who have proximal occlusion because at least some portion of the intramural segment is patent. This operation requires a microscope so that all of the abnormal tissue can be clearly seen and resected, and proper alignment of the patent residual tubal segments effected.

References

1. Greenhill JP: Evaluation of salpingostomy and tubal implantation for treatment of sterility. *Am J Obstet Gynecol* 33:39, 1937.
2. Gomel V: Tubal reanastomosis by microsurgery. *Fertil Steril* 28:59, 1977.
3. Winston RML: Microsurgical tubocornual anastomosis for reversal of sterilization. *Lancet* 1:284, 1977.
4. Diamond E: Fallopian tube circulation as it relates to microsurgery. In Philips JM (Ed): *Microsurgery in Gynecology.* Downey, CA: American Association of Gynecological Laparoscopists, 1977: p. 52.
5. Rock JA, Parmely TH, King TM, et al: Endometriosis in the development of tuboperitoneal fistula after tubal ligation. *Fertil Steril* 35:16, 1981.
6. Patton GW Jr, and Kistner RW: *Atlas of Infertility Surgery*, 2d ed. Boston: Little, Brown and Co., 1984: p. 277.
7. Gomel V: *Microsurgery in Female Infertility.* Boston: Little, Brown and Co., 1983: p. 236.
8. Winston RML, and Margara RA: Techniques for improvement of microsurgical tubal anastomosis. In Crosignani PG, Rubin BL (Eds): *Microsurgery in Female Infertility.* New York: Grune and Stratton, 1980.
9. Silber S, and Cohen MR: Microsurgical techniques for tubal reanastomosis. *Int J Fertil* 14:141, 1969.
10. Gomel V: Microsurgical reversal of female sterilization: A reappraisal. *Fertil Steril* 33: 587, 1980.
11. Verhoeven HC: Personal communication, 1980.

39

Uterotubal Implantation

Tommy N. Evans and Amir H. Ansari

Although the uterotubal junction (UTJ) seems essential for reproduction in many mammals, intrauterine pregnancies in women have been achieved following excision of this segment and implantation of the fallopian tube into the cornu or a new site. In addition, either the isthmic or ampullary segments can be implanted.

To ascertain a prognostic index, Levinson[1] suggested a point score that included the length of tube used for implantation, the technical ease of the procedure, and the type of tubal abnormality. Remaining tubal segments of at least 3 cm in length and those implanted because of the patient's desire to reverse a previous sterilization yielded the best results.

Placing one transected end of the tube into a new uterine opening is required for proximal tubal obstruction caused by extensive intraluminal or interstitial disease (i.e., salpingitis isthmica nodosa, unipolar laparoscopic sterilization). The incidence of this procedure in any large series of reported tuboplasties also depends on the surgeon's preference for either tubocornual anastomosis or implantation. When performed because of proximal obstruction caused by inflammatory disease, successful term pregnancies follow in fewer than 20 percent of patients. The percentage of women who become pregnant is probably closer to 40 percent after reversal of a sterilization.

It is sometimes difficult to select the patient for anastomosis or implantation before laparotomy because intraoperative patency testing represents the crucial deciding factor. Tubes are cut transversely about 2 cm (width of the thumb) from the uterine serosal surface with microscissors or a Beaver blade (no. 67) under optical magnification. Tubal patency testing begins by gently attempting to instill indigo carmine through a previously placed intrauterine balloon as additional segments of occluded proximal tube are removed. This maneuver requires patience. When intramural obstruction is confirmed, the decision to perform an implantation becomes inevitable. Hemostasis is obtained with bipolar coagulation under constant irrigation with heparinized lactated Ringer's solution.

The uterine opening is created either in the cornual region or in the posterior part of the corpus at the level of the ovarian ligaments after the myometrium is injected with a solution of Pitressin (20 units to 20 ml of saline). The previously

The Fallopian Tube: Basic Studies and Clinical Contributions, edited by Alvin M. Siegler, M.D. Mount Kisco, New York: Futura Publishing Company, Inc. © 1986.

placed intrauterine catheter is removed. By turning a sharp reamer and applying firm pressure, a good circular hole can be made in the endometrial cavity. There should be minimal bleeding.

The techniques of cornual excision by reamer and scalpel were compared by Rock and coworkers.[2] They analyzed results of uterotubal implantations from 1942 through 1976 and found that cornual reaming was followed by 36 percent intrauterine pregnancies while scalpel excision resulted in only 12 percent.

Once the uterine preparation is completed, attention is directed toward the tubal segment which is prepared for implantation. It is tested for patency by careful retrograde instillation of 1 to 2 ml of indigo carmine and resected until patency is established at its transected end. The implantation sutures (4-0 Vicryl® and Dexon®) are inserted through all three tubal layers at 12 o'clock and 6 o'clock positions, and the tube is incised between them for a short distance (about 1 cm) to create two flaps. About 2 cm of mesosalpinx is cut just beneath these flaps so that they are easily pulled into the uterine opening. The four sutures for implantation are threaded with an appropriately sized needle and brought individually into the uterine cavity and out onto the uterine serosal surface. These sutures, as they exit from the uterus, should be about 0.5 cm from one another, keeping in mind the desire to spread the tubal flaps within the uterine cavity. The extrauterine tubal segment is gently pushed into the new opening by grasping its serosal surface behind the transected end with a small clamp. The uterine and tubal serosa are approximated by several 5-0 absorbable sutures. The sutures on top of the uterus are tied without tension.

Various types of devices have been used as temporary splints to maintain tubal patency. Roland and Leisten[3] used a teflon tubing, anchoring one end in the uterine cavity and bringing the other end either through the abdominal skin or just beneath it with subsequent removal under local anesthesia. The implantation techniques of Madelenat et al.[4] and Cognat and Rochet[5] were performed over a splint removed subsequently either transcervically or transabdominally. The device described by Shirodkar[6] involves a circular polyethylene tubing that is placed into the uterine cavity and the lateral arms are threaded through the uterine cornua and tubes with a small probe.

Peterson and colleagues[7] described the implantation of the distal tubal segment through a posterior transverse incision placed between the insertion of the ovarian ligaments. Ostensibly this technique requires less mobilization of the tubes. Modifications of this approach have been used by Levinson[1] and the author with 50 percent intrauterine term pregnancies postoperatively. Two individual openings were made instead of the one transverse incision but in both situations, cesarean delivery is advised if a successful pregnancy results.

References

1. Levinson CJ: Implantation procedures for intramural obstruction. *J Reprod Med* 26:117, 1981.
2. Rock JA, Katayama KP, Martin EJ, et al: Pregnancy outcome following uterotubal implantation: A comparison of the reamer and sharp cornual wedge techniques. *Fertil Steril* 31:634, 1979.
3. Roland M, and Leisten D: Tuboplasty in 130 patients. *Obstet Gynecol* 39:57, 1972.
4. Madelenat P, DeBrux J, and Palmer R: Étiologie des obstructions tubaires proximales et son rôles dans le pronostic des implantation. *Gynécologie* 28:47, 1977.
5. Cognat M, Rochet Y, Gagnaire JC, et al: Notre expérience de la salpingoplastie. Á propos de 285 cases. *J Gynécol Obstét Biol Reprod* 6:839, 1977.
6. Shirodkar VN: *Contributions to Obstetrics and Gynecology*. Edinburgh: ES Livingstone, 1960.
7. Peterson EP, Musich JR, and Behrman SJ: Uterotubal implantation and obstetric outcome after previous sterilization. *Am J Obstet Gynecol* 128:662, 1977.

40

Fimbrioplasty

Maxwell Roland

Laparoscopy is essential before attempting a fimbrioplasty because in certain women who have distal tubal occlusion with partial patency, chromopertubation can be therapeutic.

Fimbrioplasty is a surgical procedure designed to restore occult fimbriae to their normal position. Sometimes they are completely hidden by a serosal scar so that the tube appears grossly like a hydrosalpinx. Careful palpation of such tubes reveals a terminal nodularity created by the inverted fimbriae. Lysis of the serosal covering along the white lines caused by scarring will reveal the delicate fimbriae. Minimal bleeding is encountered during this procedure.

Another type of fimbrioplasty requires dilatation of a phimotic ostial opening. The latter condition is a less advanced abnormality than the total terminal occlusion previously described and often no tubal incision is required. Using microsurgical techniques, the gynecologist searches for intraluminal adhesions. The special splint devised by this author has been used for both of these tubal abnormalities with excellent results. Of 220 patients who had fimbrioplasty prior to the advent of microsurgery, 51 (23 percent) had term pregnancies postoperatively. With the addition of specific microsurgical principles described elsewhere in this book, the term pregnancy rate was increased to 35 percent in the next 102 patients. Of additional significance, only two tubal pregnancies were reported in the entire series. For this procedure, ophthalmic loupes ($\times 4.5$) afford sufficient magnification and a microelectrode needle, for lysis of adhesions, eliminates the need for sutures.

The special splint is placed in the distal tubal segment after completion of the fimbrioplasty.[1] The device has the configuration of the lumen and prevents reagglutination (Fig. 40:1). One end is anchored to the anterior abdominal wall (Fig. 40:2) and peristaltic activity of the intestinal tract causes movement of the device. This action results in continual movement of the fallopian tube preventing re-formation of adhesions. The central core of this splint is made of malleable copper wire which is covered by teflon tubing.

One end is buried subcutaneously in a corner of the abdominal incision. The splint is removed by traction six to eight weeks postoperatively.

The Fallopian Tube: Basic Studies and Clinical Contributions, edited by Alvin M. Siegler, M.D. Mount Kisco, New York: Futura Publishing Company, Inc. © 1986.

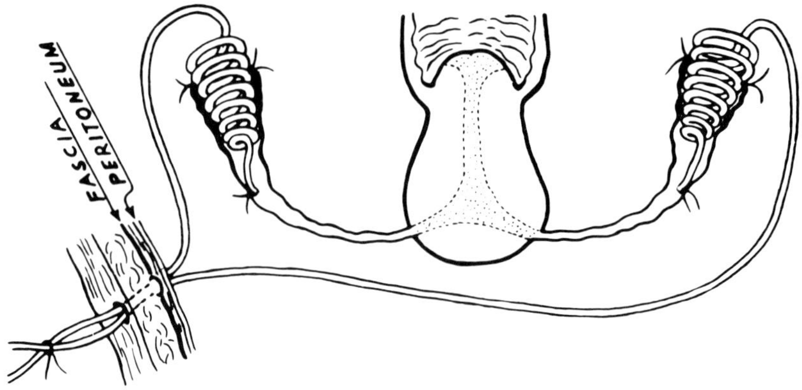

FIGURE 40:1—*The Roland stent.*

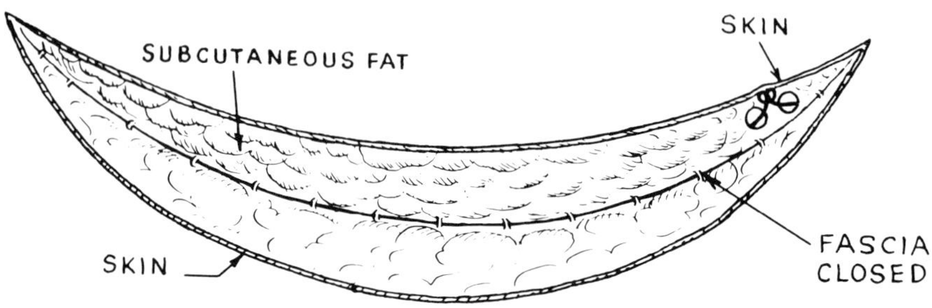

FIGURE 40:2—*One end of the Roland stent is fixed to the abdominal wall beneath the skin.*

Reference

1. Roland M, and Leisten D: New Approaches to Tuboplasty. In Phillips JM (Ed): *Microsurgery in Gynecology.* Downey, CA: AAGL, 1977: p. 96.

41

Microsutures in Tubal Surgery

Arthur Leader and
Patrick J. Taylor

The advent of gynecologic microsurgery that followed the initial work of Swolin[1] has stimulated the interest of gynecologists in the development of fine sutures. Most manufacturers restrict the term "microsutures" to 8-0 or smaller sutures. In the selection of an appropriate microsuture for gynecology, most attention has focused on the material rather than on either the needle or the suture size. The needles are curved, have a total length of 4 to 6 mm, a chord length of 3 to 5 mm, and a wire diameter of 15 to 140 μ. The curve most commonly used is 3/8 (105° to 135° arc). Taper points are less traumatic. An 8-0 or 9-0 suture size is considered optimum. Independent of the skill of the operator, a braided suture is more pliable, ties and holds a knot more readily, and is not apt to fracture as easily as a monofilament suture when grasped with instruments.[2] Controversy has focused on whether to choose an absorbable or a permanent suture and which absorbable suture is the best, polyglactin 910 (Vicryl®), polyglycolic acid (Dexon®) or polydioxanone (PDS®).

Selection of Suture Material

Suture material induces a cellular response that is generally mild but can be altered if the tissue is traumatized. Initially, in response to the suture, there is a neutrophilic infiltration that is replaced in about three days by monocytes, plasma cells, and lymphocytes. The rate at which wound healing and suture absorption occur depends on local and systemic health, suture size and type.[3] Depending on these factors, cellular enzyme activity is significant with chromic surgical gut and minimal with Vicryl® and Dexon®. Macrophagic lysosomal hydrolytic activity is important for surgical gut absorption, but it is a minor consideration for the breakdown of synthetic absorbable sutures to carbon dioxide and water[4] and of almost no consequence for nonabsorbable sutures. Vicryl® and Dexon® contain copolymers that are considered ester analogs of a glycine-alanine polyamino acid. As such, they are a structural analog of a simple protein. The hydrolysable linkages

The Fallopian Tube: Basic Studies and Clinical Contributions, edited by Alvin M. Siegler, M.D. Mount Kisco, New York: Futura Publishing Company, Inc. © 1986.

are hydrolytically degradable so that water can split the molecule into increasingly smaller fragments in a pH-dependent reaction that closely mimics the natural absorption process of catgut after lysosomal enzyme activity.[5] The proportion of the component parts and the orientation and crystallinity of the molecules can be controlled to provide predictable initial tensile strength, absorption rate,[5] and in-vivo decline of tensile strength.

Many comparative animal studies have been carried out on sutures concerning foreign body responses, tensile strength, and rates of absorption. Implantation sites in the rat gluteal muscle and rabbit and rat reproductive tissues have been used to compare sutures for these features.

In the rat gluteal muscle, the tissue response was assessed by considering cell density, the presence of neutrophils, giant cells, macrophages, and other types of cells. The absorption rate was measured by evaluating the cross-sectional area of suture remaining after given periods of implantation. The tensile strength of the suture was evaluated at 0, 50, 90, 180, and 390 days after implantation for nonabsorbable sutures and at 0, 7, 14, 18, and 21 days for the absorbable material, using an Instron Universal Materials Testing instrument to measure breaking strength.[4] In addition to changes in the physical properties of the suture and histologic reaction to the material, pregnancy rates and scanning electron microscopy were used in suture comparisons. Most studies relating to reproductive tissues focused on comparing histologic reactions to different suture materials. Clinical studies have not been conclusive because the underlying tubal disorder and surgeon's skill are more important to the outcome.

Although Khoo and Mackay,[6] and Winston[7] have described extensive tissue reactions provoked by the use of catgut suture, many university departments still teach its use for tubal repair.[8] With the introduction of Vicryl® and Dexon® about a decade ago, an alternative to catgut became available and consequently the use of catgut in infertility operations is contraindicated.

The criteria that have been used to compare absorbable and nonabsorbable microsutures, to a large extent, were established by researchers working for suture manufacturing companies. Cutright[9] and Craig[10] used a complicated system to assess tissue responses in nonreproductive animal tissue. Craig[10] noted no significant difference in the breaking strength of either Dexon® or Vicryl® after implantation at 0, 7, 14, 16, 21, 28, or 35 days. Vicryl® virtually disappeared by 70 days after implantation but Dexon® was still present at 120 days.[10] No significant difference in tensile or wound strength was demonstrated when 10-0 nylon and 7-0 Dexon® were compared.

Riddick and colleagues[11] established a sliding qualitative and quantitative scale for assessing the degree of inflammatory infiltrate and fibroblastic proliferation in reaction to sutures. Tissue blocks were fixed in 10 percent neutral buffered formalin, embedded in paraffin and tissue was stained with hematoxylin and eosin. The inflammatory response was graded from zero to 4; 1+ = minimal reaction, 2+ = mild reaction, 3+ = moderate reaction, 4+ = severe reaction. Gomel and his colleagues[12] compared polyglactin-910, polyethylene, and nylon and they prepared the tissue blocks similarly but used the Van Giesen stain in addition to the hematoxylin and eosin stain to study the degree of fibrosis. The degree of infiltration by mononuclear histiocytes was graded as follows: 0 = no infiltrate, + = minimal infiltrate, + + = moderate infiltrate, + + + = marked infiltrate. Similarly, the multinucleated giant cell reaction was graded as follows: 0 = no reaction, + = minimal reaction, + + = moderate reaction, + + + = marked reaction. No comment was made on the degree of fibrosis resulting from each type of microsuture but in a subsequent paper from this group[13] the degree of fibrosis was analyzed. Sojo and coauthors,[14] in addition, compared fertility rates. A study by Leader and colleagues compared modi-

Table 41:1

Tissue Reaction to Microsutures: Dexon® and Vicryl®

	14 days		30 days		90 days	
	Dexon®	Vicryl®	Dexon®	Vicryl®	Dexon®	Vicryl®
Riddick et al.[11]	1.89 ± 0.15	1.95 ± 0.16	Not done		1.05 ±0.18	0.77 ± 0.10
	NS				p>0.05	
Leader et al.[15]	Not done		+	0/+	0	0/+

Table 41:2

Tissue Reaction to Microsutures: Polyglactin-910 (Vicryl®), Nylon (Ethilon®), Polypropylene (Prolene®) and Polydioxanone (PDS®)

	24–30 days				80–90 days			
	Vicryl®	Ethilon®	Prolene®	PDS®	Vicryl®	Ethilon®	Prolene®	PDS®
Gomel et al[12]	++	0	0/+	Not done	0	0/+	0/+	Not done
Sojo et al.[14]	++	+	Not done	Not done	0	+	Not done	Not done
Delbeke et al.[13]	+	0	0	0/+	+	0	0	0
DeCherney et al.[16]	++	Not done	Not done	0/+	++	Not done	Not done	0

fied Vicryl® and Dexon® microsutures (Tables 41:1 and 41:2).

Riddick and coauthors[11] reported Vicryl® superior to Dexon®. The degree of fibrosis did not necessarily correspond to external tissue adhesions. Adhesions were maximal at the surgical knot regardless of the material used and polyglactic sutures produced less tissue reaction in the rabbit's uterine horn.[9] Leader and colleagues confirmed these findings at 30 days but were unable to show any significant difference at 90 days. Other reports[12–14] suggested that after 80 days polyglactin-910 resulted in less inflammation and fibrosis when compared to nylon or polypropylene. Polydioxanone (PDS®) caused less tissue reaction and fibrosis at 80 days after placement in the rabbit than did polyglactin-910.[13,16]

Based on tensile and wound strength, and tissue reaction, any of the three available absorbable microsuture materials may be used for tubal repair in the 8-0 to 10-0 range. The selection of suture material from among these three should be decided by their availability, handling properties, needle attachments, and cost.

With all of these studies, the assessment was subjective even though the slides were given to the pathologists as unknowns. The method for assessment was less rigorous than that initially outlined by Craig[10] and no statistically significant differences in results were obtained. In addition, most studies did not correlate fertility with histology.

Future Possibilities

A combination of thrombin (15 NIH units/ml) and fibrinogen in the presence of an aprotinin calcium chloride solution has been used to form a fibrin glue.[17] The tissue reaction observed when fibrin was used appeared no greater than with microsurgical sutures. Laser beams used for tissue approximation do not present any advantages over current conventional methods.[18] With further developments and modifications, these two approaches may provide better alternatives to oviductal reconstruction. Anastomosis using fine absorbable microsutures are still the most effective means for tubal reparative surgery.[19]

Conclusion

Gynecologic microsurgery has developed from an experimental technique to an integral part of clinical infertility practice and the skill of the surgeon remains the most significant factor in postoperative fertility. No significant difference exists between the absorbable sutures if tensile strength, wound strength, and tissue reaction are compared, despite the fact that Dexon® remains in the tissue longer than Vicryl® or PDS.® Recent studies with PDS® suggest that it shares the handling properties of the nonabsorbable monofilament material and the absorbable, less reactive properties of Vicryl® and Dexon®. Other methods for tissue approximation such as CO_2 laser or fibrin glue have so far not proved superior to existing microsutures.[13]

References

1. Swolin K: Fertilitätsoperationen. I. Literatur und Methodik. *Acta Obstet Gynecol Scand* 46:234, 1967.
2. Corson SL, and Smith DC: Principles and instrumentation of microsurgery. *Clin Obstet Gynecol* 23: 1201, 1980.
3. Holtz G: Adhesion induction by sutures of varying tissue reactivity and caliber. *Int J Fertil* 27: 134, 1982.
4. Allen H: Principles of wound healing and suture material. *Am Coll Obstet Gynecol*, Copenhagen, October 1983.
5. Dunlap WA, Purnell WD, and McPherson SD: A new synthetic absorbable suture for ophthalmic surgery: Laboratory and clinical evaluation. *South Med J* 69: 588, 1976.
6. Khoo SK, and Mackay EV: Reactions in rabbit fallopian tube after plastic reconstruction. I. Gross pathology, tubal patency and pregnancy. *Fertil Steril* 23:201, 1972.
7. Winston RML: Microsurgical reanastomosis of the rabbit oviduct and its functional and pathological sequelae. *Br J Obstet Gynaecol Br Commonwlth* 82:513, 1975.
8. Hartko WJ, Chanekar G, and Kemmann E: Suture materials currently used in obstetric-gynecologic surgery in the United States: A questionnaire survey. *Obstet Gynecol* 59:241, 1982.
9. Cutright DE, Beasley JC, and Perez B: Histologic comparison of polyglactic and polyglycolic acid sutures. *Oral Surg* 32:165, 1971.
10. Craig PH, Williams JA, Davis KW, et al: A biologic comparison of polyglactin-910 and polyglycolic acid synthetic absorbable sutures. *Surg Gynecol Obstet* 141:1, 1975.
11. Riddick DH, De Grazia CT, and Maenza RM: Comparison of polyglactic and polyglycolic acid sutures in reproductive tissue. *Fertil Steril* 28:1220, 1977.
12. Gomel V, McComb P, and Boer-Meisel M: Histologic reactions to polyglactin-910, polyethylene and nylon microsuture. *J Reprod Med* 25:56, 1980.
13. Delbeke LO, Gomel V, McComb P, et al: Histologic reaction to four synthetic microsutures in the rabbit. *Fertil Steril* 40:248, 1983.
14. Sojo D, Pardo JD, and Nistal M: Histology and fertility after microsurgical anastomosis of the rabbit fallopian tube with nylon and polyglactin sutures. *Fertil Steril* 39:707, 1983.
15. Leader A, Fisher A, Malkinson T, et al: A comparison of a new microsurgical suture in the rabbit model. *Fertil Steril* (in press).
16. DeCherney A, and Laufer N: The use of a new synthetic absorbable monofilament suture, polydioxanone (PDS) for surgery. *Fertil Steril* 39:401, 1983.
17. Scheidel PH, Wallweiner DR, Wiedeman RA, et al: Experimental anastomosis of the rabbit fallopian tube us-

ing fibrin glue. *Fertil Steril* 38:471, 1982.

18. Klink F, Grosspietzch R, von Klitzing L, et al: Animal in vivo studies and in vitro experiments with human tubes for end-to-end anastomotic operation by CO_2 laser technique. *Fertil Steril* 30:100, 1978.
19. Siegler AM: Microsurgery for reconstruction. In Phillips JM (Ed): *Microsurgery in Gynecology*. Downey, CA: AAGL, 1977: p 82.

42

Assessing the Results of Tuboplasty

Geoffrey Chamberlain

The results of any operation may be assessed either subjectively or objectively, the former by the contentment of the patient and the satisfaction of the surgeon. Objective assessment involves events that measure the success of the operation.

With tuboplasty, subjective evaluations are probably best not used as an audit for performance because most women are satisfied that the surgeon has operated and they feel better that something has been done. Sometimes, they have no idea of the extent of the tubal damage preoperatively or of the postoperative evaluation. Objective measurements are better for assessing results since tubal patency can be ascertained by salpingography or gas insufflation but these tests represent anatomical results; the successful outcome is the production of a viable baby. Spontaneous abortions or tubal gestations are not therapeutic triumphs.

The number of term pregnancies following tuboplasty has definitely increased during the past 20 years. Most gynecologists agree that the creation of postoperative tubal patency in a previously occluded tube is a positive objective finding, although only a successful pregnancy can be considered the hallmark of ultimate success.

Although it has been difficult to attribute a specific factor in this general improvement in outcome, certainly the advent of the microsurgical techniques and a more careful selection of patients have contributed to this progress. Nevertheless, even with the use of hysterosalpingography and laparoscopy, most women who are operated on for distal tubal obstruction do not become pregnant. Thus far, it has not been possible to predetermine which type of distally occluded tube will not permit normal transport of gametes, fertilization, and movement of the cleaving zygote into the uterine cavity.

Few gynecologists do enough tuboplasties to make a proper statistical evaluation of their work. Some of them have published results of three or four hundred operations, but during these years operative techniques changed and selection of patients was altered. Other surveys report

The Fallopian Tube: Basic Studies and Clinical Contributions, edited by Alvin M. Siegler, M.D. Mount Kisco, New York: Futura Publishing Company, Inc. © 1986.

the results of several surgeons, either at one center or diversely situated; in these, technical variations often occur. Even if the surgical procedures are similar, the pathological tubal involvement or nature and degree of pelvic adhesions vary with each woman. Finally, the selection of women who are operated on varies depending on the facilities available and the skill and interest of the surgeon. Indeed, selection of patients can change in the same hospital at different times. For these reasons, the range of successful results after tubal surgery could be ascribed to the variability of the population selected and the range of tubal pathology rather than the surgical procedures. Such factors make it difficult to assess the different techniques that might improve the outcome.

Statistically, the variability of patient selection or tubal abnormality could be reduced by performing randomized clinical trials with the same surgeons and standard techniques. Such an experiment appears unlikely.

It is feasible to standardize the degree of adnexal abnormality so that at least similar cases can be compared. Such a classification has been recommended by the American Fertility Society and it should be used. A classification can also be devised for the procedures performed and the adjuncts used.

For proximal tubal obstruction, fundotomy and tubal implantation have been common and viable pregnancies result in between 10 and 48 percent. Microsurgery has enabled a careful shaving off of the obstructed nipple of the intramural tube until patency is established with a dilute indigo carmine or methylene blue solution. After microscopic evaluation reveals that the dissection has been carried into healthy tissue, an anastomosis may be performed. The risk is then minimal for reocclusion as the fibrotic tissue is progressively resected with a scalpel or scissors. After tubocornual anastomosis, an incidence of viable pregnancies of up to 64 percent has been noted.

With the exception of microsurgery for tuboanastomosis, the success rate from tuboplasty is much less than 50 percent despite patency in over 80 percent of the operations. It becomes obvious that the opening of a closed tube does not solve the infertility problem. The infertility specialist should always check all the fertility features preoperatively by including a properly timed postcoital test and an endometrial biopsy. Too often the basic studies are bypassed in the rush to overcome mechanical, pelvic factors.

Perioperative Adjunctive Measures

Surgeons seeking to improve the results of tubal surgery are moving to microsurgical techniques, and certain perioperative medications have been used primarily to reduce the incidence of postoperative pelvic adhesions. Intraoperative use of irrigating fluids such as high-molecular Dextran and heparinized Ringer's lactate and tubal splints in selected types of tuboplasty are recommended by some authors, but their value remains unproven. The other adjuncts used to improve results include pharmacological doses of steroids and antihistamines, prophylactic antibiotics, nonsteroidal antiinflammatory agents, and hydropertubation.

Keeping in mind all the difficulties described above, comparison of conventional or macrosurgery with microsurgery shows no real difference except in the category of anastomosis. Although magnification helps a surgeon to be more precise and results in improved patency rates, the intrauterine term pregnancy rate following salpingoneostomy and fimbrioplasty has not increased significantly with the addition of microsurgical procedures.

In-vitro fertilization and embryo transplant will certainly replace tuboplasty in selected instances, such as in patients who have damaged tubes in whom previous experience has taught us to expect minimal success. The results with in-vitro fertilization and embryo transfer are going to improve so that it is only possible to propose tuboplasty in patients seeking reversal of the sterilization.

Table 42:1
Selected Published Results on Tuboplasty

Author	*Number of patients*	*Type of tuboplasty*	*Term pregnancies*
Hanton et al.[1]	32	*Salpingostomy*	1 (3%)
Siegler and Kontopoulos[2]	11		2 (18%)
Mettler et al.[3]	38		10 (26%)
Grant[4]	268	*Salpingolysis*	108 (40%)
Young et al.[5]	47		15 (32%)
Roland and Leisten[6]	135		41 (31%)
Caspi et al.[7]	57		28 (49%)
Timonen and Nieminen[8]	68	*Midtubal reanastomosis*	18 (12%)
Siegler and Perez[9]	46		14 (30%)
McCormick et al.[10]	53		26 (49%)
Gomel[11]	83		26 (31%)
Winston[12]	126	*Tubotubal reanastomosis with microsurgery*	73 (58%)
Gomel[11]	118		76 (64%)
Hanton et al.[1]	22	*Cornual reaming and implantation*	10 (48%)
Wirtz[13]	48		20 (42%)
Grant[4]	73		19 (26%)
Mulligan and Rock[14]	48	*Fundotomy and implantation*	5 (10%)
Peterson et al.[15]	16		7 (44%)

Results must always be assessed according to their source. The results reported are usually published by the more enthusiastic surgeons and from those who feel the results are good. However, most constructive or conservative operations are not being reported, possibly because of a reluctance to publish and not necessarily because the results are poor.

To assess the contributions of microsurgery, it is necessary to compare the results with conventional or macrosurgery. Even so, other variables enter into the evaluation, such as: the dexterity of the individual surgeon, the use of alternate cases, the type of operation, the nature of the tubal abnormality, the fertility potential of the couple exclusive of the tubal disease, and the histologic evaluation of the excised tissue. Obviously, therefore, scientific comparisons become extremely difficult.

Associated factors include peritubal, peritoneal, and ovarian mechanical problems, their nature and extent. The same tubal operation will not give the same result if severe periovarian adhesions are present and require removal in addition.

Interpretation of the extent of tubal damage with methods at our disposal is still unscientific. These methods yield rather little information concerning the functional capacity of the oviducts. Scanning electron microscopy and the study of cilia and their capacity to regenerate are being evaluated for their prognostic import.

Even classification of types of operations causes difficulty because of differences in terminology, borderline cases, and asymmetrical lesions.

Aside from the surgeon's experience and the type of tubal repair, other intraoperative and perioperative factors can influence the outcome, including the use of prophylactic antibiotics, their type and material, the kind of suture material, the use of splints, additional pelvic operations (e.g., uterine suspension and appendectomy), and hydropertubation.

In the evaluation of the outcome, the variability in measuring success can be affected by the number of women lost to follow-up, the duration of their follow-up, intercurrent pelvic disease, and postoperative contraception.

Results from the recent literature of tubal operations were analyzed according to the tubal segment operated on (Table 42:1). Repair of the distal end results in a 3 to 49 percent incidence of viable pregnancies. The divisions may be artificial, since the salpingoneostomy and fimbrioplasty and salpingolysis are often reported together. In this group, the degree of pathological involvement needs most careful analysis so as to make valid comments about the results. Success relates, also, to the degree and type of adhesions. Tubes damaged by infection are not so successfully repaired as those affected by endometriosis.

After conventional macrosurgery, viable pregnancies are reported in from 12 to 49 percent of patients following midsegment anastomosis (Table 42:1.) The operations for reversing sterilization are being greatly improved with the use of microsurgery because this enables precise trimming of the occluded ends, better apposition of tubal layers, and more accurate placement of the sutures. Most important, microsurgery teaches gentle handling of tissues. Term pregnancies have been reported in up to 70 percent of patients at the microsurgical reversal of nonelectric methods of sterilization.

Many try to improve their results by being more meticulous, using new techniques and paying more attention to details of surgery. These of course are important but, as a background, the results could also be improved by some of the simpler actuarial methods discussed in this chapter. Better data collection and improved patient selection would obviously improve results but would bar the potential advantages of tubal surgery to some couples. Better documentation of what we do would allow a more precise comparison from one center to another, thus highlighting any outstandingly good (or bad) points of technique which other surgeons could note.

References

1. Hanton EM, Pratt JH, and Banner EA: Tubal plastic surgery at the Mayo Clinic. *Am J Obstet Gynecol* 89:934, 1964.
2. Siegler AM, and Kontopoulos V: An analysis of macrosurgical and microsurgical techniques in the management of the tuboperitoneal factor in infertility. *Fertil Steril* 32:377, 1979.
3. Mettler L, Giesel H, and Semm K: Treatment of female infertility due to tubal obstruction by operative laparoscopy. *Fertil Steril* 32:384, 1979.
4. Grant A: Infertility surgery of the oviduct. *Fertil Steril* 22:496, 1971.
5. Young PE, Egan JE, Barlow JJ, et al: Reconstructive surgery for infertility at the Boston Hospital for Women. *Am J Obstet Gynecol* 108:1092, 1974.
6. Roland M, and Leisten D: Advances in tuboplasty. *Acta Obstet Gynecol Scand* 56:419, 1977.
7. Caspi E, Halperin Y, and Bukovski I: The importance of periadnexal adhesions in tubal reconstructive surgery for infertility. *Fertil Steril* 31:296, 1979.
8. Timonen S, and Nieminen V: Tubal pregnancy: A choice of operative method of treatment. *Acta Obstet Gynecol Scand* 46:327, 1967.
9. Siegler AM, and Perez R: Reconstruction of fallopian tubes in previously sterilized patients. *Fertil Steril* 26:383, 1985.
10. McCormick WG, Torres J, and McCanne LR: Tubal reanastomosis: An update. *Fertil Steril* 31:689, 1979.
11. Gomel VL: Microsurgical reversal of female sterilization. A reappraisal. *Fertil Steril* 33:587, 1980.
12. Winston RKL: Microsurgery of the fal-

lopian tube: From fantasy to reality. *Fertil Steril* 34:521, 1980.
13. Wirtz JW: Experience with a method for implantation of fallopian tube into the uterus. *Aust NZ J Obstet Gynaecol* 5:7, 1965.
14. Mulligan WJ, and Rock J: Surgical treatment of infertility. In Meigs J (Ed): *Progress in Gynaecology*, New York: Grune and Stratton, 1957.
15. Peterson EP, Musich J, and Behrman J: Uterotubal implantation and obstetric outcome after sterilization. In Phillips JM (Ed): *Microsurgery and Gynecology*, Downey, CA: AAGL, 1977: p. 152.

43

Techniques for Endoscopic Tubal Operations

Kurt Semm

Endoscopic tubal operations can replace the conventional procedures performed during a laparotomy in most instances. Prerequisites are a trained gynecologic surgeon, a knowledge of diagnostic and therapeutic uses of pelviscopy (laparoscopy), and the availability of a fine set of proper endoscopic instruments.

For proper observation, a good endoscope is essential. It should be at least 5 mm in diameter with a 30° angle. For extended endoscopic operations on the tubes (e.g., salpingolysis, salpingostomy), a 10 mm scope is preferable because it can also be used for full-frame slide photography, cinematography and tape recording. During diagnostic laparoscopy, chromopertubation is performed. Tubal abnormalities detected by this method include congenital malformations, proximal and distal obstructions, salpingitis isthmica nodosa, and fimbrial phimosis. Pelvic endometriosis and the type and extent of periadnexal adhesions are discerned.

Instruments for Endoscopic Intraabdominal Operations

The newly developed endoscopic instruments and optimal pelviscopic techniques can replace 80 percent of laparotomies indicated for ovarian and tubal surgery.

For several years at the Department of Obstetrics and Gynecology, University of Kiel, the diagnosis and treatment of about 79 percent of patients with tubal stenosis or occlusion have been combined during laparoscopy. The findings at laparoscopy provide the indication for tubal surgery either through the laparoscope or by laparotomy. Whenever therapeutic laparoscopy seems possible, it is performed at once. This approach has become possible since the establishment of better instruments for endocoagulation.

The operative laparoscope with lateral light insertion and direct instrument canal is not suitable for pelviscopic surgery. This monocular optic gives no

The Fallopian Tube: Basic Studies and Clinical Contributions, edited by Alvin M. Siegler, M.D. Mount Kisco, New York: Futura Publishing Company, Inc. © 1986.

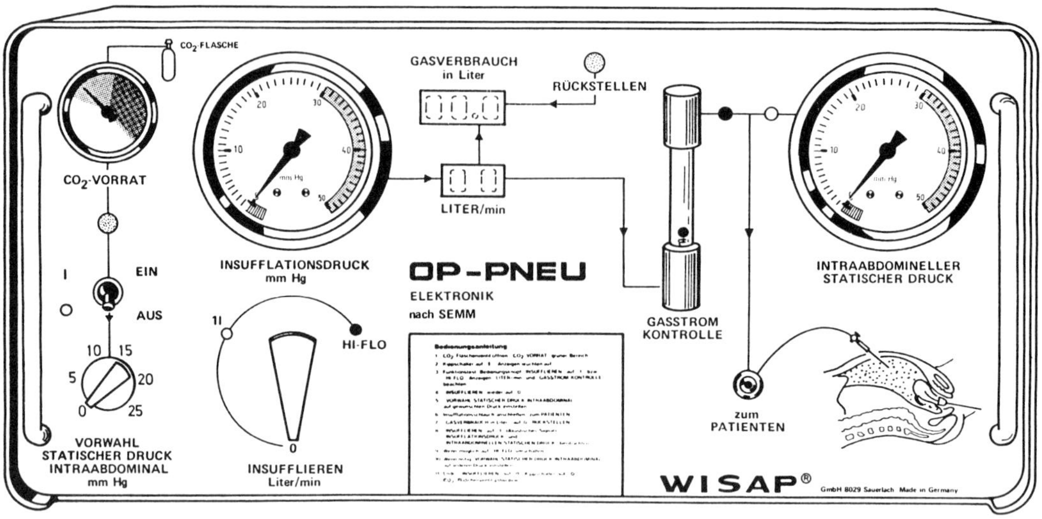

FIGURE 43:1—*OP-PNEU-Electronic® according to Semm for atraumatic CO_2 gas pneumoperitoneum for pelviscopic operations.*

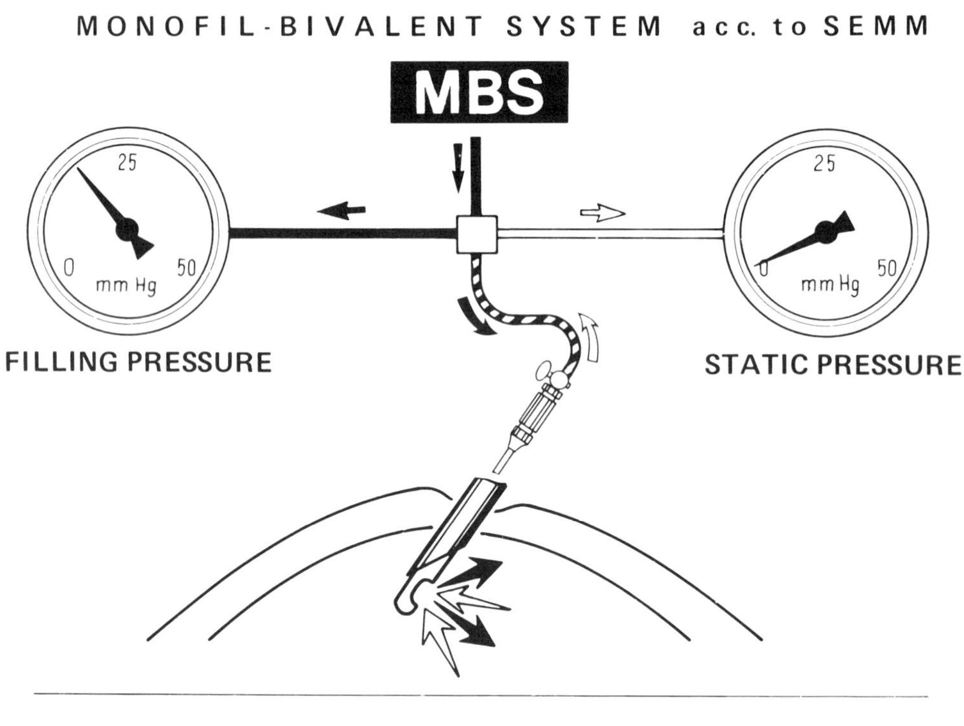

FIGURE 43:2—*Monofil-bivalent system for the electronically controlled CO_2 pneumoperitoneum: one-hole system for insufflation and measurement of the actual intra-abdominal pressure.*

stereoscopic view and operations performed parallel to the optical axis becomes dangerous because of false impressions of the size, depth, and mobility of the organs.

For extended endoscopic surgery, the electronically controlled Op-Pneu-Elektronik® is recommended (Fig. 43:1). The apparatus measures electronically and continuously the static intraabdom-

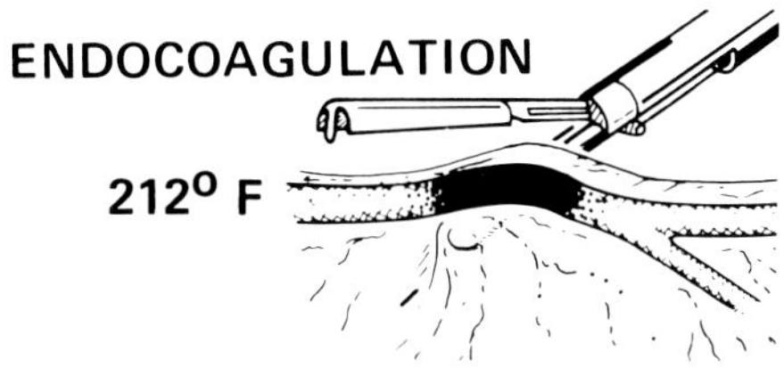

FIGURE 43:3—*Optimal protein coagulation with 212°F for secure hemostasis with the crocodile forceps.*

inal pressure (Fig. 43:2). Any necessary replacement of gas is automatically monitored, up to a flow volume of 5 L/min. Even with repeated change of instruments, and potentially considerable loss of gas, surgery is possible under the same constant conditions as having the abdomen open. Without the Op-Pneu-Elektronik, endoscopic surgical interventions are more difficult. The surgeon is obliged to measure the static pressure and to control the pneumoperitoneum, which prolongs the operation.

Endoscopic surgical procedures can be performed with minimal bleeding. A possible explanation may be that vascular dilatation provoked during laparotomy does not occur during pelviscopy. Postoperative intestinal ileus is rare following pelviscopy.

High-frequency current (monopolar or bipolar) is contraindicated for hemostasis because this current follows the path of lowest resistance and travels mainly through vessels and nerves to the ovary. These structures warm up so that ovarian hemostasis with high-frequency current at 57°C starts the destruction of the thermolabile enzymes and brings about destruction of the nutritive ovarian vessels and nerves. Since it is not our aim to damage the highly sensitive rete ovarii during diagnostic and therapeutic procedures, the use of high-frequency current should be rejected for endoscopic surgery.

Hemostasis is obtained by coagulating proteins at 100°C (Fig. 43:3). Thereafter, the proteins are not sequestered, as after high-frequency burning followed by carbonization. The endocoagulator, whose energy source is a 12 volt car battery of transformed electricity, electronically monitors the heat of the crocodile forceps, point coagulator, and myoma enucleator (Fig. 43:4). An electronic monitor gives a visual and acoustic record of the coagulation temperature.

Following ovarian biopsy, lysis of adhesions, and enucleation of ovarian cysts coagulation techniques and the endosuture set with an extracorporeal knotting can be used to effect hemostasis (Figs. 43:5–43:8).

Instruments for endoscopic abdominal surgery have been developed during the past two decades. All must be available before starting endoscopic ovarian or tubal surgery because one missing instrument may necessitate a laparotomy. The large needle for hemostasis in the abdominal wall is of utmost importance because bleeding sometimes occurs near the abdominal scars of patients who have had previous abdominal operations. The suture remains for one or two days and guarantees secure hemostasis even without a laparotomy.

The dilatation set is also helpful (Fig. 43:9). It enables an immediate, nearly atraumatic dilatation of the 5 mm trocar sheath to an 11 mm trocar following insertion of bigger endoscopes, larger forceps, and the tissue puncher.

With the Aqua-purator® and the monofilar bivalent washing grip (Fig. 43:10), irrigation of the lower pelvis with saline solution during and after operation can be carried out. It guarantees a clear operative field (e.g., in case of partially ruptured tubal pregnancy) and landmarks in the lower pelvis will be reestablished. This procedure helps to reduce formation of postoperative adhesions. Washing with one to three liters of saline is necessary when pelviscopic surgery is performed. It is very easy with the Aqua-purator. During tubal surgery, the ampulla can be washed out with the washing grip.

General Techniques for Endoscopic Intraabdominal Operations

Preoperative preparation must be carried out before starting endoscopic surgery. The patient requires a good cleansing enema so that the small intestine can

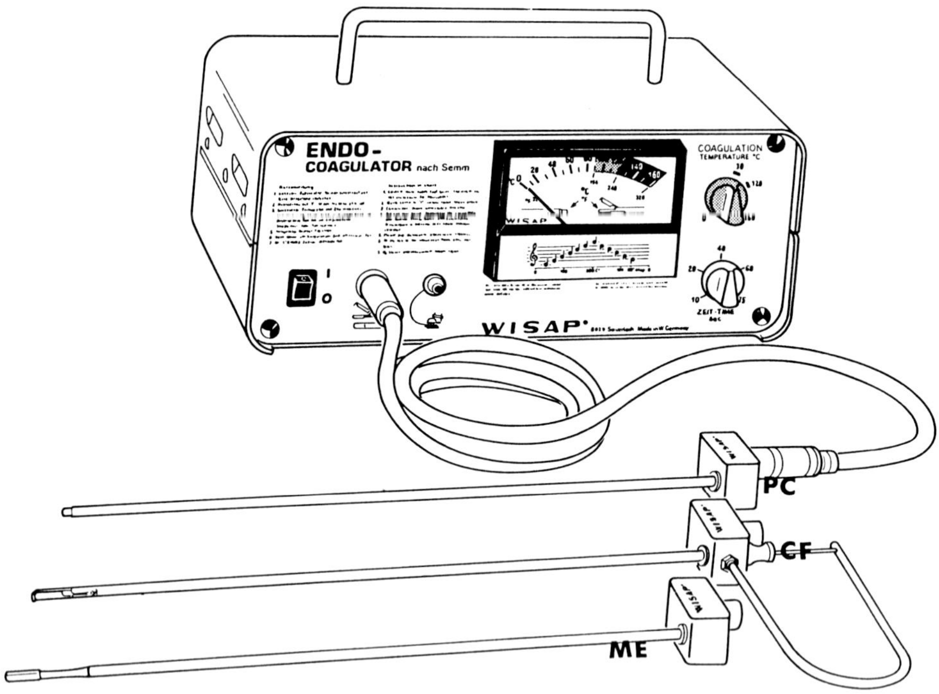

FIGURE 43:4—*Endocoagulator for secure hemostasis, ovario- and salpingolysis, myoma enucleation, etc., with the help of the following instruments: crocodile forceps (CF), point-coagulator (PC), and myoma enucleator (ME).*

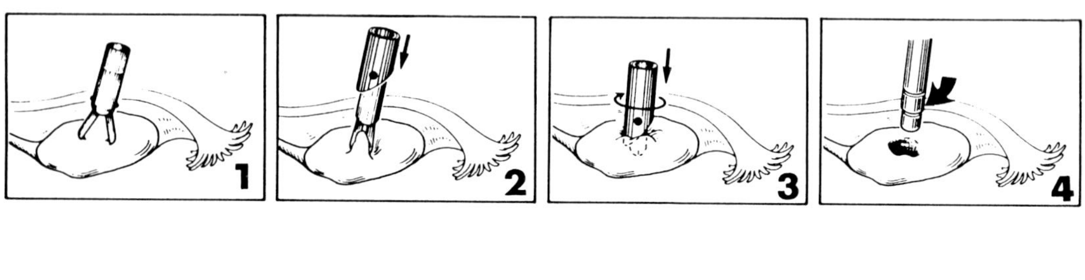

FIGURE 43:5—*After the ovarian tissue is grasped (1, 2), ovarian biopsy is performed by pushing down (arrows) the elliptical-shaped trocar sheath (2, 3). Hemostasis is secured (4) with the point-coagulator (curved arrow).*

be pushed into the upper abdomen without difficulty and the presence of a dilated sigmoid colon and rectum is avoided. When the intestines have been properly prepared and a 15° Trendelenburg position is maintained, the surgeon has a better view into the pelvis than with a laparotomy.

The point coagulator coagulates small biopsy wounds. The crocodile forceps

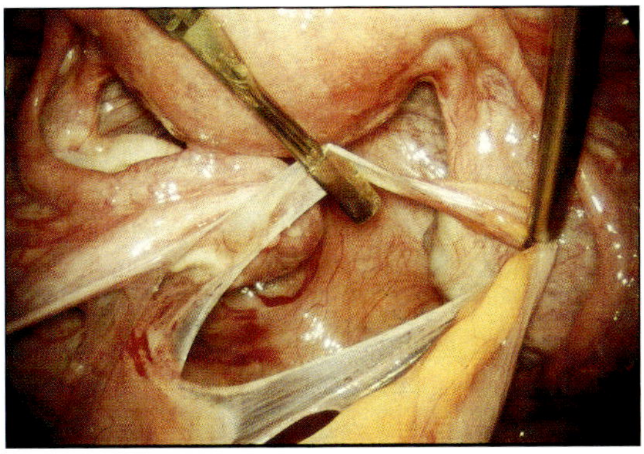

FIGURE 43:21—*Avascular adhesions are coagulated at 110°C, then cut and removed. This laparoscopic sequence prevents reformation of adhesions.*

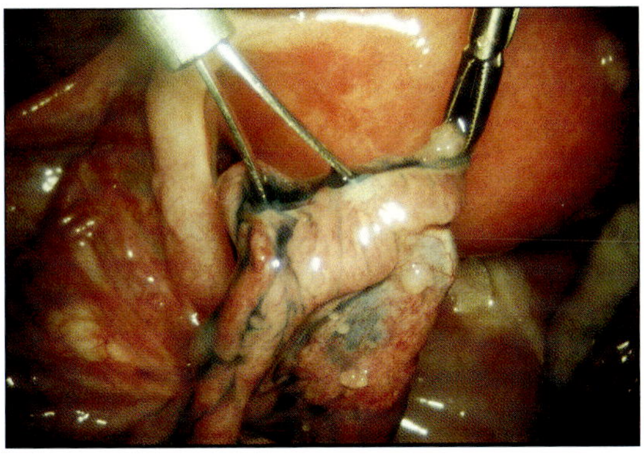

FIGURE 43:22—*Laparoscopic fimbrioplasty is accomplished after chromopertubation by holding the distal end of the tube with an atraumatic grasping forceps and inserting a tong forceps into the fimbriated end; the spreading jaws of this instrument dilate and stretch the tubal opening.*

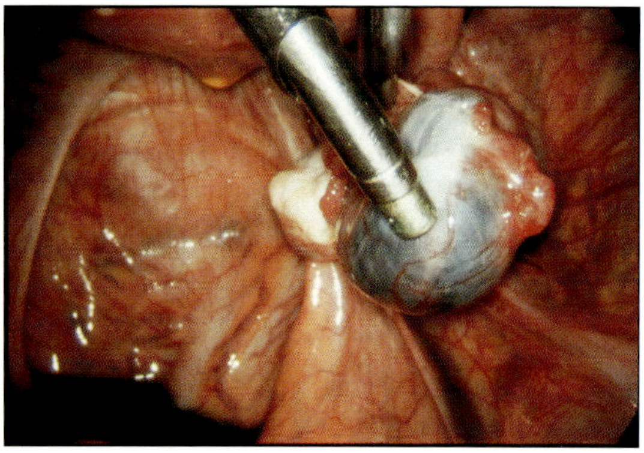

FIGURE 43:23a—*The hydrosalpinx has been dilated with colored dye and the point coagulator creates an area of coagulation from 5 mm to 15 mm in length.*

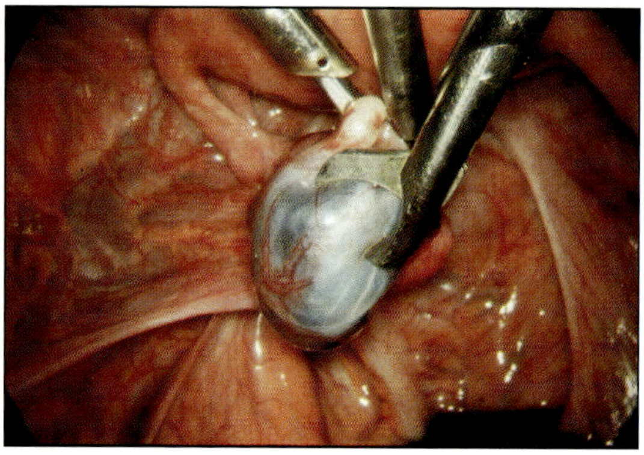

FIGURE 43:23b—*The hook scissors cuts the devascularized section while the tube is held steady with atraumatic forceps.*

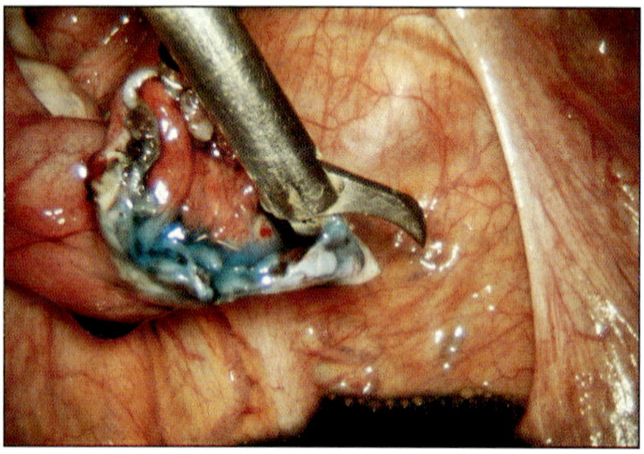

FIGURE 43:23c—*The tube is opened further and the endosalpinx appears with a good rugal pattern.*

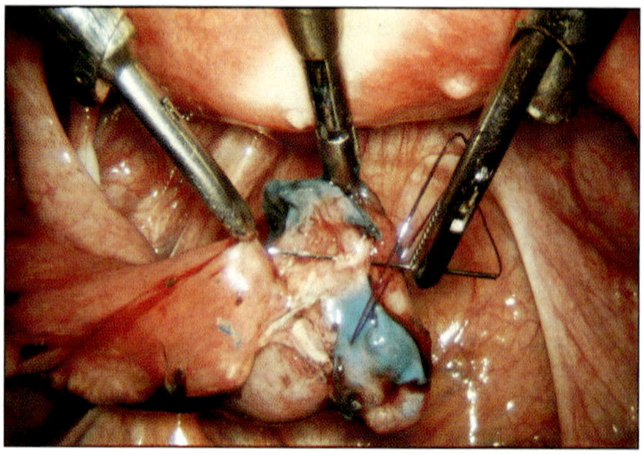

FIGURE 43:23d—*Sutures are inserted to form a cuff salpingonesotomy.*

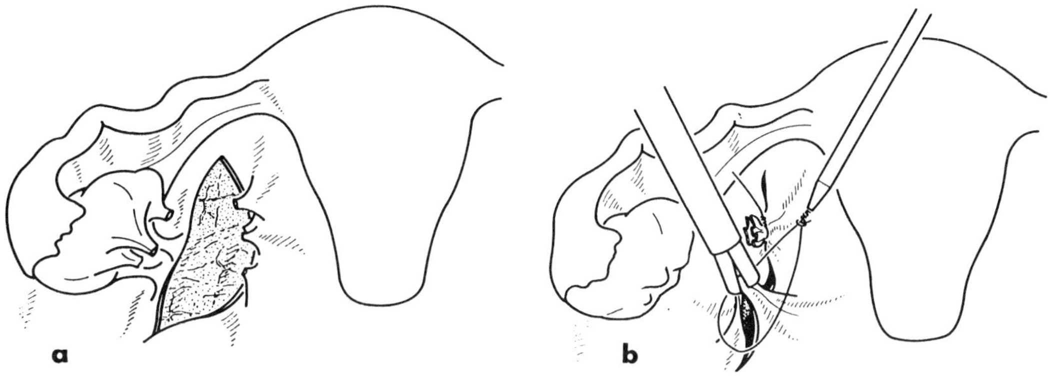

FIGURE 43:6—*Closure of parametrial wound edges after (a) ovariolysis with the help of (b) Roeder-loop ligation.*

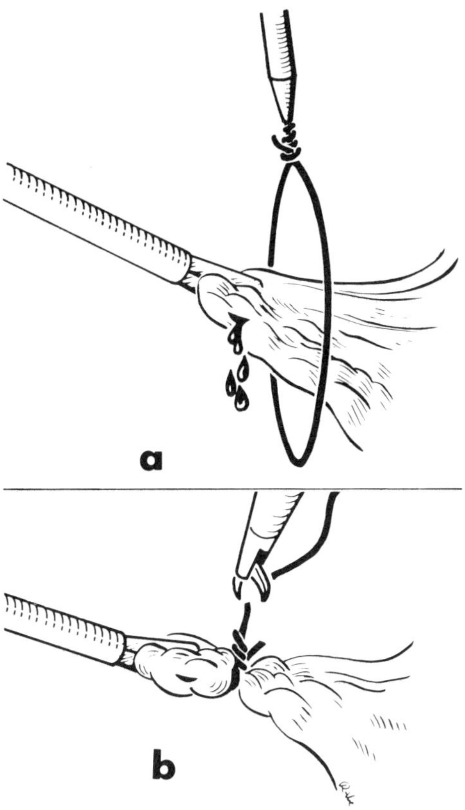

FIGURE 43:7—*The bleeding tissue is grasped (a) and pulled through a loop ligator (b) before tightening.*

stops the hemorrhage of large wound edges (e.g., after cyst wall resection). The myoma enucleator is similar to a heated knife and makes it easy to enucleate a subserous myoma bloodlessly. Wounds coagulated by endocoagulation techniques are protected by coagulated proteins. No exudation of fibrin and no immigration of histocytes and fibrocytes occurs so that no postoperative adhesions result. This is one of the main advantages of the new endocoagulation technique for hemostasis.

The Roeder-loop (Ethi-ligator®) is recommended for significant arterial bleeding, especially in the area of the mesosalpinx or in the utero-ovarian ligament, or for the occlusion of extended ovarian wounds after large cyst wall resection. This ligator can be placed with an applicator through a 5 mm trocar sheath and guarantees secure ligation of the vessels (Fig. 43:7). During 20 years of experience and following a few thousand applications of this instrument, we have never recorded any secondary hemorrhage caused by malfunction of the loop knot.

Therapeutic endoscopy should only be performed under endotracheal intubation anesthesia with assisted ventilation. This allows a second, third, and fourth incision to be made without difficulty or pain to the patient. The location for the accessory incision varies in each instance and depends on the type of pelvic abnormality.

The pneumoperitoneum is created, with awareness of the five safety steps that include palpation of the aorta, the needle test, the aspiration test, the needle insufflation pressure test, and the sounding test.

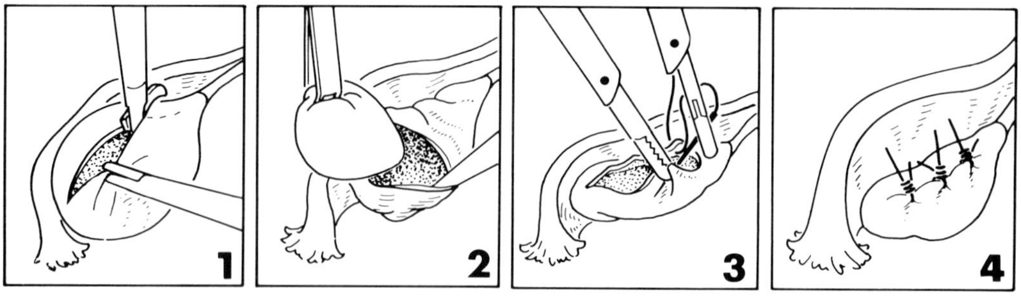

FIGURE 43:8—*Enucleation of ovarian cyst (1, 2) followed by ovarian endosuture with extracorporeal knotting (3, 4).*

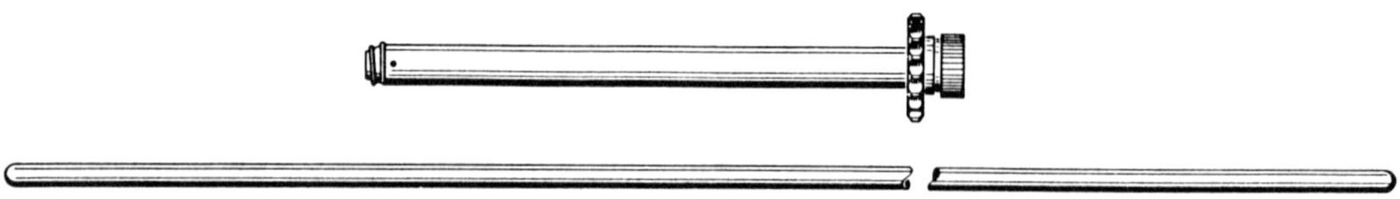

FIGURE 43:9—*Atraumatic dilatation set for changing from the 5 mm to the 11 mm trocar sheath.*

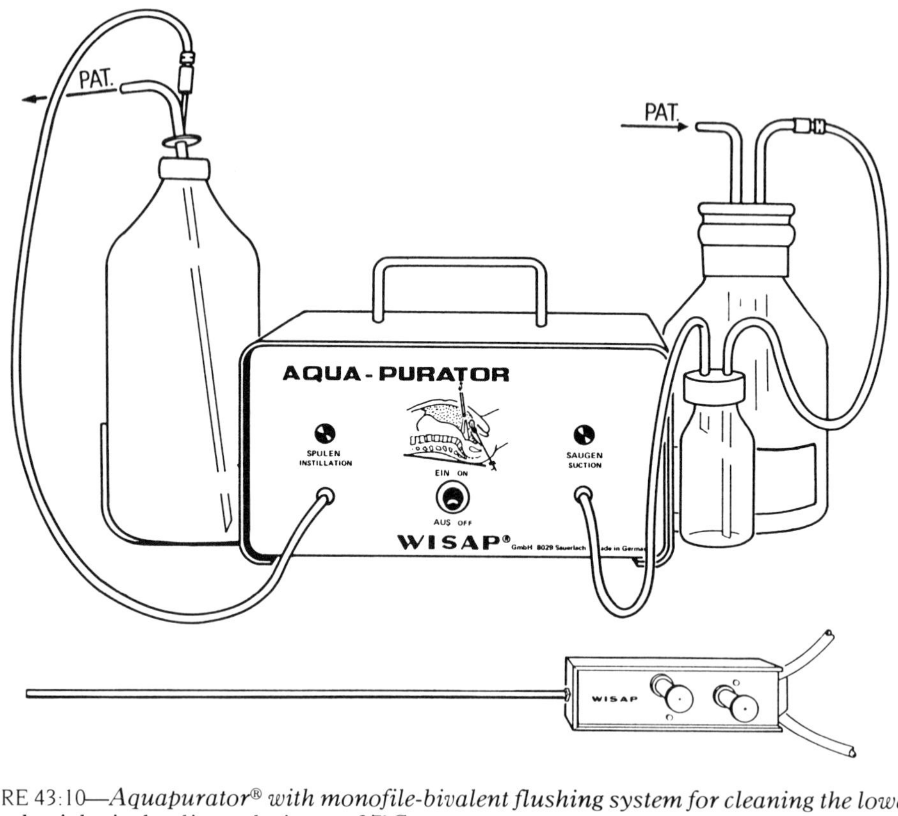

FIGURE 43:10—*Aquapurator® with monofile-bivalent flushing system for cleaning the lower pelvis with physiological saline solution at 37°C.*

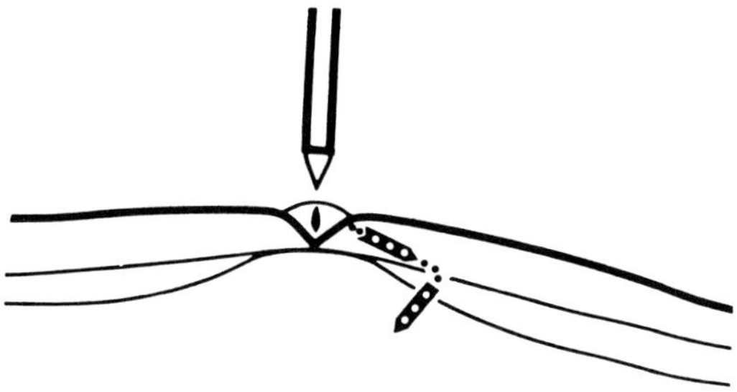

FIGURE 43:11—*Z-like puncture in the lower part of the umbilicus for an easy introduction of the trocar and sheath.*

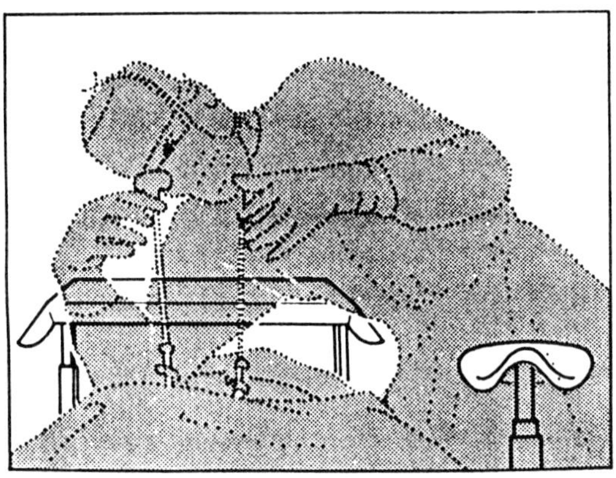

FIGURE 43:12—*Sitting and leaning position of the endoscopist.*

The filling procedure is performed up to a maximal intraabdominal pressure between 12 to 14 mmHg. This pressure is preselected on the insufflator and regulated automatically with this device. After the pneumoperitoneum is created up to the preselected pressure, the trocar is inserted according to the Z-incision technique (Fig. 43:11). This avoids later gaping wounds in the fascia of the linea alba in which omentum and intestine could be trapped postoperatively. One should never forget the anatomical sites of large blood vessels and try to avoid damage during the insertion of both the Veress needle and the trocar. Often these vessels are situated only 1 to 2 cm behind the umbilicus when patients are slim and they can be palpated. The direction of the uterine fundus should principally be followed during the insertion to avoid touching laterally the common iliac arteries and veins or their branches.

Trocar sheaths for the surgical instruments are mostly placed 1 cm below the pubic hairline. For operations on the ovaries and tubes, basically the instrument punctures the abdominal wall on the opposite sides, allowing the longest arm of a lever to be obtained. For both diagnosis and treatment, a second or third insertion in the left or right lower abdomen is necessary. With the dilatation set, the instrument or trocar sheath for the endoscope can easily be dilated from 5 to 11 mm during the diagnostic procedure. This allows for photodocumentation or a surgical procedure to remove important tissue. After removal of the endoscope or the instrument, the stump guide trocar is placed over it and with rotating movement, the wound in the abdominal wall is dilated to 11 mm without the risk of touching a vessel. This simple procedure makes an additional insertion unnecessary and an expansion of the surgical procedure possible.

When the view is not distinct from the umbilicus, one should never forget the possibility of introducing the endoscope through a trocar sheath into the lower abdomen. From this perspective, from the lower to the upper abdomen, adhesions in the upper region can easily be dissected. Often better surgery can be performed from this site than from the umbilicus.

Additional Equipment for Surgical Pelviscopic Surgery

After considerable experience, we find that the sitting position is most efficient for the surgeon to perform pelviscopy (Fig. 43:12). In this position, the endoscopist can rest a shoulder on a

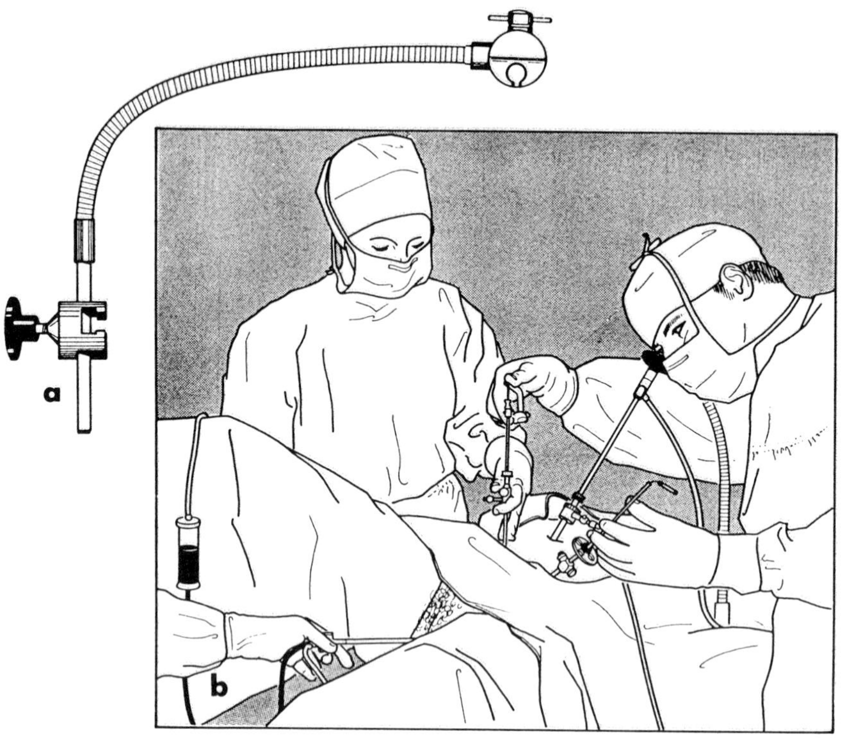

FIGURE 43:13—*Flexible cable (a) fixes the telescope to free both hands for surgery. The uterus is manipulated with the cervical cannula (b).*

bridge which can be installed over the head of the patient. The supporting sitting position of the surgeon tends to guarantee stable hands to move the instruments safely. If the endoscopic surgeon has to work without an assistant, the endoscope can easily be fixed at the operation table (Fig 43:13). This flexible device frees both hands for surgery. The assistant watches the operation, step-by-step, with the help of a flexible teaching instrument.

For tubal surgery, continuous insufflation of the tube by ascending chromosalpingography to a maintained pressure of 300 mmHG is absolutely necessary. Such continuous insufflation of the ampullary end of the fallopian tube is only possible with an insufflator used in conjunction with a vacuum intrauterine probe and a container filled with a blue dye solution (Fig. 43:14). The same system is used for repeated hydropertubation using a prolonged technique. Instead of the metal device, the flexible cervical adaptor (Fig. 43:15) is fixed to the cervix for six to eight hours to prevent reflux of the instilled mixture (streptomycin, procaine, cortisone, and alpha-chymotrypsin).

Pelviscopic Operations on the Fallopian Tube

Salpingolysis is mostly combined with intraabdominal adhesiolysis. The separation of the omentum from the peritoneum or the intestine, the uterine fundus or the ovary from the tubes is carried out carefully, in a step-by-step fashion with sharp or blunt dissection with the help of a myoma enucleator heated to 120°C. If large vessels are visible, they must be coagulated with the crocodile forceps or ligated with the Roeder-loop or with endoligation with the extracorporeal knot before operating.

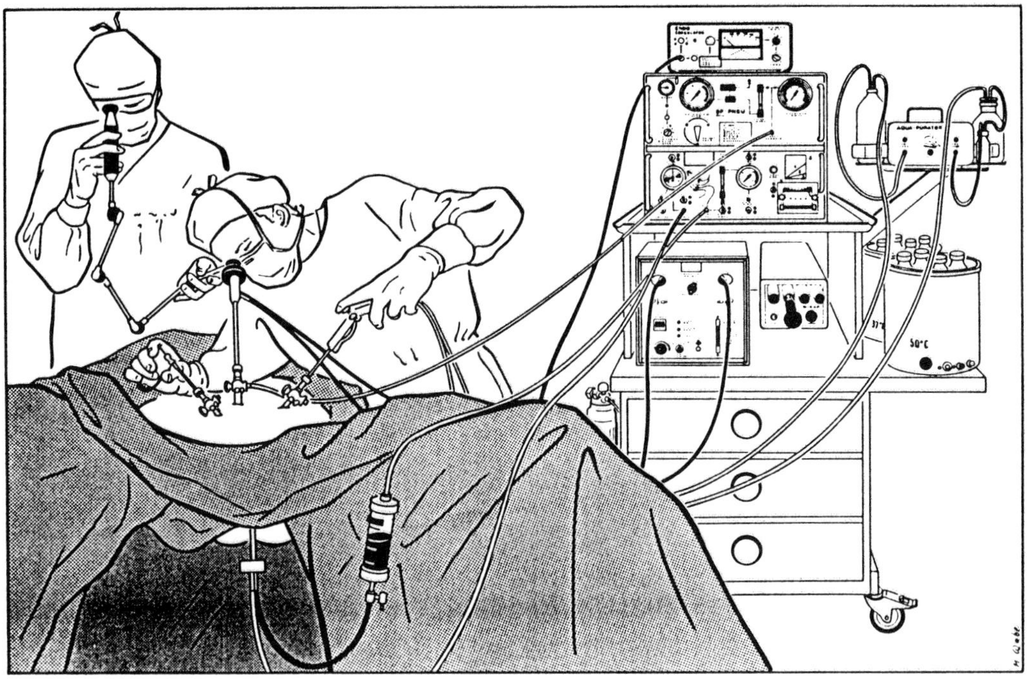

FIGURE 43:14—*Chromopertubation during laparoscopy.*

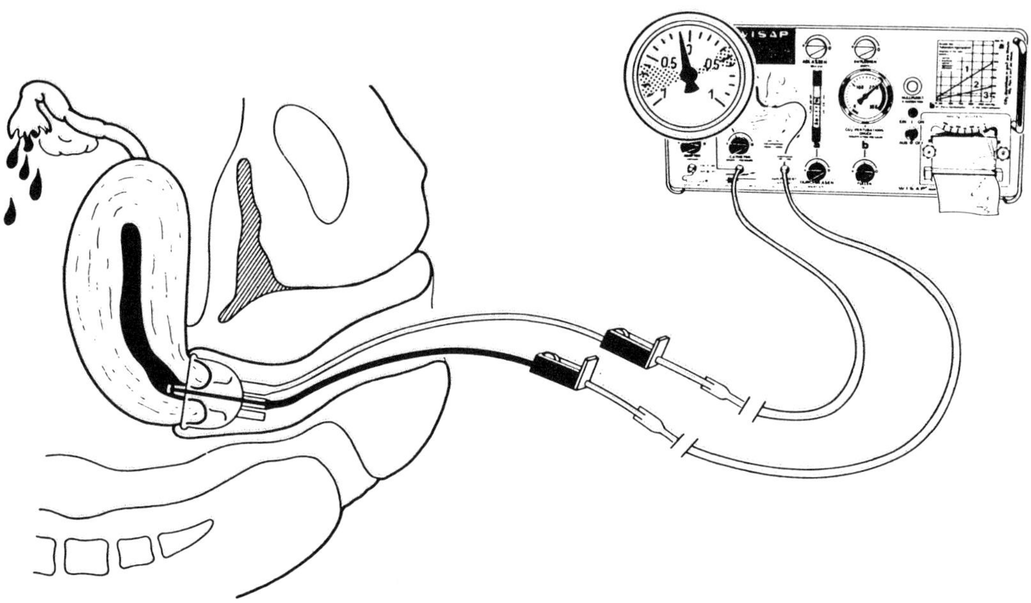

FIGURE 43:15—*A flexible atraumatic cervical adaptor is used after some endoscopic tubal operations for chromopertubation.*

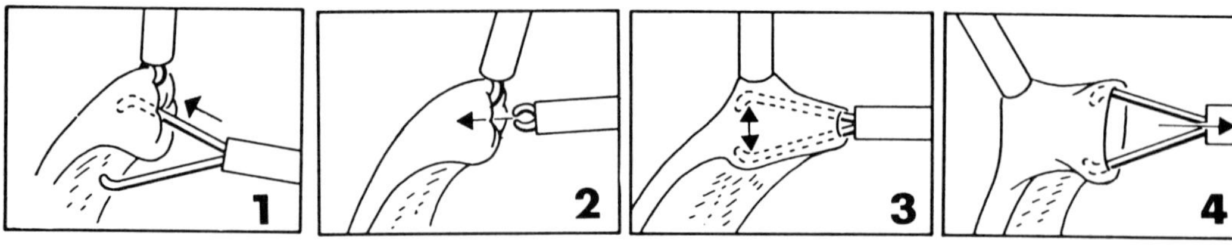

FIGURE 43:16—*Demonstration of blunt dilatation and fimbriolysis with the atraumatic forceps. (1) Tong (arrow) creates tubal opening. (2) Direction (arrow) for insertion of both tongs. (3) Arrows show stretching of tongs. (4) Tube dilated as opened tongs are removed (arrow).*

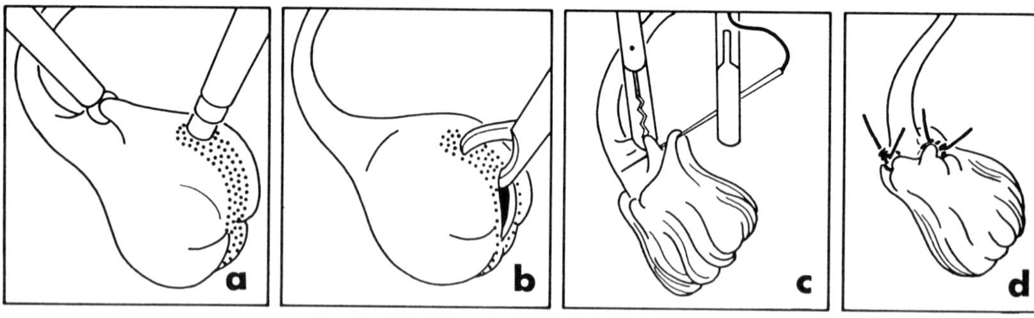

FIGURE 43:17—*Technique of opening a sactosalpinx for salpingostomy with endosutures and intracorporeal knotting after eversion of the tubal edges:* (a) *coagulation;* (b) *cutting;* (c) *eversion of endosalpinx;* (d) *completed operation.*

With two atraumatic forceps, fimbriolysis is carried out mostly in a blunt manner (Fig. 43:16). The ampullary phimosis is overcome by the introduction of the atraumatic forceps into the ampulla for a depth of 2 to 3 cm and by the extraction and simultaneous opening of the forceps. This results in a mostly atraumatic recovery of the original ampulla by blunt dilatation. During chromosalpingoscopy, the blue dye comes out into the abdominal cavity without ampullary dilatation, seen prior to the fimbrioplasty.

If there is a sactosalpinx during chromosalpingoscopy with methylene blue, it can easily be opened by surgical pelviscopy in the area of the original ampullary end. For this procedure, a coagulation strip of 2 cm length and 4 mm width is produced to obtain hemostasis with the point coagulator (Fig. 43:17).

Then the coagulated area is split using a microscissors or knife and the blue dye comes out. As during a laparotomy, the original ampullary end is everted and fixed with an extracorporeal knotted suture or with PDS® 4-0 reabsorbable suture with an intracorporeal knot (Fig. 43:17).

Because of the minimal bleeding with an endoscopic intraabdominal operation, the treatment of tubal pregnancy is facilitated. To proceed, two techniques are possible. First, blood and clots are removed with the Aqua-purator and the assistance of the electronic carbon dioxide insufflator. The point coagulator coagulates a 2–4 cm strip of tubal serosa along the antimesenteric side of the distended pregnant tube. Occasionally, pitressin is injected into the tube and mesosalpinx. After the tube has been opened in a longitudinal manner (Fig. 43:18), the gestational tissue comes out spontaneously or can be removed with either the biopsy or spoon forceps. The edges of the wound of the linear salpingotomy can be approximated with the special suture.

If a conservative operation appears to be inappropriate for the case, the fallopian tube can be grasped and ligated in a method similar to that used for an ovarian

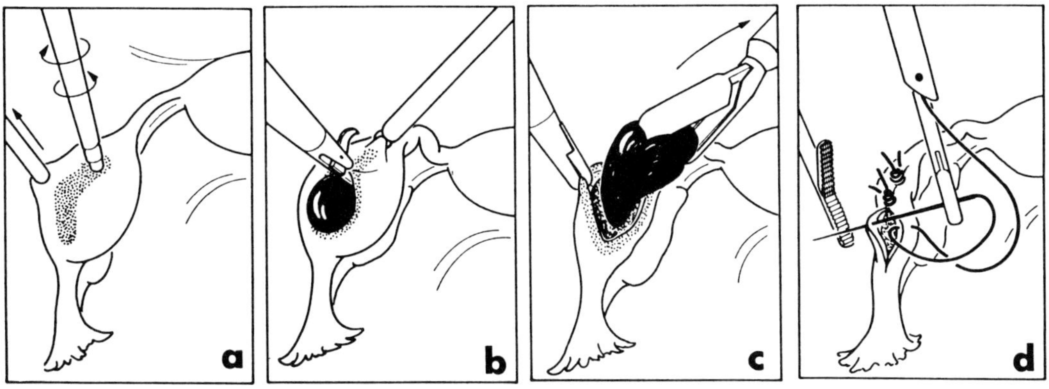

FIGURE 43:18—*Technique of salpingotomy for tubal pregnancy:* (a) *coagulation;* (b) *cutting;* (c) *removal of products of conception;* (d) *repair.*

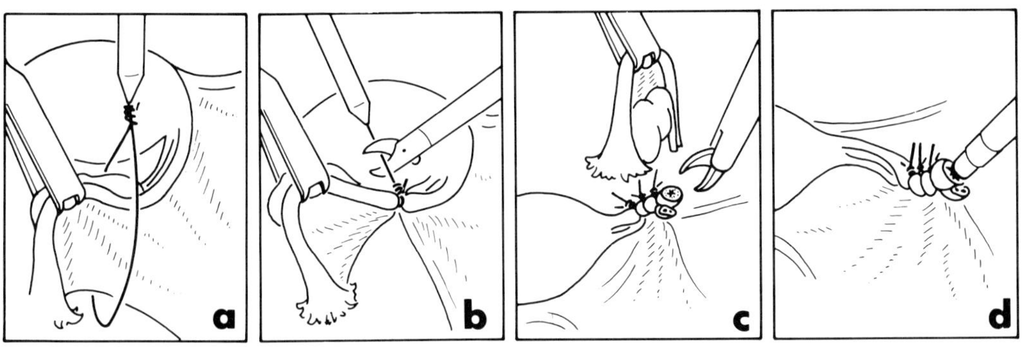

FIGURE 43:19—*Salpingo-oophorectomy by using the "3-loop-ligation" technique* (a—c)*; coagulation of the tissue stump for preventing postoperative adhesions* (d).

resection or adnexectomy by pelviscopy (Fig. 43:19). The Roeder loop ligator (endoscopic three-loop technique) should include the tube and part of the mesosalpinx for hemostasis. Finally, the remaining tissue stump must be coagulated with the point coagulator to prevent postoperative adhesions.

Postoperative Care

Following fimbrioplasty and salpingostomy, prolonged hydropertubation is carried out for a five-day period. After ovariectomy, adnexectomy, removal of a tubal pregnancy or appendectomy, five days of hospitalization are recommended. This is essentially the same postoperative regimen as for laparotomy.

These procedures are not easy to learn and we have therefore created a phantom, called a "pelvic trainer" (Fig. 43:20). It allows the physician to simulate each kind of gynecologic endoscopic operation using an extirpated uterus, tubes, and ovaries. The cervix can be grasped with a tenculum and the program involves three phases:

1. Working with both hands and controlling the manipulations by looking through the glass surface.
2. The same procedures are done through the laparoscope, occasionally "peeking" through the glass surface.
3. The "pelvic trainer" is covered with a fabric and each procedure must be done under endoscopic conditions.

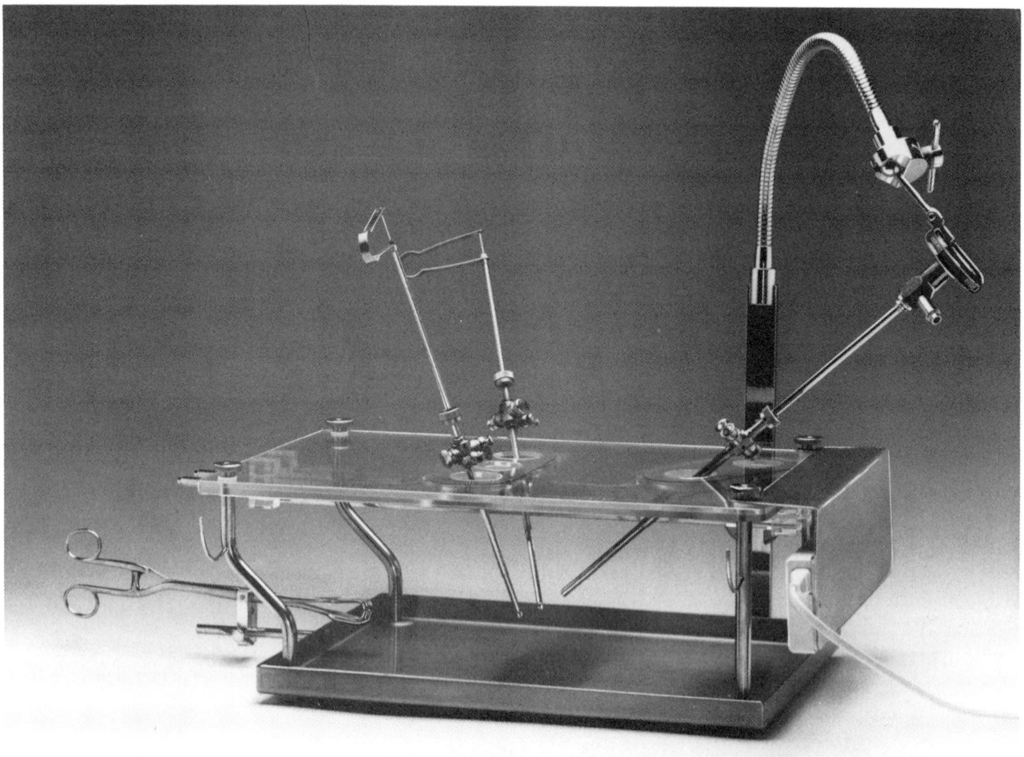

FIGURE 43:20—*"Pelvic trainer." Model for learning techniques for endoscopic surgery.*

Summary

Therapeutic laparoscopy can be repeated without severe stress to the patient. Salpingolysis (Fig. 43:21), fimbrioplasty (Fig. 43:22), and salpingostomy (Fig. 43:23)* can easily be performed in most instances so that microsurgery becomes unnecessary. The pregnancy rate (29.3 percent) for these types of tuboplasty evaluated one year after the last laparoscopy compares favorably with results obtained from a laparotomy.

The objectives of tubal reconstructive surgery remain the establishment and maintenance of tubal patency, the avoidance of postoperative adhesions, and the prevention of abortions and tubal pregnancies. All of these objectives are well met by operative laparoscopy. This chapter has emphasized the important role of endoscopic operations in patients with distal tubal obstructions. It has been conclusively demonstrated that the above-described laparoscopic technique results in a minimum of physical stress, a short hospitalization, a low operative risk, a decreased incidence of postoperative adhesions, and a possibility of being repeated or followed by laparotomy.

*Figures 43:22–43:23 are color plates and appear on pp. 431 and 432.

Reference

1. Semm K: *Operationslehre für Endoskopische Abdominal-Chirurgie Operative Pelviskopie—Operative Laparoskopie.* Stuttgart: F.K. Schattauer, 1984.

44

Prevention of Pelvic Adhesions

Bertil Larsson

Intraperitoneal adhesions are a potentially serious postoperative problem and are the most common cause of intestinal obstruction at all ages. Pelvic surgery, in particular, is the most frequent cause of postoperative bowel obstruction.[1] Adhesions may occur despite a meticulous operation and some patients require another surgical procedure to overcome the sequelae. In women of reproductive age, intrapelvic adhesions can cause lower abdominal pain, dyspareunia, and infertility.

It has been accepted that adhesions are usually formed as a result of surgical trauma.[2] The effect of the trauma depends on the severity and extent of the mechanical, chemical, thermal, and possibly bacterial damage to the peritoneum. There is a variation in the response of the peritoneum to serosal injury and in essence the precise mechanism of postoperative intraabdominal adhesion formation remains to be elucidated. Briefly, surgical trauma causes an inflammatory reaction followed by exudation of protein-rich material onto the surface of the denuded serosa, some of which remains unabsorbed. These precursors develop into collagen.[3,4]

Previous pelvic inflammatory disease (PID) is the main reason for infertility caused by the tubal factor. According to Weström, about 20 percent of all women who have had one or more episodes of PID become infertile because of tubal abnormalities.[5] Many patients who have been operated on have suffered from one or several previous undetected episodes of PID which have produced pelvic adhesions and sactosalpinges. A sequence of events similar to those described above may develop, resulting in adhesions.

Technical and pharmacological advances in tubal reconstruction, particularly since the advent of microsurgery, have reduced the incidence of postoperative adhesions.[6,7]

Numerous agents have been tried experimentally and clinically to prevent such adhesions. So far, the most effective substance is corticosteroid.[7,8] Corticosteroid medication is started on the day before the operation, high doses intraabdominally at the end of the laparotomy and continued for a week or more postoperatively.[6] However, in an experimental study in rats we observed that such a long period of corticosteroid treatment was not significantly superior to one single high dose intraabdominally at the end of the operation.[9] The corticosteroids reduce

The Fallopian Tube: Basic Studies and Clinical Contributions, edited by Alvin M. Siegler, M.D. Mount Kisco, New York: Futura Publishing Company, Inc. © 1986.

edema and prevent the growth of fibroblasts. In addition, oxyphenbutazone, an antiinflammatory agent, has routinely been given at our department. Encouraging results were recorded in a previous report in which 39 percent of patients having combined salpingostomy, salpingolysis, and ovariolysis became pregnant.[10] This drug was also effective in an experimental study.[11] A significant reduction of adhesions following a standardized trauma was noted in animals treated with ibuprofen, another type of antiinflammatory agent.[12] Dextran solutions of varying concentrations and mean molecular weights have been evaluated by several investigators.[12–14] The 32 percent solution of dextran 70 (Hyskon®) showed the greatest efficacy.[15]

Heparin inhibits clotting and fibrin formation and it is recommended in operations for fertility, based on the assumption that fibrin has an essential role in the formation of adhesions.[16,17] However, the preventive effect of heparin on the formation of adhesions is doubtful.[16]

Several authors have considered blood to be a significant factor in the formation of intraperitoneal adhesions,[17–19] whereas others believe that blood is spontaneously absorbed by the peritoneum without causing adhesions.[20] In an experimental study, we found that neither blood nor fibrinogen induced adhesions to the peritoneum or serosal surfaces.[21] These observations are in accord with those we have found in women, in whom an operation for fertility was performed and registered a blood volume in the abdominal cavity not exceeding 150 ml. We concluded that the main reason for the postoperative formation of adhesions is a surgical trauma to the serosa and adhesion is not further increased on the damaged serosa by the presence of blood.

The effectiveness of the nonwoven towels in prevention of adhesions has previously been demonstrated.[22] The influence of a drying and irrigation with saline, respectively, on the exudation of protein-rich material of an intact and an injured uterine serosa and of the cecum has been assessed after intraveous administration of fluorescin dextran (FITC-dextran) in rats.[23] Constant irrigation of the peritoneum did not inhibit exudation or prevent adhesions. However, the constant irrigation and the repeated lavages of the abdominal cavity with saline means a more gentle handling of the tissue, resulting in a reduced extent of trauma to the serosa.

In 26 patients undergoing bilateral salpingolysis, ovariolysis, and salpingostomy, without adjuvant therapy to prevent adhesions, later laparoscopy revealed adhesions at the sites of petechiae, seen at operation.

Lindenberg and coworkers[24] concluded from the results of their investigation in rats that prevention of adhesions after abdominal surgery in patients would never include routine peritoneal dialysis. My experimental and clinical investigations suggest that the presence and subsequent removal of a drain from the abdominal cavity may cause serosal trauma and induce adhesions.

Generally, suture sizes vary between 6–0 and 10–0 in gynecologic microsurgery. In essence the suture size selected for a procedure must be of adequate tensile strength for approximating and holding tissue edges together. Microsurgical procedures are performed with a minimal amount of suture material in order to minimize tissue trauma.

Nonresorbable suture may be used through operations for fertility, including the sutures placed in the circular muscles and serosa in tubal anastomosis and those used to evert a sactosalpinx.

The author's technique includes a gentle, atraumatic, and electromicrosurgical procedure with selective hemostasis. The skin is cut with a scalpel, but the subcutaneous tissues, the fascia, and the peritoneum are incised with electrocautery. Blood is prevented from escaping into the abdominal cavity by covering the edges of the abdominal incision with special nonwoven laparotomy sponges. The pouch of Douglas is packed with nonwoven sponges, soaked in saline, to keep the uterus and adnexa elevated, constantly moist, and out of contact with blood. To avoid drying of the pelvic and abdominal serosa, the peritoneal surfaces are continuously irrigated with saline and the abdominal cavity is filled to the level of the tissues undergoing electrosurgery. Adhesions attached to the abdominal wall, the pelvic wall, the bowel, the uterus, or the adnexa are excised with an isolated microelectrode. Care is taken not to denude any part of the serosa. The necrosis produced on electrosurgical dissection of the adhesions is never allowed to proceed closer than 1 mm to the normal serosa. To avoid tissue damage, clamps and forceps are not allowed to touch any tissue except for dissection of adhesions. Loose adhesions are stretched by separating the adherent tissues with the surgeon's gloved fingers and over a plastic-covered aluminum rod, then cut with the isolated epilation needle. Adherent tubes and ovaries are gently separated with a special glass rod without causing any rupture of the adhesions or the adjacent serosa, and then cut with an isolated microelectrode. Whenever blood escapes into the peritoneal cavity, it is aspirated in saline. Capillaries are identified during irrigation and hemostasis is secured by pinpoint electrocoagulation. The use of suture material is kept to a minimum.

At the end of the operation, the abdominal cavity is thoroughly lavaged with saline solution. Just before the closure of the peritoneum, 500 mg methylprednisolone dissolved in 50 ml saline is deposited in the abdominal cavity through a plastic catheter. Prophylactic antibiotics and corticosteroids are given from the day before the operation.

On the second and fourth postoperative days the patient is treated with hydropertubation. With the aid of an ordinary hysterosalpingography instrument, 250 mg hydrocortisone-succinate combined with 10 million IU benzylpenicillin in 50 ml saline are gently injected through the cervix.

Two postoperative hydropertubations are performed in cases of tuboplasties except for tubal anastomosis. Although hydropertubation remains a controversial issue, we believe it is of benefit, since we have encountered only 8 percent tubal pregnancies among our patients following tuboplasties.

References

1. Fries B: Polyphloretin phosphate, a hyaluronidase inhibitor, and hyaluronidase in the prevention of intraperitoneal adhesions. *Acta Chir Scand Suppl*, 217, 1956.
2. Ellis H: The causes and prevention of intestinal adhesions. *Br J Surg*, 69:241, 1982.
3. Ellis H, Harrison W, and Hugh TB: The healing of peritoneum under normal and pathological conditions. *Br J Surg*, 52:471, 1965.
4. Ryan GB, Grobety J, and Majno G: Postoperative peritoneal adhesions. A study of the mechanisms. *Am J Pathol*, 65:117, 1971.
5. Weström L: Effect of acute pelvic inflammatory disease on fertility. *Am J Obstet Gynecol*, 121:707, 1975.
6. Swolin K: 50 Fertilitätsoperationen. *Acta Obstet Gynecol Scand*, 46:1, 1967.
7. Sanctis A, Schatten W, and Weckesser E: Effect of hydrocortisone in the prevention of intraperitoneal adhesions. *Arch Surg*, 71:523, 1955.
8. Shikata J, and Yamaoka I: The role of topically applied dexamethasone in preventing peritoneal adhesions: Experimental and clinical studies. *World J Surg* 1:389, 1977.
9. Larsson B, Rosenborg L, Granberg-Ohman I, et al: The influence of various regimens of corticosteroid treatment on the prevention of peritoneal adhesions and on the healing of a midline incision in rats. (Work in progress.)
10. Larsson B: Late results of salpingostomy combined with salpingolysis and ovariolysis by electromicrosurgery in 54 women. *Fertil Steril*, 27:156, 1982.
11. Larsson B, Svanberg SG, and Swolin K: Oxyphenbutazone, an adjuvant to be used in prevention of adhesions in operations for fertility. *Fertil Steril*, 28:807, 1977.
12. Nishimura K, Nakamura RM, and diZerega GS: Biochemical evaluation of postsurgical wound repair: Prevention of intraperitoneal adhesion formation

with ibuprofen. *J Surg Res*, 34:219, 1983.

13. Choat WH, Just-Viera JO, and Yeager GH: Prevention of experimental peritoneal adhesions by dextran. *Arch Surg*, 88:249, 1964.
14. Soules MR, Dennis L. Bosarge A, et al: The prevention of postoperative pelvic adhesions: An animal study comparing barrier methods with dextran 70. *Am J Obstet Gynecol*, 143:829, 1982.
15. Aszodi A, Chaimoff C, and Dintsman M: Rheomacrodex in the prevention of intraperitoneal adhesions. *Int Surg*, 57:559, 1972.
16. DiZerega GS, and Hodgen GD: Prevention of postoperative tubal adhesions. *Am J Obstet Gynecol*, 136:173, 1980.
17. Knightly JJ, Domenico A, and Cliffton EE: The effect of fibrinolysin and heparin on the formation of peritoneal adhesions. *Surgery*, 52:250, 1962.
18. Levinson CJ, and Swolin K: Postoperative adhesions: Etiology, prevention, and therapy. *Clin Obstet Gynecol*, 23:1213, 1980.
19. Swolin K: Electromicrosurgery and salpingostomy: Long term results. *Am J Obstet Gynecol*, 121:418, 1975.
20. Luttwak EM, Behar AJ, and Saltz NJ: Effect of fibrinolytic agents and corticosteroid hormones on peritoneal adhesions. *Arch Surg*, 75:96, 1957.
21. Nisell H, and Larsson B: Role of blood and fibrinogen in development of intraperitoneal adhesions in rats. *Fertil Steril*, 30:470, 1978.
22. Swolin K, Bendz A, Larrson B, et al: Traumatization of the abdominal serosa. A comparison between non-woven and cotton abdominal swabs. *Acta Chir Scand*, 140:302, 1974.
23. Larsson B, Perbeck L, Fianu S, et al: The possible advantage of keeping the uterine and intestinal serosa irrigated with saline to prevent intraabdominal adhesions in operations for fertility. An experimental study in rats. (Work in progress.)
24. Lindenberg S, Moesgaard F, Vangsted M, et al: Peritoneal dialysis reduces intraperitoneal adhesion formation. An experimental study in rats. *Eur Surg Res*, 14:274, 1982.

45

Laser for Tubal Microsurgery

Dan C. Martin,
John Marlow, and
Robert W. Kelly

The use of carbon dioxide (CO_2) laser as a "light knife" offers the gynecologist and the patient many advantages. Among these are excellent hemostasis, minimal tissue manipulation, improved access to difficult sites in the pelvis, fewer instruments in the operating field, and more opportunities for therapeutic laparoscopy. The main concerns regarding the use of laser are its cost and safety. The equipment is expensive, extensive training is required to learn new concepts of this type of surgery, and many of the safety features are different from more standard techniques.

Development

The use of surgical carbon dioxide laser followed the initial development of ruby, Argon gas and combinations of Neodymium; Yittrium-Aluminum-Garnet (Nd: YAG) lasers in the early 1960s. By 1971 carbon dioxide laser had been used to perform partial hepatectomy with minimal hemorrhage and "sound healing".[1] With increasingly advanced and mobile equipment, the use of laser was extended to human beings. In gynecology, the initial report was for the treatment of cervical erosion.[2] Subsequently, with more skill and experience, the CO_2 laser was used for tubal anastomosis[3] and salpingostomy.[4] Similar preliminary work had been extended into laparoscopic laser surgery.

Laser Basics

Laser is an acronym for light amplification by stimulated emission of radiation. The high-intensity electromagnetic energy produced in this fashion is monochromatic, collimated, and coherent. All waves have the same wavelength and same energy (monochromatic waves) and they are emitted in nearly parallel fashion (collimated), resulting in a beam that maintains the same diameter and power density as it moves through space. The coherence of the wave (in phase in time

The Fallopian Tube: Basic Studies and Clinical Contributions, edited by Alvin M. Siegler, M.D. Mount Kisco, New York: Futura Publishing Company, Inc.

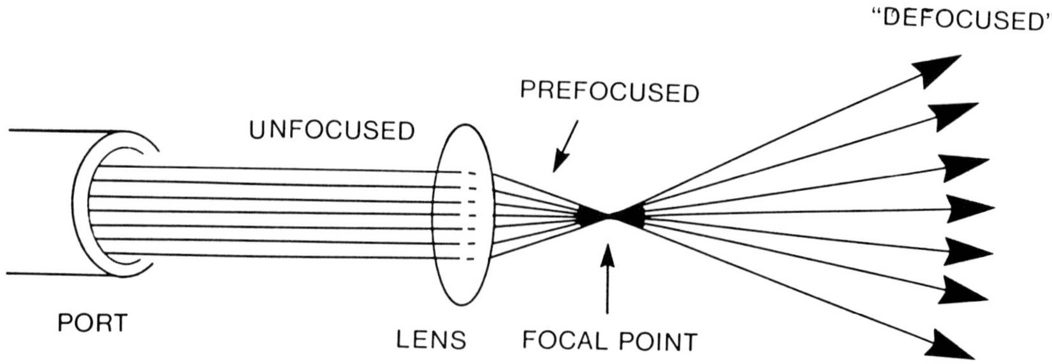

FIGURE 45:1—*The width of the laser beam changes depending on its relationship to the lens and focal point.*

and space) allows amplification to occur in a resonator cavity.

Although the power in watts produced by lasers is often less than in an ordinary light bulb, the intensity of the beam can be enormous after it is focused through a lens. The intensity of the beam is controlled by the amount of stimulation from an external source. The beam exits from a resonator cavity and is directed down hollow tubes with front surface mirrors to the operating port. The port beam is generally from 2 to 8 mm in size. A lens is used to focus this port beam to a smaller spot size with increased density (Fig. 45:1). A small spot size and high-power density are necessary for rapid incision with decreased thermal necrosis (Fig. 45:2). Thermal necrosis is related to the temperature of boiling water at the base of the crater. Higher-power densities decrease the time needed to perform an incision. The decreased time reduces the exposure to 100°C crater heat.

As the laser impacts on tissue, the beam is reflected, transmitted, absorbed, or scattered (Fig. 45:3). At high-power densities, photovaporization (flash boiling of water-containing tissues) of cells leaves a crater or incisional line (Table 45:1). Acoustic and ultrasonic shock waves are also produced during the interaction. These shock waves appear to be biologically significant with high-power-density, pulsed YAG lasers.[1] At low-power densities, photocoagulation (thermal denaturation and destruction of tissue) will occur. Photocoagulation is avoided in tubal surgery since it increases fibrosis.[5] Photocoagulation may be useful in the treatment of endometriosis, especially when using an argon or YAG laser.

Safety

A carbon dioxide laser is potentially dangerous to skin and eye surfaces. The high-power electromagnetic energy can vaporize or coagulate surfaces at a distance. Surgeons can injure their hands by passing them through previously "safe" territory. Practice should be dedicated to reduce dangers to the patient, to the operating room personnel, and to the surgeon.

Glass, pyrex, and quartz rods have been used as "backstops" to limit the penetration of the laser because they absorb energy and melt at temperatures in excess of 1,200°C. Since glass will not disperse heat well and breaks easily, and pyrex and quartz rods have also broken, water solutions, soaked pads, and etched rods are preferable. If pyrex and quartz rods are used, they should not be less than 3 mm in taper and should be changed frequently. Teflon rods commonly employed for tissue

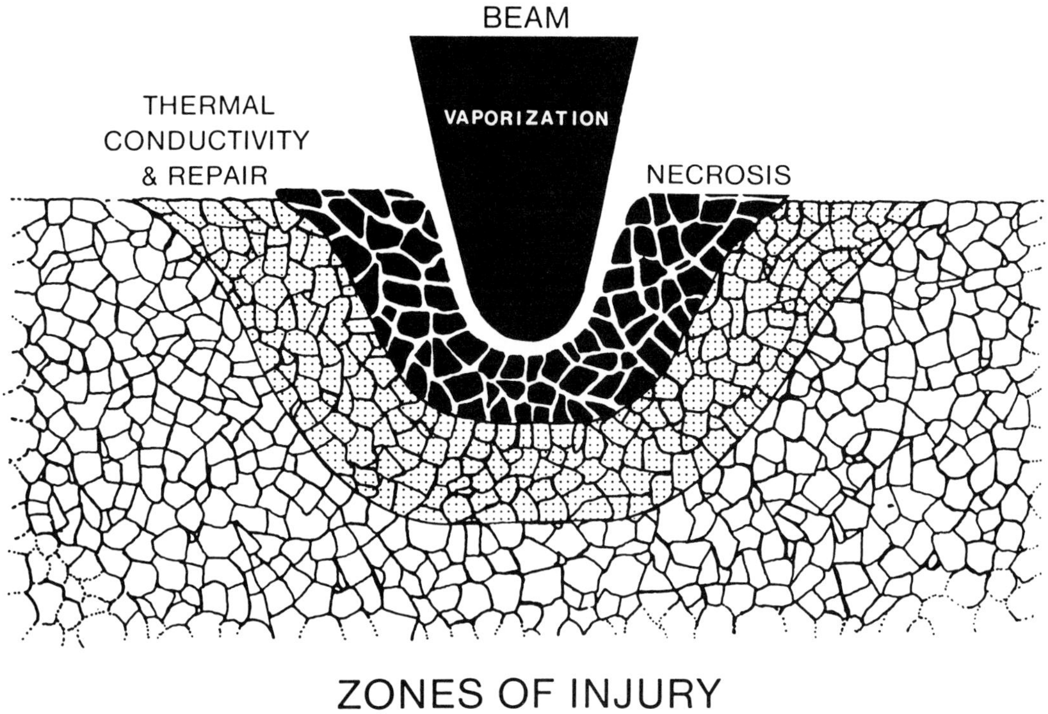

FIGURE 45:2—*The zones of injury are the thermal necrotic zone and thermal conductivity zone.*

manipulation in nonlaser cases produce a toxic fume when vaporized.

Mirrors used to direct the beam can be polished metal or rhodium front-surfaced glass. The front-surfaced glass mirrors should not be exposed to power density in excess of 12,000 W/cm^2 because higher-power densities can vaporize or shatter the front surface. Polished metal mirrors are preferable.

The smoke plume from vaporization of tissue has many of the characteristics of cigarette smoke[6] and adequate suction is needed to remove it. A filter should be kept in the suction line to protect the main hospital equipment from deposition of carbonized material.

The red helium neon aiming laser beam presents a potential danger to the human eye. The lens of the eye has the ability to focus even this low-power-density laser to a small spot size with high-power density.[7] A complete discussion of safety is available in *Laser Safety in Surgery and Medicine.*[7] It or a similar manual should be read by the surgeon who plans to use laser techniques.

Technical Considerations for Use With the Microscope

When using a carbon dioxide laser through a microscope, it is essential to parfocus the microscope. With the laser, the focal point of the microscope and the laser must coincide in order to develop the expected spot size and power density. Parfocusing is performed by focusing the microscope at its highest power. The setting is then changed to the lowest power and the oculars are focused without changing the microscope distance. To test this parfocus, move through the range of magnifications of the microscope either manually or by zoom. During the maneuver, the focus should be maintained as the power is changed.

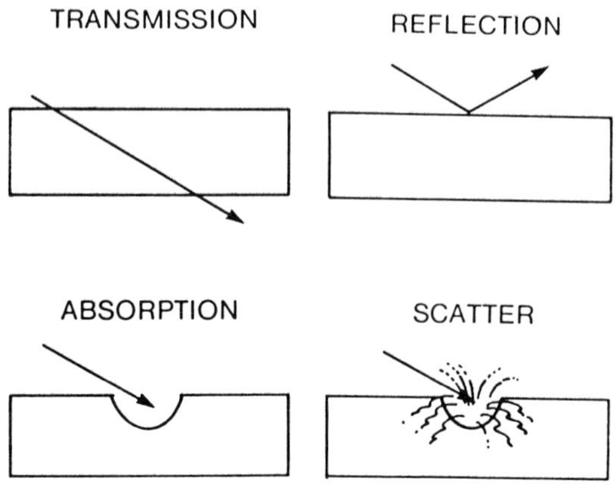

FIGURE 45:3—*The laser will interact with tissue by being transmitted, absorbed, reflected, or scattered.*

Tissue Studies

The laser causes delayed healing and increased tissue destruction, compared to a sharp knife.[8–10] The tissue destruction results in decreased resistance to bacterial infection.[8,10] The laser produces the same degree of damage as the electrosurgical unit when each is used at high-power density.[9,10]

The use of the laser pulsed mode can decrease thermal spread by using short pulses of high-power density and also can give excellent control of the laser.[11,12] The technique may drive cellular material into the deeper tissue, as a result of acoustic and ultrasonic shock waves in tissue distal to the impact site.[1] In work with tumors and condyloma, this characteristic appears to be most important but it may have no biological significance during operations on healthy tissues.

Animal Studies

Decreased postoperative adhesions have been reported by many investigators[13–19] when comparing laser with microelectric needles for incisions on peritoneal surfaces. The combination of laser and hydrocortisone gave the best results.[14] Uterine and ovarian adhesions in rabbits occurred at the same rate with carbon dioxide laser and electrocautery.[15] Statistical differences were not demonstrated in these studies.

In tubal anastomotic procedures, attempts at welding the tube have been uniformly unsuccessful thus far.[3,20–22] Attempts to use low-power density (less than 3,000 W/cm^2) and continuous mode for incisions followed by microscopic anastomoses gave poor results.[5,21–23] One group produced satisfactory results with low-power density using pulsed mode at 800 W/cm^2.[16] In a comparative study of continuous mode low-power density (1,000 W/cm^2, higher-power density (11,000 W/cm^2) and sharp incisions followed by conventional microsurgical anastomosis, a 100 percent patency rate was demonstrated with high-power density and conventional microsurgery. In this study, 28 Sprague Dawley rats were examined at intervals from 1 to 28 days. Fibrosis and hydrosalpinges were noted at 14 and 28 days in the low-power-density group.[5] A second comparative study of 500 W/cm^2, 3,000 W/cm^2, 8,000 W/cm^2, and sharp incision followed by microsurgical anastomosis resulted in 90 percent fibrosis in the 500-watt group and 10 to 30 percent fibrosis in the other groups.[33] The study was of 40 rat uterine horn anastomoses examined at 28 to 35 days following initial surgery. Based on these studies, welding techniques and low-power-density continuous mode incision techniques should be avoided in tubal surgery. Power densities of 3,000 to 12,000 W/cm^2 have been useful.[5,23,24]

When neofimbria were induced in rats and followed by cuff salpingostomy, 75 percent of the animals became pregnant after opening by the laser, in comparison with 50 percent after opening by conventional microsurgery.[25]

Clinical Experience

At laparotomy, the CO_2 laser has been most useful in the performance of

Table 45:1
Power Density and Tissue Effects

*Watts/cm^2**	*Action*
0–5	Warming
5–300	Superficial contraction/coagulation
300–1,200	Excisional vaporization
1,200–15,000	Incisional vaporization
15,000–100,000	Rapid incision

*Watts/cm^2 are calculated.

cuff salpingostomies. An initial incision is made into the tube at high-power density followed by radial incisions using backstops to limit the depth of penetration of the laser (Fig. 45:4).[24,26–28] With another technique, the microscope is set with the hydrosalpinx centered in the field of view. After an initial incision, smooth pickups are used to manipulate the tube into the area of the fixed laser point. A 0.1-second pulse of high-power density is used to incise between the folds while aiming into the tubal wall. After an initial stellate incision is made, it is continued along the antimesenteric portion until healthy endosalpingeal folds are noted or until the diameter is too small to continue. This technique results in better preservation of the endosalpingeal folds. Cautery and scissors are often needed as the incision progresses up the antimesenteric portion of the ampulla. Bruhat et al.[26] conducted a comparative study of the electroscalpel and laser cuff salpingostomy. Follow-up found 9 (24 percent) of 34 patients conceiving and progressing to term in the laser group, compared with 5 (17 percent) of 30 patients in the electroscalpel group. The abortion and ectopic rates were similar. There were no statistically significant differences in this study.[27] A separate study of 28 patients undergoing laser cuff salpingostomy resulted in a 23 percent term pregnancy rate and 7 percent ectopic pregnancy rate with two years of follow-up. [24] The patency rates for these techniques have varied from 85[24] to 91 percent.[27]

Adhesiolysis has resulted in conception rates of from 19 to 63 percent.[24,29,30] Although the laser offered technical advantages in these cases, no statistical differences were found in comparison to contemporary microsurgical techniques.[24,31] A two-year study of 210 patients was compared with an initial study of 61 patients. The uncorrected conception rate rose from 13 to 39 percent at two years of follow-up. Recently, 81 (38 percent) of 216 patients operated on for adhesive disease conceived.[29,32] A separate study of 23 patients showed 10 (63 percent) of 16 patients progressing to term when adhesions were the sole cause of infertility but only one (14 percent) of seven patients when multiple factors were present.[30]

It is reported that tubal anastomosis with the laser may be performed more rapidly, more easily, and with better hemostasis and less trauma than with microelectrosurgery.[24,33] However, three of six anastomoses resulted in tubal obstruction when low-power densities were used.[21] With higher-power densities no differences were noted in success rate following tubal anastomosis from an initial incision made by either sharp knife or microlaser technique.[24,31] Intrauterine pregnancies occurred in 8 (67 percent) of 12 patients when incisions were performed at 6,000 W/cm^2 followed by microsurgical suture anastomosis.[24]

At laparoscopy, salpingostomies have

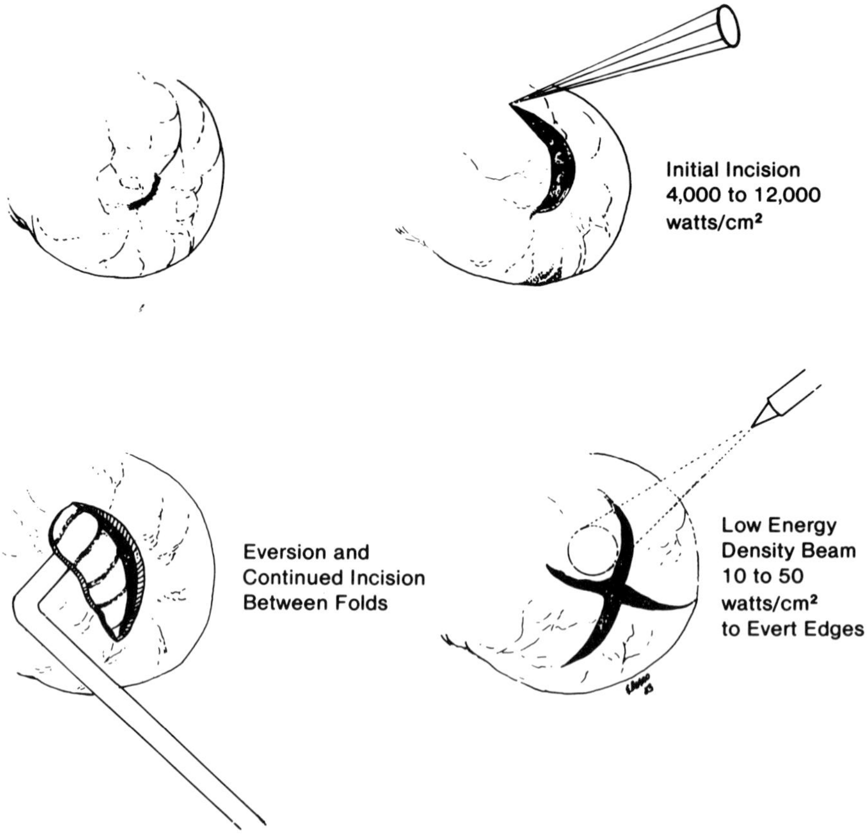

FIGURE 45:4—*The Bruhat technique involves an initial incision at high-power density followed by low-power-density contraction of serosa to evert the tubal edges.*

been performed with CO_2 laser[25–36] with techniques similar to that used at laparotomy. Pregnancies resulted in 5 of 22 patients in one series followed for 12 months but one abortion and one tubal pregnancy occurred. Patency was present in 84 percent of these patients,[37] results being similar to the laparoscopic coagulation and scissors technique.[33–40] In one study of the laparoscopic coagulation and scissors technique, two tubal pregnancies occurred in 19 patients and the tubal patency rate was 31 percent.[41]

These laparoscopic laser techniques are relevant for those patients desiring to avoid laparotomy. Technical changes that allow both hands for manipulation while a foot switch is used for cutting with the laser may improve the outcome of this procedure. In the laboratory, the results closely approximate microsurgical techniques used at laparotomy.

Tubal Sterilization

The CO_2 laser has been used with a defocused technique to perform tubal sterilization during laparoscopy in 12 patients. Three years later, one of these patients had become pregnant. There was no evidence of patency in five women studied by hysterosalpingogram.[17] The healing properties following CO_2 laser incisions militate against the use of this technique for sterilization.

References

1. Riggle GC, Hoye RC, and Ketcham AS: Laser effects on normal and tumor tissue. In Woibarsht ML (Ed): *Laser Application in Medicine and Biology,* vol. 1. New York: Plenum Press, 1971: p. 35.
2. Kaplan I, Goldman J, and Ger R: The treatment of erosions of the uterine cervix by means of the CO_2 laser. *Obstet Gynecol,* 41:795, 1973.
3. Klink F, Grospietzsch R, Klitzing L, et al: Animal in vitro experiments with human tubes for end to end anastomotic operations by CO_2 laser technique. *Fertil Steril,* 30:100, 1978.
4. Bruhat MA, Mage G, and Manhes M: Use of the CO_2 laser via laparoscopy. In Kaplan I (Ed): *Proceedings of the Third International Congress for Laser Surgery.* Tel-Aviv: Ot-Paz, 1979: p. 271.
5. Martin DC, McCoy TD, and Poston WM: Reanastomosis of rat uterine horn following sharp and laser microincisions. Presented at the World Congress of Tubal Surgery, West Palm Beach, Florida, 1983.
6. Mishashi S, Ueda S, Harino M, et al: Problems about condensates induced by CO_2 laser irradiation. In Atsumi K, Nimsakul N (Eds): *Proc Fourth Cong Int Soc Laser Surg.* Tokyo: Japanese Society for Laser Medicine, 1981, p. 25.
7. Rockwell J (Ed): *Laser Safety in Surgery and Medicine.* Cincinnati: Rockwell Associates Incorporated, 1983.
8. Masterson BJ, Nealon N, and Sowas D: Tissue effects of lasers on wound healing. *Lasers in Surg Med,* 3:153, 1983 (Abstr).
9. Nishimura N, Tinino R, and Miyasha N: Comparative study of CO_2 laser scalpel with electroscalpel. In Atsumi K, Nimsakul N (Eds): *Proc Fourth Cong. Int. Soc. Laser Surg.* Tokyo: Japanese Society for Laser Medicine, 1981: p. 21.
10. Madden JE, Edlich RF, and Custer JR: Studies in the management of contaminated wound: Resistance to infection of surgical wounds made by knife, electrosurgery and laser. *Am J Surg,* 119:222, 1970.
11. Oshiro T, Etoh E, and Kato Y: Multi and one shot laser therapy: Which is better in clinical use? In Atsumi K, Nimsakul N (Eds): *Proceedings of the Fourth Congress of the International Society for Laser Surgery.* Tokyo: Japanese Society for Laser Medicine, 1979: p. 5.
12. Yamamoto T, Fukamoto I, and Satio M: Dynamic characteristics of the light reflected from the living tissue under laser irradiation. In Atsumi K, Nimsakul N (Eds): *Proceedings of the Fourth Congress of the International Society for Laser Surgery.* Tokyo: Japanese Society for Laser Medicine, 1981: p. 8.
13. Schiedel P, Wallwiemer G, and Hepp H: CO_2 laser in treatment of pelvic adhesions—Experimental results. In Kaplan I (Ed): *Proceedings of the Third International Congress for Laser Surgery.* Tel Aviv: Ot-Paz, 1979: p. 269.
14. Tadir Y, Ovadia J, Magara R, et al: Intraperitoneal adhesiolysis by CO_2 laser microsurgery. In Atsumi K, Nimsakul N (Eds): *Proceedings of the Fourth Congress of the International Society for Laser Surgery.* Tokyo: Japanese Society for Laser Medicine, 1981: p. 27.
15. Pittaway DE, Maxson WS, and Daniell JF: A comparison of the CO_2 laser and electrocautery on postoperative intraperitoneal adhesion formation in rabbits. *Fertil Steril,* 40:366, 1983.
16. Choe JK, Dawood MY, and Andrews AH: Conventional versus laser reanastomosis of rabbit ligated uterine horns. *Obstet Gynecol,* 61:689, 1983.
17. Tadir Y, Kaplan I, Zuckerman Z, et al: New techniques for laparoscopic carbon dioxide operations: A preliminary report. *Obstet Gynecol,* 63:582, 1984.
18. Choe JK, Dawood MY, Bardawil WA, et al: Clinical and histologic evaluation of laser reanastomosis of the uterine tube. *Fertil Steril,* 41:754, 1984.
19. Bellina JH, Hemmings R, Voros JI, et al: Carbon dioxide laser and electrosurgical wound study with an animal model: A comparison of tissue damage and healing patterns in peritoneal tissue. *Am J Obstet Gynecol,* 148:327, 1984.
20. Grospietzsch R, Inthraphuvasak J, Klink F, et al: Experiments on operative treatment of tubal sterility by CO_2 laser techniques. In Kaplan I (Ed): *Proceedings of the Third International Congress for Laser Surgery.* Tel Aviv: Ot-Paz, 1979: p. 256.
21. Baggish MS, and Chong AP: Carbon dioxide laser microsurgery of uterine tube. *Obstet Gynecol,* 58:111, 1981.
22. Fayez JA, McComb JS, and Harper NA:

Comparison of tubal surgery with CO_2 laser and unipolar electrode. *Fertil Steril,* 40:476, 1983.

23. Archer RW, Martin DC, and Poston WM: Comparative study of rat uterine horn microsurgical anastomosis following laser and sharp incision. Presented at Resident's Research Day, University of Tennessee Center for the Health Sciences, Memphis, May 25, 1984.
24. Kelly RW, and Roberts NK: Experience with the carbon dioxide laser in gynecologic microsurgery. *Am J Obstet Gynecol,* 146:585, 1983.
25. Inoue N, Shinozuka R, Kuroshima Y, et al: Microsurgery of the rabbit oviduct by CO_2 laser technique. In Atsumi K, Nimsakul N (Eds): *Proceedings of the Fourth Congress of the International Society for Laser Surgery.* Tokyo: Japanese Society for Laser Medicine, 1981.
26. Bruhat MA, Mage G, and Pouly JL: The use of the CO_2 laser in neosalpingostomy. In Kaplan I (Ed) *Proceedings of the Third International Congress for Laser Surgery.* Tel Aviv: Ot-Paz, 1979: p. 271.
27. Mage G, and Bruhat MA: Pregnancy following salpingostomy: Comparison between CO_2 laser and electrosurgical procedure. *Fertil Steril,* 40:472, 1983.
28. Bellina JH: Microsurgery of the fallopian tube with the carbon dioxide laser: Analysis of 230 cases with a 2 year follow-up. *Lasers Surg Med,* 3:225, 1983.
29. Bellina JH: Lasers in gynecology. *World J Surg,* 7:692, 1983.
30. Feste JR: Laser laparoscopy: A new modality. *Lasers Surg Med,* 3:170, 1983 (Abstr).
31. Taylor SN: The carbon dioxide laser in the practice of infertility. Presented at the Ortho Symposium Luncheon, American Fertility Society, New Orleans, 1983.
32. Bellina JH: Reconstructive microsurgery of the fallopian tube with carbon dioxide laser. *Reproduction,* 5:1, 1981.
33. Intraphuvasak J, Grospietzsch R, Klink F, et al: CO_2 laser beam in gynecologic microsurgical operations—A preliminary report. In Kaplan I (Ed): *Third Int Cong Laser Surg.* Tel-Aviv: Ot-Paz, 1979: p. 263.
34. Bruhat MA, Manhes H, Drisa M, et al: Laparoscopy and CO_2 laser. In Atsumi K, Nimsakul N (Eds): *Fourth Cong Int Soc Laser Surg.,* Tokyo: Japanese Society for Laser Medicine, 1981: p. 28.
35. Daniell JF, and Pittaway DE: Use of the CO_2 laser in laparoscopic surgery: Initial experience with the second puncture technique. *Infertility,* 5:15, 1982.
36. Daniell JF: CO_2 laser in infertility surgery. *J Reprod Med,* 28:265, 1983.
37. Daniell JF, and Herbert CM: Laparoscopic salpingostomy utilizing the CO_2 laser. *Fertil Steril,* 41:558, 1984.
38. Swolin K: Laparoscopy as an operative tool in female sterility. *J Reprod Med,* 19:167, 1977.
39. Gomel V: Salpingostomy by laparoscopy. *J Reprod Med,* 18:265, 1977.
40. Mettler L, Giesel H, and Semm K: Treatment of female infertility due to tubal obstruction by operative laparoscopy. *Fertil Steril,* 32:384, 1979.
41. Fayez JA: An assessment of the role of operative laparoscopy in tuboplasty. *Fertil Steril,* 39:476, 1983.

46

Laser Laparoscopy

Yona Tadir and
Jardena Ovadia

Laser beams have been applied in gynecologic surgery using different operating mechanisms and wave lengths. The most commonly used is the carbon dioxide laser (10.6 μm), but the argon laser (0.5 μm) is also used. Each of these lasers has different characteristics and tissue effects.

The Nd:YAG and the argon laser beams can be delivered via flexible fibers and passed through fluids, which is an advantage over the CO_2 laser regarding the ease of delivery. The CO_2 laser beam is highly absorbed in water and allows vaporization and precise incision of tissue. Because human tissues are poor conductors of thermal energy, damage can be limited to a very narrow zone when the laser beam exposure is brief. The CO_2 laser is an invisible beam and therefore a low-power helium neon (He-Ne) laser aiming beam is needed.

The CO_2 laser was first used in gynecology by Kaplan and colleagues[1] in 1973 for the treatment of cervical erosion and intraabdominally for female reconstructive pelvic surgery by Bellina[2] in 1974. The use of the CO_2 laser through a laparoscope was first reported by Bruhat et al.[3] using the single puncture technique and by Tadir and coauthors[4] through a second trocar using a diagnostic laparoscope. Numerous therapeutic laparoscopic procedures have been performed with the CO_2 laser.

Development of Instruments

Advanced technology has changed basic concepts in medicine, mainly with regard to diagnostic equipment such as ultrasonography and magnetic resonance imaging, while in surgery, scissors and scalpels are still the basic instruments. Improvements in laser equipment are making new applications possible, and this form of a "light scalpel" might replace the conventional one. The physical characteristics of the laser enable this fine beam of light to be delivered to locations that would be unreachable by contact techniques. The laser does not take up crucial space in the operative field and allows continuous unobstructed vision. The different wavelengths of laser beams

The Fallopian Tube: Basic Studies and Clinical Contributions, edited by Alvin M. Siegler, M.D. Mount Kisco, New York: Futura Publishing Company, Inc. © 1986.

require different delivery systems and produce different effects on live tissue. As with advances in conventional operating techniques, developments in contemporary laser instrumentation will improve operative results.

Several different delivery systems are used in gynecology:

1. "free-hand end-piece" attached to a mirrored articulated arm;
2. micromanipulator-connected to an operative microscope or colposcope, allowing precise aiming of the beam;
3. computerized micromanipulator allowing automatic homogeneous tissue vaporization within preselected boundaries used mainly on the cervix;
4. rigid endoscopes;
5. flexible fibers for endoscopic and "free-hand" use.

The diameter of the collimated laser beam emitted from the oscillator in parallel fashion is too large for most surgical applications, and the power contained is not of sufficient intensity, unless transmitted through a special lens and focused at a point distal to the instrument. This provides a beam small enough to limit the size of the surgical incision and it also increases the effective use of the laser power. The power concentration, or power density (PD) is a measure of the laser power (in watts) per square centimeter (W/cm^2), and this information is important to the surgeon for predicting the beam effect. The beam energy is controlled with a foot pedal or by an electronic shutter. The CO_2 laser is typically delivered through a zinc selenide focusing lens with a focal length that is suitable for each application. Free-hand laser surgery does not require any special device for beam alignment. In microsurgery and laparoscopy, beam aiming is achieved by manipulating a joystick. A special endoscope coupler (Fig. 46:1) was designed for connecting the laparoscope to the articulated arm (Fig. 46:2). It has a 300 mm focusing lens, a movable mirror, and a joystick. This has special importance because of the length of the laparoscope and the narrow port for the beam. This long focal length lens produces a spot with a diameter of 0.6 mm.

The first reported laser laparoscope by Bruhat[3] allowed the aiming of a focused CO_2 beam through the operating channel of a single-puncture laparoscope. Tadir and coworkers[4,5] developed a variety of second-puncture laparoscopes of different lengths (200–300 mm) and diameters (6–9 mm), allowing a standard laparoscope to be used and solving the problem of limited visibility. They also introduced an annular channel around the main cannula tubing for smoke dissipation by suction, a guard at the lower end for protecting adjacent tissues from inadvertent damage, and the coupler (Fig. 46:3). (This set of instruments was developed in collaboration with the Laser Industries Ltd.-Israel, manufacturer of the Sharplan surgical lasers.) An automatic suction device, generated synchronously by the main laser instrument during operation, collects smoke produced by the beam when it is focused on tissue. This combination allows a clear intracavitary view and a clean central channel to further simplify the procedure. The interrupted suction also prevents deflation of carbon dioxide from the abdominal cavity. A constant intracavitary pressure is maintained using an automatic gas-regulating device.

Preliminary laparoscopic experience using the Nd:YAG laser by Lomano,[6] and the argon laser by Keye and associates,[7] also demonstrates the potential of laser laparoscopy. Their technique involves passing 0.6 mm flexible quartz fibers through a second-puncture trocar.

Clinical Applications

Gynecologists face new possibilities that require a changing of attitude toward classic surgical treatments. The possibility of fertilizing human oocytes in vitro to bypass damaged fallopian tubes, or the routine use of sensitive beta HCG test and ultrasonography for the early diagnosis of unruptured tubal pregnancy

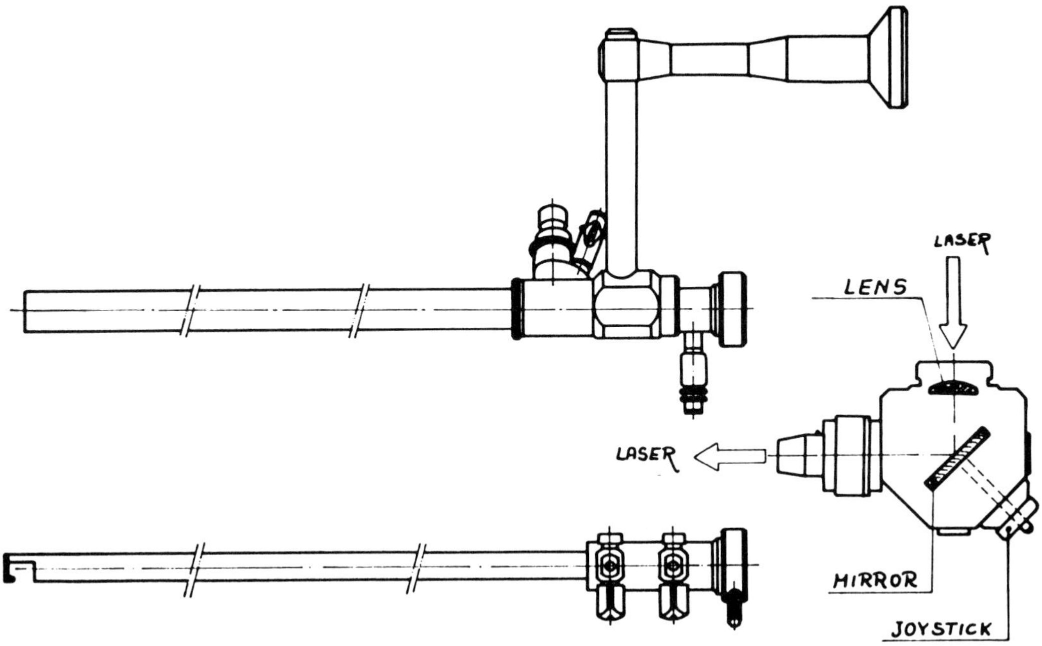

FIGURE 46:1—*The carbon dioxide laser endoscope coupler can be attached to single- or double-puncture laparoscopes. The laser beam is delivered through a zinc selenide focusing lens. A joystick is connected to a movable mirror for beam alignment.*

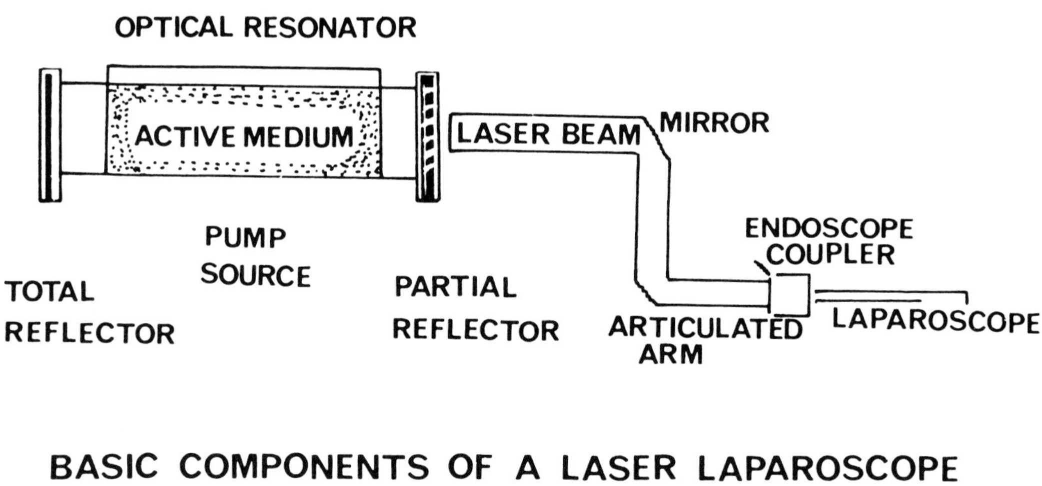

FIGURE 46:2—*Basic components of a laser system with laparoscope.*

enables laparoscopic treatment and short hospitalization. Laser laparoscopy offers the surgeon access to abnormalities that previously could not be treated endoscopically but the potential superiority of any new method must be proved by the accumulation of data. Several authors have reported success with the CO_2 laser laparoscope used for various indications:

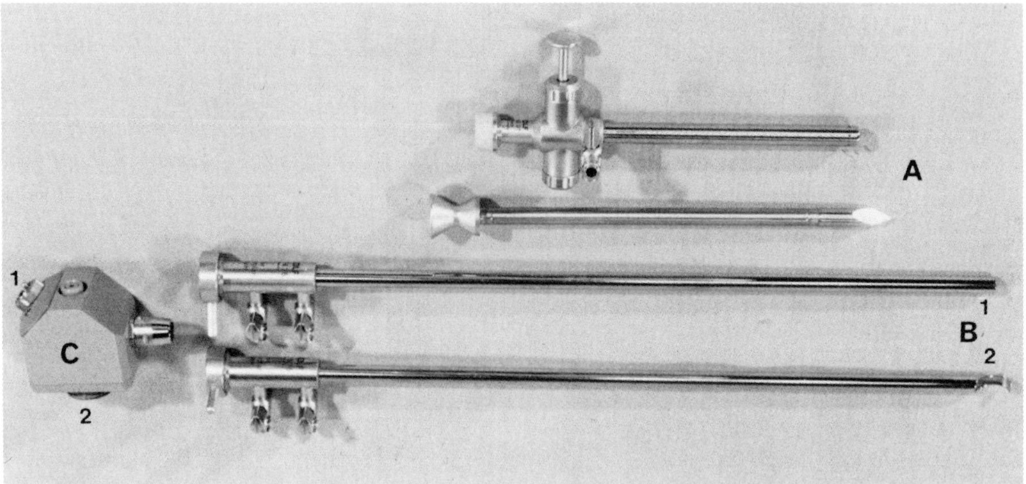

FIGURE 46:3—*Double-puncture CO_2 laser laparoscope set.* (A) *Trocar and sheath 9 mm outside diameter.* (B) *Laser cannula 8 mm outside diameter, 32 cm long with open end (1), protecting hook (2).* (C) *Endoscope coupler with joystick (1) and connector to delivery system articulated arm (2). (Adapted from Tadir et al.[5])*

1. pelvic adhesiolysis[3,5]
2. vaporization of endometriosis[5,16–19]
3. terminal neosalpingostomy[23,24]
4. ablation of sacrouterine ligaments[25]
5. vaporization of small uterine and ovarian fibromas[32]
6. linear salpingotomy for tubal pregnancy removal[31,32]
7. tubal sterilization[3–5]

Pelvic adhesiolysis was the first application performed laparoscopically using CO_2 laser in the single-[3] and double-[4] puncture routes. The tissue to be removed is bloodlessly vaporized and adjacent organs are unaffected. The second-puncture technique seems to be superior because of its safety and relative simplicity. The aiming He-Ne beam offers better visibility and the probe with a built-in backstop is suitable for adhesions that can be grasped prior to firing the laser.[8]

Avascular filmy adhesions can easily be dissected with endoscopic scissors, but other forms of laparoscopic adhesiolysis do not allow such a precise procedure. The superiority of laser adhesiolysis with respect to adhesion reformation has not yet been proven. Several investigators claim better results in animal[9–11] and human studies[12,13] using the CO_2 laser compared to other methods. However, Diamond and his collaborators,[14] in a multicenter study, found that nonlaser infertility surgery prevented adhesion formation equally. In adhesiolysis by laparoscopy, the relevant questions are which procedure leads to fewer reformed adhesions and which is the safest and simplest method for dealing with the pelvic abnormalities laparoscopically. That is dependent on location of the adhesions, the surgeon's experience, and familiarity with the available instruments.

The CO_2 laser directed through the microscope or the freehand piece of the articulated arm was used to vaporize focal endometrial implants and to excise endometrial cysts. Chong and Baggish[15] reported a conception rate of 60.8 percent in treating endometriosis. Mild and moderate endometriosis can more effectively be removed through a laparoscope with the laser than cautery and scissors. The depth of vaporization is limited to 1 to 2 mm and with skilled application of the beam there is no injury beyond the visible tissue destruction. Daniell and Pittaway[16] reported their initial experience in 15 patients with endometriosis, but who had no adhesions. The procedure was carried out without complications. In three to six months follow-up, three women conceived. Kelly and Roberts[17] reported a conception rate of 67 percent for treatment of Stage I (mild) and 14 percent for Stage II (moderate) endometriosis, with laparoscopic application of the CO_2 laser. Keye et al.[7] performed photocoagulation of peritoneal implants with argon laser during laparoscopy with a 600 μm flexible quartz fiber. Although long-term follow-up is not yet possible, they asserted that this technique may be an important therapeutic modality because of the selective absorption of the argon laser by the hemoglobin of the endometriotic implants. A third form of laser energy has also been used laparoscopically to treat pelvic endometriosis: Lomano[16] evaluated Nd:YAG laser transmitted through fibers in a similar fashion to the argon. The Nd:YAG produces coagulation to a depth of 4–5 mm and the beam scatters significantly from the impact site.

The CO_2 laser has been applied for performing terminal salpingostomy with different techniques[18] and results are similar to conventional microsurgery as reported by Mage and Bruhat[19] and by Tulandi et al.[20] The "central dimple" of the occluded fimbrial end was identified by hydrotubation, and radial incision with a focused beam (PD:10,000 to 30,000 W/cm^2) followed by reducing the power and defocusing the laser (PD:1000 W/cm^2) and directing the beam 2 to 3 mm along the margin. Retraction of the serosal flap creates a "spontaneous laser eversion." Daniell and Herbert[21] modified the technique and found the CO_2 laser laparoscope an ideal instrument for opening a mobile, thin-walled hydrosalpinx with minimal blood loss and minimal tissue trauma. Two grasping forceps are used for traction and the beam is aimed at right angles to the end of the hydrosalpinx through either the second-puncture laser probe, or the operative, single-puncture instrument. A hysterosalpingogram documented a tubal patency rate of 75 percent postoperatively, and five pregnancies resulted (including one ectopic gestation and one miscarriage) in the first 22 patients. With a second year of follow-up, this group of patients achieved a 30 percent pregnancy rate. These encouraging, and somewhat surprising results, highlight the potential of laparoscopic surgery and should be analyzed in view of reported in-vitro fertilization pregnancy rates. A combination of the two procedures can be considered in some women with distal tubal occlusion. Feste[23] performed a modified Doyle procedure[24] by incising the Frangenheim ganglion in the uterosacral ligament with a CO_2 laser laparoscope. He reported a moderate or complete relief of dysmenorrhea following this procedure in 73 percent of the women.

A significant rise in tubal pregnancy has been seen in the last two decades.[25] Because of the routine use of the sensitive beta HCG test, ultrasonography, and laparoscopy, most tubal pregnancies are detected in an early, unruptured stage. Laparoscopic treatment of tubal pregnancy has been reported by several authors.[26–28] Bruhat[29] and Tadir[30] have removed the gestational mass through a linear salpingotomy performed with the laser laparoscope. A short hospitalization of 24 hours and the immediate serum beta HCG regression, result from this kind of treatment for small unruptured tubal pregnancies.

Small uterine and ovarian fibromas can be ablated with a defocused beam. Tubal transection as a method of contraception was performed bloodlessly in a similar approach.[5] One tube recanalized, and it seems that the other available methods of laparoscopic sterilization are more suitable.

Intraperitoneal smoke accumulation, loss of pneumoperitoneum from gas leakage, fogging of lens and mirrors, and maintenance of beam alignment are technical problems.

The best instrument diameter and length are in each instance learned in the early stages of using these techniques. Experience using the proper equipment and, matching the right instrument to each procedure will lead to a less cumbersome operation and improved results.

Prospects for the Future

Nearly every cavity in the human body can be studied endoscopically as an outpatient procedure and abnormalities detected in early stages. Most new designs in endoscopes have led to further developments in ancillary equipment and the availability of "light scalpels" has brought about the logical conjunction of both modalities. Lasers require development of delivery systems, miniaturization, and flexibility of instruments for outpatient clinical use, and improvements of additional equipment for the most commonly used beams.

Of critical importance in reproductive surgery is delicate tissue handling with minimal scar formation. These objectives have led to the investigation of laser tissue interaction in different wave forms[31] (continuous wave versus electronically pulsed). Preliminary results revealed different zones of injury and detailed analysis of new systems is necessary for clarifying the optimal mode and its endoscopic potential. A combination of CO_2 and Nd:YAG is already being used[32] and a coaxial endoscopic operating improvement will increase the scope of laser surgery. Hysteroscopic laser applications[33,34] will be routinely used when some of the above-mentioned refinements are integrated with hysteroscopes. The application of high-powered argon, Nd:YAG, and tunable dye lasers (400–1000 μm), all of which can be propagated through fine fibers, and the development of CO_2 laser transmitting fibers, offers operative capabilities that endoscopists have anticipated for years. It becomes apparent that operating rooms of the future will have fibers hung from the ceiling for direct attachment to endoscopes. Photoradiation therapy (PRT), a technique developed by Dougherty,[35] has been useful in treating early preinvasive cancer. Hematoporphyrine derivatives (HPD) are given parenterally, the area is scanned for fluorescent identification of the tumor, and a laser beam (630 nm) is transmitted to the tumor area. Laser-induced fluorescence stimulates the development of singlet oxygen, which is cytotoxic. The endoscopic application of these principles, and research into other derivatives that are sensitive to specific laser intensity and wavelengths for early cancer cure are exciting. Lasers will probably be coupled to precise imaging systems for the same purpose.

References

1. Kaplan I, Goldman J, and Ger R: The treatment of erosion of the uterine cervix by means of CO_2 laser. *Obstet Gynecol*, 41:795, 1973.
2. Bellina JH: Gynecology and the laser. *Contemp Obstet Gynecol*, 4:24, 1974.
3. Bruhat M, Mage C, and Manhes M: Use of the CO_2 laser via laparoscopy. In Kaplan I (Ed): *Laser Surgery III, Proceedings of the Third International Society for Laser Surgery*. Tel Aviv: Ot-Paz, 1979: p. 275.
4. Tadir Y, Kaplan I, Zuckerman Z, et al: Laparoscopic CO_2 laser sterilization. In Semm K, Mettler L (Eds): *Human Reproduction*. Amsterdam: Excerpta Medica, 1981: p. 429.
5. Tadir Y, Kaplan I, Zuckerman Z, et al: New instrumentation and technique for laparoscopic carbon dioxide laser operations: A preliminary report. *Obstet Gynecol*, 63:582, 1984.
6. Lomano JM: Laparoscopic ablation of endometriosis with the Nd:YAG laser. *Lasers Surg Med*, 3:179, 1983 (Abstr).
7. Keye WR Jr, and Dixon J: Photocoagulation of endometriosis by the argon laser through the laparoscope. *Obstet Gynecol*, 62:383, 1983.
8. Daniell JF, and Pittaway DE: Use of the CO_2 laser in laparoscopic surgery:

Initial experience with the second puncture technique. *Infertility*, 5:15, 1982.
9. Tadir Y, Ovadia J, Margara R, et al: Intraperitoneal adhesiolysis by CO_2 laser microsurgery. In Atsumi K, Nimsakul N (Eds): *Laser Tokyo 81*. Tokyo: Inter Group Corp, 1981: p. 13.
10. Scheidel P, Wallwiener G, and Hepp H: Microsurgery adhesiolysis: A comparative study of the CO_2 laser with the microelectrode in experimental animals. *Eur J Obstet Gynecol Reprod Biol*, 14:55, 1982.
11. Bellina JH, Hemmings R, Voros JI, et al: Carbon dioxide laser and electrosurgical wound study with an animal model: A comparison of tissue damage and healing patterns in peritoneal tissue. *Am J Obstet Gynecol*, 148:327, 1984.
12. Bellina JH, Voros JI, et al: Carbon dioxide laser microsurgery in gynecology. In Kaplan I (Ed): *Laser Surgery II*. Jerusalem: Academic, 1978: p. 15.
13. Baggish MS, and Chong AP: Carbon dioxide laser microsurgery of the uterine tube. *Obstet Gynecol*, 58:111, 1981.
14. Diamond MP, Daniell JF, Martin DC, et al: Tubal patency and pelvic adhesions at early second look laparoscopy following intraabdominal use of the carbon dioxide laser: Initial report of the intraabdominal laser study. *Fertil Steril*, 42:717, 1984.
15. Chong AP, and Baggish MS: Management of pelvic endometriosis by means of intraabdominal carbon dioxide laser. *Fertil Steril*, 41:14, 1984.
16. Daniell JF, and Pittaway DE: Use of the CO_2 laser in laparoscopic surgery: Initial experience with the second puncture technique. *Infertility*, 5:15, 1982.
17. Kelly RW, and Roberts DK: CO_2 laser laparoscopy: A potential alternative to danazol in the treatment of stage I and II endometriosis. *J Reprod Med*, 28:638, 1983.
18. Bellina JH: Microsurgery of the fallopian tube with the carbon dioxide laser: Analysis of 230 cases with a two years follow up. *Laser Surg Med*, 3:255, 1983.
19. Mage G, and Bruhat MA: Pregnancy following salpingostomy: Comparison between CO_2 laser and electrosurgery procedures. *Fertil Steril*, 40:472, 1983.
20. Tulandi T, Farag R, McInnes RA, et al: Reconstructive surgery of hydrosalpinx with and without the carbon dioxide laser. *Fertil Steril*, 42:839, 1984.
21. Daniell JF, and Herbert CM: Laparoscopic salpingostomy utilizing the CO_2 laser. *Fertil Steril*, 41:558, 1984.
22. Daniell JF: The role of lasers in infertility surgery. *Fertil Steril*, 42:81, 1984.
23. Feste JR: CO_2 laser neurectomy for dysmenorrhea. *Laser Surg Med*, 3:327, 1984 (Abstr).
24. Doyle JB: Paracervical uterine denervation by transection of the cervical plexus for the relief of dysmenorrhea. *Am J Obstet Gynecol*, 70:1, 1955.
25. Beral V: An epidemiological study of recent trends in ectopic pregnancy. *Br J Obstet Gynaecol*, 82:775, 1975.
26. Bruhat MA, Manhes H, Mage G, et al: Treatment of ectopic pregnancy by means of laparoscopy. *Fertil Steril*, 33:411, 1980.
27. DeCherney AH, Romero R, and Naftolin F: Surgical management of unruptured ectopic pregnancy. *Fertil Steril*, 35:21, 1981.
28. Shapiro HI, and Adler DH: Excision of an ectopic pregnancy through the laparoscope. *Am J Obstet Gynecol*, 117:290, 1973.
29. Bruhat MA: Personal communication, 1984.
30. Tadir J: Unpublished data, 1984.
31. Bellina JH, Meandzija MP, Schillt V, et al: Analysis of electronically pulsed versus quasi-continuous wave carbon dioxide laser in an animal model. *Am J Obstet Gynecol*, 150:934, 1984.
32. Fasano VA: The use of the laser in neurosurgery. *J Neurosurg Sci*, 26:245, 1981.
33. Goldrath M, Fuller T, and Segal S: Laser photovaporization of endometrium for the treatment of menorrhagia. *Am J Obstet Gynecol*, 140:14, 1981.
34. Tadir Y, Raif J, Dagan J, et al: Hysteroscope for CO_2 laser application. *Laser Surg Med*, 4:153, 1984.
35. Dougherty TJ, Kaufman JE, Goldfarb A, et al: Photoradiation therapy for the treatment of malignant tumors. *Cancer Res*, 38:2628. 1978.

Index